AF413005

Director of Publications: Nancy M. Perrin, M.A., CAE
Publications Project Manager: Wendi S. Kishi, B.A.
Copy Editor: S. Jane Thomas, B.S.
Desktop Publisher: Michele L. Rook, B.A.
Editorial Assistant: Scott M. Faubion, B.A.

For order information or questions, write or call:
Pharmacogenomics: Applications to Patient Care
American College of Clinical Pharmacy
3101 Broadway, Suite 650
Kansas City, MO 64111
816-531-2177
816-531-4990 (Fax)
accp@accp.com

Library of Congress Control Number: 2004100941
ISBN: 1-880401-80-0

Test Completion Information
If you are completing any of these chapters for ACPE credit, you have until March 1, 2007, 3 years from the date of publication, to return test sheets to ACCP.

Acknowledgments
Development and publication of *Pharmacogenomics: Applications to Patient Care* was assisted by an educational grant from Amgen, Inc. ACCP gratefully acknowledges their support.

Welcome

Pharmacogenomics, or the study of how an individual genetic variation affects the body's response to drugs, is likely the next revolution in how we diagnose, define, and treat disease. Right now, randomized, clinical trials are ongoing, where many patients derive little or no benefit from a treatment regimen and no thought is given to why this drug is wrong for them. Every day, we select drugs and their dosages by trial and error. Pharmacogenomics may change all this, allowing us to eliminate our "one size fits all" treatment approach and to move toward a customized drug therapy regimen. By using genetic traits to select the right drug for an individual patient, pharmacogenomics may help us both increase the efficacy and decrease the toxicity of a regimen.

Pharmacogenomics represents both an opportunity and a challenge. It is an opportunity for clinicians to dramatically improve the health outcomes of the millions receiving drug therapy by understanding how and why particular individuals benefit or experience toxicity and by using that information to select a drug that is right for them. It is a challenge because of the seemingly limitless amount of genetic information assembled over the past decade, although there is still so much to learn in this rapidly advancing area.

To meet this challenge, the American College of Clinical Pharmacy (ACCP) served as the springboard for the development of the first edition of *Pharmacogenomics: Applications to Patient Care*. This three-module textbook combines the basics of pharmacogenomics with disease-specific applications and is designed to give students and practitioners a solid foundation for understanding the basic science of pharmacogenomics and the skills to integrate pharmacogenomics into their daily clinical practice.

Completion of this textbook has truly been a long and winding road, combining the skills of individuals from many different practice areas, disciplines, and research environments. Conventional wisdom declares it is the journey that is important, rather than the destination. And, although we have enjoyed this journey, we, on the editorial board, are glad to have reached our destination and hope that you enjoy your travel along the way.

Pharmacogenomics: Applications to Patient Care
Editorial Board

Pharmacogenomics: Applications to Patient Care

Editorial Board

Howard L. McLeod, Pharm.D.
Associate Professor
School of Medicine
Washington University
Saint Louis, Missouri

H. Trent Spencer, Ph.D.
Assistant Professor
Division of Hematology/Oncology and BMT
Department of Pediatrics
School of Medicine
Emory University
Atlanta, Georgia

Joseph A. Tami, Pharm.D.
Director, Clinical Drug Development
ISIS Pharmaceuticals
Carlsbad, California

Module I Panel

Authors

William L. Allen, M.Div, J.D.
Associate Professor
College of Medicine
University of Florida
Gainesville, Florida

Ronald G. Davidson, M.D., FRCPC
Professor Emeritus
Program in Human Genetics
Department of Pediatrics
McMaster University
Ancaster, Ontario, Canada

Austin L. Hughes, Ph.D.
Director of the Biotechnology Institute
Department of Biological Sciences
University of South Carolina
Columbia, South Carolina

Daren L. Knoell, Pharm.D., FCCP
Associate Professor of Pharmacy and Internal Medicine
Director of the Dorothy M. Davis Heart and Lung Research Institute
Lung Cell Isolation Program
The Ohio State University
Columbus, Ohio

Taimour Y. Langaee, MSPH, Ph.D.
Director of the Center for Pharmacogenomic Genotyping Core Laboratory
Research Assistant Professor
Department of Pharmacy Practice
College of Pharmacy
University of Florida
Gainesville, Florida

Joseph D. McInerney, M.A., M.S.
Executive Director
National Coalition for Health Professional Education in Genetics
Lutherville, Maryland

Wolfgang Sadee, Ph.D.
Professor and Chair
Department of Pharmacology
Director, Ohio State University Program in Pharmacogenomics
Director, School of Biomedical Sciences
The Ohio State University
Columbus, Ohio

H. Trent Spencer, Ph.D.
Assistant Professor
Division of Hematology/Oncology and Bone Marrow Transplants
Department of Pediatrics
School of Medicine
Emory University
Atlanta, Georgia

Issam Zineh, Pharm.D.
Assistant Professor
Department of Pharmacy Practice
College of Pharmacy
University of Florida
Gainesville, Florida

Reviewers

The American College of Clinical Pharmacy, the editorial board, and the authors would like to thank the following individuals for their careful review of Module 1.

Ronald Bachman
Chief, Department of Genetics
Kaiser Permanente Hospital
Oakland, California

Lee Ann Baxter-Lowe, Ph.D., diplomate A.B.H.I.
Professor in Residence
Department of Surgery
Director
Immunogenetics and Transplantation Laboratory
University of California, San Francisco
San Francisco, California

Jennifer Beall, Pharm.D.
Assistant Professor
McWhorter School of Pharmacy
Samford University
Clinical Coordinator
Healthsouth Metro West Hospital
Birmingham, Alabama

Timothy L. Brenner, Pharm.D.
Assistant Professor
Department of Pharmacy Practice and Science
University of Arizona College of Pharmacy
Tucson, Arizona

Roger S. Klotz, R.Ph., BCNSP, FASCP, FACA, FCPhA
President and CEO
Specialized Clinical Services, Inc.
Irvine, California

Howard P. Levy, M.D., Ph.D.
Assistant Professor
Department of Medicine
Johns Hopkins University
Baltimore, Maryland

James W. McAuley, R.Ph., Ph.D.
Associate Professor of Pharmacy Practice and Neurology
College of Pharmacy
The Ohio State University
Columbus, Ohio

Pilar N. Ossorio, Ph.D., J.D.
Assistant Professor of Law and Bioethics
University of Wisconsin Law School
Madison, Wisconsin

Robert B. Parker, Pharm.D., FCCP
Associate Professor
Department of Clinical Pharmacy
College of Pharmacy
University of Tennessee
Memphis, Tennessee

Marisel Segarra-Newnham, Pharm.D., MPH, BCPS
Clinical Pharmacy Specialist, Infectious Diseases
Veterans Affairs Medical Center
West Palm Beach, Florida

Peter W. Swaan, Ph.D.
Associate Professor
Department of Pharmaceutical Sciences
University of Maryland
Baltimore, Maryland

Module 2 Panel

Authors

Reginald F. Frye, Pharm.D., Ph.D.
Associate Professor
Department of Pharmacy Practice
Associate Director
UF Center for Pharmacogenomics
College of Pharmacy
University of Florida
Gainesville, Florida

Julie A. Johnson, Pharm.D.
Professor and Chair
Department of Pharmacy Practice
Professor of Pharmaceutics and Medicine (Cardiology)
Director
UF Center for Pharmacogenomics
University of Florida
Gainesville, Florida

Werner Kalow, M.D., F.R.S.(C)
Professor Emeritus
Department of Pharmacology
University of Toronto
Toronto, Ontario, Canada

Deanna L. Kroetz, Ph.D.
Associate Professor
Department of Biopharmaceutical Sciences
School of Pharmacy
University of California San Francisco
San Francisco, California

Tan D. Nguyen, Ph.D.c
University of California, San Francisco
San Francisco, California

Pilar N. Ossorio, Ph.D., J.D.
Assistant Professor of Law and Bioethics
University of Wisconsin Law School
Madison, Wisconsin

John M. Valgus, Pharm.D., BCOP
Clinical Pharmacogenetics Fellow
GlaxoSmithKline
Clinical Assistant Professor
University of North Carolina Hospitals and Clinics
University of North Carolina School of Pharmacy
Chapel Hill, North Carolina

Reviewers

The American College of Clinical Pharmacy, the editorial board, and the authors would like to thank the following individuals for their careful review of Module 2.

Karen E. Bertch, Pharm.D., FCCP
Director, Formulary Development and Director, Product Planning
Premier, Inc.
Oak Brook, Illinois
Clinical Associate Professor
University of Illinois College of Pharmacy
Chicago, Illinois

Jack J. Chen, Pharm.D., BCPS, CGP
Assistant Professor
College of Pharmacy
Western University of Health Sciences
Pomona, California

Michael B. Cockerham, M.S., Pharm.D., BCOP
Associate Professor of Clinical Pharmacy
ULM School of Pharmacy
LSU Health Sciences Center
Christus Schumpert Health System
Shreveport, Louisiana

Mary Ann G. Cutter, Ph.D.
Professor
Department of Philosophy
University of Colorado
Colorado Springs, Colorado

Ray Dingledine
Professor and Chair
Department of Pharmacology
School of Medicine
Emory University
Atlanta, Georgia

Lea S. Eiland, Pharm.D.
Assistant Clinical Professor of Pharmacy Practice
Harrison School of Pharmacy
Auburn University
Huntsville, Alabama

Kevin M. Sowinski, Pharm.D., FCCP, BCPS
Associate Professor of Pharmacy Practice
School of Pharmacy and Pharmacal Sciences
Purdue University
Indianapolis, Indiana

Brian B. Spear, Ph.D.
Director of Pharmacogenomics
Abbott Laboratories
North Chicago, Illinois

Grant R. Wilkinson, Ph.D., D.Sc.
Professor of Pharmacology
Division of Clinical Pharmacology
Vanderbilt School of Medicine
Nashville, Tennessee

Module 3 Panel

Authors

Jeffrey R. Bishop, Pharm.D.
Psychopharmacology and Pharmacogenomics Fellow
Clinical and Administrative Division
College of Pharmacy
University of Iowa
Iowa City, Iowa

Gilbert J. Burckart, Pharm.D., FCCP
Professor and Chairman
Department of Pharmacy
Co-Director
Clinical Pharmacogenomics Laboratory
University of Southern California
Los Angeles, California

Larisa H. Cavallari, Pharm.D., BCPS
Assistant Professor
Section of Cardiology
Department of Pharmacy Practice
College of Pharmacy
University of Illinois at Chicago
Chicago, Illinois

Vicki L. Ellingrod, Pharm.D., BCPP
Assistant Professor
Clinical and Administrative Division
Director
Pharmacogenetics Laboratory
College of Pharmacy
University of Iowa
Iowa City, Iowa

Jill M. Kolesar, Pharm.D., FCCP, BCPS
Associate Professor of Pharmacy
University of Wisconsin School of Pharmacy
Director
Analytical Instrumentation Laboratory for Pharmacokinetics,
Pharmacodynamics and Pharmacogenetics
University of Wisconsin Comprehensive Cancer Center
Madison, Wisconsin

John J. Lima, Pharm.D.
Director
Centers for Clinical Pediatric Pharmacology and Pharmacogenetics
Nemours Children's Clinic
Jacksonville, Florida

P. David Rogers, Pharm.D., Ph.D.
Assistant Professor of Pharmacy, Pharmaceutical Sciences, and Pediatrics
Colleges of Pharmacy and Medicine
University of Tennessee Health Science Center
Children's Foundation Research Center of Memphis
Le Bonheur Children's Medical Center
Memphis, Tennessee

Jianwei Wang, M.D.
Research Scientist
Centers for Clinical Pediatric Pharmacology and Pharmacogenetics
Nemours Children's Clinic
Jacksonville, Florida

HongXia Zheng, M.D., Ph.D.
Co-Director
Clinical Pharmacogenomics Laboratory
University of Southern California
Los Angeles, California

Reviewers

The American College of Clinical Pharmacy, the editorial board, and the authors would like to thank the following individuals for their careful review of Module 3.

Tamara Adams, Pharm.D., BCPS
Clinical Pharmacist
University of Louisville Hospital
Louisville, Kentucky

Sharyn D. Baker, Pharm.D.
Assistant Professor of Oncology
The Sidney Kimmel Comprehensive Cancer Center (SKCCC) at Johns Hopkins
Baltimore, Maryland

Allison M. Chung, Pharm.D.
Assistant Professor
Department of Pharmacy Practice
Harrison School of Pharmacy-Auburn University
Department of Pediatrics
University of South Alabama Children's and
Women's Hospital
Mobile, Alabama

Michael Czop, B.S., BCPS
Clinical Coordinator
Department of Pharmacy Services
Broward General Medical Center
Fort Lauderdale, Florida

David W. Dyer, Ph.D.
Professor
Department of Microbiology and Immunology
Director
Laboratory for Genomics and Bioinformatics
Oklahoma University Health Sciences Center
Oklahoma City, Oklahoma

Emilie Karpiuk, Pharm.D., BCOP, BCPS
Clinical Manager
St. Joseph Regional Medical Center/Cardinal Health
Milwaukee, Wisconsin

Deanna L. Kroetz, Ph.D.
Associate Professor
Department of Biopharmaceutical Sciences
School of Pharmacy
University of California San Francisco
San Francisco, California

Gary M. Levin, Pharm.D., BCPP, FCCP
Professor and Chairman
Department of Pharmacy Practice
School of Pharmacy
South University
Savannah, Georgia

William J. McIntyre, Pharm.D.
Dean and Professor
College of Health Sciences and Human Services
University of Texas - Pan American
Edinburg, Texas

James E. Tisdale, Pharm.D., FCCP, BCPS
Associate Professor
School of Pharmacy and Pharmacal Sciences
Purdue University
Indianapolis, Indiana

Dennis Williams, Pharm.D, FCCP, BCPS
Associate Professor of Pharmacotherapy and Experimental Therapeutics
University of North Carolina
Chapel Hill, North Carolina

Julie Wright, Pharm.D., FCCP, BCPS
Associate Professor
University of Missouri - Kansas City
School of Medicine
Kansas City, Missouri

CONTINUING EDUCATION AND PROGRAM EVALUATION INSTRUCTIONS

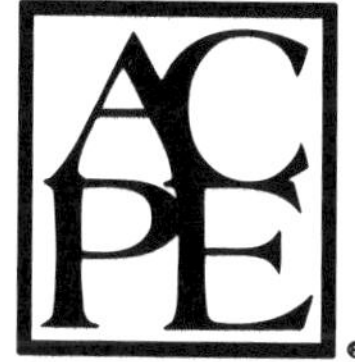 **Continuing Education Credit:** The American College of Clinical Pharmacy (ACCP) is accredited by the Accreditation Council for Pharmacy Education as a provider of continuing pharmacy education. *Pharmacogenomics: Applications to Patient Care* (PG) subscribers can earn 31.5 contact hours of continuing education credit for successfully completing Fundamentals of Applied Human Genomics (Module 1), Fundamentals of Pharmacogenomics (Module 2), and Pharmacogenomics: Applications in Patient Care (Module 3) modules of PG. Continuing education credit is available for individual chapters.

The Universal Program Numbers for Module 1 are: Principles of Genetic Medicine 217-000-04-011-H04, 2.0 contact hours; Applied Molecular and Cellular Biology 217-000-04-012-H01, 3.0 contact hours; Analysis of the Human Genome and Proteome 217-000-04-013-H01, 1.5 contact hours; Bioinformatics 217-000-04-014-H04, 1.5 contact hours; Applications of Genomics in Human Health and Complex Disease 217-000-04-015-H01, 1.5 contact hours; Ethical, Legal, and Social Issues in Genomics 217-000-04-016-H04, 1.5 contact hours.

The Universal Program Numbers for Module 2 are: Pharmacogenetics: A Historical Perspective 217-000-04-017-H04, 1.0 contact hour; Pharmacogenetics of Oxidative Drug Metabolism and Its Clinical Applications 217-000-04-018-H01, 2.0 contact hours; Drug Transporter Pharmacogenetics 217-000-04-020-H01, 1.5 contact hours; Drug Target Pharmacogenetics 217-000-04-021-H01, 2.0 contact hours; Pharmacogenomics in Drug Discovery and Drug Development 217-000-04-022-H01, 1.0 contact hour; Societal and Ethical Issues in Pharmacogenomics 217-000-04-023-H04, 2.5 contact hours.

The Universal Program Numbers for Module 3 are: Oncology and Hematology 217-000-04-024-H01, 1.5 contact hours; Infectious Diseases 217-000-04-025 H01, 1.0 contact hour; Cardiovascular Diseases 217-000-04-026-H01, 2.0 contact hours; Central Nervous System/Psychiatry 217-000-04-027-H01, 2.0 contact hours; Respiratory Diseases 217-000-04-028-H01, 2.0 contact hours; Transplantation 217-000-04-029-H01, 2.0 contact hours.

To receive Continuing Pharmacy Education credit, an answer sheet must be submitted online for scoring. *Pharmacogenomics: Applications to Patient Care* purchasers receive an e-mail confirmation with a URL address, user name and password. If you have not received an e-mail confirmation, please contact ACCP. Continuing education (CE) credit is awarded for test scores 60% or greater. The answers to each CE test are made available electronically to each participant after he or she has successfully completed the CE test. The deadline for submitting tests is March 1, 2007.

To receive the explained answers to the self-assessment questions without submitting a test for CE credit, submit a blank test and the answers are made available electronically.

Self-Assessment Questions

Directions: The self-assessment questions (items) are found after each chapter. Each item consists of a question followed by four lettered answers. Please read each carefully and select the one lettered answer that is best in each case.

Subscriber Evaluation

The American College of Clinical Pharmacy would like your assistance in evaluating the quality and usefulness of the Fundamentals of Applied Human Genomics (Module 1), Fundamentals of Pharmacogenomics (Module 2), and Pharmacogenomics: Applications in Patient Care (Module 3) modules of PG. For each chapter, please complete this evaluation in addition to the self-assessment questions. Indicate your response to the following questions by choosing the corresponding number in the evaluation area of the online answer sheet that best represents your assessment.

1 = Definitely agree 2 = Moderately agree 3 = Cannot decide 4 = Moderately disagree 5 = Strongly disagree

Subscriber Evaluation-Fundamentals of Applied Human Genomics (Module 1)

1. I was satisfied with the content of the program.
2. I was satisfied with the administration of the program.
3. The program achieved its stated educational objectives.

Questions 4-8 apply to the chapter on Principles of Genetic Medicine

4. The information presented was accurate and timely.
5. The material provided new information.
6. The material was clearly written.
7. The learning objectives were adequately assessed by the self-assessment questions.

8. The self-assessment questions were written clearly.

Questions 9-13 apply to the chapter on Applied Molecular and Cellular Biology

9. The information presented was accurate and timely.
10. The material provided new information.
11. The material was clearly written.
12. The learning objectives were adequately assessed by the self-assessment questions.
13. The self-assessment questions were written clearly.

Questions 14-18 apply to the chapter on Analysis of the Human Genome and Proteome

14. The information presented was accurate and timely.
15. The material provided new information.
16. The material was clearly written.
17. The learning objectives were adequately assessed by the self-assessment questions.
18. The self-assessment questions were written clearly.

Questions 19-23 apply to the chapter on Bioinformatics

19. The information presented was accurate and timely.
20. The material provided new information.
21. The material was clearly written.
22. The learning objectives were adequately assessed by the self-assessment questions.
23. The self-assessment questions were written clearly.

Questions 24-28 apply to the chapter on Applications of Genomics in Human Health and Complex Disease

24. The information presented was accurate and timely.
25. The material provided new information.
26. The material was clearly written.
27. The learning objectives were adequately assessed by the self-assessment questions.
28. The self-assessment questions were written clearly.

Questions 29-33 apply to the chapter on Ethical, Legal, and Social Issues in Genomics

29. The information presented was accurate and timely.
30. The material provided new information.
31. The material was clearly written.
32. The learning objectives were adequately assessed by the self-assessment questions.
33. The self-assessment questions were written clearly.

Subscriber Evaluation-Fundamentals of Pharmacogenomics (Module 2)

1. I was satisfied with the content of the program.
2. I was satisfied with the administration of the program.
3. The program achieved its stated educational objectives.

Questions 4-8 apply to the chapter on Pharmacogenetics: A Historical Perspective

4. The information presented was accurate and timely.
5. The material provided new information.
6. The material was clearly written.
7. The learning objectives were adequately assessed by the self-assessment questions.
8. The self-assessment questions were written clearly.

Questions 9-13 apply to the chapter on Pharmacogenetics of Oxidative Drug Metabolism and Its Clinical Applications

9. The information presented was accurate and timely.
10. The material provided new information.
11. The material was clearly written.
12. The learning objectives were adequately assessed by the self-assessment questions.
13. The self-assessment questions were written clearly.

Questions 14-18 apply to the chapter on Drug Transporter Pharmacogenetics

14. The information presented was accurate and timely.
15. The material provided new information.
16. The material was clearly written.
17. The learning objectives were adequately assessed by the self-assessment questions.
18. The self-assessment questions were written clearly.

Questions 19-23 apply to the chapter on Drug Target Pharmacogenetics

19. The information presented was accurate and timely.
20. The material provided new information.
21. The material was clearly written.
22. The learning objectives were adequately assessed by the self-assessment questions.
23. The self-assessment questions were written clearly.

Questions 24-28 apply to the chapter on Pharmacogenomics in Drug Discovery and Drug Development

24. The information presented was accurate and timely.
25. The material provided new information.

26. The material was clearly written.
27. The learning objectives were adequately assessed by the
    self-assessment questions.
28. The self-assessment questions were written clearly.

Questions 29-33 apply to the chapter on Societal and Ethical Issues in Pharmacogenomics

29. The information presented was accurate and timely.
30. The material provided new information.
31. The material was clearly written.
32. The learning objectives were adequately assessed by the
    self-assessment questions.
33. The self-assessment questions were written clearly.

Subscriber Evaluation-Pharmacogenomics: Applications in Patient Care (Module 3)

1. I was satisfied with the content of the program.
2. I was satisfied with the administration of the program.
3. The program achieved its stated educational objectives.

Questions 4-8 apply to the chapter on Oncology and Hematology

4. The information presented was accurate and timely.
5. The material provided new information.
6. The material was clearly written.
7. The learning objectives were adequately assessed by the
   self-assessment questions.
8. The self-assessment questions were written clearly.

Questions 9-13 apply to the chapter on Infectious Diseases

9. The information presented was accurate and timely.
10. The material provided new information.
11. The material was clearly written.
12. The learning objectives were adequately assessed by the
    self-assessment questions.
13. The self-assessment questions were written clearly.

Questions 14-18 apply to the chapter on Cardiovascular Diseases

14. The information presented was accurate and timely.
15. The material provided new information.
16. The material was clearly written.
17. The learning objectives were adequately assessed by the
    self-assessment questions.
18. The self-assessment questions were written clearly.

Questions 19-23 apply to the chapter on Central Nervous System/Psychiatry
   19. The information presented was accurate and timely.
   20. The material provided new information.
   21. The material was clearly written.
   22. The learning objectives were adequately assessed by the self-assessment questions.
   23. The self-assessment questions were written clearly.

Questions 24-28 apply to the chapter on Respiratory Diseases
   24. The information presented was accurate and timely.
   25. The material provided new information.
   26. The material was clearly written.
   27. The learning objectives were adequately assessed by the self-assessment questions.
   28. The self-assessment questions were written clearly.

Questions 29-33 apply to the chapter on Transplantation
   29. The information presented was accurate and timely.
   30. The material provided new information.
   31. The material was clearly written.
   32. The learning objectives were adequately assessed by the self-assessment questions.
   33. The self-assessment questions were written clearly.

For any question you answered 4 or 5, please provide additional information in the Notes section of the online answer sheet.

If you would like to provide additional comments, please provide them in the Notes section of the online answer sheet.

TABLE OF CONTENTS

Module I

BIOINFORMATICS

APPLICATIONS OF GENOMICS IN HUMAN HEALTH AND COMPLEX DISEASE

ETHICAL, LEGAL, AND SOCIAL ISSUES IN PHARMACOGENOMICS

Module 2

PHARMACOGENETICS: A HISTORICAL PERSPECTIVE

PHARMACOGENETICS OF OXIDATIVE DRUG METABOLISM AND ITS CLINICAL APPLICATIONS

DRUG TRANSPORTER PHARMACOGENETICS

DRUG TARGET PHARMACOGENETICS

Module 3

ONCOLOGY AND HEMATOLOGY

Principles of Genetic Medicine

Ronald G. Davidson, M.D.
Joseph D. McInerney, M.A., M.S.

Key Words

Genomics, proteomics, genotype, phenotype, anticipation, imprinting, uniparental disomy, X inactivation, complex (multifactorial) disorders, genetic counseling, gene therapy, mitochondrial disorders, Southern blot.

Abstract

The world is changing for the entire health care community. The basic principles of genetics, the vocabulary used to discuss these principles, and the need to understand genetic laboratory testing have become essential parts of practitioners' knowledge bases. This introductory chapter presents the basic principles and basic assumptions pertinent to genetic medicine, as it emphasizes the persistence of far more questions than answers. All personnel involved in health care must become lifelong learners; the references and the list of pertinent Web sites should help provide on-going access to new information as it is presented, developed, and adapted to therapeutics. Pharmacists and pharmacologists are at the forefront of the new genetics, probably working much more closely than in the past with physicians in the often difficult process of helping patients understand the nature of their illness and the new approaches to individualized therapy. These approaches include elucidation of the genetics of the individual, uncovering the possibly numerous mutations of, for example, a particular malignancy, and devising ways to match the genomes of both in order to ascertain the proper dose of the proper drug, as well as for providing techniques to get the drug efficiently and safely to the proper site.

Outline

Learning Objectives

1. Understand the central assumptions of genetics and genetic medicine.
2. Recognize and apply the basic vocabulary of genetics and the basic principles of inheritance.
3. Understand and apply the basic principles of molecular biology as they relate to genetic medicine.
4. Understand and know how to access new genetic technologies as appropriate.
5. Recognize the ethical, legal, and social issues that arise from the application of genetic knowledge and technology.

Abbreviations in this Chapter

A	Adenine
C	Cytosine
cDNA	Complementary deoxyribonucleic acid
DNA	Deoxyribonucleic acid
FGFR	Fibroblast growth factor receptor
G	Guanine
mRNA	Messenger ribonucleic acid
mtDNA	Mitochondrial deoxyribonucleic acid
OI	Osteogenesis imperfecta
PCR	Polymerase chain reaction
rDNA	Recombinant deoxyribonucleic acid
RNA	Ribonucleic acid
rRNA	Ribosomal ribonucleic acid
T	Thymine
tRNA	Transfer ribonucleic acid
U	Uracil
UPD	Uniparental disomy

Central Assumptions of Genetics and Genetic Medicine

What is Genetics?

If asked to define genetics, most nongeneticists likely would use the terms heredity, genes, deoxyribonucleic acid (DNA), and perhaps chromosomes. Although those entities and concepts are central to understanding the discipline, genetics at its heart is the study of biological variation.

Variation is the rule rather than the exception in the living world. Without it, species would neither evolve nor survive. In *Homo sapiens*, as in other species, some variation is advantageous, contributing to survival in certain environments. Some variation is disadvantageous in certain environments, resulting in disease, and some variation is neutral, contributing to the seemingly limitless human differences observed, for example, in facial features and behavioral characteristics. The latter, of course, may not be neutral; some behaviors are species specific and likely have adaptive value, whereas others may be highly detrimental.

Genetics in medicine is the study of the variation associated with illness and death. In health care, the practitioner must try to find the point of entry in the pathway from gene(s) to disease that presents the best chance of benefit or cure. That point may vary according to heterogeneity both of genes and precipitating environmental factors.

Premendelian Concepts

Possibly the first documentation of concepts relating to human genetics occurred in Greek civilization 500 BCE, when Pythagorus, the mathematical genius, recognized that some individuals who ate fava beans became sick; others suffered no adverse effects. Pythagorus, of course, had no concept of patterns of inheritance and there is no evidence that the familial nature of the phenomenon was observed. However, this example is probably the first observation of some sort of inborn predisposition that required an environmental factor for its expression. Curiously, this famous mathematician apparently recorded nothing about his observations or accomplishments; there are no written documents.

The Romans, a few centuries later, observed the adverse effects on an unborn fetus of alcohol ingested during pregnancy, and they promulgated warnings for pregnant women in relation to drinking wine.

The Talmud, the collection of Jewish law and tradition written circa AD 500, contains notations pertaining to circumcision of newborn males. It is noted that if a woman's first male offspring was circumcised, and he died as a result of exsanguination, and a second child died similarly, she must not have her third child circumcised. Furthermore, if two sisters' sons were circumcised and both died from exsanguination, the third sister should not

4

have her sons circumcised. The explanation offered is that members of some families have "loose blood," whereas normally the blood is "held fast" (i.e., it coagulates). This situation is a clear recognition of the pattern of X-linked inheritance and the nature of the disease. In addition, it could be considered the first known example of genetic counseling.

There were two notable observant physicians, both of whom lived in the 19th century, one in France, Pierre de Maupertuis, and the second in England, Joseph Adams. Both noted the familial and probably noninfectious occurrence of diseases. Adams, an apothecary, learned dispensing as an apprentice to his father. Subsequently, Adams attended the lectures in medicine at Bartholomew's Hospital in London and wrote a book titled, "A Treatise on the Supposed Hereditary Properties of Disease." Adams noted that some conditions were confined to one generation, whereas others were passed from generation to generation. Adams also recognized different types of congenital conditions, some of which were familial and others environmental, the latter including infections, such as maternal syphilis. Adams recognized familial predispositions and also noted that some of these familial, noninfectious conditions had an onset later in life (i.e., were not necessarily congenital).

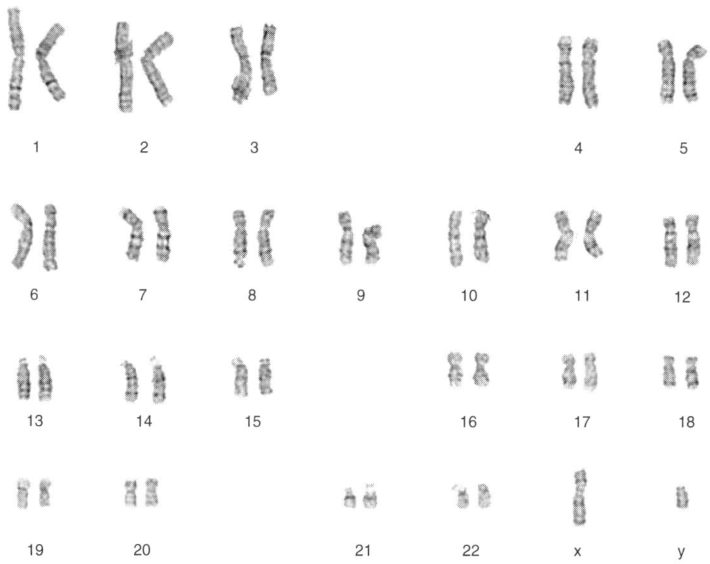

Figure 1. Pictoral display of normal human chromosomes. Reprinted with permission from the Harvey Institute for Human Genetics, Greater Baltimore Medical Center.

The Location of the Genetic Material

In *Homo sapiens* and all other eukaryotes, the genetic material is located primarily in the cell nucleus, in the familiar structures called chromosomes. Human beings have 46 chromosomes, in 23 pairs. One pair comprises the sex chromosomes; women have two X chromosomes; men have an X and Y. Figure 1 displays a normal male karyotype designated 46, XY. A normal female karyotype would have two X chromosomes and, of course, no Y chromosome. The designation would be 46, XX. A karyotype of a male with Down syndrome, trisomy 21, would include an extra chromosome 21 and would be designated 47, XY, +21.

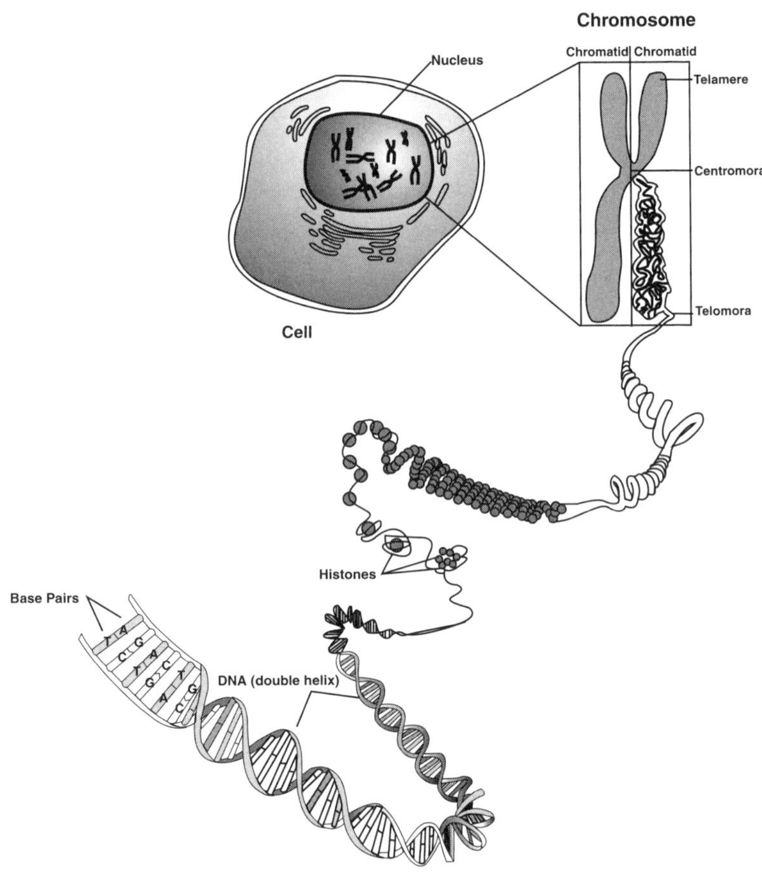

Figure 2.   Normal chromosome structure. Reprinted with permission from the National Institutes of Health (NIH) *www.genome.gov.*
DNA = deoxyribonucleic acid

Each chromosome (Figure 2) probably contains a single continuous DNA double helix, existing in a complex with proteins known as histones, as well as nonhistone proteins. The DNA plus the complex of histone and nonhistone proteins constitute the chromatin. In addition, there is a protein scaffold of nonhistone proteins in each chromosome.

Each gene occupies a particular place on a chromosome, a locus. A gene can have two or more alternative forms, called alleles, but only one allele at a time can occupy any given locus on a chromosome.

Additional genetic material resides in mitochondria. The majority of cells contain hundreds of these organelles, each with a circular mitochondrial chromosome made up of about 16 kilobases of DNA. What explains the presence of DNA in mitochondria? According to the endosymbiont hypothesis, mitochondria (and chloroplasts) were once free-living prokaryotes—aerobic or photosynthetic bacteria—that contained their own DNA and came to live inside eukaryotic cells, providing a selective advantage in terms of energetics.

Mitochondrial DNA (mtDNA) encodes only a few dozen genes, all of which produce proteins that function within the mitochondria. However, most of the proteins that are found in mitochondria are encoded by nuclear genes, and they find their way into the mitochondria by various mechanisms.

The organization of the human genome is not well understood. Some areas of the genome responsible for related characteristics are clustered in the same region; others may be widely separated. Other notable aspects of the human genome include the following:

- Some regions of chromosomes are high in gene content; some are low.
- Less than 10 percent of the DNA in the human genome encodes functional genes.
- Some repeating sequences of DNA occur even millions of times.
- There are "families" of repeats, some of which are known as satellite DNA, others as the Alu family. Some are clustered in a few locations; others are scattered. Together these repeated sequences add up to an estimated 10-15 percent of the genome. The precise reason for this is unknown, but some may play a role in centromere function, ensuring proper chromosome segregation during cell division. Alu sequences have been implicated as the cause of mutations in some genetic diseases.

What is a Gene?

This brief introductory chapter cannot include the details of molecular genetics that are readily available in any textbook of human genetics (favored by this author are References 1 and 2). However, it is important to include some of the highlights, beginning with the definition of a gene. Basically, a gene is a sequence of DNA encoding the information for production of a functional polypeptide chain or a ribonucleic acid (RNA) molecule. The vast majority of the polypeptides are proteins.

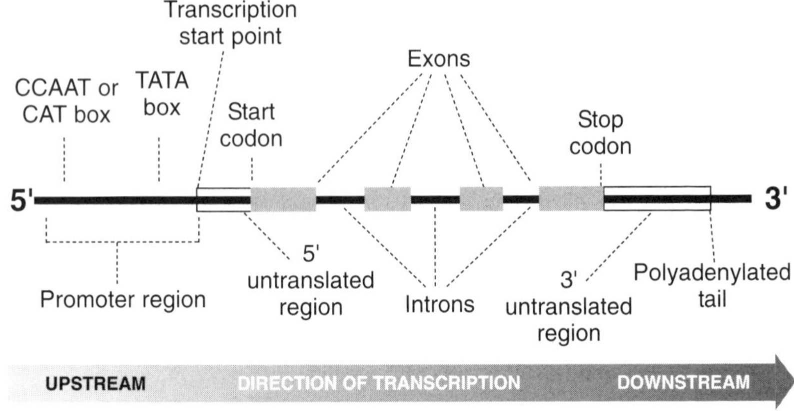

Figure 3. Diagrammatic representation of a gene.
A = adenine; C = cytosine; T = thymine

Obviously, this definition is incomplete, at least for higher organisms, including mammals. Figure 3 illustrates some of the main components of the gene in modern terms.

Deoxyribonucleic acid, which takes the form of the well-known double helix (Figure 4), is a digital information molecule in which the information is stored in the form of four nitrogenous bases: adenine (A), thymine (T), cytosine (C), and guanine (G). In the complementary pairing of the bases, A always pairs with T and C always pairs with G. As was noted in the classic paper of 1953, "the specific pairing immediately suggests a possible copying mechanism for the genetic material." Replication of DNA occurs during the cell cycle (see Figure 5 for cell cycle and Figure 6 for replication).

The strands from which the complementary bases extend are made of phosphates and five-carbon sugars. As Figure 4 illustrates, these strands run in opposite directions. That is, at the end of one strand, the 5' sugar is exposed, whereas the 3' sugar is exposed at the end of the other strand. Molecular biologists refer to the 5' direction as "upstream" and 3' direction as "downstream."

Processes known as transcription and translation transform the digital information in DNA into protein. As Figure 7 illustrates, in virtually all biological systems the flow of this information proceeds as follows: DNA → RNA → protein.

Transcription uses complementary base pairing, with a single strand of DNA as a template to produce single-stranded RNA, as shown in Figure 8 (part a). Note that in RNA uracil (U) replaces T as the base that is complementary to A.

The promoter region of the gene includes sequences responsible for the proper initiation of transcription. This region interacts with transcription

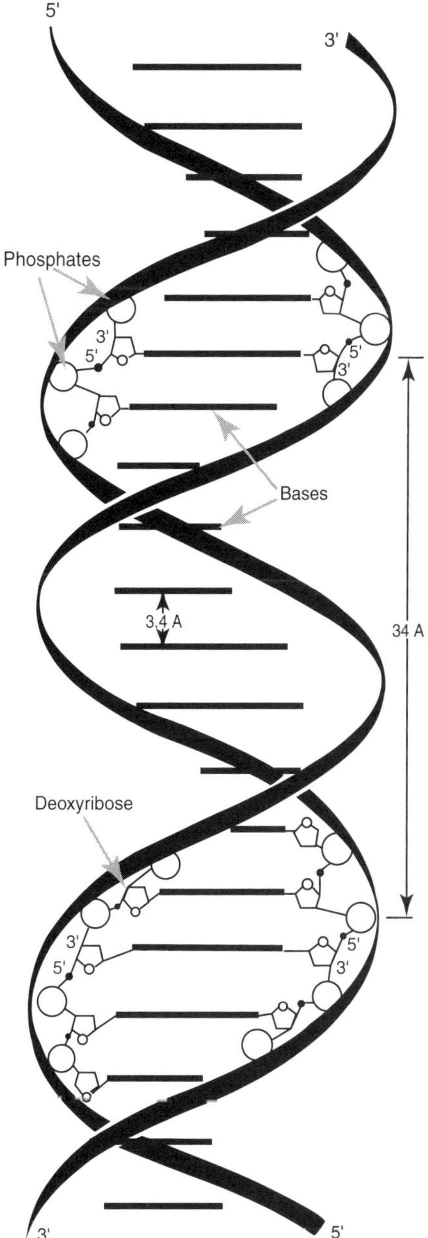

Figure 4. Diagrammatic representation of DNA.
DNA = deoxyribonucleic acid

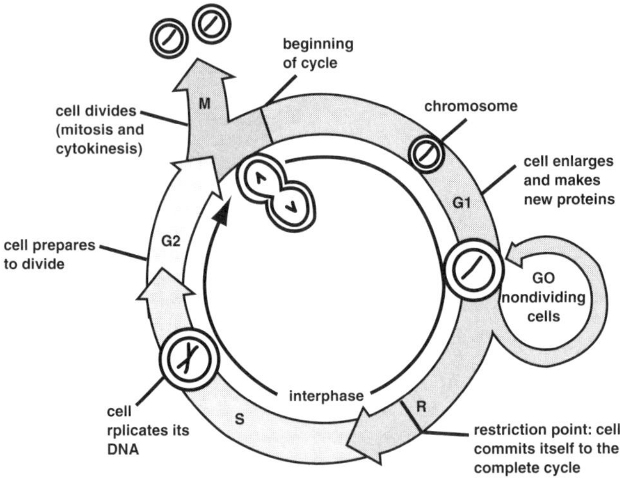

Figure 5. Diagram of the cell cycle. Reprinted with permission from Biological Sciences Curriculum Study *www.bscs.org*.
DNA = deoxyribonucleic acid; G1 = Gap1-prereplication; G2 = Gap2-premitosis; R = restriction point; S = DNA synthesis.

factors (specific proteins) that regulate transcription; that is, they turn the process on or restrict activation to specific cells (brain cells, for example, do not make hemoglobin). Genes that specify transcription factors may be upstream from the start of transcription. Mutations in these sites can, for example, greatly decrease the rate of transcription.

There are also "enhancers," another type of activating sequence that may be at a considerable distance from the transcription site and can be either 5' or 3'. They seem to be involved in tissue specificity and may affect expression of several genes. Sometimes several enhancers work together.

The transcribed RNA is modified (Figure 8 parts b-d) by the addition of a polyA sequence at the 3' end of the RNA and by the excision of segments called introns (intervening sequences), which occur in almost all living organisms evolutionarily above bacteria. Introns do not code for protein. The remaining segments, called exons (expressed sequences), which ultimately are expressed as protein, are spliced together. So, this messenger RNA (mRNA), which at first was collinear to its DNA template, is not so when it leaves the nucleus for translation into protein.

For translation to occur (Figure 10), the digital information encoded into mRNA, the sequence of bases, must be decoded into the building blocks of proteins, amino acids. There are 20 amino acids and four bases, and some

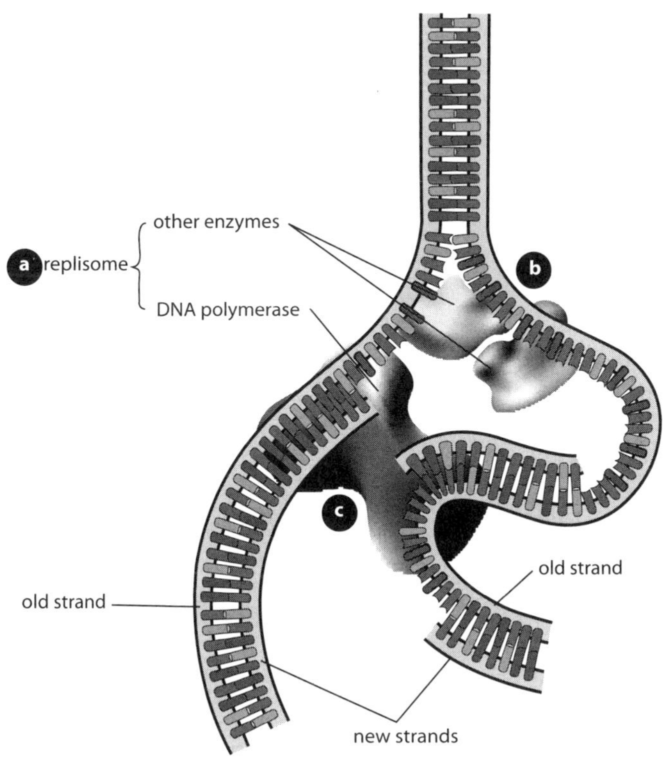

Figure 6. Diagram depicting replication of DNA. Reprinted with permission from Biological Sciences Curriculum Study *www.bscs.org*.
DNA = deoxyribonucleic acid

basic arithmetic demonstrates that the code must be at least three bases long to provide enough combinations of the bases to code for all possible amino acids ($4^1 = 4$; $4^2 = 16$; $4^3 = 64$).

This triplet code, written in RNA bases, is displayed in Figure 9. Each triplet is called a codon and each codon specifies a particular amino acid. Because there are only 20 amino acids and 64 codons, most amino acids are specified by more than one codon.

Translation always is initiated by the codon that specifies methionine, which is, therefore, the first encoded amino acid of each polypeptide chain, although it is usually removed before protein synthesis is complete. That codon establishes the reading frame of the mRNA, and each subsequent codon is read in turn to specify the amino acid sequence of the protein. Three of the codons are called stop or nonsense codons because they designate the termination translation at that specific point.

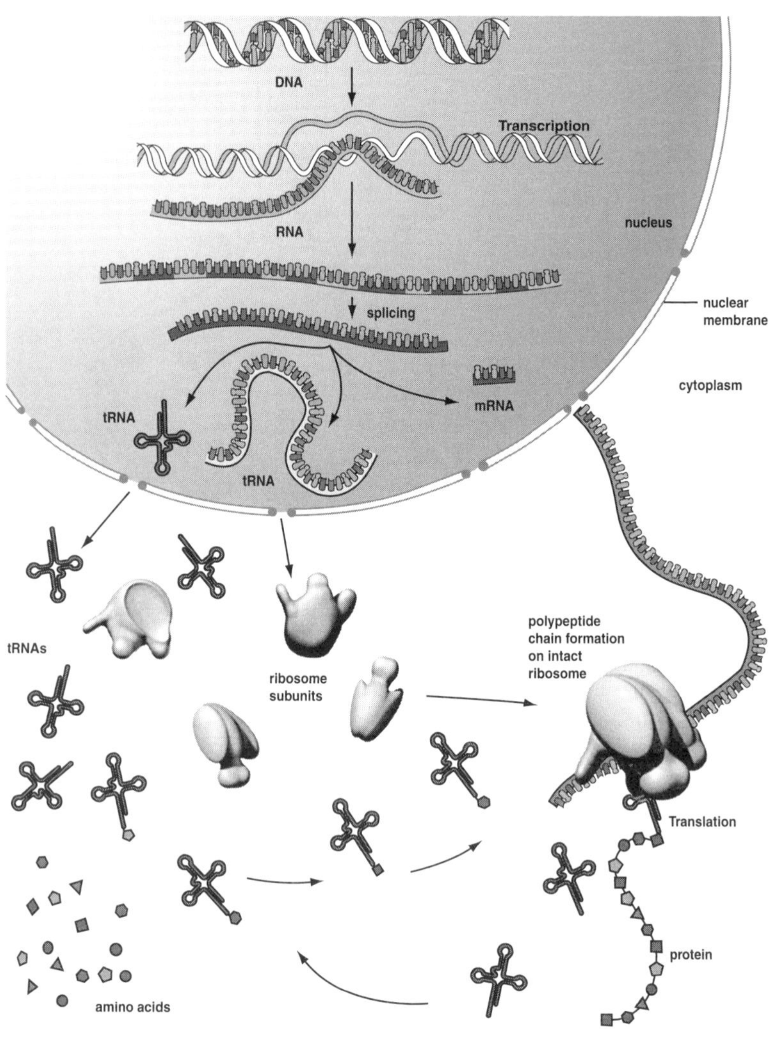

Figure 7.   Diagrammatic representation of the steps from DNA to protein. Reprinted with permission from Biological Sciences Curriculum Study *www.bscs.org*.
DNA = deoxyribonucleic acid; mRNA = messenger ribonucleic acid; rRNA = ribosomal ribonucleic acid; RNA = ribonucleic acid; tRNA = transfer ribonucleic acid

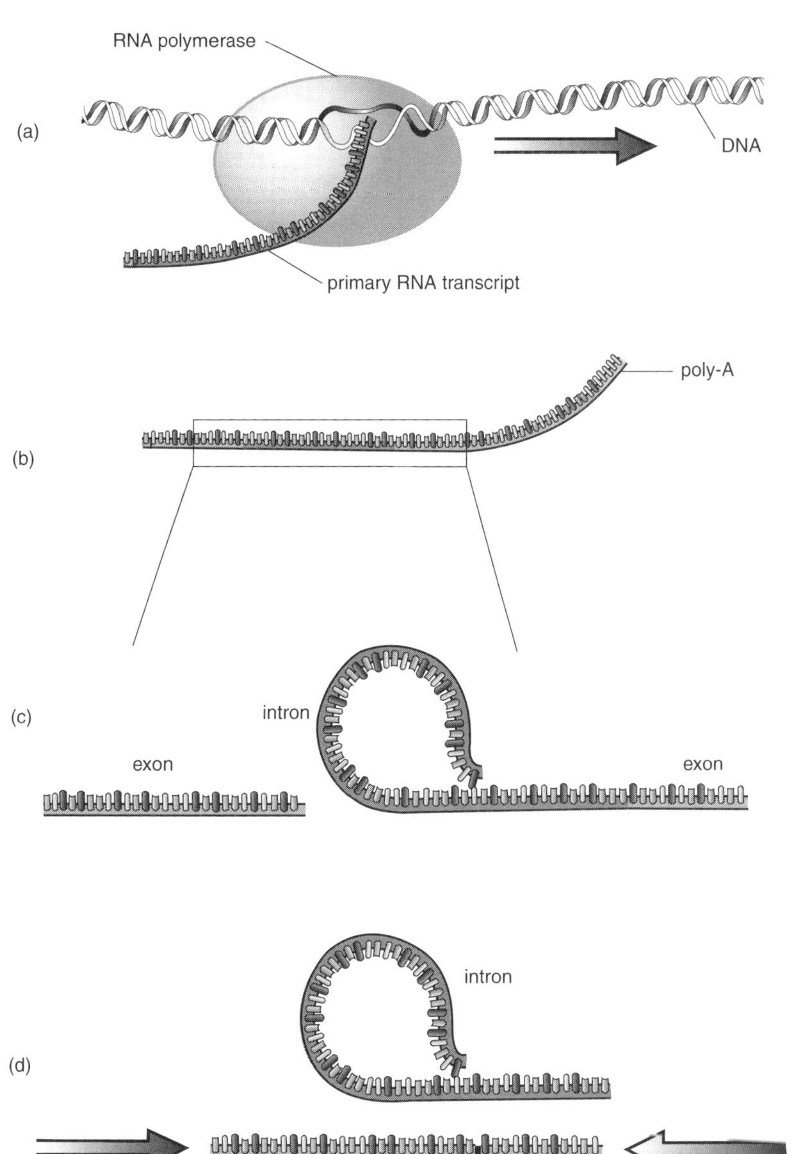

Figure 8. Transcription to mRNA. Reprinted with permission from Biological Sciences Curriculum Study *www.bscs.org*.
DNA = deoxyribonucleic acid; RNA = ribonucleic acid.

First Base	Second Base				Third Base
	U	**C**	**A**	**G**	
U	phenylanine	serine	tyrosine	cysteine	U
	phenylanine	serine	tyrosine	cysteine	C
	leucine	serine	stop	stop	A
	leucine	serine	stop	tryptophan	G
C	leucine	proline	histidine	arginine	U
	leucine	proline	histidine	arginine	C
	leucine	proline	glutamine	arginine	A
	leucine	proline	glutamine	arginine	G
A	isoleucine	threonine	asparagine	serine	U
	isoleucine	threonine	asparagine	serine	C
	isoleucine	threonine	lysine	arginine	A
	(start) methionine	threonine	lysine	arginine	G
G	valine	alanine	aspartate	glycine	U
	valine	alanine	aspartate	glycine	C
	valine	alanine	glutamate	glycine	A
	valine	alanine	glutamate	glycine	G

Figure 9. The triplet code written in RNA bases. Reprinted with permission from Biological Sciences Curriculum Study *www.bscs.org*.
A = adenine; C = cytosine; G = guanine; U = uracil

Translation, the production of protein, occurs on the ribosomes, in the cell cytoplasm, using the processed mRNA as the template. Ribosomes are themselves composed of RNA (ribosomal RNA [rRNA]) and protein.

Protein synthesis involves yet another type of RNA. This transfer RNA (tRNA) has two business ends, as it were (Figure 10). One end contains an anticodon-a sequence of three bases complementary to a specific mRNA codon. The other end contains the specific amino acid represented by that codon. Translation proceeds as the ribosome moves along the mRNA strand, reading each codon in turn. As each successive tRNA matches its anticodon to the appropriate mRNA codon, the appropriate sequence of amino acids is assembled, resulting in the polypeptide chain specified by the original sequence of DNA in the nucleus. The amino acids are joined by peptide bonds into a complete protein.

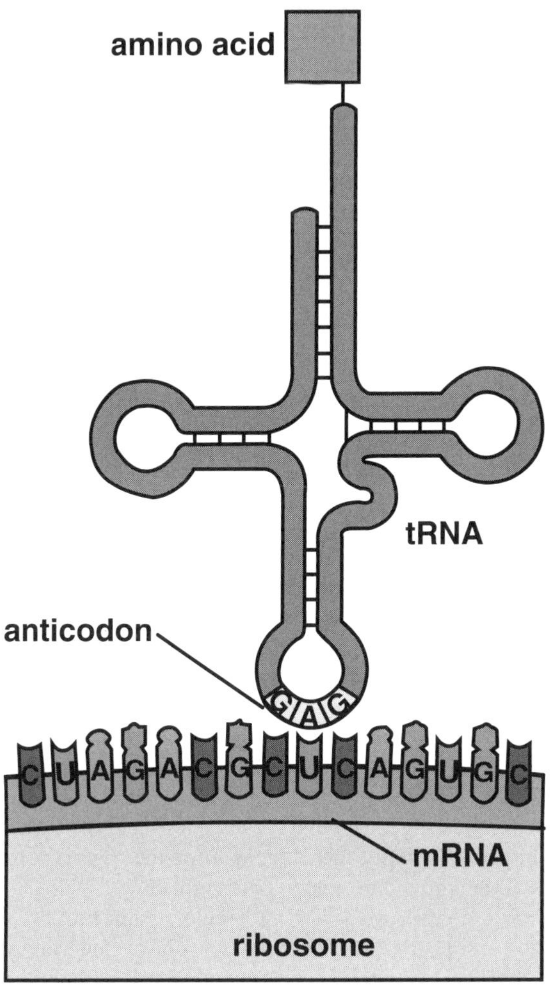

Figure 10. Translation from mRNA to protein. Reprinted with permission from Biological Sciences Curriculum Study *www.bscs.org*.
A = adenine; C = cytosine; G = guanine; mRNA = messenger ribonucleic acid; tRNA = transfer ribonucleic acid; U − uracil

Post-translational processing includes many steps:
- The polypeptide chain folds, presumably as a result of the specific sequence of its amino acids; this is the beginning of the development of the protein's three-dimensional structure.
- Two, three, or more polypeptide chains may come together to form a protein; examples include the four chains of the human hemoglobin molecule and the six chains of connective tissue molecules.
- Phosphates and carbohydrates may be added to the molecule.
- Portions of the polypeptide chain may be cleaved off (e.g., amino terminal sequences that will result in directing a protein to a specific cell, or to a specific location/organelle within the cell).
- Sometimes a molecule is split into smaller polypeptide chains (e.g., proinsulin starts out as a molecule with 82 amino acids and in maturing is broken down into two chains—one of 21 amino acids and the other of 30).

At this point, it is a good idea to look back at Figure 3 to note that the 3' to 5' strand of DNA actually serves as the template for transcription. However, the 5' to 3' strand corresponds to the 5' to 3' sequence of the mRNA identical to it, except for substituting U for T, the difference between DNA and RNA.

What do Genes do?

The pathway from gene to trait or phenotype can be considered as a component of gene action. Gene action is distinguished by outcome (i.e., the specification of a structural protein or a functional protein [e.g., an enzyme]).

Historically, there have been opposing points of view in relation to the pathway from gene to a phenotype:

Proponents of "the supremacy of the gene" say that the gene is central within the cell, literally and figuratively. From the time of conception, according to this view, the genes make the decisions and the elements of the cytoplasm (in humans, initially the cytoplasm of the ovum) respond. This viewpoint came to be known as genetic determinism.

Proponents of "the gene as an inert molecule" claim that the genome is the blueprint (the architect's plan), but the cytoplasm undertakes the main mission of the cell. That is, nothing can happen in a cell without the interplay of the other factors—signal proteins, tRNAs, and rRNA—all going forward with no further reference to the genes.

For medicine, genes certainly do have special meaning. Clearly, nothing happens without the cytoplasm, but genes are with human beings from conception to death, supplying the information to keep humans going, usually in health, occasionally in illness. Genes reflect who individuals are and where they come from, and to a considerable extent, where they are going.

The pathway from DNA to protein has been discussed; up to that point, it is accurate to state that there are "genes for" the specificity of the product and its function (e.g., the structural genes for gamma globulin). However, those are just the first few steps in the pathway from gene to phenotype. Next come the derivation of metabolites, organs, tissues, systems, and finally the phenotype, normal or otherwise. But after the specification of the primary gene product, there is a major change in the relationship. To continue the gamma globulin analogy, each immune globulin has to function within the homeostatic system, of which it is only one component. It has to react to certain antigenic stimuli, its actual structure varies depending on the invader, and it must interact with other elements of host resistance.

In conclusion, in the action of the gene—the path from a gene to a phenotype—it is not simply the gene or its protein product that actually produces the phenotype, but the coming together of many events. In some instances, the gene effect overrides everything else and produces disease, although often with individual variation (see the example of hemochromatosis below). Much more frequently, intervening events create variability, sometimes to the extent of escaping the disease phenotype entirely in one person, whereas its manifestations are inevitable in another, despite the presence of precisely the same causative mutation in each individual.

The Basic Vocabulary of Genetics and the Basic Principles of Inheritance

Some Key Definitions

As with any discipline, genetics has a specialized vocabulary. See Table 1 for a list of key terms and their definitions. The use of genetics-related jargon has been limited in this introductory chapter, but the terms in Table 1, some already encountered in the previous section, are essential to understanding the application of genetics to health care, particularly as genomic perspectives become more prevalent.

Mendelian Genetics and Single-gene Inheritance

Gregor Mendel, an Augustinian monk working in what is now the Czech Republic during the mid-19th century, uncovered the basic principles of heredity through his now-famous investigations of pea plants. Mendel did painstaking experiments, looking primarily for an explanation for the nature of hybrids.

In addition to unearthing the principles of dominance and recessiveness (see the Mendel and Darwin section), Mendel demonstrated the particulate nature of inheritance. That is, he showed that some biological entity—he called them factors, we now call them genes—could carry hereditary

Table 1.   Key Terms and Their Definitions

Autosome	a chromosome that is not a sex chromosome; in humans, chromosomes 1-22.
Sex chromosome	the chromosomes involved in sex determination, in humans designated X and Y.
Expressivity	the extent to which a trait is manifest. That is, the trait can vary in expression from mild to severe. Compare with penetrance.
Genomics	the study of the organization and function of the complete genetic material of an organism (i.e., the genome is the entire DNA sequence).
Proteomics	the study of the structure and function of the complete set of proteins encoded by the genome.
Genotype	for a given trait, the gene(s) associated with that trait.
Phenotype	the observable expression of the genotype as a morphological, clinical, biochemical, or molecular trait.
Homozygous	the presence of two identical alleles for a given trait.
Heterozygous	the presence of two different alleles for a given trait.
Mitosis	somatic cell division. In humans, the somatic cell chromosome number, or diploid number, 46, generally is maintained, ensuring the genetic continuity of somatic cells during development.
Meiosis	cell division that forms gametes; the chromosome number is halved to the haploid number, 23, with one representative of each chromosome pair going to each reproductive cell, ovum or sperm. The process also results in increased variation through the exchange of genetic material (crossing over) between the paired maternally and paternally derived chromosomes.
Mutation	any change in nucleotide sequence or arrangement of DNA. Mutations can be broadly classified as: • affecting the *number* of chromosomes in the cell • altering the *structure* of chromosomes • altering individual genes
Penetrance	an all-or-none term indicating the frequency of expression of a genotype. If there is no detectable manifestation of the genotype, the trait is said to be nonpenetrant or to show lack of penetrance. If there is even a minor detectable manifestation, the gene is penetrant. This term is often used incorrectly in reference to expressivity (see above).

DNA = deoxyribonucleic acid.

information, and, therefore, traits, intact from one generation to the next, even though their effects (the traits or phenotypes) might be blurred in some generations. He also noted that these hereditary factors segregate independently, one from the other, and brilliantly was able to work out the various ratios that allow prediction of the segregation of different phenotypes from generation to generation.

It is important to note that Mendel was lucky in his choice of traits to study. The patterns of inheritance that Mendel identified, and the ratios of the resulting traits, are directly related to the behavior of the chromosomes during meiosis. Mendel knew nothing about chromosomes, but completely by chance chose to study traits that were associated with genes on different chromosomes. His work lay unappreciated for some 35 years, until it was rediscovered independently by three botanists about 1900.

Mendel and Darwin

Mendel's work provided the answers to important questions that plagued Charles Darwin throughout his life. Darwin knew that differential selection based on phenotypic variation is the key to evolution by natural selection. He also realized that the only type of variation that matters for evolution is variation that can be inherited. However, he could not propose supportable hypotheses for the ultimate location of that variation (the genes) or for its transmission from one generation to the next. Mendel's work contained the answers to both problems, and although he and Darwin were contemporaries (Darwin published The Origin of Species in 1859), it appears that Darwin was unaware of Mendel's work. The rediscovery of Mendel's work led ultimately to the Modern Synthesis of Evolution, the reconciliation of Darwinism and Mendelism, in the 1930s and 1940s. That intellectual structure is the basis for all of modern biology, including genetics and genomics and their application to health care.

In reviewing the brief summary of dominant and recessive inheritance that follows, it is important to remember that it is not the genes that are dominant or recessive. It is their protein products that have a dominant effect in a single dose or no obvious effect unless present in a double dose. (Obvious is a key word; as illustrated in the following sections, the so-called recessive nature of a gene may depend on how hard one looks at the phenotype and with what tools.)

Autosomal Dominant Inheritance

In autosomal dominant inheritance, the trait in question is expressed in the homozygote and in the heterozygote. That is, only one copy of the allele associated with the trait is necessary for expression.

With respect to disease, the thoughtful student might ask why, given that genes come in pairs, one abnormal member of a pair would have any effect at all on the phenotype of the individual possessing it? The other member of that pair (i.e., the other allele) ought to be able to make enough product to allow normal function. That certainly is the case for individuals who carry the mutant gene for cystic fibrosis, Tay-Sachs disease, and literally thousands of others (see the Autosomal Recessive Inheritance section).

Part of the explanation for the dominant effect lies in the fact that many dominant conditions involve structural proteins, whereas many recessive conditions involve enzyme deficiencies. If a mutation results in a totally nonfunctional allele, half of a product may not be enough, as in some cases of osteogenesis imperfecta (OI), fragile bone disease.

Another possibility to consider in relation to dominance is the abnormal polypeptide chains mixed in with normal chains, even in a roughly 50-50 ratio, may simply weaken the structure, as epitomized in the old adage, a chain is only as strong as its weakest link. Osteogenesis imperfecta is a good example for that as well; the poor quality of the connective tissue matrix of bone results in poor mineralization and, hence, the fragility of the bone. Similarly, the poor quality of connective tissue making up tendons and joint capsules is responsible for the overly extensible joints and dislocations that may occur in some affected individuals.

Furthermore, the structure of the protein involved may be important. In one type of OI, for example, the mutation affects type 1 collagen, a tissue that is composed of two alpha 1 (I)-chains and one alpha 2 (I)-chain (i.e., it is a trimer). A mutation in the alpha 1 (I)-chain results in the abnormal type 1 collagen, even if the alpha 2 (I)-chain is normal, because a mutation in the alpha 1 (I)-chain affects more than half of the molecule. This is referred to as a dominant negative effect.

Finally, there are gain-of-function mutations as well, in which a mutation causes a product to have a different function than it normally exhibits. In achondroplasia, the most common type of autosomal dominantly inherited bone dysplasia, the causative mutation is in a fibroblast growth factor receptor (FGFR)3 gene. The mutations activate the negative growth control exerted by *FGFR3*, which causes constitutive activation of the FGFR and a negative regulation of bone growth. The net result is impaired bone growth. In addition, mutations in oncogenes cause typical gain-of-function: mutations allow suppressed cellular growth genes to reactivate.

Variability is virtually the rule for dominant conditions. Some of the variability seen in OI have been discussed previously, but there is much more. The characteristic blue sclerae are simply due to the poorly developed, thin connective-tissue layer through which the underlying vessels show a blue-grey discoloration. The teeth are often dysplastic with opalescent enamel and increased susceptibility to decay. Add to this tissue heterogeneity some of the genetic components, for example, the complexity of the connective-tissue molecule whose structural components are encoded not in one but in several gene loci. Furthermore, there are various combinations of the polypeptide chains that contribute to variability. To make the situation more complex, the various structures affected by the mutant collagen chains of OI also are functioning in a milieu of other gene products that will vary from individual to individual even within the same family. And, of course, there are environmental and societal influences; a sedentary person with the more mild types of OI may never have a fracture; an athletically inclined sibling may suffer dozens of them.

Other examples are easy to find. Some individuals with neurofibromatosis have almost nothing to show for it—perhaps a few café-au lait spots with freckling in the axillae and groin. Others have multiple small subcutaneous tumors or even quite massive deforming neurofibromas with involvement of many other organ systems. As with OI, a variety of explanations may account for this genetic heterogeneity, including multiple mutant alleles with different effects and influences from other genetic loci.

The prediction of risk for autosomal dominant disorders is analogous to tossing a coin. An affected individual has one mutant and one normal allele; because genes are passed to offspring one member of a pair at a time, the risk of an affected parent having an affected child is 0.5 (50 percent). However, beware, each toss of the coin is an independent event. Sometimes coin tossing will result in two, three, four, or even more heads in a row, but no matter how many heads have been tossed, the chance of tossing a head on the next throw is still 0.5.

The pedigree for a family expressing an autosomal dominant disorder typically is quite straightforward (Figure 11). The number of affected men and women ought to be equal, and the trait in question usually does not skip generations. Exceptions to these rules abound, as could be predicted from the previous discussion. The reasons for these exceptions include:

- sex limited disorders—although such conditions as male pattern baldness are unquestionably complex disorders, some families show apparent autosomal dominant segregation with lack of expression in women, some of whom do indeed develop postmenopausal partial alopecia. Presumably female sex hormones exert a protective effect on scalp hair follicles.
- lack of penetrance (see Table 1 for a definition).
- decreased expressivity—in some cases expression of a gene may be so mild as to be entirely missed, especially if the health care professional is

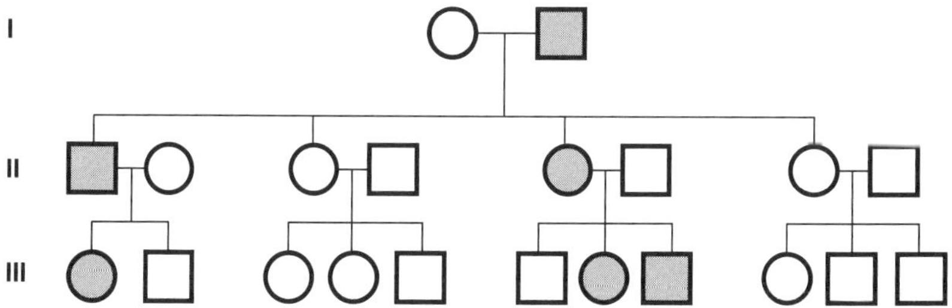

Figure 11. Autosomal dominant pedigree.

not thoroughly familiar with the total spectrum of the condition, including the minor manifestations.

Autosomal Recessive Inheritance

In this type of inheritance, the trait is present only in the homozygote, that is, only in those who carry two copies of the allele associated with the trait. Those who have one copy of the allele do not show the trait, but they are carriers. If two carriers mate, the probability that they will conceive an affected offspring (homozygous recessive—two mutant alleles) is 0.25 with each conception. The probability is 0.5 that they will conceive a carrier (heterozygous—one normal and one mutant allele) and 0.25 that they will conceive an offspring who is homozygous. Note that carriers can transmit the mutant allele to their offspring.

Figure 12 is a stylized pedigree showing the well-known 1-2-1 segregation ratio of the phenotype for a mating of two carriers (two heterozygotes). The parents are heterozygous for a mutant allele at the same gene locus and are unaffected phenotypically by the mutation in a single dose. However, whether a carrier is considered "normal" often depends on how hard the situation is examined and by what means. For example, the carrier of the sickle cell mutation is symptom free, but examination of a blood smear usually reveals scattered sickle cells. After exposure to a reducing agent, widespread sickling occurs.

That the parents in Figure 12 are unaffected illustrates another important characteristic of autosomal recessive inheritance: the trait may seem to disappear or skip generations. Although the trait may not be evident, the mutant alleles are still present in the family.

The risk that two carries will have a homozygous affected offspring is one in four, but keep in mind that people's understanding of odds is often surprisingly primitive. Some will conclude that because they have one affected child, the next three children are unaffected. The deck-of-cards analogy will usually work; there is a one-in-four chance of drawing a heart, spade, diamond or club, but there is a game called poker and a hand known as a flush (five cards of the same suit). When using the card-game analogy,

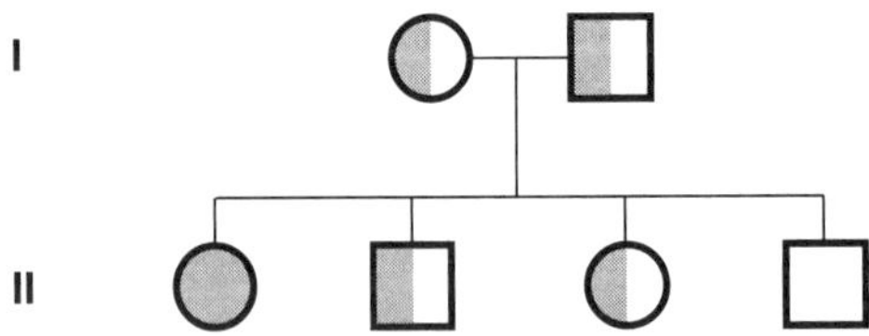

Figure 12. Autosomal recessive pedigree.

if the person to whom you are explaining the risks suggests that the analogy works only if you replace the drawn card into the deck each time and then reshuffle before drawing again, then the point has been made. Obviously, with a one-in-four risk, two or even more affected offspring in a sibship are not so unlikely.

Note that among the unaffected offspring of carrier parents, two out of three are carriers, on the average, and one is homozygous normal. This seems to be a bit difficult for some people to grasp and if involved in explaining this, the clinician needs to point out that the affected individual is usually obvious. That leaves two possibilities for the remaining three hypothetical offspring in the pedigree in Figure 12, carrier or homozygous normal, and usually a distinction between them cannot be made unless there is a biochemical, molecular, or other test.

Consanguinity—genetic relatedness—plays a role in autosomal recessive inheritance. Obviously, the chance that both parents carry a mutant allele at the same locus is increased if the parents are related and could both have inherited the mutant allele from a single common ancestor. An example is the incidence of congenital malformations, many of which are due to homozygosity for a recessive mutation. For first cousin marriages, the incidence is 3–5 percent, which is about double that for offspring born to unrelated parents. The risk falls off for less close parental relationships, and consanguinity is not considered to be of significance for relationships at the level of third cousins or more remote, except in populations where inbreeding has been occurring for many generations.

As with dominant conditions, variability is the rule, not the exception. Hemochromatosis (see the Single-gene Disorders as Complex Diseases—Hemochromatosis section) exemplifies many of the causes of this variability.

X-linked Disorders

As the designation indicates, X-linked disorders are associated with genes carried on the X chromosome. X-linked recessive disorders are much more common than X-linked dominant disorders, but both do occur.

Figure 13 shows a typical pedigree in which an X-linked recessive trait is present. Males are most often affected and receive the gene through their carrier mothers who, typically, are phenotypically "normal." On *average*, half the sons of a carrier mother are affected and half of the daughters are carriers.

Women can be *affected* on the basis of the following:
- having a carrier mother and an affected father (i.e., the female [marked by the arrow] is homozygous for an X-linked mutation, as illustrated in Figure 13, generation IV);
- nonrandom X inactivation (see the Exceptions to Mendelian Inheritance section); and
- partial dominance/manifesting carrier.

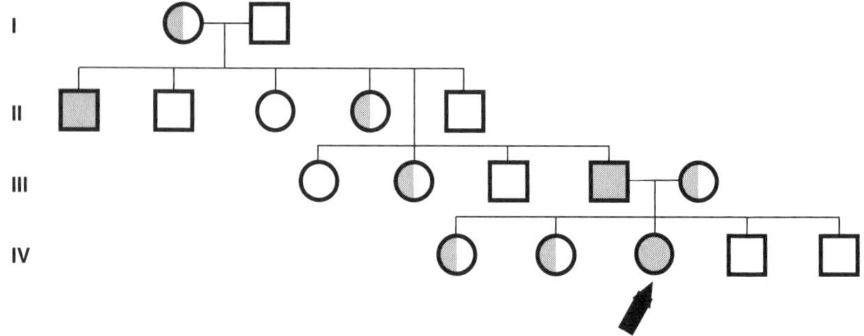

Figure 13. A typical X-linked recessive pedigree.

Some additional points to note are:
- father-to-son transmission of an X-linked trait is impossible; if a man passes his one and only X to an offspring, the child is female, except under rare circumstances involving, for example, chromosome translocations;
- unless dealing with a common recessive condition, such as color blindness, the vast majority of affected individuals are males, in contrast to X-linked dominant conditions (see paragraph below); and
- whereas consanguinity is a factor in autosomal recessive inheritance, it is irrelevant for X-linked recessive inheritance.

X-linked dominant conditions occur much more frequently among women because women have twice as many X chromosomes as men. For an affected woman, the pedigree appears identical to that for an autosomal dominant trait. On average, half of the daughters and half of the sons are affected. However, for an affected man, things are different, as shown in Figure 14. All of his daughters and none of his sons are affected. Often, as would be expected, the manifestations of an X-linked dominant condition in affected men are more severe than in affected women because of the mitigating influence of the normal allele on the woman's second X. In fact, many X-linked dominant mutations are apparently lethal in males during intrauterine life.

Exceptions to Mendelian Inheritance
X-inactivation and the Lyon Hypothesis

When biologists realized that the sex-determining pair of chromosomes in mammals, the X and Y, contain important genes having nothing to do with sex determination (literally thousands of them on the human X, for example), a puzzle emerged. How can a species tolerate a situation where one sex, the woman, has twice as many of these genes as the man and at least the potential for producing twice as much gene product for each of them? Without some compensatory mechanism, one sex would almost certainly

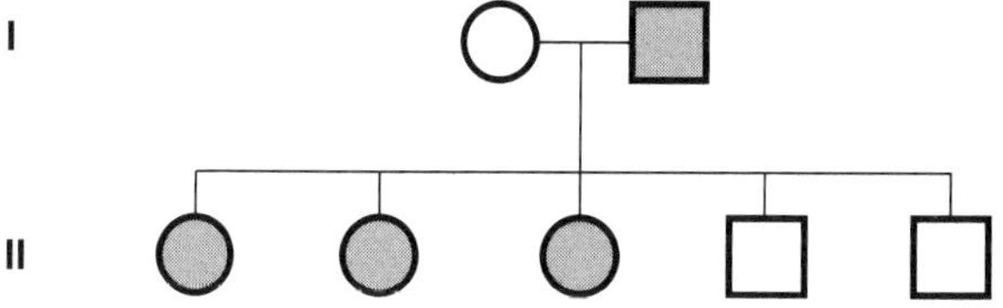

Figure 14. An X-linked dominant pedigree.

have a significant advantage over the other, and the disadvantaged sex would, over the eons of evolution, disappear, and with it, the entire species.

Mary Lyon, an English mouse geneticist, first proposed, on the basis of studies of X-linked coat-color variants, that in the normal mammalian female, one of the two X chromosomes is genetically inactivated. This, she suggested, is the mechanism for equalization of gene-dosage effects between the sexes.

Lyon went on to hypothesize that:

- the inactivation must occur early in the life of the embryo;
- in each embryonic cell, it is a matter of chance as to which of the two X chromosomes (the paternally or maternally derived one) is inactivated; and,
- once an X is inactivated in an embryonic cell, all of the progeny of that cell maintain the same inactive X.

Research has demonstrated that Lyon's hypotheses are correct. The normal mammalian female, therefore, is a mosaic of X-chromosome gene expression, with patches of cells expressing the genes of the paternally derived X and patches expressing those of the maternally derived X. On average, the split is 50-50, but because the inactivation event is random, considerable variation can and does occur. Continued research has shown that many genes escape inactivation and that the process is not entirely random (Reference 3).

The significance of X inactivation is profound. It was the first example of "genomic imprinting" (see the Genomic Imprinting section), and there are clear clinical implications. For example, in many X-linked recessive disorders, heterozygotes have a remarkable range of expression, from being phenotypically normal to manifesting characteristics of the disorder almost as severely, or even as severely, as affected men. In most instances this results from the randomness of X inactivation, a phenomenon referred to as skewed inactivation.

Further, in X chromosome aneuploidy (males and females with multiple X chromosomes [e.g., Klinefelter syndrome], 47, XXY; and the triple X female, 47, XXX), affected individuals are often phenotypically normal or have relatively minor anomalies, in sharp contrast to autosomal aneuploidy (e.g., trisomies 13 and 18) where devastating effects are the rule. Obviously, inactivation of all X chromosomes in excess of one accounts, in large part, for these comparatively mild effects of X chromosome aneuploidy. However, as the number of additional X chromosomes increases, the phenotypic anomalies become more severe. There is little doubt that some of the genes that escape inactivation play a role in the abnormal features of the phenotypes of individuals with X chromosome aneuploidy, as does the period in embryogenesis from conception to the time of X inactivation, during which all of the X chromosomes are active.

Mitochondria and Maternal Inheritance

As discussed in the Location of the Genetic Material section, mitochondria, the important energy-producing cytoplasmic organelles, contain DNA. Mutations in mtDNA also can cause disease.

Figure 15, a stylized pedigree for mitochondrial inheritance, shows a unique pattern: only affected women transmit the trait; all of the daughters and all of the sons of an affected woman are affected, as shown in generations I and II. Generation III is where things get interesting, but readily explicable. Again, all the offspring of an affected woman are affected regardless of their sex, but none of the offspring of affected men are affected. This "maternal inheritance" results from mitochondrial mutations. With only rare exceptions, mitochondria in humans are transmitted exclusively by women. Mitochondria present in sperm are confined to the tail piece and are shed at fertilization. However, only rarely is such a typical pedigree found for any given family with any given mitochondrial disorder. A variety of factors contributes to the heterogeneity.

For example, when a mitochondrial mutation first arises within a cell, it creates an intracellular mixture of mutant and normal molecules, which is called heteroplasmy. As a heteroplasmic cell divides, chance determines the relative number of mutant and normal DNAs that end up in the daughter cells. The proportion can differ from pure mutant to pure normal mitochondrial populations, a phenomenon known as homoplasmy. All variations of heteroplasmies are seen between the two homoplasmies. As would be expected, this random distribution of differing populations of

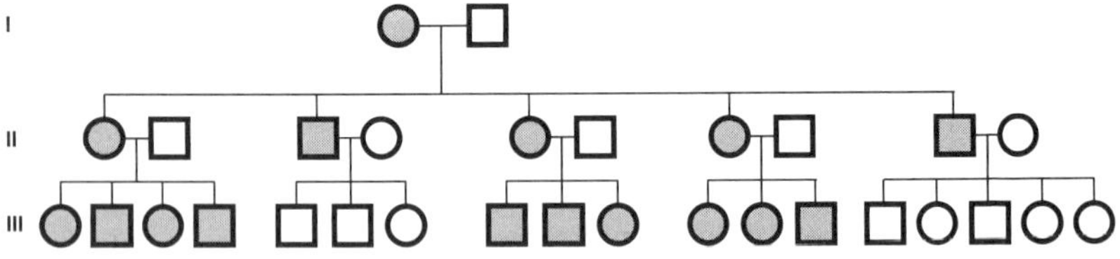

Figure 15. Maternal inheritance.

mitochondria creates great variability among offspring, even within the same sibship.

Sometimes mutations accumulate in mtDNAs of *post*mitotic tissues as humans age, and they may interfere with normal organ and tissue function. Their potential importance in organ senescence associated with aging and with the diseases of aging, such as Parkinson's and Alzheimer's disease, is a subject of exciting current research (Reference 4).

Organ systems that have the highest energy requirements (e.g., the brain, skeletal muscle, and heart muscle) are most susceptible to damage from mitochondrial mutations, and mitochondrial diseases, therefore, often are associated with those systems. More than 40 mitochondrial disorders have been described in humans. Each is quite rare, but epidemiological studies have shown that collectively mitochondrial disease is far more common than previously believed (Reference 5).

Involvement of multiple systems is typical, with unusual combinations of brain and/or neuromuscular disorders, with or without defects in vision or hearing. All manifestations are usually progressive in nature (e.g., muscle weakness, myoclonia, loss of muscle control or lack of coordination, developmental delay, and visual and/or hearing impairment).

Laboratory findings include elevated blood lactate and blood sugar (diabetes is not uncommon in mitochondrial disorders), along with aberrations of a variety of metabolites detectable by amino acid and organic acid screening. Definitive diagnosis depends on biopsy findings and molecular analysis.

Genetic Anticipation

One of the basic concepts established in Mendel's experiments with plant hybridization is that genetic "factors," as he dubbed them, pass unchanged from generation to generation, although the phenotypes may vary dramatically. But there was a confounding observation that in some medical conditions, mostly dominantly inherited neurological or neuromuscular diseases, the age at onset decreases and the severity of the symptoms increases as the gene passes from generation to generation.

This phenomenon is known as a genetic "anticipation." The first clear demonstration of anticipation was in families with myotonic dystrophy, an autosomal dominant disorder characterized by myotonia (prolonged spasm or slow relaxation of skeletal muscle after contraction), muscle weakness, and cataracts (Reference 6). All of the manifestations are progressive, although the rates of progression may vary considerably even within families.

In some recorded pedigrees, individuals with isolated cataracts and no detectable muscle disorder produced descendants with, in addition to cataracts, progressive myotonia and muscle weakness. The first attempt at a detailed study was in 1947, in which a worsening of clinical signs and earlier ages at onset from generation to generation was clearly shown, with statistical analyses to back up those conclusions.

The observation was ignored as simply a statistical aberration due to ascertainment bias, that is, families with the most severe cases were more likely to be discovered than those with mildly affected individuals. In addition, it seemed totally inexplicable on a biological basis. How could a single mutant gene change as it passed from generation to generation?

The first indication of a biological explanation for anticipation in myotonic dystrophy was documented in 1960, with the first clear descriptions of *congenital* myotonic dystrophy. The affected infants were invariably the offspring of affected *mothers*. The nature of the biological factor responsible for this phenomenon was unknown at the time, but some investigators proposed that a maternal metabolite might cross the placenta during intrauterine development.

Detailed family studies of myotonic dystrophy in the mid 1980s eventually refuted the explanation of anticipation as entirely a statistical phenomenon. The studies showed clear and unequivocal intergenerational differences. In 1989, similar family studies done for fragile X disease (an X-linked syndrome characterized by mild to moderate intellectual impairment and specific facial features) also showed similarly remarkable intergenerational differences. In 1991, unstable DNA sequences were demonstrated in fragile X families. The underlying molecular phenomenon consisted of variable length CCG repeat sequences. By the end of that same year, unstable DNA sequences in myotonic dystrophy also were demonstrated and confirmed by additional studies in 1992.

Now there are more than a dozen neurodegenerative diseases known to be caused by the expansion of triplet repeat sequences in DNA (e.g., Huntington disease, many of the cerebellar ataxias, myotonic dystrophy, fragile X, and Friedreich ataxia, Friedreich ataxia being the only autosomal recessive in the group so far; the rest are autosomal dominants, except for fragile X). Anticipation occurs in Huntington disease only when the gene expansion is passed from the father to a child. The reverse is true for myotonic dystrophy; the congenital form occurs only when the myotonic dystrophy expansion originates from an affected mother. In both disorders, the sex of the affected offspring is irrelevant (i.e., males and females are affected equally frequently).

Numerous models have been proposed to explain how the expansion of triplet repeats leads to human disease. At the DNA level, expansions in one of the two alleles can cause misalignment at meiosis, resulting in both deletions and further expansions. As a result, sometimes the gene can become completely disabled and fail to produce an mRNA transcript. These expansions may even affect adjacent genes. When expanded segments are transcribed, the repeat triplets might affect protein folding and cause varying degrees of impairment of the action of the gene product.

Genetic Imprinting

This term describes the differing phenotypes of some syndromes, depending on the sex of the parent from whom the mutant allele is inherited (Reference 7). Most autosomal genes are expressed from both the maternal and the paternal alleles. However, imprinted genes are expressed from only one chromosome, in a manner that depends on the parent of origin, on the basis of imprints that are laid down in the parental germ cells.

Genetic imprinting in mammals was discovered in the early 1980s as a result of experiments in mice where, for example, nuclear transplantation was used to produce embryos that had only one of the two sets of parental chromosomes. In other experiments, techniques were used to create embryos that inherited specific single chromosomes from one parent only. Data from both types of experiments showed that mammalian genes could function differently depending on whether they came from the mother or the father. Research during the early 1990s produced the discovery of a relationship between imprinted genes and human disease: Mutations in the proximal part of the long arm of chromosome 15 cause Prader-Willi syndrome when the mutated allele originates from the paternally derived chromosome, but when the same mutation is inherited from a maternal allele, the result is Angelman syndrome, an entirely different condition.

Research also demonstrated that DNA methylation is a key molecular mechanism of imprinting. The methylation marks the imprinted genes differently in egg and sperm, and inheritance of these marks leads to differential gene expression.

Further aberrations related to imprinting include:

- imprinted genes are rarely found on their own. Most are physically linked in clusters with other imprinted genes, and for some of the clusters, imprinting centers or imprinting control elements have been discovered. These centers or elements are needed for the regional control of imprinting or imprinted expression.
- as a rule, paternally expressed genes enhance fetal growth and maternally expressed genes suppress fetal growth. In addition, there is evidence that imprinted genes influence brain development or function, as exemplified by the surprisingly large number of neurological and psychiatric disorders in which parent-of-origin expansions are differentially involved.

Uniparental Disomy

Uniparental disomy (UPD) is a fascinating phenomenon wherein an individual inherits both chromosomes of a homologous pair or segments of both chromosomes solely from one parent (Reference 8). Depending on which parental chromosome is involved, the result can be devastating even though no single-gene mutations are present.

In humans, many UPDs are derived from a trisomic conceptus where postzygotic nondisjunction leads to chromosomal mosaicism.

(Nondisjunction is the term for failure of pairs of homologous chromosomes to separate during meiosis.) The trisomic cell line may be lost and the remaining diploid cells can have that one chromosome pair as both of paternal origin, both of maternal origin, or one of each. In the case of *maternal* UPD for chromosome 15, for example, the affected person will have Prader-Willi syndrome; *paternal* UPD for the same chromosome results in Angelman syndrome. Both syndromes are characterized by mental retardation but otherwise are completely different. Uniparental disomy actually accounts for about 30 percent of cases of Prader-Willi syndrome but for less than 5 percent of cases of Angelman syndrome. The cause for the difference in proportions is unknown. For other chromosomes, UPD apparently causes no adverse effects.

There also can be UPD for only a portion of a chromosome pair as a result of chromosomal rearrangements such as translocations or duplications. Some cases of Beckwith-Wiedemann syndrome, for example, are due to partial UPD for a section of chromosome 11, with paternal imprinting. Overgrowth disorders such as Beckwith-Wiedemann syndrome typically include varying degrees of tall stature, enlarged internal organs, and often a predisposition to malignancies.

Another puzzle solved by the discovery of UPD is the observation that occasionally a child with molecularly categorized cystic fibrosis has only one parent who is a heterozygote. False paternity was suspected in families where it was the father who was the noncarrier, but others showed the mother as the noncarrier. Recent studies have shown unequivocally that UPD is sometimes the explanation.

How Do Disorders Caused Primarily by Single-gene Mutations Differ from Multifactorial or Complex Disorders?

Terms and Definitions

The majority of human traits, normal and abnormal, fall into the category of multifactorial or complex. Complex disorders include atherosclerotic heart disease, hypertension, most congenital anomalies, most types of cancer, the psychiatric disorders, and even infections. An infectious disease can be viewed as the result of a conflict between two genomes: that of the host and that of the invading organism, each of which has opportunities for variability and each of which is affected by environmental circumstances operating at the time. Complex disorders are far more common than those caused by single-gene mutations and they constitute the bulk of the health care burden in developed countries.

The term "multifactorial" is still widely used but is being replaced by the more inclusive term "complex disorders." "Multifactorial etiology" is the correct phrase, and it means that there is more than one predisposing gene whose products interact with factors in the environment to overcome the homeostatic equilibrium of the organism; the end result is disease. The term, complex diseases, requires one to think not only about causative agents but also about physiological mechanisms that include evolution, development, and homeostatic processes, all operating within specific societies and cultures. (Homeostasis can be defined simply as the status quo—a steady state of lifelong stability of one's individuality in face of the variety of experiences of a lifetime. It implies access to the environment, as well as protection from it, and it serves an evolutionary purpose, maintaining individuals as fit to reproduce [i.e., it includes development—those devices that promote growth, differentiation, and maturation].)

Complex disorders show familial aggregation without clear segregation, a key concept that tends to escape the casual observer. The *genes* of complex diseases certainly segregate; it is the *phenotypes* that do not, or at least they do not in any predictable ratios, as do single-gene defects. In other words, complex disorders cluster within families more frequently than can be accounted for by chance, but not in the predictable ratios of affected to nonaffected that are characteristic of Mendelian conditions.

Uncertainties Regarding Risks

Most of the time, complex conditions are so highly variable from a causal point of view that even for a given population, risk figures for close relatives provided in texts and journal articles mean little. When facing an *individual* to discuss the probability of a given complex disorder, whatever risk figure is found, it is *not* that person's risk. THE INDIVIDUAL RISK SIMPLY IS NOT KNOWN. It might be as low as 2 percent or even zero; but it also might be 50 percent if the condition were due to a new dominant mutation in one of the parental germ lines. It is OK for geneticists or other health care providers to present the usual 2-5 percent risk for offspring of affected parents or siblings of affected individuals as long as the person with whom the risks are being discussed *understands* the limitations of the stated risk in relation to the individual.

The uncertainties of risks and susceptibilities in complex disorders are going to be a challenge for physicians and counselors for some time. They vary from family to family with the same apparent disease and vary to some extent even within families. For example, a disease may involve five predisposing genes, any three of which can, but will not always, cause it to become manifest. Each member of a given family may inherit different sets of predisposing genes from his or her parents. And again, the effects of the genes will be influenced differently by the modifying effects of genes at other loci and by differing environmental factors. When it becomes possible to test for some of the specific susceptibility alleles, as it already has for a handful of diseases (e.g., some of the early-onset types of Alzheimer's disease), careful and clear discussion will be essential for patients and their families to address the true meaning of genetic susceptibility and complex causation, and the limited predictive value of both positive and negative test results.

Single-gene Disorders as Complex Diseases—Hemochromatosis

Papers have been written describing single-gene traits as complex diseases (Reference 9 and 10). How can this be? Consider individuals with glucose-6-phosphate dehydrogenase deficiency. It is an X-linked condition wherein affected individuals may go through life without realizing that they have it if they never eat fava beans or never are exposed to the oxidizing drugs (e.g., phenacetin, sulfonamides, and antimalarial drugs) that precipitate hemolysis. Similarly, the autosomal recessive metabolic disease, hemochromatosis (Reference 10), is remarkably complex. Hemochromatosis is by far the most common autosomal recessive disease in people of northern European descent, with a carrier frequency of about one in 10 and a disease incidence between one in 250 and one in 400. Hemochromatosis causes increased gastrointestinal absorption of iron, with potentially fatal iron deposition in multiple tissues and organs. Manifestations include cirrhosis, hepatoma, cardiomyopathy, diabetes, arthritis, sexual dysfunction, and dark pigmentation or bronzing of the skin. Early diagnosis followed by regular therapeutic phlebotomies can prevent iron overload and give homozygous affected individuals a normal life expectancy; even therapy later in the course of the disease improves the symptoms and prolongs life.

The cause is a mutation in the *HFE* gene that is responsible for producing a protein in the deep crypts of the duodenum, where gastrointestinal iron absorption is at its highest. *HFE* in normal amounts modulates iron absorption according to need; insufficient amounts result in the characteristics of iron overload. The majority of individuals with hemochromatosis have an identical point mutation called C282Y, although an additional mutation, H63D, accounts for a small proportion of cases. A third small group of patients has non-*HFE*-associated hemochromatosis.

Why would this classical autosomal recessive disorder be considered a complex disease? A recent, admittedly controversial, paper (Reference 11) showed that an astonishingly small proportion (less than 1 percent) of homozygous affected individuals develop frank clinical hemochromatosis. What factors could be responsible for this extraordinary observation? Consider the following:

- major environmental factors are involved in the etiology (e.g., diet [intake of foods such as red meats that are rich in iron] and vitamin C supplementation increases iron absorption);
- for all homozygous affected individuals, sufficient iron storage takes time (i.e., childhood cases are rare, and the usual onset of manifestations occurs during middle age);
- half of the population of homozygous individuals treats itself— menstruation in women is therapeutic and women affected before menopause are rare unless other risk factors are present;
- similarly, regular blood donors may never develop manifestations even though homozygous for the mutant gene;

- pathological blood loss is therapeutic (e.g., inflammatory bowel disease—one disease correcting another);
- manifestations of hemochromatosis in homozygous affected individuals often require the simultaneous presence of another disease (e.g., hepatitis or other types of liver disease);
- curiously, given the low penetrance of the *HFE* mutations, even heterozygotes occasionally develop overt clinical disease, but again, in association with other risk factors, including hepatitis, alcoholism, and diseases requiring transfusion;
- mutations at other genetic loci (e.g., individuals with hemochromatosis are more likely to develop diabetes if they have a family history of diabetes even among relatives who do not have hemochromatosis). Thus, a better example of a multifactorial or complex disorder could hardly be found.

It was not long ago that many were advocating screening of all children or young adults of northern European descent for the hemochromatosis mutations with the goal of instituting early intervention and, thus, preventing the development of serious disease later in life. The "complexity" of the disorder is now giving them pause.

Well then, how *do* complex diseases differ from single-gene disorders? In spite of the previously discussed examples, most of the single-gene disorders are expressed regardless of the environment. If individuals inherit a mutation responsible for achondroplasia, they will be dwarfs regardless of where they live or what they eat. If an infant is homozygous for the mutant gene responsible for deficient hexosaminidase A activity, that infant will have Tay-Sachs disease and inevitably manifests progressive physical and mental deterioration with death by 3-4 years of age.

The difference boils down to understanding that complex diseases differ from single-gene disorders *quantitatively* in that for the former, the multiple contributing genes specify proteins whose effects combine to produce a phenotype, whereas in the latter, the proteins encoded by *one* locus override the effects of those from other loci. In addition, in complex disorders, multiple environmental variables interact with the various proteins to modify their effects in a variety of ways, and expression is influenced by the products of these multiple genes interacting throughout development, maturation, and aging. The environmental factors are broadly defined and most of the time we do not know what these environmental factors are or how they interact with gene products. In fact, most of the so-called predisposing *genes* have yet to be worked out.

Although single-gene and complex diseases differ quantitatively, they do not differ qualitatively (i.e., the relationship among genes, proteins, and biological processes is the same for both). However, for single-gene problems, it is usually easier to discern the relationship between the gene and the phenotype, and we know the details of that relationship for many of these disorders. The relationship is less easily determined in complex disorders, and we know only a few of the details for a few such diseases.

Age at Onset

Age at onset merits consideration when thinking of differences between single-gene and complex disorders. The former tend to disrupt homeostasis early in development, whereas the effects of the multiple alleles of the latter culminate in onset later in life.

Yet, complex diseases demonstrate a declining heritability of disease with age. Schizophrenia is a good example. If a person is at risk because of affected close relatives who typically showed signs of disease in the late teens or 20s, the older that person gets (beyond the usual ages at onset) without showing signs of the disease, the less likely he or she is to develop the disease.

Environmental Issues

What does environment really mean? Understanding complex disease requires an expanded view of the "environment" that goes well beyond teratogens, toxins, radiation, and other carcinogens. The environment begins with the intracellular milieu at conception, progresses to the interaction of the individual (embryo and fetus) with the intrauterine environment and then, the outside world. The environment for a given single gene could include the effects of its products interacting with the products of other genes, as previously discussed for hemochromatosis.

Furthermore, consideration of "environment" requires recognition of the unique developmental history and experiences of a given disease through a unique series of events particular to that one individual. Again, the many environmental factors influencing the eventual expression or lack of expression of hemochromatosis are illustrative.

Population Genetics

Population genetics merits a brief discussion. There are no sharp boundaries between human populations around the globe but clearly, certain populations have accumulated specific mutations (e.g., sickle cell disease in blacks and cartilage-hair hypoplasia among the Amish). Nevertheless, there is far more variation within populations than between them. Thus, the designation of biological races blurs, just as the boundaries between complex and Mendelian disorders blur, as previously discussed.

Table 2 summarizes the similarities and differences between single-gene and complex disorders.

Table 2. Complex vs. Single-Gene Disorders

Characteristics	Complex	Single-Gene
Gene(s)	segregates	segregates
Disorder	aggregates	segregates
Gene products involved	multiple	primarily one
Role of environment	important	often over-ridden by effect(s) of gene mutation
Age of onset	older	younger
Risks for relatives of probands	smaller, less predictable	larger, more predictable
Health care burden	high	low

Understanding and Learning How to Access New Genetic Technology

Advances in Technology

Modern molecular techniques essential to pharmacy are detailed in subsequent Pharmacogenomics modules. However, to comprehend the new, it is important to have some appreciation of the pioneering research that tends to get lost in the admittedly appropriate excitement over cloning, microarrays, and gene sequencing.

The Southern Blot

The discovery in the early 1970s of bacterial restriction endonucleases, or restriction enzymes, was a major advance. These enzymes recognize specific double-stranded complementary DNA (cDNA), usually about a dozen nucleotides in length, and cleaves the complementary DNA at or near these specific sequences. Two fragments usually are generated at each cleavage site, each with single-stranded identical tails, as shown in Figure 16. These tails often are referred to as "sticky" ends because in subsequent reactions to create recombinant DNA (rDNA), cDNA sequences adhere to each other, nucleotide by complementary nucleotide (C $\rightarrow$ G, A $\rightarrow$ T, and vice versa).

Different restriction enzymes recognize different sequences of nucleotides, and there are more than a thousand known restriction enzymes. Because there are hundreds of thousands of sequences scattered through

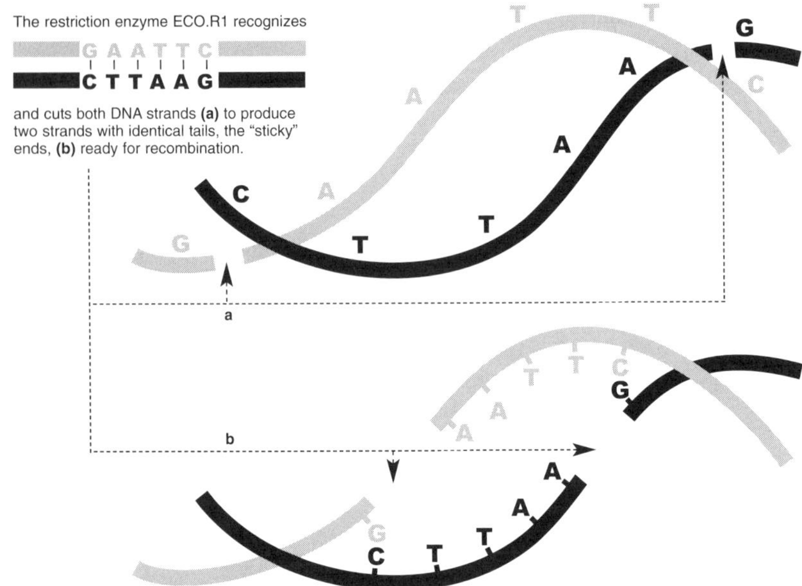

Figure 16. The action of restriction endonucleases.

the genome that are recognized by each restriction endonuclease, each breaks up the DNA into characteristic and reproducible fragments reflecting the frequency and location of specific cleavage sites, each with identical single-stranded sticky ends.

The important feature to keep in mind is that even a single base-pair change in a potential cleavage site abolishes its recognition by the restriction enzyme and a unique larger fragment is created as a result. These unique fragments may reflect specific disease-causing mutations or simply DNA polymorphisms, but in any case the fragments can be identified by the technique known as Southern blotting. The basic details of the procedure are diagrammed in Figure 17.

Genomic DNA is first isolated from any accessible cells or tissues and then exposed to restriction enzyme digestion. The resulting fragments— about 1 million of them—are separated by size on gel electrophoresis; the smaller the fragment, the more quickly it migrates through the gel. The double-stranded fragments are denatured to separate the two cDNA strands and the now single strands are transferred from the gel to a piece of nitrocellulose filter paper by simple blotting; hence, the word "blot." The technique was named for the person who invented it; it has nothing to do with the compass direction.

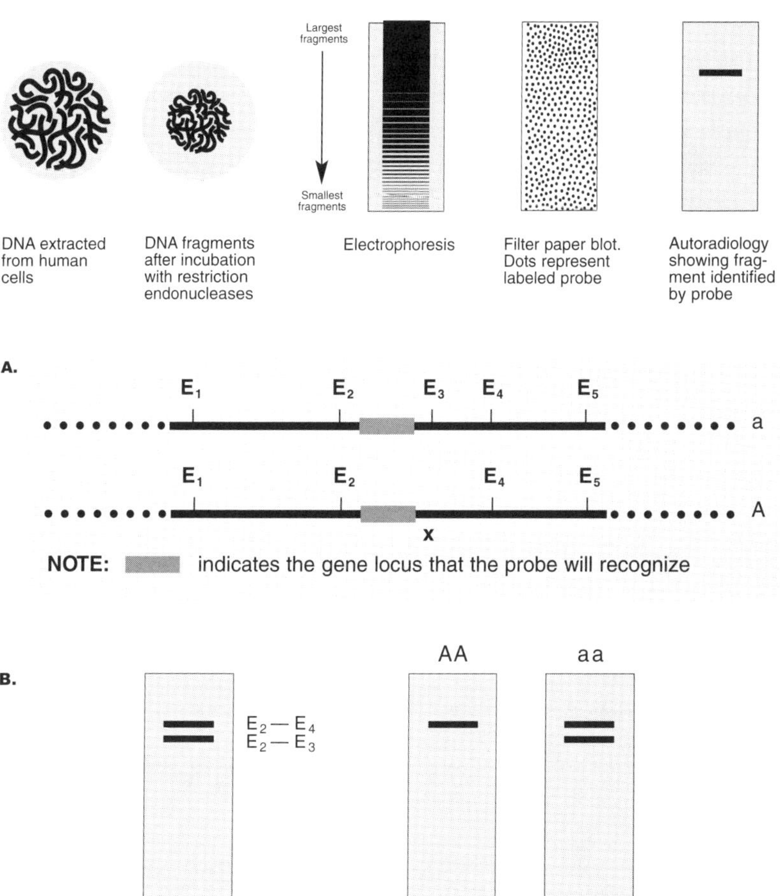

Figure 17. Diagram of the Southern blot technique. In the DNA strand A, the recognition site is mutated (x) and the DNA fragment recognized by the probe will be larger than for strand a. At the bottom of the diagram, B is shown the results after electrophoresis: the gel on the left is from a heterozygote. AA is homozygous for the mutant and aa, homozygous normal.

To identify specific fragments of interest among the millions, a specific labeled probe is used, usually a piece of cloned DNA that has been radioactively or fluorescently labeled. Probe and filter paper are incubated together and because of the specificity of cDNA base pairing, the probe anneals stably only to its complementary strand on the filter paper. Thus, usually only one or two fragments are labeled. Unbound probes are washed off the filter, which is then placed onto radiograph film (if a radioactive label is used) with its bound probe, and specific bands are produced by the radioactivity, as shown in the diagram (Figure 18).

Southern blotting continues to be a standard procedure for diagnostic purposes in molecular laboratories but is frequently replaced by polymerase chain reaction (PCR)-based methodology.

Expansion of this technique finds the molecular biology community guilty of etymological obfuscation. The minor modification of the Southern blot to use RNA in the place of DNA is referred to as a "Northern blot," and when antibodies are used as probes to detect protein molecules after gel electrophoresis, it is called a "Western blot." Believe it or not, there is also a "Far Western blot" (protein to protein) and "South Western blot" (protein to DNA). The punning has apparently stopped; there is no Eastern blot … at least, not yet.

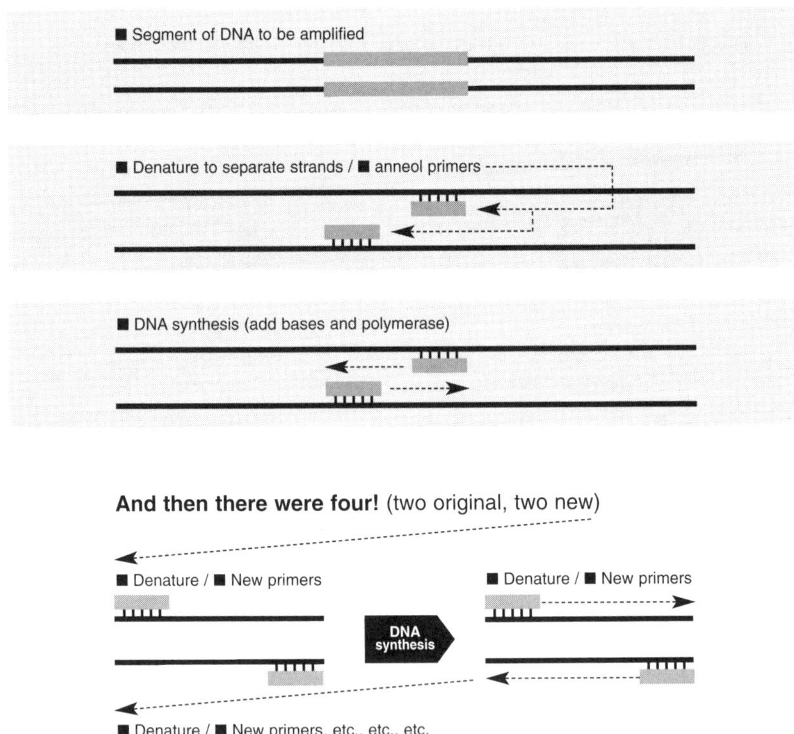

Figure 18. Polymerase chain reaction.

Vectors

The concept of vectors is important for understanding many of the past, present, and future uses for rDNA. A vector is a DNA molecule that can replicate autonomously (e.g., in bacterial or yeast cells), and from which specific DNA sequences can later be isolated in pure form. Vectors include bacterial plasmids, bacteriophage, and both bacterial and yeast artificial chromosomes. For instance, the specific human gene responsible for encoding insulin can be inserted into a bacterium by means of restriction enzymes. The same enzyme is used to produce the human DNA fragment as to fracture the host cell DNA; the sticky ends thus created are complementary and permit the insertion.

The host cell then replicates and can produce huge numbers of copies of the human gene, which can then be separated from bacterial gene products. This is a mechanism for cloning human genes, and the cloned genes can be used for further study and for therapeutic purposes. For example, virtually all human growth hormone for use in treating short stature is now derived through these techniques. In the past, there was no way to obtain the hormone other than by extraction from human anterior pituitary glands obtained at autopsy and gathered at great effort and expense by The Human Growth Foundation, a voluntary organization dedicated to patients and families with growth-hormone deficiencies and other growth disorders.

Genetic Libraries

Various laboratories now have generated large quantities of human gene sequences as sets of clones of bacteria or yeast that contain a vector into which fragments of DNA have been inserted. These collections of clones are called libraries. The next step in the application of such DNA libraries to molecular diagnosis and further research is to identify clones of interest using a variety of screening methods.

Reverse Transcriptase

Another extremely important discovery relevant to libraries also goes back several decades, to the discovery of reverse transcriptase, isolated from a retrovirus (retroviruses are simple RNA viruses). This enzyme can synthesize a cDNA strand from an RNA template; that is, it reverses the standard flow of genetic information. Single-stranded cDNA can be converted to a double-stranded molecule, ligated into a suitable vector, and be used to produce a cDNA library that represents the original mRNA transcripts from the starting cells or tissue. Why would researchers bother to do this? Complementary DNA libraries are invaluable resources for gene cloning. A major advance over DNA libraries is the absence of intron sequences (the introns were spliced out in the original transcription of nuclear DNA to mRNA); cDNA contains only the exons.

Polymerase Chain Reaction

Figure 19 diagrams the molecular technique whereby a short DNA or RNA segment can be amplified almost indefinitely by repeated doublings. It requires the sequence of interest to be flanked by two oligonucleotide primers, one complementary to one strand of the DNA molecule on one side of the target sequence, and the other complementary to the DNA molecule on the opposite side of the target sequence. The primers are oriented so that they initiate two new strands of DNA that are themselves complementary and form a second copy of the original target sequence. The cycles of denaturation, hybridization of primers, and enzymatic DNA synthesis initiated by DNA polymerase result in cycles of amplification as shown. The process has been automated and can generate literally billions of copies of a starting sequence within just a few hours.

Stem Cells

Stem-cell research is still in an embryonic stage (pun intended) and there are far more questions than answers at this time. A series of "Insight" articles on the subject was published recently; the following, brief comments are based on that overview (Reference 12).

The impetus for the current excitement about stem cells arose primarily from two important reports. The first, in 1997, showed that an adult cell nucleus can be reprogrammed to produce a whole animal; that was the cloning of a lamb, the now famous "Dolly." The second was the derivation of embryonic stem-cell lines from human blastocysts, in 1998. The latter provided a potential source of cells for a potentially wide spectrum of stem cell-based therapies for human diseases.

Perhaps more interesting has been the possibility of therapeutic cloning, whereby stem cells could be derived from the actual patient, grown up into large colonies, and then used in that same patient to cure the disease. This technique already is available in a handful of centers for clinical purposes. For example, stem cells have been isolated from the peripheral blood of patients with leukemia or lymphoma who are no longer responsive to the standard therapeutic gamut. The stem cells are grown in vitro. The patient's bone marrow then is destroyed by chemotherapy, followed by infusion of the cultured stem cells. When the implantation is successful, the disease is cured. This approach, of course, avoids the problem of immune rejection.

Among the many remaining questions related to the use of either adult or embryonic stem cells are:
* What defines a stem cell in molecular terms?
* What are the signaling events that control stem-cell differentiation?
* How does an adult cell become "reprogrammed"?
* Is it really possible that adult stem cells are so plastic that they can in some circumstances contribute to cell types totally different from those in their tissue of origin (or do adult tissues contain mixtures of stem cells from several sources)?

Politically and ethically, the use of early embryos as a source of stem cells has precipitated intense debate. However, most ethicists believe that the use of human embryos, produced initially for in vitro fertilization and that would be discarded, pose no ethical problems. These societal and moral issues are discussed in detail in one of the "Insight" papers.

The concluding paragraph of the overview is an excellent forecast:

> "The next few years no doubt will bring great advances in understanding of stem cells at the molecular level. New techniques will aid in identifying critical genes involved in controlling their self-renewal and differentiation. Perhaps these will allow us to manipulate stem cells in vivo in a useful way. Similarly, genes involved in reprogramming will be found. So far the only even remotely reliable way of reprogramming an adult cell type into another is by transferring its nucleus into the cytoplasm of an oocyte. This presumably reflects the normal ability of the egg to reprogram the incoming sperm DNA to behave like its own. But is this due to one or many cytoplasmic factors? Identifying these and understanding how they can restore totipotentiality will be a substantial but worthwhile challenge."

Perspectives on Gene Therapy

Gene therapy is the delivery of functional copies of a relevant gene to targeted cells to improve a patient's health by correcting or repairing a DNA mutation. The normal gene is delivered to the appropriate *somatic* cells. Introduction of genes into the *germ line* is unnecessary and undesirable for both ethical and technical reasons. For example, any attempt to integrate a normal copy of a gene into a reproductive cell could create a significant risk of causing new mutations.

Several general purposes have been put forward in relation to somatic-cell gene therapy, the most obvious being to compensate for a mutant cellular gene. ß-Thalassemia is a good example to illustrate the approach. A sample of the patient's bone marrow is removed and exposed to an aliquot of the purified normal ß-chain gene. Techniques have been developed to facilitate entry of DNA into cells in vitro; the "corrected" bone marrow cells then could be injected back into the patient. If the implantations were successful and sufficient numbers of corrected cells survived, the disease would be cured.

Another potential approach is the inactivation of the mutation, which is useful in dominant conditions where an abnormal gene product causes the disease phenotype. Obviously, inactivating the abnormal gene allows the normal one to produce normal product unimpeded; thus, the disease is cured. It sounds easy, but in practice it is technically difficult. In the gene-expansion conditions, for example (see the Genetic Anticipation section), destroying the mutant RNA, rather than the gene that caused it, would work. Selective degradation of the mutant RNA encoding a dominant negative protein, as previously discussed (see the Autosomal Dominant Inheritance section) for OI, also would work.

Furthermore, and of much interest to pharmacists, is the use of gene therapy as a pharmaceutical approach—an attempt to counter the *effects* of a mutant cellular gene(s). For example, it might be possible and therapeutically beneficial to introduce a tumor necrosis gene into a malignant tumor, thereby destroying it. Similarly, and much in the news at this time, is the possibility of inserting DNA that leads to the production of growth factors into a heart that has undergone infarction to stimulate the growth of blood vessels in the damaged area.

Finally, words of caution: all of the previously discussed goals and approaches are fraught with problems and pitfalls. To date there has been no long-term success for gene therapy and there has been at least one death in a volunteer with a relatively benign genetic disease. The ethical issues are legion and include such issues as the patenting of genes and privacy of DNA data in relation to insurance and employment, all of which are discussed in detail in subsequent Pharmacogenomics modules.

On the other hand, it is completely inaccurate to assume that there is no hope simply because a condition is genetic. A wide variety of treatment and preventive modalities have been available since antiquity. Tales of approaches to prevention from Pythagorus and from biblical days are discussed in the Central Assumptions of Genetics and Genetic Medicine section. In addition, surgeons have dealt with disfiguring and potentially lethal congenital malformations with increasing sophistication and success, and metabolic diseases such as phenylketonuria, diabetes, and galactosemia yielded to environmental manipulations long before any notion of the basic DNA mutations were uncovered. Enzyme replacement therapy has worked remarkably well for some of the inherited lysosomal diseases such as Gaucher disease and in severe immune deficiency due to adenosine deaminase deficiency. Some exciting glimpses into the future are found in the other chapters of this module and other Pharmacogenomics modules.

Geneticists have been among the leaders in advocating and then implementing preventive screening programs. Such programs include the newborn screens for metabolic diseases and hyperthyroidism, prenatal testing for chromosome anomalies and other genetic disorders, and preoperative screening for carrier detection of some of the common mutant alleles, such as in Tay-Sachs disease, thalassemia, sickle cell disease, and cystic fibrosis.

Genetics in Medicine Today—The New Genetics

Genetic Counseling

Until recently, the physician's involvement with genetic disorders has been restricted mainly to the relatively rare single-gene disorders and chromosome anomalies. Observations of single-gene disorders segregating within families led to a few books on the subject in the late 19th century and the first half of the 20th century, but little interest resulted because of the perceived lack of satisfactory treatment or prevention.

With Lejeune's pivotal 1959 paper on the cause of Down syndrome, trisomy 21, followed by the descriptions of anomalies of many other chromosomes, geneticists finally had an anatomical tissue of their own. These discoveries emerged at about the same time as the almost geometric increase in elucidation of the enzyme defects responsible for the metabolic diseases, along with preventive techniques and even treatment. The training of physicians in genetics began after World War II, along with the establishment of genetics as a subject in medical school curricula, and the founding of genetic counseling centers, usually in association with medical schools. A complete listing of centers in North America, Europe, and Australia is available on the Web sites listed in the Reference section.

Genetic counseling combines the provision of risk information to individuals and families with appropriate psychological and educational support. It was carried out as a specific referral service, but that approach is changing as complex disorders such as heart disease and cancer capture the interest of medical practitioners, including virtually all specialties and subspecialties within medicine. Predisposing mutations for complex disorders are being uncovered, and with them comes, before long, new approaches to diagnosis, prevention, and therapeutic intervention.

Pharmacists and pharmacologists are in the forefront of the new genetics, probably working much more closely than in the past with physicians in the often difficult process of helping patients understand the nature of their illness and the new approaches to individualized therapy. These include elucidation of the genetics of the individual, uncovering the possibly numerous mutations (e.g., of a particular malignancy) and devising ways to match the genomes of both to ascertain the proper dose of the proper drug, as well as for providing techniques to get the drug most efficiently and safely to the proper site.

References

1. Motulsky AG, Vogel F. Human Genetics: Problems and Approaches. 3rd ed. Berlin: Springer Verlag, 1997.

2. Nussbaum RL, McInnes RR, Willard HF. Thompson & Thompson Genetics in Medicine. 6th ed. Toronto: W.B. Saunders, 2001.

3. Brown CJ, Robinson WP. The causes and consequences of random and non random X chromosome inactivation in humans. Clin Genet 2000;58:353–63.

4. Wallace CD. Mitochondrial DNA variation in human evolution, degenerative disease, and aging. 1994 William Allan Award Address. Am J Hum Genet 1995;57:210–23.

5. Spellberg B, Carroll RM, Robinson E, Brass E. mtDNA disease in the primary care setting. Arch Intern Med 2001;161:2497–2500.

6. Harper PS, Harley HG, Reardon W, Shaw DJ. Anticipation in myotonic dystrophy: new light on an old problem. Am J Hum Genet 1992;51:10–16.

7. Reik W, Walter J. Genomic imprinting: parental influence on the genome. Nat Rev Genet 2001;2:21–32.

8. Engel E. Uniparental disomies in unselected populations. Am J Hum Genet 1998;63:962–6.

9. Scriver CR, Waters PJ. Monogenic traits are not simple: lessons from phenylketonuria. Trends Genet 1999;15:267–72.

10. McCarthy GM, McCarthy CJ, Kenny, D, Crowe J, Eustace S. Hereditary hemochromatosis: a common, often unrecognized, genetic disease. Cleve Clin J Med 2002;69:224–37.

11. Beutler E, Felitti VJ, Koziol JA, Ho NJ, Gelbart T. Penetrance of 845G*A (C282Y) *HFE* hereditary haemochromatosis mutation in the USA. Lancet 2002;359:211–18.

12. Lovell-Badge R. The future for stem cell research. Nature 2001;414:88–91.

Web Sites
Genetics Societies

1. American Society of Human Genetics: *http://www.faseb.org/genetics/ashg/ashgmenu.htm.*

2. American College of Medical Genetics: *http://www.acmg.net/.*

3. Canadian College of Medical Geneticists: *http://ccmg.medical.org/.*

4. European Society of Human Genetics: *http://www.eshg.org/.*

5. Australasian Human Genetics Society: *http://www.hgsa.com.au/main.html.*

Additional Useful Sites

1. New York State Department of Health Web site. Available at *http://www.health.state.ny.us/nysdoh/dpprd/main.htm#fulldoc.*

This is a useful site designed primarily as a guideline for evaluation of the newborn with congenital malformations. In addition, it contains, in appendices, useful references, Web sites, and a list of genetics centers in the United States.

2. National Coalition for Health Professional Education in Genetics Web site. Available at *http://www.nchpeg.org/*.

   The mission of the National Coalition for Health Professional Education in Genetics is to promote health professional education and access to information about advances in human genetics to improve the health care of the nation.

3. The Genetic Alliance Web site. Available at *http://www.geneticalliance.org/*.

   This site offers support groups for patients/families with genetic disorders.

Self-Assessment Questions

1. Which one of the following best defines a gene?

    A. A segment of DNA that encodes the amino acid sequence for an enzyme (i.e., one gene → one enzyme).
    B. A segment of DNA that encodes the amino acid sequence for a polypeptide chain.
    C. A segment of DNA that has a coding sequence flanked by a start codon and a termination codon.
    D. A segment of DNA that encodes the amino acid sequence of one, and only one, specific polypeptide chain.

2. There is a genetic polymorphism in the acetylation of isoniazid, the major mechanism for its inactivation. Some individuals are rapid inactivators, some are slow, and the rest are intermediate. Marked differences are found among global populations. For Europeans and blacks, about half are slow inactivators but among several Asian populations, the prevalence of the allele for rapid inactivation is close to 70 percent. Which one of the following is the best approach for drug management of this antituberculous drug?

    A. Test members of the Asian races for rapid activators and use a drug regimen with higher doses given more frequently.
    B. Use the usual recommended dose schedule since there is no mention of problems with rapid acetylators in the information sheet provided by the manufacturer.
    C. Use a different antituberculous drug for Asians even though it may not be quite as effective or as free of complications as isoniazid.
    D. Monitor blood levels of isoniazid for all patients regardless of race.

Questions 3 and 4 pertain to the following case.

A 25-year-old man has been informed that his older brother had been diagnosed with an inherited, adult-onset, slowly progressive neuromuscular disorder. Clinical and molecular studies have been completed on the family and the pedigree is shown on the following page. All family members shown have been tested except for the one mentioned above (indicated by a question mark) and the affected individuals are shown as darkened symbols.

3. Which one of the following is the most likely mode of inheritance?

    A. Autosomal dominant.
    B. X-linked dominant.
    C. X-linked recessive.
    D. Mitochondrial.

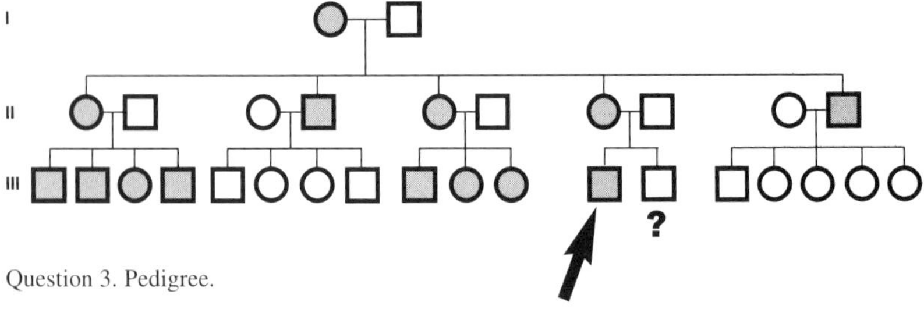

Question 3. Pedigree.

4. Which one of the following is the chance that the untested 25-year-old brother has inherited the gene that is the cause of the disease in this family?

    A. 100 percent.
    B. 50 percent.
    C. 2-5 percent.
    D. 0.

5. A 3-year-old boy is brought to the emergency department with a 2-day history of increasing fatigue and pallor. He has had no previous serious illnesses. The previous week, he was found to have an ear infection and was being treated with a sulfonamide as well as "Tylenol" for the fever. He is now extremely lethargic and the mother, as would be expected, is nearly frantic. In giving the history she blurts out that she is Italian and that could be important but she cannot remember why. Laboratory test results revealed a severe hemolytic anemia. Which one of the following is the most likely cause of the acute hemolytic anemia?

    A. Thalassemia major (Mediterranean anemia).
    B. Glucose-6-phosphate dehydrogenase deficiency (favism).
    C. Hemolysis due to a bacterial toxin from the organism that caused the ear infection.
    D. An idiosyncratic reaction to the sulfonamide.

6. A 22-year-old woman has epilepsy that is well controlled with hydantoin (Dilantin). She is anxious to have children but is concerned because she has heard that the drug is teratogenic. Which one of the following is the best approach to managing the patient?

    A. Advise her not to have children of her own in spite of her desire to do so.
    B. Stop the drug as soon as she has a confirmed pregnancy.
    C. Switch her to a different anticonvulsant that might be less teratogenic.
    D. Reassure her by informing her that the incidence of congenital anomalies in the offspring of women taking hydantoin is low.

7. Before the availability of molecular testing for Huntington's disease, a late-onset autosomal dominant disease, a 40-year-old man with a clinically affected father was tested in a family linkage study and told that he had an 80 percent chance of having inherited the Huntington's disease gene. He put his affairs in order and prepared for the worst. Ten years, later he was still free of any manifestations of the disease and was retested using DNA mutation analysis. The typical Huntington's disease gene expansion was not present. Which one of the following is the most likely cause for the misleading linkage information?

A. A cross-over between a marker locus and the Huntington's disease gene.
B. The mother and other affected family members had some other form of presenile dementia.
C. A laboratory reporting error.
D. False paternity.

Questions 8 and 9 pertain to the following case.
A 20-year-old healthy Caucasian woman with no history of any respiratory or gastrointestinal problems is planning to start a family. She is worried about her risk of having a child with cystic fibrosis, an autosomal recessive condition, since both her 15-year-old sister and 13-year-old brother have the disease.

8. Which one of the following is her risk of being a carrier of the cystic fibrosis gene?

A. 1 in 2.
B. 1 in 3.
C. 1 in 4.
D. 2 in 3.

9. The prevalence of the cystic fibrosis gene in the general population of European descent is about 1 in 20. Prior to any molecular testing and assuming her partner has a negative family history for cystic fibrosis, which one of the following is closest to her chance of having a child with cystic fibrosis?

A. 1 in 1,600.
B. 1 in 400.
C. 1 in 120.
D. 1 in 30.

10. Which one of the following diseases, each inherited as autosomal recessive traits, is most likely to be among the first to be 'cured' by gene replacement therapy?

A. Tay-Sachs disease, a progressive neurodegenerative disease that leads to death usually before age 5 years.
B. Thalassemia, a lethal form of anemia due to severe deficiency of normal hemoglobin production in the bone marrow.
C. Cystic fibrosis, a usually lethal defect in a membrane transport molecule that causes thickened secretions in the respiratory and gastrointestinal tracts, the vas deferens, and other parts of the organism.
D. Walker-Warburg (HARD+E) syndrome, with manifestations that include hydrocephalus, agyria, retinal dysplasia, and sometimes encephalocele.

11. A 30-year-old woman has myotonic dystrophy with relatively mild manifestations—cataracts, myotonia (e.g., difficulty relaxing a hand grasp), slowly progressive muscle weakness. It is one of the gene expansion disorders that shows anticipation. Her three children, ages 8, 5, and 2 are free of any detectable signs of the disease. When the mother found out about molecular testing, she wanted her children tested immediately, even though she realized that no preventive measures are available to delay the age of onset and there are no treatments for the manifestations (other than surgery for the cataracts). Which one of the following is the best way to deal with this request?

A. Go ahead and test because the mother has the right and the responsibility to make what she feels is the best decision for her children and family.
B. Refuse to arrange the testing because there is no preventive management and no treatment for the disease.
C. Refuse to test because the molecular laboratory policy and the recommendations of the American Society of Human Genetics are not to test asymptomatic children until after age 12.
D. Suggest that testing be postponed until each child reaches an age where he or she can participate maturely and rationally in the decision as to whether to test or not.

12. An 18-year-old woman has a severe, autosomal recessive disease that has caused progressive physical and mental deterioration; the age of onset is between 10 and 20 years. The patient has an 11-year-old sister who is asymptomatic. The family (parents and both children) has participated in a research study to identify the mutant gene; their participation has been totally voluntarily with appropriate written consent. The family doctor receives a call from the researcher to announce that the gene has been identified and mapped and the younger sister is also homozygous affected and will develop the disease. In fact, he observed some subtle signs of it in the sibling at the time of obtaining

the last blood specimen. Which one of the following is the best course for the physician to take?

A. Inform the parents of the results and let them decide how they are going to deal with a second affected child.
B. Explain the achievement of the researcher to the younger sibling and, with the parents, pose the question as to whether the child herself would like to know her result.
C. Withhold the information entirely from the family since it is a research project and this possibility should have been discussed in detail as consent for participation was being obtained.
D. Contact other relatives as soon as possible to let them know that a molecular test has been discovered and that testing will be made available to them and their children if they wish.

52

Applied Molecular and Cellular Biology

Taimour Y. Langaee, MSPH, Ph.D.
Issam Zineh, Pharm.D.

Key Words

Nucleus, cytoplasm, organelles, deoxyribonucleic acid (DNA), ribonucleic acid (RNA), DNA replication, DNA polymerase, RNA polymerase, transcription, protein synthesis, promoter, transcriptional activator and repressor, gene regulation, cell signaling, G protein-coupled receptors, enzyme-linked receptors.

Abstract

Ongoing research in molecular and cellular biology has resulted in tremendous advances in the basic, translational, and clinical sciences. Specifically, application of molecular and cellular biology principles has furthered human health through improved diagnosis, prevention, and treatment of diseases. Molecular and cellular biology also has played an important role in pharmacogenomics, a fairly new discipline aimed at novel drug development and rational therapeutics based on human genetic variability. As this discipline continues to grow, it becomes increasingly important for clinician-scientists to become familiar with eukaryotic cell structure and function, gene processing and regulation, and cell signaling processes. This chapter highlights fundamentals for practical application.

Outline

Learning Objectives

1. Define the cellular functions of the nucleus and cytoplasmic organelles.
2. Describe the effects of regulatory sequences and proteins on transcription.
3. Synthesize a timeline of the events in ribonucleic acid (RNA) processing and messenger RNA (mRNA) translation.
4. Understand the role of cell signaling molecules, receptors, and intracellular signaling in cell signal transduction.
5. Apply molecular and cellular biology principles to explain the possible genetic basis of variability in drug responses.

Abbreviations in this Chapter

A	Adenine
ATP	Adrenosine 5'-triphosphate
bp	Base pair
C	Cytosine
CDK	Cyclin-dependent kinase
CO_2	Carbon dioxide
CoA	Coenzyme A
CTD	Carboxy terminal domain
dNTP	Deoxyribonucleoside 5'-triphosphate
DNA	Deoxyribonucleic acid
EGF	Epidermal growth factor
EIF	Eukaryotic initiation factor

ER	Endoplasmic reticulum
FADH$_2$	Flavin adenine dinucleotide, reduced
G	Guanine
GPCRs	G Protein-coupled receptors
GTP	Guanosine triphosphate
H$_2$O	Water
H$_2$O$_2$	Hydrogen peroxide
HRE	Hormone response element
IRE	Iron-responsive element
KDEL	Lysine aspartic acid-glutamic acid-leucine
MAPK	Mitogen-activated protein kinase
mRNA	Messenger RNA
NADH	Nicotinamide adenine dinucleotide, reduced
O$_2$	Oxygen
PCNA	Proliferating cell nuclear antigen
PDGF	Platelet-derived growth factor
Pol	Polymerase
RFA	Replication factor A
RFC	Replication factor C
RNA	Ribonucleic acid
rRNA	Ribosomal RNA
RTK	Receptor tyrosine kinase
SRP	Signal recognition particle
SSB	Single-stranded binding protein
T	Thymine
TBP	TATA box binding protein
TF	Transcription factor
TfR	Transferrin receptor
tRNA	Transfer RNA
UTR	Untranslated region
XP	Xeroderma pigmentosum
XP-V	XP-variant

Introduction

Molecular and cellular biology is the cornerstone of all biological sciences and has wide applications in different scientific disciplines including medicine, drug development, and pharmacotherapy. New methods for diagnosis, prevention, and treatment of human diseases are made possible by understanding and applying the principles of this science. The importance of molecular and cellular biology in pharmacogenomics, for example, cannot be understated. Many drugs used in clinical practice show significant differences in therapeutic efficacy and toxicity, likely partially mediated through genetic, molecular, and cellular variability.

Pharmacogenomics applies molecular and cellular biology to develop tests that improve the efficacy and safety of drugs used in patients. Consideration of a polymorphism's potential impact on the protein product may help translational scientists and clinicians determine the likelihood for efficacy and/or toxicity of a drug in a patient. Current examples include genotype/protein expression-guided therapy with azathioprine (thiopurine methyltransferase gene) in leukemia and trastuzumab human epidermal growth factor receptor-type 2 (Her2 protein) in metastatic breast cancer.

In the first part of this chapter, the structure and functions of eukaryotic cells are described with emphasis on nuclear and cytoplasmic organelles. The second part of this chapter provides the essential information on eukaryotic gene processing and regulation, starting with deoxyribonucleic acid (DNA) replication—regulation of the initiation of DNA transcription by cell cycle machinery, close association of DNA replication with cell division. Transcription (the transfer of genetic information from DNA to messenger ribonucleic acid [mRNA], ribonucleic acid [RNA] processing, and regulation of eukaryotic gene by transcription) and translation or protein synthesis (processes of translation, regulation of translation, and the post-translational modification of proteins) are subsequently described. Finally, cell signaling processes are described. In this section different cell signaling molecules, receptors, and cell signaling pathways are covered. Throughout the chapter, wherever appropriate, molecular-based drug therapy used to treat diseases associated with the eukaryotic cell system is discussed. The purpose of this chapter is to enhance the reader's knowledge to be used as a background for practical applications.

Structure and Function of Eukaryotic Cells

To develop an understanding of molecular and cellular bioprocesses, it is important to review the functions of various organelle structures that are found in nearly all eukaryotic cells. The organization of eukaryotic cellular components can be broadly divided into *nuclear* and *cytoplasmic* (see Figure 1). The nucleus is divided into substructures essential for DNA replication and RNA synthesis and processing. Cytoplasmic organelles are described as those involved in protein processing (e.g., endoplasmic reticulum, Golgi apparatus, and lysosomes) and those metabolic organelles involved in cellular bioenergetics, namely the mitochondria. Following is an overview of relevant cell structures and their molecular and genetic functions (see Table 1).

The Nucleus
The nucleus is the largest cellular organelle in eukaryotes and serves as a storage structure for DNA. In addition, the nucleus is crucial in DNA replication, RNA synthesis and processing, and the assembly of ribosomes which are necessary for RNA translation or protein synthesis (Reference 1).

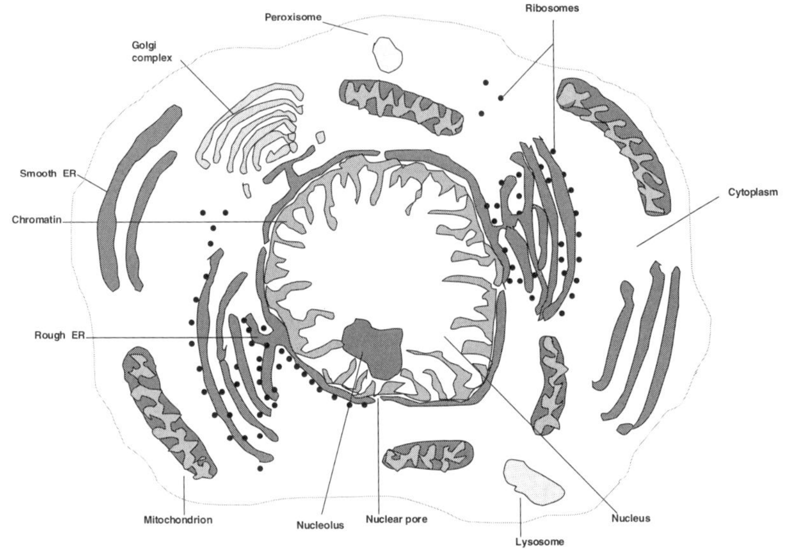

Figure 1. The eukaryotic cell.
The major nuclear and cytoplasmic organelles are depicted. Organelles are not drawn to scale.
ER=endoplasmic reticulum.

The nucleus' integrity is mainly maintained by a phospholipid bilayer that separates the nucleus from the surrounding cytoplasm. These nuclear membranes, collectively termed the nuclear envelope, are divided into an inner membrane and an outer membrane separated by a narrow lumen. The inner membrane faces the nucleus, whereas the outer membrane is associated with the endoplasmic reticulum and is exposed to the cytoplasm. Because it extends into the endoplasmic reticulum, the outer membrane exhibits protein processing functions similar to the endoplasmic reticulum.

Even though the nucleus and cytoplasm are structurally distinct, it is imperative that molecules be able to be transported from the nucleus to the cytoplasm and vice-versa. This transport is mediated through pores located in the nuclear envelope (References 2, 3). These nuclear pores are found at the junction of the concentric inner and outer membranes, and are instrumental in both the passive and active transport of ribonucleotides and proteins across the cell membrane. For example, although transcription (mRNA synthesis) occurs in the nucleus, transcription factors and RNA polymerases (required for nuclear transcription) must be transported from the cytoplasm. In addition, once mRNA is synthesized in the nucleus, it must be shuttled to the cytoplasm for protein synthesis. Depending on the polarity and size of the molecule, nuclear pores facilitate transfer through either passive diffusion or energy-dependent active transport (Reference 4).

Table 1. Structure and Function of Eukaryotic Cellular Organelles

Organelle	Molecular composition	Properties and functions
Nucleus	Approximately 4–6 mm in diameter surrounded by a nuclear membrane. The genetic material in the nucleus consists of chromatin, DNA combined with histones.	Major organelle of eukaryotic cells which serves as storage structure for DNA and is crucial for DNA replication and RNA synthesis and processing.
Endoplasmic reticulum (ER)	Membrane network extending from the nuclear membrane into the cytoplasm. May be smooth or rough (studded with ribosomes).	Protein and lipid synthesis, carbohydrate metabolism, detoxification.
Ribosomes	Two subunits, each composed of RNA and proteins. May be found free in cytoplasm or bound to rough ER.	Site of protein synthesis.
Golgi complex	Flattened, stacked membranous vesicles.	Sorting, packaging, and secretion of proteins received from the ER.
Lysosomes	Spherical single membrane-bound cytoplasmic bodies about 0.2–0.5 mm in diameter containing hydrolytic enzymes such as proteases and nucleases.	Break down biomolecules, cellular debris, and foreign bodies.
Mitochondria	Rod-shaped, about 1 mm in diameter with an outer and inner membrane. The inner matrix is rich in enzymes.	Energy production and cellular respiration. Synthesize most ATP used in eukaryotic cells through oxidative phosphorylation.
Peroxisomes	Similar to lysosomes.	Energy production through oxidation of fatty acids, amino acids, and other bio molecules. Convert H_2O_2 to H_2O.

ATP = adenosine 5'-triphosphate; DNA = deoxyribonucleic acid; H_2O = water; H_2O_2 = hydrogen peroxide; RNA = ribonucleic acid.

Nuclear translocation, although mechanistically not fully elucidated, also has important implications for drug therapy since there is potential to affect target activity of certain drugs that work at the nuclear level such as antineoplastics, corticosteroids, and activated protein C.

The interior of the nucleus is organized into several structural and functional domains. The nuclear genetic architecture consists of nucleosomes, complexes of DNA and histones, which are the basic structural subunits of chromatin. Chromatin, a fiber-like arrangement of DNA, is assembled into chromosomes that contain many genes. The human genome is organized into 46 chromosomes in the nucleus of most human cells, the exceptions being red blood cells and germ cells. Cells also can have abnormal numbers of chromosomes, such as in Down syndrome, where some cells have an extra copy of chromosome 21. In addition, there appear to be several discrete regions where specific nuclear functions such as DNA replication, pre-mRNA splicing, and mRNA transport take place.

With the exception of translation, all preparation and processing of genetic material occurs in the nucleus. The nucleolus, involved in ribosomal RNA (rRNA) transcription and subsequent ribosome production, is another important nuclear substructure. The nucleolus essentially functions to bridge nuclear and exonuclear activities through the production of ribosomes, the organelles responsible for the translation of mRNA into proteins.

Although the nucleolus is characterized as a structure within the nucleus, it does not possess a plasma membrane that distinguishes it from other nuclear components. Instead, nucleoli are organized along chromosome regions that contain genes for the synthesis of ribosomes and are comprised of these genes as well as rRNA and ribosomes in various stages of assembly (Reference 5). Ribosomal RNA is transcribed and associated with proteins which produce ribosomal subunits.

The Cytoplasm
Protein Processing Organelles
Ribosomes

The ribosome is an intricate organelle responsible for the translation of mRNA into proteins by facilitating the complicated interplay between mRNA, transfer RNA (tRNA), and initiation, elongation, and releasing factors (Reference 6). The ribosome consists of two subunits manufactured in the nucleoli of the cell. These ribosomal subunits are formed from rRNA molecules and proteins. Depending on the amount of rRNA in the subunit, they are classified as either large (with three rRNA molecules) or small (with one rRNA molecule) subunits. The eukarytoic ribosome consists of one large and one small subunit (Reference 7).

After individual ribosomal subunits are formed in the nucleolus, they are transported into the cytoplasm through nuclear pores. Once in the cytoplasm, a large and small ribosomal subunit come together to form a full ribosome that becomes functional. Formed ribosomes cannot be transported back into the nucleus because of their relatively large size. Ribosomes form complex with mRNA and scan the nucleotides of the mRNA in order to sequentially add appropriate amino acids in the synthesis of a specific protein. The small subunit serves as the main genetic processing unit. Along with mRNA and an initiator tRNA, the small subunit forms a translation initiation complex. The small subunit then scans the mRNA nucleotide sequence one codon at a time (a codon being three consecutive mRNA nucleotides that code for a specific amino acid) and promotes the interaction between mRNA codons and tRNA anticodons (three nucleotides on tRNA complimentary to the codon on mRNA). The large subunit facilitates the formation of peptide bonds between amino acids necessary for polypeptide chain elongation (Reference 8).

Functional ribosomes are either bound to the membrane of the endoplasmic reticulum (i.e., rough endoplasmic reticulum) or freely circulating in the cytoplasm. Cytoplasmic ribosomes are found as single units or in groups with mRNA serving to attach the ribosomes together (polyribosomes). Generally, cytoplasmic ribosomes are more abundant in cells that retain their proteins, while membrane-bound ribosomes are more numerous in cells that secrete their manufactured proteins (e.g., pancreatic and digestive enzymes). Regardless whether free or membrane-bound, the main role of the ribosome is to serve as the formational locus for mRNA-tRNA interaction and translation of nuclear mRNA into proteins also described in the section Translation (Protein Synthesis).

Endoplasmic Reticulum

The endoplasmic reticulum (ER) is a continuous membrane network that extends from the nuclear membrane into the cytoplasm and occupies a large proportion of intracellular space. Morphologically and functionally, the ER appears as two distinct regions: the rough ER, which is studded with membrane-bound ribosomes and the smooth ER, which is devoid of ribosomes. The rough ER is involved in ribosome-mediated protein synthesis. These include both secretory and membrane proteins. The smooth ER is involved in the synthesis of lipids, carbohydrate metabolism, and detoxification (References 9, 10).

The interplay between the ribosome and the ER membrane is rather complex in the rough ER. The ribosome begins the process of translation of the mRNA nucleotide sequence into a polypeptide chain (protein). The initial few peptides of proteins to be synthesized and sorted by the ER act as a signal sequence directing the ribosome-mRNA complex to the ER. This signal sequence is recognized by a signal recognition particle (SRP) which binds the large subunit of the ribosome to a SRP receptor on the ER membrane (Reference 11). Translation of mRNA into a protein occurs in the normal fashion. As the polypeptide chain is elongated, it extends into the lumen of the rough ER. These proteins are subsequently sent to the Golgi apparatus through vesicular transport for further processing and are either secreted outside the cell or are incorporated into cell membranes.

The smooth ER has unique biosynthetic and metabolic functions (References 12, 13). A major role of the smooth ER is to facilitate the synthesis of phospholipids, the major lipid in cell membranes (Reference 14). This is done through a series of catalytic reactions that occur at the ER-cytosol interface. The smooth ER also is involved in the synthesis of glycolipids and cholesterol. Smooth ER function is diverse and largely depends on cell type. For example, the smooth ER serves as the site of cholesterol biosynthesis in male and female reproductive organs and functions in the hepatic detoxification of drugs through the cytochrome P450 and other pathways (References 9, 15).

Golgi Complex

The Golgi complex, or Golgi apparatus, is comprised of a series of flattened, closed membranous stacks in close proximity to the ER whose main purpose is the sorting and packaging of proteins produced in the ER. Conventionally, the Golgi complex is described as having three distinct domains: the *cis* region, which is proximal to the ER; the *medial* region, also referred to as the Golgi stack, which serves as the site of many enzymatic modifications of proteins; and the *trans* region which is the final site of sorting and packaging before the modified proteins are sent to their respective cellular loci (Reference 16).

Once proteins are formed in the rough ER, they are transported in vesicles from the ER to the Golgi complex. These protein-filled vesicles fuse with the surface of the *cis* region of the Golgi complex and release the proteins into the Golgi lumen. The proteins are enzymatically modified and sequentially transported, through shuttle vesicles, through the *cis*, *medial*, and *trans* regions and repackaged into secretory vesicles that bud off from the *trans* region of the Golgi complex (Reference 17). The ultimate destination of these secretory vesicles which transport the modified proteins include: 1) intracellular locations (e.g., lysosomes, peroxisomes); 2) the plasma membrane surface to be incorporated into the cell membrane; 3) the cell surface for secretion into the extracellular space; or 4) return to the ER in the case of recyclable enzymes (Reference 9).

The metabolic activities of the Golgi complex are largely comprised of modification of glycoproteins received from the ER as well as lipid synthesis. Proteins undergo a wide array of enzymatic modifications with the common molecular theme being addition or subtraction of biochemical groups to these proteins. These modifications occur as the proteins are transported through shuttle vesicles from *cis* to *medial* to *trans* Golgi compartments. These modifications may include sulfation, acetylation, phosphorylation, addition of fatty acid groups, peptide cleavage, and importantly, glycosylation. It is largely glycosylation that determines the final destination of respective proteins (e.g., lysosomes, plasma membrane, and secretion) (Reference 18). After protein modification, the Golgi complex sorts proteins for delivery to their respective final destinations through a multifarious identification system.

The putative method for transport of proteins both between the regions of the Golgi complex and beyond the Golgi complex to other organelles and cellular regions is vesicular transport. Simply stated, vesicular transport is a series of events that entails: 1) invagination of the membrane at the site of vesicle origin; 2) gradual formation of the vesicle; 3) budding of the vesicle from the membrane; 4) transport to the intracellular target; and 5) fusion of the vesicle to the target membrane. Vesicle budding is a common mode for transport of proteins, and the mechanism for transport of protein-containing vesicles is quite complex.

Conserved structural motifs on the various proteins themselves are involved in protein sorting in the Golgi complex and targeting of proteins to their post-translational destinations. One of the best-elucidated examples is that of proteins targeted for return to the ER. For example, the enzyme protein disulfide isomerase, by virtue of its crucial role in protein folding, requires return transport to the ER from the Golgi complex. Protein disulfide isomerase (as well as other proteins targeted for return to the ER) possesses a C-terminal amino acid sequence comprised of Lys-Asp-Glu-Leu (or KDEL) that serves as a signal for ER return (Reference 19). These ER-targeted proteins are transported to the *cis* region of the Golgi apparatus along with other proteins through transport vesicles that have KDEL receptors associated with the vesicle membrane. The KDEL motifs on the ER-targeted proteins, such as disulfide isomerase, bind to transport vesicle KDEL membrane receptors. Consequently, when the transport vesicles fuse with the *cis* Golgi, all proteins except those attached to the KDEL receptors are released into the Golgi complex lumen for further processing and targeting. These KDEL-KDEL receptor complexes are then repackaged in vesicles that return from the Golgi complex back to the ER (References 20, 21). In addition to this example, there are other structural components which direct proteins to lysosomes, mitochondria, and the nucleus.

Proteins sorted and packaged in the Golgi complex may be secreted into the extracellular environment. Depending upon the cell's function, this secretion is either constitutive (i.e., unregulated and continuous) or regulated as a result of stimuli outside the cell (Reference 22). The current theory is that regulated proteins contain structural signals that divert their processing in the *trans* Golgi network from the constitutive pathway. On the other hand, constitutive proteins do not possess these signals and are transported directly to the cell membrane for exocytosis (release of intracellular molecules to the extracellular environment). Proteins that are secreted through the regulated pathway are stored in cytoplasmic storage vesicles until an extracellular stimulus triggers their release. Examples of proteins that undergo regulated secretion include histamine, insulin, and pancreatic digestive enzymes.

Lysosomes

Lysosomes are membrane sacs that contain degradative enzymes and circulate in the cytoplasm of the cell. These hydrolytic lysosomal enzymes are capable of degrading proteins, carbohydrates, lipids, DNA, RNA, and essentially all major components of biomolecules. For lysosomal enzymes to be active, they must be in an environment with a pH of approximately 5. Therefore, lysosomes possess proton pumps that decrease the pH of the interior, making the milieu more acidic. As such, this pH-sensitive mode of activity protects the intracellular environment from the destructive actions of lysosomal enzymes. Since cytoplasmic pH is neutral, lysosomal enzymes that accidentally leak out of the lysosomes would have no activity and could not affect other organelles and cell components.

Lysosomes are integral in the degradation of molecules from three processes: 1) endocytosis; 2) phagocytosis; and 3) autophagy (Reference 9). In endocytosis, extracellular components are internalized through vesicles. These vesicles, or endosomes, then fuse with lysosomes whereby their contents are exposed to lysosomal enzymes. In addition, certain cells, such as macrophages and neutrophils, are capable of internalizing microorganisms, cell debris, and insoluble particles by attaching to the particle and ingesting it into a phagosome. This phagosome joins with the lysosome through a similar mechanism of fusion as described. Lysosomal enzymes are released into the phagosome thereby digesting the foreign products. Finally, in autophagy lysosomes fuse with autophagosomes that contain the cell's own components (e.g., mitochondria). This occurs during development and physiologic stress and is a normal cellular activity. Lysosomes, then, are responsible for the degradation of biomolecules, foreign particles, and cellular components as part of intracellular and extracellular homeostasis.

Metabolic Organelles

Mitochondria

The mitochondria are referred to as the powerhouses of the eukaryotic cell. Their primary role is the production of energy in the form of adenosine 5'-triphosphate (ATP) which is used to drive the bioenergetic processes of the organism. Through oxidative phosphorylation and electron transfer, the mitochondria serve to maintain critical supplies of free energy essential for functions compatible with life (Reference 23).

Morphologically, the mitochondrion is comprised of two membranes, an inner and outer membrane. The outer membrane, a smooth, porous membrane, surrounds the inner membrane. The inner membrane is continuous and exhibits many folds, called cisternae, which extend into the central compartment of the organelle. The inner membrane is the location of ATP synthesis in the mitochondria. The space between the inner and outer membranes is called the intermembrane compartment. The internal compartment of the mitochondrion, which is enclosed by the inner membrane, is referred to as the matrix and houses the enzymes necessary for oxidative phosphorylation (References 24, 25).

Mitochondria are distinct from other organelles in that they contain their own genome. Mitochondria are composed of proteins that are coded in the nucleus and contain extranuclear genes that encode for electron carriers vital in reduction and oxidation reactions and ATP synthesis. They contain, in their matrix, all the machinery necessary for these reactions as well as for transcription and protein synthesis. This distinct mitochondrial genome suggests that these organelles are the evolutionary product of bacteria that lived symbiotically within other cells that later became eukaryotes.

The mitochondria are the sites of carbohydrate, protein, and lipid metabolism and ATP synthesis. The production of ATP occurs through oxidative phosphorylation and electron transfer. In the example of carbohydrate metabolism, glucose is broken down in the cytoplasm in a series of reactions to form pyruvate. The early steps in glycolysis require energy expenditure in the form of two molecules of ATP. However, four ATP molecules are formed further downstream. Consequently, the breakdown of glucose to pyruvate in the cytoplasm yields a net of two ATP molecules.

Under aerobic conditions, pyruvate is transported to the mitochondria where it is converted to carbon dioxide (CO_2) and acetyl coenzyme A (CoA). Acetyl CoA enters the citric acid cycle (or Kreb's cycle) where further oxidation yields CO_2 molecules and two ATP molecules. As such, each molecule of glucose provides four molecules of ATP (two from glycolysis and two from the citric acid cycle). In addition, glycolysis and oxidation in the citric acid cycle results in the formation of nicotinamide adenine dinucleotide, reduced (NADH) and flavin adenine dinucleotide, reduced ($FADH_2$) molecules. These molecules are essential in electron transfer and energy production in oxidative phosphorylation.

The majority of ATP molecules produced in the mitochondria are produced through the oxidation of NADH and $FADH_2$ molecules (e.g., oxidative phosphorylation) which occurs in the inner membrane. In oxidative phosphorylation, electrons are transferred in a series of steps from NADH and $FADH_2$ through a chain of protein complexes referred to as the electron transport chain. The ultimate reaction is the reduction of oxygen (O_2) to water (H_2O). The sequential transfer of electrons across the complexes results in free energy release used to synthesize ATP. In general, oxidative phosphorylation yields 34 molecules of ATP for each molecule of glucose metabolized.

Peroxisomes

Along with mitochondria, peroxisomes are the second major organelle involved in bioenergetics. Peroxisomes are structurally similar to lysosomes in that they are single membrane-bound cytosolic organelles containing large amounts of enzymes. Peroxisomal enzymes are involved in the metabolism of fatty acids, amino acids, and other biomolecules through oxidation. In this way, peroxisomes contribute to the production of free energy. However, the breakdown of these compounds (e.g., fatty acids) results in the formation of hydrogen peroxide (H_2O_2). Peroxisomes also contain the enzyme catalase which further converts cytotoxic H_2O_2 to H_2O (Reference 24). Peroxisomes are abundant in hepatocytes. They are believed to be important in cholesterol, phospholipid, and bile acid synthesis. In fact, the number of peroxisomes increases in the presence of the lipid-lowering agent colestipol, highlighting their importance in lipid homeostasis and suggesting the activity of these organelles might be altered in response to certain pharmacologic agents.

Gene Processing and Regulation

DNA Replication

DNA exists as a condensed and compact double helical structure in the nucleus and is composed of subunits called nucleotides. Each nucleotide is comprised of a sugar, a phosphate, and either a purine (adenine [A] or guanine [G]) or pyrimidine (cytosine [C] or thymine [T]) nitrogenous base. The deoxyribose sugar of DNA is more resistant to chemical degradation than the ribose sugar of RNA. This stabilizes the sugar-phosphate backbone of DNA, making the DNA molecule more durable than RNA.

Each strand of the DNA double helix has a 5' end and a 3' end. At the 5' end of a DNA strand, a phosphate group is attached to carbon 5 of deoxyribose. At the 3' end, DNA has a hydroxyl group on carbon 3 of deoxyribose that is free to bind to other molecules (Reference 26). The double helix DNA strands are bound together by A-T and C-G base pairing in a head to tail or antiparallel form (5'→3' and 3'→5'). The bases of DNA molecules are concealed within the DNA helix which protects them from chemical attack.

The transfer of genetic information from parent to daughter cells requires the accurate and strict replication of genomic DNA (Reference 27). DNA replication is semi-conservative in that one parent strand always serves as the template for the new complementary daughter strand (Reference 28). In a newly synthesized DNA molecule, the double helix is composed of an old (parent) and a new (daughter) strand. For DNA replication, several proteins are required to help facilitate the unwinding and separation of the double-stranded DNA molecule. These proteins are essential since DNA replication can only occur when DNA is single-stranded (References 26, 29).

Proteins Involved in DNA Replication
Topoisomerases

Topoisomerases are enzymes that act on DNA to isomerize, or convert, one topological form of DNA into another. Topoisomerases decrease the degree of DNA supercoiling (the form that DNA naturally takes in vivo) by cutting DNA strands, and are involved in primary cellular functions such as replication, transcription, chromosome condensation, and maintenance of genomic stability. There are two types of topoisomerases in eukaryotic cells, designated as type I (IA and IB) and II. Type I topoisomerase cuts and rejoins one strand of duplex DNA in a reversible and non-ATP-dependent process, resulting in relaxation of supercoiled DNA. Type II topoisomerase cleaves and rejoins the two strands of double helix DNA in a reversible, ATP-dependent process (References 30, 31).

Since these enzymes are able to relieve the torsional stress in DNA molecules, they are involved in both DNA replication and transcription. Topoisomerase initiates the unwinding of the DNA double helix, which is normally kept in a coiled and supercoiled state, by cleaving a phosphodiester bond in one strand. This creates a gap in the strand, relieving the conformational tension intrinsic to double-stranded DNA. This is a crucial first step in replication. These broken DNA strands are rejoined as the phosphodiester bond forms again (References 30, 31). Without topoisomerase enzymes, DNA helical unwinding and subsequent DNA replication could not occur. In fact, many commonly used antineoplastic agents, such as daunorubicin, doxorubicin, etoposide, irinotecan, and others, exploit the necessity of topoisomerases and work by interfering with the actions of topoisomerases, preventing DNA replication of malignant cells.

DNA Helicases

DNA helicases are responsible for unwinding double-stranded DNA into single-stranded DNA, a perquisite for processes such as RNA synthesis, discussed in this section, and homologous DNA recombination. After uncoiling the DNA supercoil by topoisomerase, helicases separate the double-stranded DNA by an energy-dependent process. To inhibit the separated strands from reannealing, DNA single-stranded binding proteins (SSBs) bind to both separated strands of DNA and stabilize the single-stranded structure generated by helicases (References 32–34).

DNA Polymerases

DNA polymerases (pols) are enzymes that catalyze the synthesis of new strands of DNA. DNA pols bind to the DNA template (parent strand) and synthesize DNA in the 5'→3' direction by adding a deoxyribonucleoside 5'-triphosphate (dNTP), a molecule composed of a sugar, three phosphates, and a deoxygenated purine or pyrimidine, to the 3'-hydroxyl group of the growing chain. In addition to DNA replication, DNA pols are involved in cell cycle regulation, DNA repair, DNA recombination, and teleomere maintenance (References 35, 36).

There are five DNA pols (α, β, γ, δ, and ϵ) in eukaryotic cells designated as classical polymerases which share a similar active site. DNA pols α, δ, and ϵ are believed to be responsible for nuclear genomic DNA replication. The classical pols are grouped into five different families (A, B, C, X, and Y) based on their structural similarities and sequence homology, with the replicative pols (α, δ, and ϵ) grouped in family B (References 35, 37).

New pols (ζ, η, θ, ι, κ, λ, μ, σ, φ, and rev1) that recently were discovered are referred to as novel or lesion-replicating polymerase enzymes. While the classical pols show high accuracy and fidelity during DNA synthesis, the novel pols are not as accurate in their performance. The presence of lesions in DNA during the replication process can interfere with DNA synthesis (References 35, 38, 39).

Many pols have an associated proofreading exonuclease responsibility for excising mismatched nucleotides that, if uncorrected, may manifest as clinical disorders. For example, xeroderma pigmentosum (XP) is a rare genetic disorder that renders a patient highly prone to ultraviolet-induced skin cancer and is associated with defective DNA repair. In contrast to many XP patients who have defective nucleotide excision repair, XP-variant (XP-V) patients have normal nucleotide excision repair, but because of a mutation in their DNA pol η, replicate ultraviolet-damaged DNA (References 35, 37–40).

Origins and Initiation of Replication

In eukaryotic cells, the replication of DNA begins at a unique sequence called the origin of replication. In order to replicate DNA in a biologically timely fashion, multiple origins of replication are necessary. For example, for mammalian cells to replicate their genome within a few hours, multiple replication origins in these cells are essential. It is estimated that the human genome may contain around 30,000 origins of replication (References 26, 28, 41).

Recent studies suggest that the initiation of DNA replication is regulated by cell cycle machinery. Even though DNA replication occurs in the S phase (DNA synthesis) of the cell cycle, the initiation complex may form at the origin of replication during the transition from M (mitosis) to G1 (G stands for gap in DNA synthesis) and await the signal to start replication. When cells progress from the G1 to S phase, the initiation complex is activated and replication begins (Reference 28). One of the major regulators of this transition is the level of cyclin-dependent kinase (CDK) activity in the cell. Cells in the G1 phase show low CDK activity which is essential for the assembly of the pre-replication complex at the origins of DNA replication. The activation of CDK results in the transition from the G1 to S phase, initiation of DNA replication, and disassembly of the pre-replication complex at the origin of replication. The inhibition of CDK activity resets the cell cycle to the G1 phase (References 29, 35). While the details of eukaryotic DNA replication are not as well understood as those of DNA transcription and protein synthesis, it is clear that multiple origins of replication are necessary, and that the process of DNA replication is closely related to the progression of the cell cycle.

The DNA Replication Fork

The DNA replication fork is another component of the DNA replication machinery, containing several proteins with different functions. Helicase proteins unwind the DNA double helix to generate the replication fork. Accessory proteins (e.g., replication factor C [RFC], proliferating cell nuclear antigen [PCNA], and replication factor A [RFA]) regulate the interaction of pols with DNA. Finally, DNA pols synthesize the new DNA strands, and exonucleases have 3'→5' proofreading activity (References 34, 42).

DNA replication starts at the specific chromosomal origin of replication and proceeds to the terminus. Since the two strands of DNA double helix are antiparallel, one strand needs to be synthesized in the 5'→3' direction and the other in the 3'→5' direction. Because all DNA pols catalyze the polymerization of dNTPs only in the 5'→3' orientation, one strand designated as the leading strand can be synthesized continuously in the direction of the replication fork. The other strand, or lagging strand, is synthesized backwards in relation to the movement of the replication fork (see Figure 2). Because DNA pol cannot initiate synthesis of a new DNA chain *de novo* and requires a 3'-OH terminus of an oligonucleotide primer, a short fragment of RNA-DNA hybrid (10 RNA bases followed by 20–30 base pairs [bps] long DNA) is synthesized by pol α/primase (an RNA primase enzyme that catalyzes the synthesis of short RNA primer molecules).

Then this RNA-DNA hybrid oligonucleotide is taken over by DNA pol δ and ε for elongation on both leading and lagging strands. On the lagging strand, short discontinuous segments of DNA (about 200 bps) called Okazaki fragments, are synthesized from the RNA primers created by primase These RNA primers are removed by exonuclease activity of DNA pol I/α, and the gaps between Okazaki fragments are then filled by DNA pol I/α polymerase activity. Finally, the completed Okazaki fragments are joined together by DNA ligase (References 29, 32, 34, 43, 44).

Transcription

For cells to carry out their essential life processes such as reproduction, growth, and metabolism, they must continuously synthesize proteins. Protein synthesis requires precise transfer of information from DNA strands into amino acid sequences in proteins. The first step in this process of gene

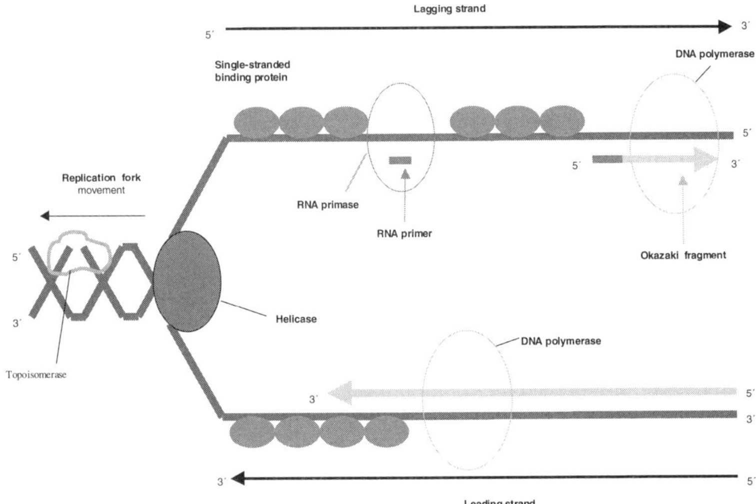

Figure 2. DNA replication in eukaryotic cells.
DNA replication occurs in the S phase of the cell cycle. Topoisomerase relieves the stress intrinsic to the DNA double helix. Part of the double helix is unwound by helicase. DNA polymerase binds to one template strand and moves in the 3'→5' direction, creating the complimentary leading strand and reforming a double helix. Since DNA synthesis only occurs in the 5'→3' direction, a second DNA polymerase binds to the other template strand and creates discontinuous polynucleotide strands (Okazaki fragments). DNA ligase then joins these fragments together into the lagging strand.
DNA=deoxyribonucleic acid; RNA=ribonucleic acid.

expression and protein synthesis is called transcription. Transcription is the process of synthesizing RNA from the information in DNA nucleotide sequences. RNA is synthesized in the 5'→3' direction from a DNA strand that runs in the 3'→5'direction. In a eukaryotic gene, only one strand of DNA, the complementary or antisense strand, is used for DNA replication and mRNA synthesis. The sequence of the RNA transcript is the same as the top (sense) strand in double-stranded DNA. Transcription can be either constitutive where genes are transcribed in a continuous permanent manner, or regulated in which many different extracellular and intracellular signals control RNA synthesis (References 45, 46).

RNA Polymerases

RNA pols are huge multisubunit protein complexes that catalyze the assembly of RNA from their DNA templates. There are three different nuclear DNA-dependent RNA pols in eukaryotic cells that transcribe various classes of genes. RNA pol I transcribes rRNA genes for the precursors of the 28S, 18S, and 5.8S molecules which represent the majority of the RNA synthesized in transcription. RNA pol II is a megadalton-sized holoenzyme complex whose exact composition and structure are not fully elucidated. RNA pol II transcribes all the protein-coding mRNA and several small nuclear RNA genes. RNA pol II cannot initiate transcription without the presence of several transcriptional factors. RNA pol III transcribes the 5S rRNA and all the tRNA genes involved in translation (References 47–49).

Basal Promoter

Promoters are sequences on DNA that determine the site of transcription initiation and the direction of transcription. They are sites on DNA that are upstream (5') of the coding region to which RNA pol (and other molecules such as transcription factors) binds in order to initiate transcription. The basal or core promoter, which determines the precise transcription start site, consists of an initiator sequence. The consensus initiator sequence is 5'-YYA^{+1}NA/TYYY-3', where A is the start point (+1), Y stands for pyrimidine (C or T), and N is any base. The basal promoter of many genes also consists of a 7-base sequence (5'-TATWAW-3', where W=A or T) called the TATA box located about -25 bases from the start point; this sequence binds the multiprotein transcription factor (TF) IID which is the TF complex that must bind for transcription to begin. All protein-encoding genes have a basal or core promoter (References 45, 50–52).

Upstream Promoter Elements

A number of upstream promoter elements exist in eukaryotic genes whose structures and respective binding factors vary. The GC box (GGGCGG), found within 200 bp upstream of the TATA box and usually associated with "house-keeping" genes (constantly expressed genes), and the CAT box (CCAAT), located approximately 50 bp upstream from the TATA box, are two examples of these elements. Upstream promoter elements function by binding specific transcription factors that increase the frequency of initiation of transcription at a particular promoter (References 45, 53).

Stages of Transcription

The process of transcription in eukaryotes can be divided into initiation (pre-initiation complex assembly, promoter clearance), elongation, and termination. Initiation of transcription is complex and takes place at the promoter. Since RNA pol II cannot recognize the promoter or initiate transcription by itself, several general TFs—TFIIA, TFIIB, TFIID, TFIIE, TFIIF, and TFIIH—assist RNA pol II in recognition of its target. The TFs first form a complex with DNA and then recruit RNA pol II to the DNA at the transcription initiation site (References 45, 53, 54).

In the pre-initiation step, the TATA box binding protein (TBP) of TFIID recognizes and binds to the TATA element of the promoter. This interaction may be regulated by another TF, TFIIA, which interacts with the TBP and other TBP-associated factors in TFIID. These TBP-associated factors, or TAFs, are co-factors that associate with TBP and help in DNA unwinding and transition from transcription initiation to elongation of the RNA transcript. At first, different TFs bind to the upstream promoter and form a multiprotein complex with DNA. Then RNA pol II is recruited to the DNA at the transcriptional initiation site. TFIIB promotes the binding of TFIID-TBP complex to the promoter, subsequently establishing a site for RNA pol II association with the DNA template. Binding of TFIIF to the latter complex results in recruiting TFIIE and TFIIH into the complex,

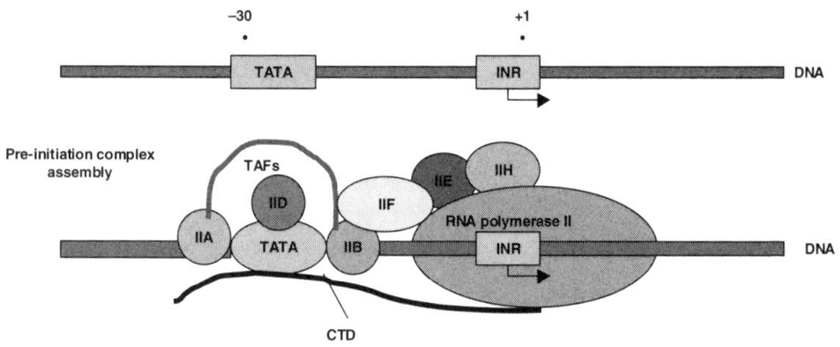

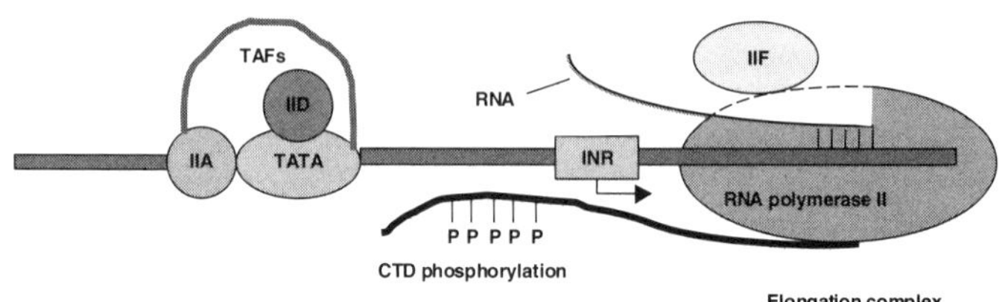

Figure 3. Transcription by RNA polymerase II.
In eukaryotes, protein-encoding genes are transcribed by RNA pol II to produce mRNA. The promoter is the site of transcription initiation. However, RNA pol II has no affinity for DNA and only can be recognized and bind to the promoter after transcription factors (TFs) bind to the promoter. The TFIID complex recognizes and binds to the TATA box of the promoter. Other TFs subsequently bind. TFIIF is bound to RNA pol II, allowing RNA pol II to recognize the TFII complex. Unphosphorylated RNA pol II enters the initiation complex. Its carboxy terminal domain (CTD) is then phosphorylated by TFIIH, signaling RNA pol II to dissociate from the initiation complex and begin transcription.
+1=first nucleotide to be transcribed; DNA=deoxyribonucleic acid; INR=initiator region; mRNA=messenger RNA; P=phosphorylated residues; RNA=ribonucleic acid; TAFs=TATA box binding protein-associated factors.

which are necessary for RNA elongation (see Figure 3) (References 45, 52, 54, 55).

Elongation

The synthesis of the RNA transcript is not a nonstop process where nucleotides are added at a constant rate. There are different transcription elongation blocks that RNA pols must overcome for efficient RNA synthesis. After forming the pre-initiation complex (promoter, RNA pol II, and TFs), DNA helicase activity of TFIIH unwinds the DNA template at the transcriptional start site through an ATP-dependent process. The DNA melting begins at about -10 bp upstream from the first nucleotide to be transcribed. The pre-initiation complex is believed to convert the closed DNA configuration to an open complex before initiation of RNA synthesis by RNA pol II. The carboxy terminal domain (CTD) of the large subunit of RNA pol II, which is rich in proline, serine, and threonine residues, plays an important role in elongation. Regions rich in these amino acids are found in transcriptional activation domains (References 46, 52, 56).

TFIIF is bound to unphosphorylated RNA pol II, allowing RNA pol II to recognize the TFII complex. During the initiation step, the unphosphorylated CTD becomes phosphorylated by TFIIH, resulting in the release of the RNA pol II from the initiation complex, clearance from the promoter, and initiation of transcription. RNA pol II uses nucleoside triphosphates for RNA synthesis. These nucleoside triphosphates are assembled onto the strand by complimentary base pairing. Since there is no T in RNA, each A on the DNA guides the insertion of the pyrimidine uracil (U, from uridine triphosphate). RNA pol II, in conjunction with transcription elongation factors, proceeds down the DNA template strand in the 3'→5' direction at about 30 bp per second, continually assembling the strand of RNA in a 5'→3' fashion. RNA pol II transcription continues until a termination signal on the template DNA strand is read, resulting in both the release of the enzyme and the RNA transcript from the DNA strand (References 46, 57–60).

Termination

The processed eukaryotic mRNA contains a poly (A) addition signal (AAUAAA), located downstream of the last exon at the 3' end followed by a series of As. The poly (A) signal is responsible for polyadenylation (addition of adenylate residues during RNA processing), termination of transcription, and release of RNA pol II from the DNA template molecule. While the upstream RNA transcript undergoes post-transcriptional modification after cleavage at the poly (A) site, the unstable downstream RNA transcript will be degraded soon after synthesis (References 56, 60, 61).

RNA Processing

In eukaryotes, all nuclear pre-mRNA transcripts must undergo processing, and change into functional mRNA before being exported to the cytoplasm. The primary precursor of mRNA transcripts is called heterogeneous nuclear RNA which contains exons and introns (coding and noncoding regions, respectively). The maturation process of heterogeneous nuclear RNA takes place in three steps (5'-capping, 3'-polyadenylation, and mRNA splicing) in the nucleus (see Figure 4). After RNA processing, the mature and functional mRNAs are transported to the cytoplasm to be translated into proteins by ribosomes (References 56, 62, 63).

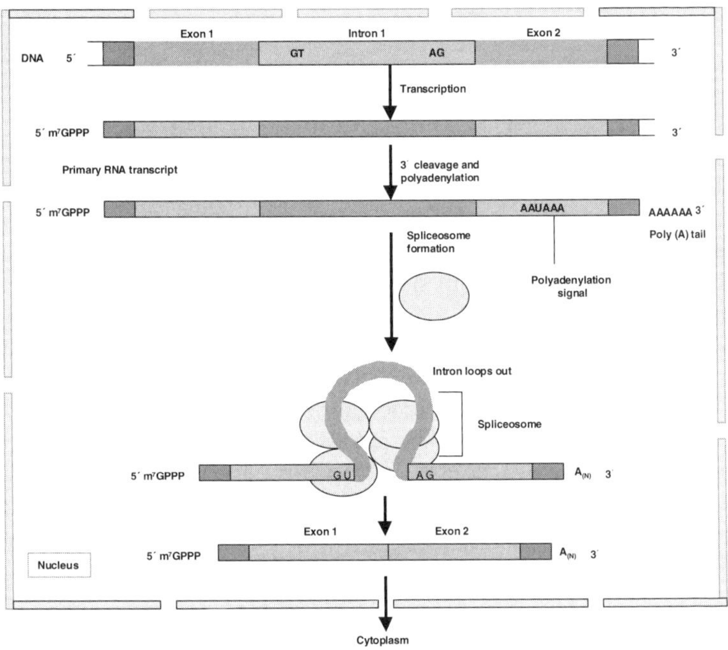

Figure 4. RNA processing in eukaryotes.
Primary RNA transcripts undergo processing to become functional RNA before export to the cytoplasm. A guanine cap is attached to the 5'-end of pre-mRNA as it emerges from RNA pol II during transcription, protecting the pre-mRNA from degradative enzymes. A series of adenine (A) nucleotides (the poly (A) tail) is attached to the 3'-end of the RNA transcript when transcription is complete. Introns are excised from the pre-mRNA and exons are spliced together by spliceosomes. The completed mRNA is transported to the cytoplasm where it interacts with ribosomes during protein synthesis.
5'm7GPPP=5'-guanine cap; A(N)=poly (A) tail; DNA=deoxyribonucleic acid; exon=coding region; intron=noncoding region; mRNA=messenger RNA; RNA=ribonucleic acid

5'-Capping

In all eukaryotes, mRNA synthesized by RNA pol II has a cap structure at its 5' end, which consists of a 7-methlyguanosine linked with the first nucleotide of the mRNA. The 7-methlyguanosine is added to the 5' end when the length of the RNA transcript reaches 25-30 nucleotides by RNA pol II. A capping enzyme associated with the phosphorylated CTD of RNA pol II catalyzes this process. 5'-capping is specific only for RNA transcripts synthesized by RNA pol II. The 5' cap is believed to be important in mRNA stability, initiation of translation (protein synthesis), and protection of the end of mRNA from exonuclease attack (References 56, 64).

3'-Polyadenylation

The 3' ends of most eukaryotic mRNAs are modified by adding a long chain of adenosine residues called a poly (A) tail. The poly (A) tail is not coded for in DNA and its length may vary from 30 to 200 A nucleotides. The AAUAAA sequence found near the 3' end of most eukaryotic mRNAs act as a signal for the site of 3' trimming and poly (A) tail addition. Whereas most mRNAs have a poly (A) tail, some normal mRNAs without poly (A) tails also are found the in cytoplasm. Since poly (A) tails do not exist in histone mRNA, it is assumed that they are not essential for translation. The presence of a poly (A) tail at the 3' end of mRNA, like 5' capping of mRNA, protects the mRNA molecules from degradation by nucleases (References 56, 64).

Splicing

One of the most important steps in RNA processing is RNA splicing. Most eukaryotic genes are divided into exons and introns. The parts of DNA that are transcribed into RNA but not translated into protein are known as introns (noncoding regions), whereas the stretches of DNA that code for amino acids in the protein are called exons (coding regions). In most genes, introns are interspersed among exons. The process by which introns are removed and exons are joined together is called RNA splicing. RNA splicing is carried out on pre-mRNA by large ribonucleoproteins called spliceosomes. In a protein-coding gene the intron-exon junctions, or splice sites, have consensus sequences. Most introns start with GU and end with AG sequences in the 5'→3' direction, referred to as splice donor and acceptor sites, respectively. Variation in splice sites can result in different isoforms of a polypeptide from a single gene. This process, termed "alternative splicing," is believed to occur in about 30 percent of all human genes. Excision and splicing of mRNA requires great precision because the removal of a nucleotide from an exon or carry over of a nucleotide from an intron may cause a shift in the reading frame (the codons read during translation) and result in a premature stop codon and other alterations (see Figure 4). Many genetic diseases, which result from defective proteins in a specific tissue system, involve misreading of a splice signal due to a mutation. (References 56, 62, 63, 65).

Dysfunction of splicing mechanisms can result in protein abnormalities causing dire clinical consequences. For example, hemoglobin consists of two molecules of α and β globin polypeptides. The β globin gene has three exons and two introns. The introns start with GT sequences that ensure the removal of introns and correct exon splicing during β globin mRNA synthesis. The resulting mRNA is translated into β globin polypeptide. In some individuals, a mutation from GT to AT in DNA at the beginning of the first or second intron sequences of the β globin gene results in an alternate splice site. Consequently, they are not capable of producing β globin polypeptides and suffer from $β^0$ thalassemia, which is a severe form of anemia (Reference 66).

Transcriptional Gene Regulation

Regulation of eukaryotic gene expression originally takes place at the transcription initiation step. The transcriptional activity of single genes, for example through altering the efficiency of initiation, is regulated by the transcriptional regulatory components in response to environmental changes. Protein coding genes are usually regulated by *cis*-acting transcription control elements which are located near the start site (basal promoter), or farther upstream or downstream from the promoter (enhancer). The regulation of expression of many genes is based on the interactions between the *cis*-acting transcription control elements and the *trans*-acting regulatory proteins. *Cis*-acting elements are sequences of a gene that *directly* affect the gene, while *trans* acting elements act on a gene but are encoded for by *other* genes. The majority of regulatory proteins that directly attach to DNA contain at least two functional domains. While one domain is responsible for recognizing and binding to the *cis* elements in the DNA, the other domain is involved in the activation of transcription (References 45, 64, 67).

Transcriptional Activators and Repressors

Almost all eukaryotic genes are in the inactive state and require transcriptional activators for expression. The change from an inactive to active state results from a response to an external stimulus. There are short sequence motifs upstream and downstream of promoters that are used as binding sites for transcriptional factors (transcriptional activators and repressors). Regulatory transcriptional proteins may function constitutively, act positively as transcriptional activators and increase the rate of transcription, or function as repressors of transcription (References 45, 68–70).

Transcriptional activators are proteins that bind regulatory elements in the upstream promoter and enhancer regions to regulate gene expression. Transcription activators have a single DNA-binding domain and one or several activation domains. Transcriptional repressors resemble activators in having a single DNA-binding domain and one or several repression domains. Repressors and activators can regulate transcription by binding to a site that is hundreds to thousands of nucleotides away from the start site. Repressors may simply interfere with the function of activators by competing for the activator binding site. These transcriptional regulatory proteins have different structural forms or domains. This section includes a description of a few of the DNA-binding domains: helix-turn-helix, zinc-finger, and leucine-zipper (see Figure 5) (References 45, 69).

The helix-turn-helix motif has two α-helical fragments bound to each other by a short segment of amino acids forming a bend or turn (see Figure 5). One of the helices, designated as the recognition helix, locates itself in the major or minor DNA groove and the amino acid side chains facing the groove bind to the specific sequence in the DNA. Then the second helix, called the stabilization helix, supports and stabilizes the recognition helix. The DNA-binding domains usually form dimers (two helix-turn-helix molecules) and fit into the major DNA groove (References 71, 72).

The zinc-finger proteins are formed by the interaction of one or two zinc atoms with two cysteines and two histidines, or in some cases with four cysteines. The cysteine and histidine residues are bound to a zinc atom in a way that forms a fingerlike loop pointing into the major DNA groove (see Figure 5). There are many regulatory proteins (e.g., TFIIIA that

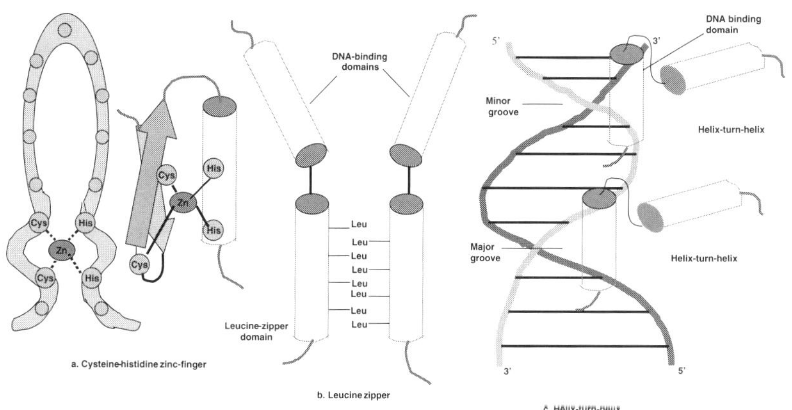

Figure 5. DNA binding domains.
a. Zinc-finger;
b. Leucine-zipper;
c. Helix-turn-helix bound to major groove of DNA.
DNA binding domains are regions of transcriptional activators or repressors that bind regulatory elements in the upstream promoter and enhancer regions to regulate gene expression.
Cys=cysteine; DNA=deoxyribonucleic acid; His=histidine; Leu=leucine; Zn=zinc.

activates 5S rRNA genes, and steroid hormone receptors) that have zinc-finger motifs (References 71, 73).

The third DNA-binding motif is called the leucine-zipper. Because leucine amino acids are hydrophobic, they are attracted when facing each other on the outer surface of two opposing α-helices and form the teeth of the zipper that joins the two helices together (see Figure 5). The leucine-zipper maintains the α-helices in a position that fits exactly into the major DNA groove (References 71, 74).

Enhancers, Silencers, and Insulators

Enhancers are transcriptional regulatory nucleotide sequences ranging from 50 to 200 bps in length to which TFs bind and increase gene expression. They are not part of the promoter and could be located from 200 bps to 10 kilobases upstream or downstream, or within an intron of a gene. Many genes require enhancers for differential expression. Besides the DNA-binding site, the enhancer-binding proteins have other sites that bind to TFs at the promoter of the gene (see Figure 6). The binding of an enhancer to the promoter makes the DNA form a loop. Enhancers interact even in the opposite orientation, and can still be functional. In contrast to enhancers, promoters are both position- and orientation-dependent in their activity (References 45, 64, 68).

Silencers are DNA sequences or control regions that repress the expression of genes when bound to TFs. Silencers, like enhancers, are located thousands of bps away from the transcribed gene and still be effective. In contrast to transcriptional activators, which can only control

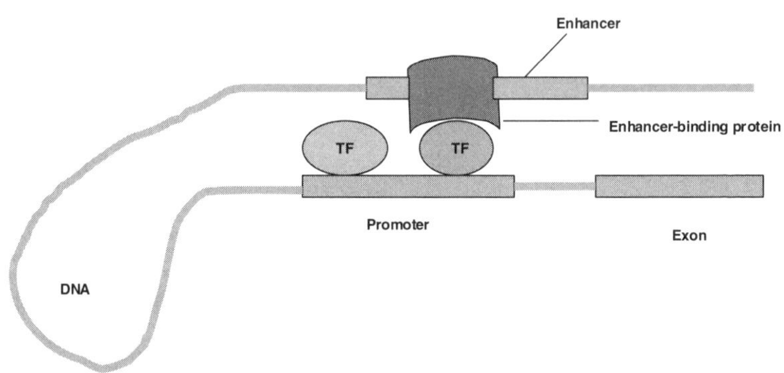

Figure 6. Diagram of an enhancer.
Enhancers are just one of several control mechanisms for gene transcription. Enhancers stimulate the rate of transcription initiation.
DNA=deoxyribonucleic acid; TF=transcription factor.

one gene, enhancers and silencers can control the expression of more than one gene (References 45, 75).

Insulators are short stretches of DNA sequences that are located between enhancers and promoters, or silencers and promoters, and function as blocking elements to prevent the activation or repression effects of adjacent genes. Insulators need to bind a protein called CTCF, an 11-zinc-finger DNA-binding protein, to become functional (Reference 75).

Steroid Hormone Receptors and Transcription Regulation

Steroid hormones (e.g., glucocorticoids, estrogen, progesterone, and testosterone) are small lipid molecules that cross the plasma and nuclear membranes of the cell and bind to steroid hormone receptors. Hormones act as cell signaling molecules and control the activity of many TFs. It is shown that steroid hormones (mostly located in the nucleus) selectively regulate the transcriptional activity of a specific group of genes through binding to steroid hormone receptors and associating with hormone response elements (HREs) on the gene. The hormone receptors in the steroid, thyroid, and retinoid supergene family act as transcription factors that bind to target sequences in the regulatory regions of hormonally regulated genes to enhance or suppress their transcription. Eukaryotic cells may have several thousand receptor proteins for a single hormone. These receptors are members of the zinc-finger DNA-binding protein family (References 76–79).

Nuclear receptors bind small lipophilic hormones that are produced by the endocrine system. In general, the nuclear receptors are classified according to the type of hormones they bind to: steroids (glucocorticoids, mineralocorticoids, androgens, progestins, and estrogens), steroid derivates (vitamin D3), nonsteroids (thyroid hormone, prostaglandins, and retinoids), and receptors without a known ligand (orphan receptors). Through evolution, these receptors have conserved structural similarities such as a ligand-binding domain, a DNA-binding domain, a dimerzation domain, and one or more trans-activation domains (References 68, 76–80).

In steroid hormone receptors, the N-terminal domain is involved in transcription activation, and the C-terminal region is the hormone-binding domain. The center part of the receptor contains a cysteine-cysteine zinc motif and is responsible for recognizing and binding to HREs (References 77, 79).

The binding of a hormone receptor to the HRE activates mRNA transcription or inhibits the transcription of previously activated genes. Some hormone receptors, such as glucocorticoid receptors, are able to bind two different types of response elements and activate or repress the transcription of a gene by inhibiting the binding of other TFs to the promoter site. HREs, like other DNA sequences that are identified by regulatory proteins, are palindromes or consensus sequences that consist of two repeats (e.g., 5'-AGAACANNNTGTTCT-3', 3'-TCTTGNNNACAAGA-5') (References 76, 77, 79).

All hormone receptors, except androgen receptors, exhibit recessive patterns. Mutations in hormone receptor genes affect DNA binding affinity, ligand binding capacity, homo/heterodimer formation, and trans-activation functions. These mutations are associated with various human diseases such as breast and prostate cancer, osteoporosis, and Kennedy's disease (X-linked recessive spinal and bulbar muscular atrophy). Further understanding of receptors in the hormone superfamily may promote the development of agonists or antagonists for the treatment of diseases associated with hormone receptor dysfunction (References 78–80).

DNA Methylation

Modification of DNA (methylation) and histones (acetylation) is related to genetic regulation and plays a role in transcription selection. DNA methylation is one of the most common forms of DNA modification in eukaryotic cells that alters gene expression without changing the nucleotide sequencing. DNA methylation occurs through addition of a methyl group to carbon 5 of a C ring by DNA methyltransferase. The methylation of C usually takes place next to a G in a 5'-CG-3' sequence called the CpG dinucleotide. DNA methylation can be reproduced during DNA replication and transferred to the next generation. In eukaryotes, the Cs of many genes in the inactive state of transcription are highly methylated (modified to 5'-methlycytosine). The change from inactive to active state of transcription occurs through removal of a methyl group from the C specially located in the 5'-flanking region of the gene. It is proposed that DNA methylation suppresses gene transcription by keeping the chromatin in the condensed 30 nanometer (nm) fiber form that protects the DNA from being exposed to RNA polymerase and TFs. Studies show that DNA methylation plays a vital role in transcription repression, neoplasia, and silencing specific genes during development and cell differentiation. *De novo* methylation also serves as a cellular defense mechanism to inactivate integrated foreign DNA. A complete understanding of methylation and demethylation make these processes potential targets for the development of drugs for prevention and treatment of malignancies and viral infection (References 68, 81).

Histone Acetylation

Histone acetylation plays an important role in the regulation of transcription. In eukaryotic cells, chromosomes are packaged in such a way that DNA is wrapped around histones approximately every 200 bps to form complexes called nucleosomes. One hundred forty-six bps of DNA are wound around a histone octamer with the remaining 54 bps intervening between each nucleosome. This organization impacts levels of transcription. The association between histone and DNA blocks the access of transcription factors and RNA pol II to the promoter (References 68, 82–85).

While histone acetylation in many cases increases transcription, a lack of acetylation or histone deacetylation represses transcription. Histone acetylation is a reversible process catalyzed by histone acetyltransferases, and histone deacetylation is catalyzed by histone deacetylases. Histone acetyltransferases function by transferring an acetyl group from acetyl CoA to the amino group of specific lysine side chains in the N-terminal region of the histone. This removes positive charges and results in the reduction of affinity between the histone and DNA and generates more open DNA conformation. After relieving the bond between histone and DNA, RNA pol II and TFs access the promoter on the DNA, initiating the expression of the corresponding genes (References 68, 82–85).

Histone acetylation plays an important regulatory role during development, proliferation, differentiation, and gene expression. Abnormal acetylation or deacetylation results in various disorders such as leukemia, epithelial cancers, and genetic diseases associated with physical and cognitive abnormalities. Recent studies show that inhibition of histone acetyltransferases is the primary cause of cellular pathogenesis in polyglutamine diseases such as Huntington's disease (References 83, 86, 87).

The association between histone acetylation and human diseases raised the possibility that pharmacologic manipulation of histone acetylation (e.g., with histone deacetylases inhibitors) could be used as a treatment strategy for several disorders. Several different classes of histone deacetylases inhibitors are identified: short chain fatty acids (e.g., butyrates), hydroxamic acids (e.g., trichostatin A, oxamflatin, and suberoylanilidehydroxanic acid), cyclic peptides (e.g., trapoxin A and apicidin), and benzamides. A few of these inhibitors like phenylbutyrate, pyroxamide, and suberoylanilidehydroxanic acid are being investigated in clinical trials (References 82, 83, 85, 86).

Translation (Protein Synthesis)

Translation is the process of decoding the genetic information on mRNA and synthesizing a protein based on that sequence information. The protein synthesis machinery includes mRNA as the template containing the genetic codes for translation into protein; ribosomes, the large ribonucleoproteins that are the sites of protein synthesis; tRNA, the adaptor molecules that carry the correct amino acids to the ribosome for synthesis of the polypeptide chain; and the accessory proteins that are involved in the initiation, elongation, and termination of protein synthesis (References 88, 89).

Ribosomal RNA

Ribosomal RNAs associate with certain proteins to form small and large ribosomal subunits that serve as the site for protein synthesis. There are four kinds of rRNA in eukaryotic cells. One molecule of 18S rRNA along with 50 different protein molecules makes the small subunit of the ribosome.

One molecule each of 28S, 5.8S, and 5S rRNA with more than 50 different protein molecules make the large subunit of the ribosome (References 57, 58).

Transfer RNA

Transfer RNAs are located in the cytoplasm where they pick up and transfer activated amino acids to mRNA for protein synthesis. There are as many as 50–100 different kinds of tRNA in a typical eukaryotic cell. Transfer RNAs are small and contain between 70-90 nucleotides. The paired bases in tRNA form a section of double helix while the unpaired bases form three loops. Transfer RNAs exist for each of the 20 amino acids. Some of the amino acids have more than one tRNA designated to them. The three unpaired bases at one loop form the anticodon which are the complementary bps of the codon on a mRNA molecule. This consequently ensures that the right amino acid is added to the growing polypeptide chain coded for by mRNA (see Figure 7) (References 88–90).

Initiation of Translation (Formation of the Initiation Complex)

Initiation of protein synthesis starts with separation of the two ribosomal subunits (40S and 60S). Then a ternary complex, the pre-initiation complex, is formed which consists of initiator tRNA (tRNA$^{met\ [methionine]}$, the initiator tRNA carries and incorporates the initiator methionine in all proteins), guanosine triphosphate (GTP), eukaryotic initiation factor 2 (eIF-2), and the 40S ribosomal subunit. First, GTP binds to eIF-2 which is composed of α,β, and γ subunits. This binary complex then binds to the initiator tRNA forming the ternary complex, which subsequently binds to the 40S ribosomal subunit, ultimately forming the 43S pre-initiation complex. The pre-initiation complex is then stabilized by the association of eIF-3 and eIF-1 to the 40S subunit. The binding of the 5' cap on mRNA to the pre-initiation complex is accomplished by the eIF-4F initiation factor which is made of 3 proteins: eIF-4A, eIF-4E, and eIF-4G. eIF-4A hydrolyzes ATP and has RNA helicase activity. EIF-4G assists in binding of the mRNA to the 43S pre-initiation complex.

After binding of the pre-initiation complex to the 5'-end of mRNA, the complex scans mRNA until it reaches an initiator AUG codon. The binding of initiator tRNA to the initiator AUG codon is facilitated by eIF-1. Hydrolysis of eIF-2-bound GTP by eIF-5 results in the release of eIF-2 from the 40S complex and leaves the initiator tRNA in the P (peptidyl)-site of the 40S ribosomal subunit. The 60S ribosomal subunit then attaches to the 40S subunit and forms the 80S initiation complex. The energy for formation of the 80S complex is provided by hydrolysis of the GTP bound to eIF-2. Now that the initiator tRNA is bound to the mRNA in the P-site of the ribosome, protein synthesis begins (References 91–97).

Elongation of Polypeptide Chain (New Protein)

In protein synthesis, tRNA acts as a translator between mRNA and the new protein by bringing the correct amino acid to mRNA. Each tRNA has an amino acid acceptor or attachment site and a nucleotide triplet (anticodon) that binds to the complementary sequence (codon) on mRNA. The codon is composed of three nucleotides and starts near the 5' end of mRNA. The tRNA carries the amino acid attached to its 3'-terminal OH group (see Figure 7). There are 61 codons for 20 different amino acids, and the codons for some amino acids only vary in the third position of the codon (e.g., phenylalanine; UUU and UUC). The base pairing at the first and

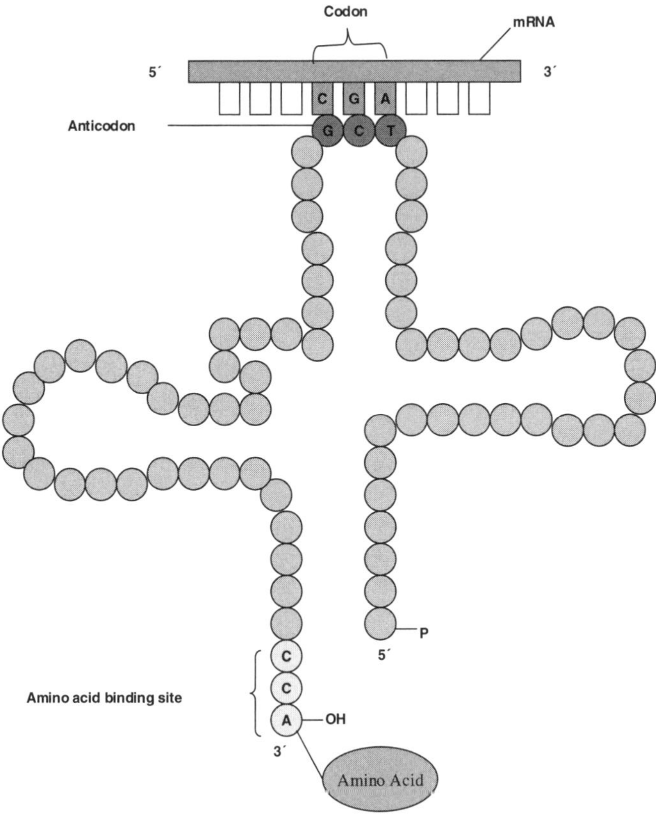

Figure 7. Diagram of transfer RNA (tRNA).
In translation (protein synthesis), tRNA is responsible for matching the appropriate amino acid to the nucleic acid codons on mRNA. At one end, tRNA possesses an anticodon that recognizes the codon, and at the other end it carries the amino acid for that codon. The appropriate amino acid is added to the tRNA via the actions of the enzyme amino-acyl tRNA synthetase. Amino acids are added to the growing peptide chain at the ribosome.
A=adenine; C=cytosine; G=guanine; mRNA=messenger RNA; U=uracil.

second position in the codon and anticodon follows standard rules (A-U and C-G), but in the third position both U and C of the codon can form hydrogen bonds with a G of the anticodon. In this case only one tRNA is needed for two codon sequences, indicating a redundancy in some tRNA functioning.

The binding of an amino acid to its correct tRNA occurs through interaction with the aminoacyl tRNA synthetase enzyme. First, the enzyme attaches the amino acid to the α-phosphate of ATP, resulting in the release of pyrophosphate. Then tRNA synthetase catalyzes the transfer of the amino acid to the 3'-terminal adenosine residue of tRNA which generates activated aminoacyl-tRNA. For each amino acid and its tRNA, there is at least one aminoacyl tRNA synthetase enzyme (References 88, 89, 98).

Translation continues along the mRNA in the 5'→3' direction that corresponds to the amino terminal (N-terminal) to carboxy terminal (C-terminal) direction of amino acid sequences in proteins. In the large ribosomal subunit there are two sites, the A-site which accepts the new tRNA carrying an amino acid and the P-site that sustains the tRNA bound to the growing chain. After the AUG start codon and Met-tRNA are positioned in the P (peptidyl) site of the ribosome, the new aminoacyl-tRNA carrying a second amino acid enters the A (aminoacyl) site or decoding site of the ribosome. Then its anticodon pairs with the mRNA codon, and their recognition is mediated by eEF-1 associated with GTP (References 88, 89, 98).

The mRNA codon designates which aminoacyl-tRNA should come next to the A site. The covalent bond between the amino acid (Met) and initiator tRNA (Met-tRNA) in the P-site is broken, and a peptide bond is formed by the peptidyl transferase enzyme between the methionine and the second amino acid in the A-site. This process is called transpeptidation. The empty tRNA in the P-site dissociates from the ribosome and the peptidyl tRNA (the tRNA carrying two amino acids) in the A-site is translocated into the P-site. This process of translocation is catalyzed by eIF-2 coupled to GTP hydrolysis. Another aminoacyl-tRNA carrying the third amino acid enters the A-site and the addition of new amino acids to the growing polypeptide chain continues in this fashion until the ribosome reaches the stop codon (References 88, 89, 98).

Termination of Protein Synthesis

In general, the termination of protein synthesis is similar to the elongation process in that the stop (nonsense) codon is decoded at the ribosomal A-site. There are three stop codons (UAA, UAG, and UGA) that have no complementary anticodon or aminoacyl-tRNA to bind to mRNA. The termination of translation occurs on the ribosomes and requires two polypeptide release factors designated as eRF-1 (a codon-specific RF) and eRF-3 (a noncodon specific RF) (References 88, 89, 99, 100).

The release factor recognizes and binds to the stop codon at the A-site and begins the process of translation termination. The stop codon at the A-site causes the release factor to bind to the A-site with GTP instead of aminoacyl-tRNA. After binding of release factor to the stop codon, the bond that holds the polypeptide chain to the tRNA at the P-site is hydrolyzed. Because there is no amino acid at the A-site, the hydrolysis permits the newly synthesized polypeptide chain to be released from the ribosome (Reference 99).

Following the release of the polypeptide chain, the tRNA at the P-site along with the release factor from the A-site are expelled. The large and small ribosomal subunits separate but can reassemble with mRNA and Met-tRNA to make a new initiation complex and proceed with the translation process to produce more copies of the protein (References 99, 100).

Regulation of Translation

The second level in the regulation of gene expression involves the regulation of translation. Translational regulation can occur by controlling individual initiation factors, altering activity of translational factors, or through interaction between the *cis*-acting sequences on mRNA and the *trans*-acting factors. One of the most common mechanisms of translation regulation is binding of repressors to specific mRNA sites, thereby inhibiting protein synthesis by direct blockade of translation. In eukaryotic cells, translational repression is well described in the regulation of the synthesis of ferritin, the ubiquitous iron storage protein that chelates iron in the cytosol. The quantity of iron present in the cell controls the translation of ferritin mRNA (References 101, 102).

The regulatory system of ferritin mRNA translation consists of the iron-responsive element (IRE), the ferritin repressor protein or IRE-binding protein, and an inducer (iron). The IRE that is located at the 5' untranslated region (UTR) of ferritin mRNA contains a 28-nucleotide fragment responsible for the stimulation of ferritin synthesis by iron. The translation of ferritin mRNA is controlled by binding of IRE-binding protein to the IRE sequence at the 5' end of ferritin mRNA which prevents the mRNA from forming an initiation complex with the ribosomal subunits. In the presence of low iron concentration, IRE-binding protein binds to the IRE and the translation of ferritin mRNA is inhibited. In the presence of sufficient amounts of iron, the IRE-binding protein does not bind to IRE and the translation of ferritin proceeds (see Figure 8) (References 101, 102).

Interference with translation and regulation is a major mode of action of several drug therapies. For example, many antibiotics block protein synthesis in both prokaryotes and eukaryotes. The inhibition of bacterial protein synthesis by antibiotics has been an effective means of fighting infectious diseases. This strategy is effective because of the structural differences between prokaryotic and eukaryotic ribosomes, initiation factors, elongation factors, release factors, and also the fact that protein translation plays an important role in the overall metabolism of the cell (Reference 103).

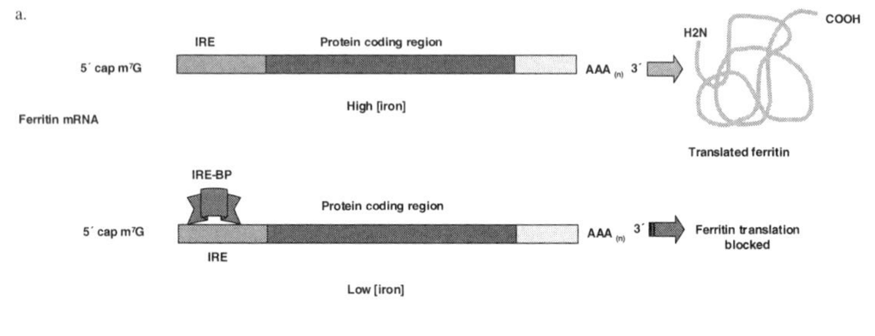

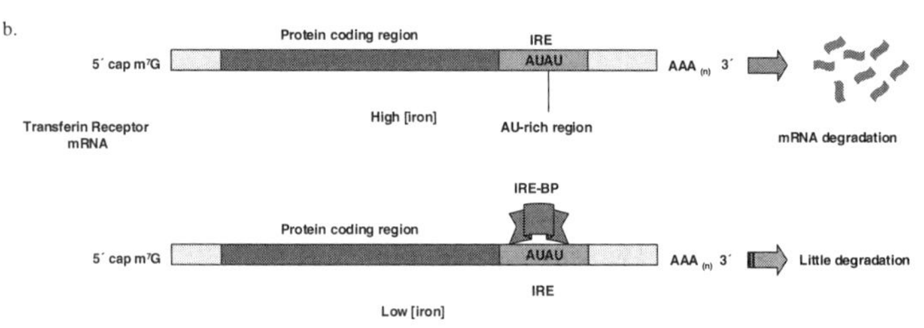

Figure 8. Translational regulation of ferritin (a.) and transferrin (b.). See text for description.
A=adenine; COOH=carboxy terminus; H^2N=amino terminus; IRE=iron-responsive element; IRE-BP=IRE-binding protein; mRNA=messenger RNA; U=uracil.

Stabilization of mRNA

Stabilization and selective degradation of mRNA play important roles in regulating gene expression at the translational level. Rapid degradation of mRNA after entering the cytoplasm results in the synthesis of less protein, while stabilization of mRNA increases its half-life and results in the production of more protein. The stability of different mRNA transcripts within a cell varies to a certain extent based on the cell's activities, differentiation, and development. While mRNAs for some growth factors have half-lives of less than 30 minutes, other mRNAs (e.g., β globin) could be stable for more than 15 hours (References 104, 105).

Messenger RNA decay is triggered by different events such as poly (A) tail shortening, translational arrest caused by a premature stop codon, and endonucleolytic cleavage. The 3' UTR of mRNA plays a crucial role in the stabilization of mRNA. The 3' UTR promotes rapid deadenylation of the 3' poly (A) tail, which results in the decapping of the 5' end of mRNA, and 5'→3' degradation (References 104, 105).

Expanding on the example of iron homeostasis, transferrin is a serum protein that transports iron to the cells that need it. Transferrin plays an important role by binding to iron and preventing the possible damage caused by free iron. Regulation of iron uptake and metabolism is mediated by a plasma membrane protein receptor called the transferrin receptor (TfR). The 3' UTR of TfR mRNA contains a few sets of IREs that are rich in AU sequences. It has been shown that the AU rich elements promote the degradation of mRNA (References 104, 105).

The regulation of TfR is controlled by the 3' UTR of TfR mRNA and the cytoplasmic IRE-binding protein. In the presence of low concentrations of iron, the IRE-binding protein binds to the IREs in the 3' UTR, and inhibits the degradation of TfR mRNA. This results in the accumulation of TfR, and more iron is transferred to the cell. At high iron concentrations, the IRE-binding protein does not bind to the IREs, and the AU rich sequences stimulate the degradation of TfR mRNA (see Figure 8) (References 104, 105).

Post-translational Modification

To become active proteins, newly synthesized polypeptides undergo post-translational modification. For polypeptides to become functional proteins, they must fold correctly in a three-dimensional conformation. Proteins acquire the necessary information for folding from their amino acid sequences. For proper folding, newly synthesized proteins require the assistance of other proteins called molecular chaperones. Chaperones stabilize and support the partially folded polypeptide into a correct and stable three-dimensional protein (References 106–108).

Misfolded and unfolded protein molecules tend to attach to each other and form insoluble aggregates. These aggregates resemble amyloid protein deposits found in several diseases such as Alzheimer's. A complete understanding of the protein folding process may help develop therapies which inhibit protein aggregation in diseases such as Alzheimer's (References 106, 109).

Proteins may be cleaved by proteolytic (protein-cutting) enzymes at a specific amino acid. Proteolysis is an irreversible process that regulates and controls enzyme activation. For example, the post-translational cleavage of initiator methionine from the N-terminal of many polypeptides, which is followed by addition of fatty acid chains or acetyl groups, plays an important role in translocation of proteins to different targets such as lysosomes, mitochondria, and the plasma membrane (References 110, 111).

The lifespans of different proteins vary greatly. In contrast to long-lived structural proteins, regulatory proteins are short-lived and quickly degraded. Misfolded and abnormal proteins are eliminated in a selective protein degradation process by the ubiquitin/proteasome pathway (nonlysosomal proteolytic system). Ubiquitin is a small and stable protein that binds to the internal lysine residues of the substrate through its C-terminus. Ubiquitins (multiubiquitin chains) are used for tagging proteins that are to be degraded by proteasomes (Reference 112).

Some amino acids of the polypeptide chain are altered by phosphorylation and dephosphorylation. Protein phosphorylation is a reversible process catalyzed by protein kinases. Phosphorylation occurs through transfer of phosphate groups from ATP to the -OH groups of the side chains of serine, threonine, and tyrosine. Dephosphorylation of proteins is carried out by protein phosphatases that are specific for serine, threonine, and tyrosine. The processes of phosphorylation and dephosphorylation play important roles in activation and deactivation of proteins involved in signal transduction pathways in eukaryotic cells (References 113, 114).

One of the most significant post-translational modifications that occurs in eukaryotic secretory and membrane-bound proteins is the attachment of sugar chains to an amino acid containing a hydroxyl group, a process called glycosylation. Sugars are naturally added to many proteins during and after protein synthesis. The importance of glycosylation is so great that it caused the creation of a new field in biology called "glycobiology." Serine, threonine, asparagine, tyrosine, hydroxyproline, and hydroxylysine are amino acids that contain a hydroxyl functional group and are involved in glycosylation. There are two major kinds of protein glycosylation designated as N- and O-glycosylation. The N-glycans are linked to asparagine and O-glycans are attached to serine and threonine residues. The N-linked glycans are involved in the folding of glycoproteins by acting as mediators in interactions between ER chaperone proteins calnexin and calreticulin and nascent glycoproteins (References 114–117). Glycosylation can change stability, uptake, solubility, hydrophobicity, immunological properties, and electrical charge of proteins, thus, changing the protein confirmation and its biological activity (References 114, 117).

Defects in glycosylation are responsible for a number of human diseases. In a brain with Alzheimer's disease, the abnormal glycosylation of tau protein, which is one of the major microtubule-associated proteins in neurons, results in an early abnormality of neurofibrillary degeneration. The progress in elucidating the role of proteins and lipid-linked carbohydrates in various biological processes has shifted the attentions toward drugs that target the enzymes involved in glycosylation. Drugs such as glycosidase inhibitors are shown effective in the treatment of viral infections, such as hepatitis B and C in animal models (References 114–116, 118, 119).

Cell Signaling

Cells in multicellular organisms are constantly interacting with the surrounding environment. The reaction of cells to environmental stimuli is determined by the receptors displayed on the cell's surface. Cells respond to changes in their environment by altering patterns of gene expression, regulating the activity of proteins. Cell signaling refers to the mechanism by which an external change (usually in the form ligand-receptor binding) initiates an intracellular cascade that results in a specific cellular response.

Cell Signaling Molecules

Cells respond to changes in the environment and facilitate appropriate adaptations to these changes through extracellular signals. Cell signaling molecules are diverse and range from light particles to odorants and pheromones to ions and peptides. Binding of these molecules to their respective receptors initiates the signaling cascade that transduces the extracellular signals into intracellular biochemical reactions, eliciting the specific cellular response. Not only are the signaling molecules varied, but so are their receptors, including cell surface and intracellular receptors. Extracellular signaling molecules can propagate their signals in various ways including through: plasma membrane diffusion, ion channels, G protein-coupled receptors (GPCRs), and enzyme-linked receptors.

Plasma Membrane Diffusion

Although the majority of signaling molecules initiate the signaling process through binding with a plasma membrane-associated receptor, this is not true for all molecules. Several hydrophobic molecules are able to diffuse through the lipid bilayer of the plasma membrane and bind to intracellular receptors found in the cytoplasm or on the nucleus. Examples of these signaling molecules include steroids, nitric oxide, and arachadonic acid.

Steroids such as estrogen, progesterone, testosterone, and the glucocorticoids and mineralocorticoids are derived from cholesterol. They initiate cellular changes by diffusing across the plasma membrane and binding to intracellular receptors (Reference 120). These receptors serve as transcription factors. Once steroids bind to their respective receptors and associate with regulatory DNA sequences (previously described HREs) in the nucleus, activation of transcription occurs. Although important in a wide array of homeostatic functions, hormone-hormone receptor binding can be pathological as in the case of metastatic breast cancer where estrogen-mediated transcription results in tumor proliferation. In fact, several pharmacological agents used in current practice interrupt estrogen's effects at the receptor level. For example, tamoxifen directly binds to the estrogen receptor causing a conformational change that blocks the transcription of estrogen-dependent genes implicated in breast cancer.

Nitric oxide is another example of a signaling molecule that exerts its effects by diffusing across the cell membrane. Nitric oxide, which is produced from L arginine through nitric oxide synthase, diffuses from the cell in which it was produced and across the plasma membrane of neighboring cells to activate guanylyl cyclase which increases the production of cyclic guanosine-5'-monophosphate (Reference 121). The actions of cyclic guanosine-5'-monophosphate are diverse resulting in smooth muscle relaxation and vasodilation. In clinical practice, organic nitrates like nitroglycerin are converted to nitric oxide and result in vasodilation, a beneficial treatment modality for acute and chronic angina.

Another commonly prescribed drug, sildenafil, potentiates the vasodilatory effects of nitric oxide by inhibiting type 5 phosphodiesterase-mediated breakdown of cyclic guanosine-5'-monophosphate in the corpus cavernosum, thereby making it a commonly prescribed agent for the treatment of erectile dysfunction.

Ion Channels

Cell signaling molecules also include small ions such as calcium, potassium, and sodium. These molecules affect cellular changes through ion channels in the plasma membrane. Ion channels are ubiquitous proteins and are crucial in many signaling processes that regulate electrolyte homeostasis, smooth muscle contraction, cell and intravascular volume, insulin release, neuronal activity, and cardiac function (Reference 122). In general, ion channels are specific to ionic molecules and are described as either voltage-gated or ligand-gated (Reference 123). These terms refer to the mechanism by which the ion channels are opened to allow for passage of the ions into the intracellular space. In the case of voltage-gated ion channels, the membrane potential of the cell determines whether the ion channel is open or closed. In ligand-gated ion channels, binding of a molecule to a receptor that is associated with the channel results in conformational changes in the ion channel that regulate the flux of ions into the cell.

G Protein-coupled and Enzyme-linked Receptors

The most common initiation of signaling pathways by extracellular signaling molecules is through direct binding of membrane-bound receptors. By binding to membrane-associated receptors such as GPCRs and enzyme-linked receptors like receptor tyrosine kinases, ligands initiate a series of intracellular events that modify intracellular proteins and elicit appropriate cellular responses to a given stimulus. These receptors are discussed in further detail in the next two sections.

G Protein-coupled Receptors

G protein-coupled receptors represent the most numerous class of signaling receptors. Their ubiquitous nature (it is estimated that approximately 1 percent of the vertebrate genome is comprised of genes that encode GPCRs) (Reference 124) and diversity have made them the focus of decades of study. In addition, their importance in human disease is underscored by the fact the majority of pharmacological agents exert their effects at GPCRs (see Table 2).

The field of GPCR research has progressed since the identification of the first G protein, G_s, and the first GPCR, the β-adrenergic receptor, was characterized in the early 1980s (References 125, 126). The classical linear paradigm of ligand-induced conformational changes in the receptor, G protein activation, and downstream signaling events leading to

Table 2. Examples of Drugs that Work at G Protein-coupled Receptors

Receptor	Drug
Muscarinic acetylcholine	Atropine, ipratropium
$GABA_A$	Benzodiazepines, zolpidem, zaleplon
$\beta_1 AR$	Atenolol, metoprolol
$\beta_2 AR$	Albuterol
$\alpha_1 AR$	Terazosin, doxazosin
$\alpha_2 AR$	Clonidine
D_2	Antipsychotics, metoclopromide, prochlorperazine
D_2/D_4	Olanzapine, clozapine
5-HT_{1A}	Buspirone
5-HT_{1D}	Sumatriptan, zolmitriptan
5-HT_2	Quetiapine, olanzapine, risperidone, ziprazadone, aripiprazole, clozapine
5-HT_3	Ondansetron, granisetron
H_1	Diphenhydramine, loratidine, cetirizine
H_2	Ranitidine, cimetidine, famotidine, nizatidine
AT_1	Losartan, valsartan, eprosartan, telmisartan
μ opioid	Morphine, oxycodone, methadone
Prostaglandin	Misoprostol, epoprostenol
Somatostatin	Octreotide
Vasopressin	Desmopressin
Leukotriene	Montelukast, zafirlukast
Endothelin	Bosentan

5-HT=serotonin; α=aminobutyric acid; AR=adrenergic receptor; AT=angiotensin; D=dopamine; GABA=gamma aminobutyric acid; H=histamine.

physiological responses to stimuli has been expounded. It appears that the interactions between the various proteins in the signaling cascade are more complex than originally thought (Reference 127), thereby allowing for insights into the specificity of GPCR activity and complicating the field of receptor pharmacology.

G Protein-coupled Receptors and G Protein Structure

The GPCRs contain common structural motifs that form the basis of their conserved functional activity. These receptors possess seven membrane-spanning regions comprised of approximately 30 amino acids each (Reference 128). The transmembrane domains are connected by three intracellular and three extracellular loops. In addition, the amino terminus of the receptor is located on the extracellular tail while the carboxy terminus is located intracellularly (see Figure 9) (Reference 129). Agonist binding to the GPCR leads to a series of intracellular signaling events mediated by G

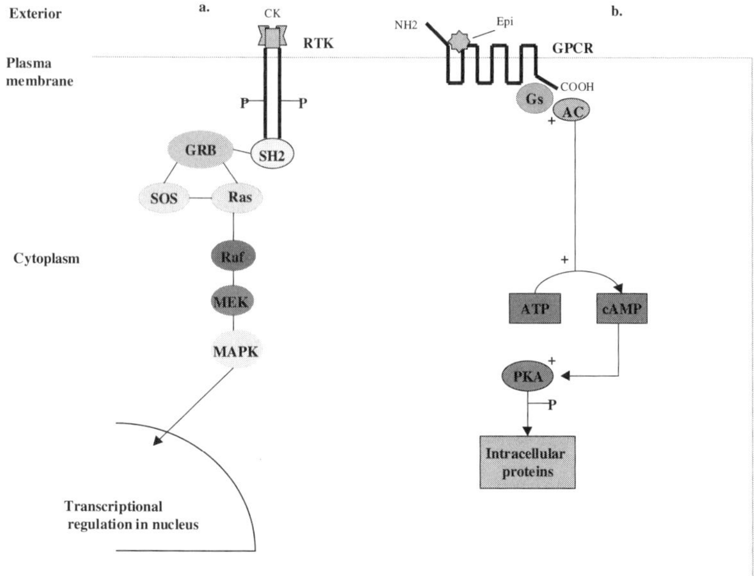

Figure 9. Receptor tyrosine kinase and G protein-coupled receptor signaling pathways.
a. RTKs are bound by an extracellular ligand such as insulin or growth factors, resulting in RTK dimerization. This allows the receptor to activate itself through autophosphorylation. In this example, GRB recognizes phosphorylated tyrosines on the RTK and binds to the receptor through the SH2 portion of the GRB. Ras, a major protein in RTK signaling, is associated with GRB and SOS, a Ras-activating protein. Ras is then activated and further phosphorylates MEK, which in turn activates MAPK. MAPK then phosphorylates various transcription factors to alter gene expression and elicit a particular biological response.
b. In this case, epinephrine binds to the β-adrenergic receptor, which is coupled to the Gs protein. The Gs protein is activated and subsequently stimulates AC. AC converts ATP to cAMP, cAMP activates PKA, and PKA phosphorylates various intracellular proteins resulting in vasodilation, bronchodilation, increased heart rate, and other effects.
C=adenylyl cyclase; ATP=adenosine triphosphate; cAMP=cyclic adenosine monophosphate; CK=cytokine; COOH=carboxy terminus; Epi=epinephrine; G_s=G stimulatory; GPCR=G protein-coupled receptor; GRB=growth factor receptor binding protein; MAPK=mitogen-activated protein kinase; MEK=MAPK/ERK kinase; NH2=amino terminus; P=phosphorylated residue; PKA=protein kinase A; RTK=receptor tyrosine kinase; SOS=son of sevenless protein.

proteins and facilitated through effectors, such as adenylyl cyclase and phospholipase C.

The structure of G proteins is well characterized. These proteins are divided into four classes: G_s and G_i, which activate and inhibit adenylyl cyclase, respectively; G_q, which activates phospholipase C; and G_{12}/G_{13} whose functions are not well understood (Reference 130). These G proteins are responsible for transduction of extracellular signals into intracellular responses.

G proteins are structurally heterotrimeric (Reference 131). They are comprised of three subunits: α, β, and γ. Physiologically, the β and γ subunits are associated and act as one functional unit ($\beta\gamma$) (Reference 132). The α subunit has two important domains, the G domain and the helical domain. The G domain is the site of GTP binding and also exhibits intrinsic GTPase activity (i.e., hydrolysis of GTP). The helical domain is important for GTPase activity and effector binding (Reference 133). The propeller-like structure of the β subunit and the α-helix of the γ subunit allow for complementary association at their N termini regions, forming a functional unit that only is dissociated through denaturation (Reference 130). When the GPCR is not activated, the α and $\beta\gamma$ subunits are associated, with the α subunit also bound to GDP. It is not until an agonist activates the GPCR that the α subunit dissociates from $\beta\gamma$ and both subunits activate their respective effectors (Reference 131).

G Protein-coupled Receptor Signaling

G protein-coupled receptors are integral in facilitating the physiological responses to a myriad of stimuli including (but not limited to) adrenergic amines, ions (e.g., calcium), light, and protein hormones. These extracellular signals bind to their respective GPCRs. Once binding occurs, the GPCR undergoes a conformational change (References 133, 134). Since the α subunit of the G protein (G_α) is associated with the GPCR, it also undergoes a change in its conformation. This change decreases the binding affinity of guanosine diphosphate for G_α, and guanosine diphosphate dissociates from the subunit. Once the G domain of G_α is unoccupied, GTP binds to G_α. This is accomplished competitively since GTP is present in higher concentrations intracellularly than guanosine diphosphate. The binding of GTP confers activity on G_α, and this subunit dissociates from the receptor and from $G_{\beta\gamma}$. Consequently, both G_α and $G_{\beta\gamma}$ are free to interact with their respective effectors. Effectors are enzymes (e.g., adenylyl cyclase and phospholipase C) or ion channels (e.g., calcium and potassium channels) that alter second messenger and ion concentrations, respectively, resulting in cellular and physical responses (Reference 130).

The active state of G proteins, and consequently the signaling cascade, is dependent on the binding of GTP to G_α. The activity of G_α is intrinsically regulated since this subunit possesses GTPase activity. The α subunit hydrolyzes GTP to guanosine diphosphate at variable rates. Once GTP is hydrolyzed to guanosine diphosphate, the G_α and $G_{\beta\gamma}$ subunits reassociate and return to the receptor until further agonist stimulation (References 135–137).

To illustrate the integration of the components of GPCR signaling (i.e., stimulus, GPCR, G protein, effector, and second messenger) take the example of stimulation of the β-adrenergic receptor by epinephrine. The β-adrenergic receptor is coupled to the G protein, G_S. On stimulation of the β-adrenergic receptor by the binding of epinephrine, the receptor undergoes a conformational change resulting in a concomitant conformational change in $G_{s\alpha}$. This alteration facilitates guanosine diphosphate dissociation and GTP binding to $G_{s\alpha}$. The $G_{s\alpha}$ subunit then activates the effector adenylyl cyclase. Adenylyl cyclase subsequently catalyzes the conversion of ATP to cyclic adenosine monophosphate, the second messenger in this cascade. In turn, cyclic adenosine monophosphate activates protein kinase A, an enzyme responsible for the phosphorylation of intracellular proteins (see Figure 9). Since β-adrenergic receptors are located on various cells, different intracellular proteins are available for phosphorylation, leading to a wide range of physiologic responses to epinephrine including increased chronotropy and inotropy ($β_1$-adrenergic receptor stimulation), arteriolar vasodilation, bronchodilation, and increased glycogenolysis ($β_2$-adrenergic receptor stimulation).

G Protein-coupled Receptor Diversity and Specificity

The complexity of GPCR-mediated cell signaling becomes apparent when one considers that there are more than 1,000 GPCRs, four classes of G_α units (with subclasses within each), multiple isoforms of β and γ subunits, and finally subtypes among the effectors themselves (Reference 132). This raises the following fundamental question: what are the cellular components and/or processes that result in a specific cellular response to a given external stimulus? A comprehensive review of proposed structural and chemical regulatory points of cellular signaling is beyond the scope of this section. However, this section briefly outlines some current considerations.

There are several proposed mechanisms that explain the specificity of cell signaling through G proteins (Reference 130). The first is that GPCRs contain G protein recognition sequences that allow for the receptor to interact with the appropriate G protein. In addition, cytoplasmic regions of the GPCR outside of the G protein recognition site help to ensure specificity in GPCR-G protein interaction. This is evidenced by research that demonstrates decreased selectivity in adrenergic and cholinergic receptor binding to appropriate G proteins on alteration of these cytoplasmic regions (Reference 138). In addition to receptor-G protein surface interactions, G proteins also are largely specific for their effectors. However, the above two control mechanisms do not completely account for the specificity of ligand-induced cellular response when considering that individual receptors interact with more than one G protein simultaneously.

As previously discussed, the active state of G_α, and consequently $G_{\beta\gamma}$ and effectors, are limited by the GTPase activity of the G_α subunit (Reference 139). Therefore, the rate of GTP hydrolysis serves as another control mechanism in cell signaling. In addition, there is growing evidence that effectors themselves, perhaps in conjunction with $G_{\beta\gamma}$, can alter the rate of G_α ATPase activity, thereby limiting their own activity and achieving specificity in cellular response (Reference 140).

Other purported mechanisms by which binding of given agonists to their respective GPCRs results in unique cellular responses include modification of α and $\beta\gamma$ subunits through phosphorylation or lipid modification, regulatory protein (e.g., calmodulin and regulator of G protein signaling) effects on G protein subunits, and localization of GPCRs, G proteins, and effectors into lipid rafts and caveolae (References 137, 141).

Implications for Drug Therapy

The elucidation of GPCR signaling pathways has several important implications for pharmacotherapy. These are broadly described in terms of current drug therapy, drug development, and variability in drug response.

The majority of pharmacological agents currently on the market exert their effects at the level of GPCRs (see Table 2). There are many examples of agents whose mechanism of therapeutic benefit is mediated through agonism or antagonism of certain G protein pathways. For example, the selective β_1-adrenergic receptor antagonists metoprolol and bisoprolol and the nonselective $\beta_1/\beta_2/\alpha_1$-adrenergic receptor antagonist carvedilol mediate their effects largely through interruption of GPCR signaling pathways, resulting not only in beneficial hemodynamic and cardio-structural effects, but also in reductions in mortality and morbidity in patients with systolic heart failure.

It is not mandatory for pharmacological agents to bind directly with the GPCR to exert their effects. Modulation of second messengers also result in demonstrable cellular and clinical changes. For example, milrinone exerts its positive inotropic and vasodilatory effects by inhibition of type III phosphodiesterase. Type III phosphodiesterase is responsible for degrading cyclic adenosine monophosphate to adenosine monophosphate. By inhibiting type III phosphodiesterase, milrinone increases cyclic adenosine monophosphate concentrations near the sarcoplasmic reticulum, leading to activation of protein kinase A and protein kinase G. Consequently, phosphorylation of cellular proteins results in increased cardiac contractility and decreased pulmonary pressure and systemic vascular resistance.

An understanding of the components of GPCR signal transduction also has implications for drug development. For example, compounds which target GPCRs that are currently in development or in late phase clinical trials include dual endothelin receptor antagonists, vasopressin receptor antagonists, a central cannabinoid receptor antagonist for the treatment of obesity and smoking cessation, a cholecystokinin receptor agonist for the treatment of obesity and an antagonist for pancreatic cancer, CC chemokine receptor 5 and CX chemokine receptor 4 and inhibitors for the treatment of human immunodeficiency virus, a purinergic receptor P2Y agonist, and many others.

Other elements of the signaling cascade besides the GPCRs themselves, specifically regulatory proteins serve as novel drug targets. For example, the regulator of G protein signaling proteins dramatically increase the

GTPase activity of G_α thereby resulting in GTP hydrolysis and termination of the cell signal (References 142, 143). As such, both regulator of G protein signaling antagonists and agonists may prove to be important therapeutic agents in a plethora of clinical conditions. Notably, regulator of G protein signaling antagonists could potentiate the effects of endogenous agonists (similarly to benzodiazepines at the gamma aminobutyric acid A receptor) or block receptor desensitization to exogenously administered agents to which rapid desensitization occurs (e.g., opioid analgesics). On the other hand, blocking cell signaling in specific tissues (through a regulator of G protein signaling agonist) also could be beneficial. Since inflammatory cytokines, epinephrine, endothelin, and angiotensin all mediate their effects through GPCRs, regulator of G protein signaling agonists may diminish the cellular responses to these agonists and be useful in a broad range of inflammatory and cardiovascular conditions (Reference 144).

Another area of opportunity for drug development, although specialized, is G protein disease. Numerous endocrine and malignant diseases such as pituitary, thyroid, adrenal, and ovarian adenomas, pseudohypoparathyroidism, obesity, diabetes, and essential hypertension are linked to variant alleles in the genes that encode the α or β subunits of G proteins (Reference 145). These are candidate diseases for nontraditional approaches to treatment such as gene therapy.

Perhaps the most interesting opportunity for drug discovery and development is that of orphan GPCRs. These orphan receptors are GPCRs with no identified endogenous ligands or known physiological role. To date, more than 100 orphan GPCRs have been identified, and these receptors represent a new subclass of receptors as they share little amino acid homology with known GPCRs (about 30 percent) (References 146–148). The current approach to identifying orphan GPCRs and their ligands involves bioinformatic screening and analysis of cDNA libraries for signature motifs of GPCRs; full-length cloning and receptor expression studies; performance of functional assays (e.g., measurement of intracellular cyclic adenosine monophosphate changes); and "ligand fishing" by attempting to stimulate the receptors with known and novel ligands (Reference 149). This strategy could potentially identify orphan GPCRs that would be targets for drug discovery.

Finally, G proteins and their receptors are the focus of research in the field of pharmacogenomics. For example, polymorphisms are identified in many GPCRs and their G protein subunits including β- and α-adrenergic, dopaminergic, and opioid receptors. These polymorphisms could potentially help personalize drug therapy by identifying patients most likely to respond to specific agents or experience side effects to those drugs. Genetic variations in GPCRs and their G protein subunits may be future predictors of drug response in areas of cardiovascular, pulmonary, neuropsychiatric, and other areas of pharmacotherapy.

Enzyme-linked Receptors

In addition to GPCRs, enzyme-linked receptors represent a major class of surface receptors that are not only important in cell regulation, but also serve as future targets of pharmacological intervention for a vast array of diseases. Enzyme-linked receptors vary from GPCRs in structure and in many functions. However, the paradigm of ligand stimulation, putative domain alteration, modification of intracellular proteins, and cellular response is the same.

Enzymatic alteration of key proteins in response to biological signals through enzyme-linked receptors is a fundamental mode of cell communication. Receptor tyrosine kinases (RTKs), a class of membrane protein receptors that are responsible for the phosphorylation of tyrosine residues, play an instrumental role in metabolic processes (e.g., the insulin receptor is a RTK) and cell development and division (Reference 150). Dysregulation of RTK signaling is implicated in various malignancies and in type 2 diabetes. Given their importance in mediating the molecular events that lead to specific cellular responses, RTKs are of interest in biochemistry and clinical pharmacology.

Receptor Tyrosine Kinases and RTK Structure

Receptor tyrosine kinases possess an extracellular domain that binds various peptide hormones important in cell proliferation, differentiation, migration, and metabolism. These hormones include insulin, epidermal growth factor (EGF), fibroblast growth factor, nerve growth factor, platelet-derived growth factor (PDGF), and vascular endothelial growth factor (Reference 151).

Like GPCRs, RTKs have an amino terminal extracellular region that serves as the site for ligand binding. The RTK also has a membrane-spanning region. However, rather than seven spanning regions interpolated within the plasma membrane, RTKs are generally comprised of a single helix that links the extracellular region with the intracellular region. The intracellular region is comprised of a tyrosine kinase catalytic domain and a carboxy terminus. The tyrosine kinase domain is the functional component of RTKs. It is here that autophosphorylation occurs, activating the receptor and priming the receptor for phosphorylation and regulation of downstream signaling proteins that perpetuate the signal initiated by extracellular input stimuli (Reference 151).

Ras, Raf and RTK Signaling

Receptor tyrosine kinases serve as major membrane receptors that help regulate bioprocesses associated with the major aspects of cell cycling. Ligands for RTKs include many growth factors as well as insulin. These ligands bind to the extracellular domain of the RTK and cause receptor dimerization. This conformational change allows for the intrinsic tyrosine kinase activity of the receptor to phosphorylate key tyrosine residues in the receptor's intracellular domain (autophosphorylation). Once in the phosphorylated or activated form, the RTK binds cytoplasmic proteins at specific binding domains on these proteins. This results in signal propagation with the ultimate effect being activation of transcription factors in the nucleus and cell-specific response.

With the exception of the insulin receptor, RTKs exist as monomers in the inactivated state. The purported view of receptor activation is that, upon binding of the hormone peptide, two monomers become a dimeric receptor unit (References 152, 153). In fact, many of the RTK ligands are dimeric in nature, capable of binding two receptors at once. Because of their constitutive enzymatic activity, this dimerization allows for the receptors to reciprocally phosphorylate one another's tyrosine residues and, therefore, activate each other.

The following is an example of events subsequent to autophosphorylation that illustrates how the tyrosine kinase activity of RTKs mediates further downstream signaling using the Ras pathway, the main pathway for RTK signaling. Ras is a small, membrane-bound G protein not entirely unlike the G proteins associated with GPCRs. In fact, like those on GPCRs, Ras is inactive when bound to guanosine diphosphate, active when bound to GTP, and possesses intrinsic GTPase activity that hydrolyzes GTP to guanosine diphosphate. The difference between Ras and the GPCR G proteins is that Ras is monomeric as opposed to trimeric (Reference 150). When the RTK is activated by ligand binding and autophosphorylation, a protein called growth factor receptor-binding protein recognizes the phosphorylated tyrosines on the receptor and binds to them through a domain on the growth factor receptor-binding protein called SH2. This binding domain is not exclusive to growth factor receptor-binding protein. In fact, many signaling proteins possess SH2 domains that promote binding to the receptor. Ras is associated with growth factor receptor-binding protein and a Ras-activating protein called SOS (References 154, 155). Therefore, when the growth factor receptor-binding protein-SOS complex binds to the activated RTK, Ras exchanges guanosine diphosphate for GTP and becomes activated. Ras then initiates a cascade that activates a series of serine/threonine protein kinases. First, Raf is phosphorylated which, in turn, phosphorylates mitogen-activated protein kinase kinase. Mitogen-activated protein kinase kinase then phosphorylates mitogen-activated protein kinase (MAPK). Finally, MAPK phosphorylates various transcription factors leading to the altered transcription that causes the specific cellular response (i.e., cell proliferation, differentiation, etc. [see Figure 9]) (Reference 156).

Thus, RTKs are membrane-bound proteins that function as receptors for various ligands such as growth factors and insulin. As a result of their tyrosine kinase activity, they are able to phosphorylate, and consequently activate various downstream signaling proteins which possess protein kinase activity. The signal ends at the nucleus in the phosphorylation of transcription regulating proteins that govern such cell activities as proliferation, growth, apoptosis, motility, and metabolism.

Implications for Drug Therapy

Since RTKs are important in cell differentiation and proliferation, it is not surprising that irregular signal modulation through these receptors are implicated in various human cancers (Reference 157). Therefore, inhibitors of RTK-mediated signal transduction are available, or in development, for the treatment of many malignant diseases (Reference 158). There are several strategies to inhibit RTK cell signaling. These include inhibition of the receptor-ligand interaction, interfering with the tyrosine kinase intracellular domain, inhibiting Ras activity, and targeting RTK mRNA to inhibit translational processes (Reference 159).

The RTK-ligand binding interaction is successfully blocked by monoclonal antibodies against the RTK of interest. For example, trastuzumab is a monoclonal antibody against the HER2 RTK. HER2, when overexpressed, is associated with a subset of breast cancers (Reference 160). Trastuzumab binds to the HER2 receptor and is thought to have a dual mechanism of action: inhibition of ligand-mediated cell signaling and tumor proliferation, as well as cell opsonization and cytotoxicity through natural killer cells and monocytes.

Receptor tyrosine kinase cell signals also can be interrupted at the level of the tyrosine kinase domain. Tyrosine kinase inhibitors predominantly exert their effects by binding to a specific ATP binding region on the cytoplasmic domain of RTKs, blocking tyrosine kinase activity (Reference 159). Other tyrosine kinase inhibitors block the intracellular protein binding sites on the RTK, preventing the interaction between the receptor and downstream signaling molecules. The net effect is to prevent propagation of the cell signal from ligand-bound RTKs. Currently, several pharmaceutical companies are conducting early phase clinical trials with tyrosine kinase inhibitors against EGF receptor for use in various cancers.

Another strategy to inhibit RTK signals is to develop antisense oligonucleotides against RTK mRNA (Reference 159). These nucleotides bind to RTK mRNA through complementary base pairing, thus, inhibiting proper translation, and consequently expression, of RTKs. Farnesyl transfer inhibitors inhibit the enzyme involved in post-translational modification of Ras. The result is the inability of Ras to associate with the plasma membrane essentially making this key G protein nonfunctional (Reference 161). Antisense oligonucleotides and farnesyl transfer inhibitors are examples of inhibition of RTK signaling at the level of protein expression. There are several compounds in both classes under development for the suppression of tumor growth.

As with GPCRs, an understanding of the pathways of RTK signaling is important in the identification of novel compounds for the treatment of human diseases. For the clinical scientist, knowledge of signal transduction mediated through this receptor class may provide opportunities for drug development, clinical trial experiences, pharmacogenomic study, and other scientific endeavors. For the clinician, a broad awareness of cell transduction is used to bridge the gap between molecular biology and clinical practice.

Janus Family Tyrosine Kinase/Signal Transducer and Activator of Transcription Signaling Pathway

The Janus family tyrosine kinase/signal transducer and activator of transcription pathway was first identified as a major pathway for cytokine-initiated signal transduction which regulates many phases of hematopoiesis, inflammation, and immune response. Cytokines are intercellular messenger molecules that regulate many cellular functions in the hematopoietic and inflammatory systems. The intercellular signals that cytokines transmit are either autocrine (the cell that produces the cytokine also responds to it) or paracrine (cytokine is produced by one cell and acts on another cell). The Janus family tyrosine kinase/signal transducer and activator of transcription pathway plays important roles in cell signaling and regulation of cellular development and survival. This pathway is the center of much attention, and in the past few years, more than 1500 articles were published on Janus family tyrosine kinase and signal transducer and activator of transcription (References 162, 163).

The Janus family tyrosine kinase/signal transducer and activator of transcription pathway rapidly transmits extracellular polypeptide signals through transmembrane receptors directly to the target gene promoters in the nucleus. The Janus family tyrosine kinase/signal transducer and activator of transcription pathway is the major signal transduction pathway for ligands that include erythropoeitin, thrombopoeitin, granulocyte colony-stimulating factor, granulocyte-macrophage colony-stimulating factor, growth hormone, and prolactin; interleukins such as IL-2, IL-6, IL-7, IL-10, and others; and interferons α, β, and γ (References 162–165).

Much like with RTKs, an important step in signal transduction through the Janus family tyrosine kinase/signal transducer and activator of transcription pathway is tyrosine phosphorylation. The Jaks are receptor-associated protein kinases comprised of four nonreceptor tyrosine kinases (designated as Jak1, Jak2, Jak3 and Tyk2). The Jaks were named Janus kinases (after Janus, the mythologic Roman god of gates with two faces) for having both true kinase and pseudokinase domains. Upon binding of a cytokine to its receptor, these kinases selectively phosphorylate and activate Stat proteins, which are ultimately responsible for regulating gene expression and bringing about cellular responses to stimuli. While Jak1, Jak2, and Tyk2 are expressed ubiquitously, Jak3 is mostly expressed in cells of the myeloid and lymphoid lineages. Seven conserved Jak homology (JH1-JH7) domains exist among Jaks (see Figure 10), including the JH1 and JH2 domains which are the respective tyrosine kinase and pseudokinase domains. The functions of the remaining homology domains (JH3-JH7) are not fully elucidated but are thought to be important in Jak association with its receptor (References 162–165).

The Stat proteins are seven structurally and functionally related proteins designated as Stat1, Stat2, Stat3, Stat4, Stat5a, Stat5b, and Stat6. The Stats reside as clusters on chromosomes and range from 750 to 800 amino acids in length except for Stat2 and Stat6 which are approximately 850 amino acids in length. The seven members of the Stat family of transcription

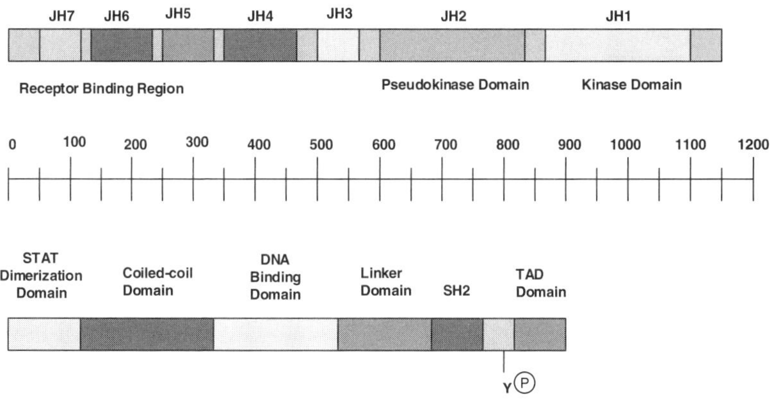

Figure 10. Structures of Jak and Stat proteins.
Jaks are comprised of seven conserved homology domains (JH1-JH7). JH1 and JH2 are the kinase and pseudokinase domains, respectively, while the remaining domains are thought to be important in receptor binding. Stats are comprised of the tyrosine activator domain (TAD), an SH2 domain, a linker domain, the DNA-binding domain, a coiled-coil region, and the Stat dimerization domain on the amino terminus. The scale represents the size of each protein/domain in number of amino acids.
DNA=deoxyribonucleic acid; Jak=Janus Kinase; P=phosphorylated residue; SH2=a domain on the growth factor receptor-binding protein; Stat=signal transducers and activators of transcription; Y=tyrosine residue.

factors share five conserved domains that include the N-terminal domain, the coiled-coil domain, the DNA binding domain, the linker domain, and the SH2 tyrosine activation domain (see Figure 10). Stat specificity is determined by a SH2 domain whose sequence is quite divergent among Stat proteins and recognizes different phosphorylated motifs (References 162–166).

In the absence of specific receptor activation, Stat proteins exist as inactive transcriptional factors in the cytoplasm of the target cells. The binding of a cytokine to its cognate receptor induces receptor tyrosine phosphorylation by Jak kinases that specifically bind to the intracellular domains of cytokine receptors. The phosphorylated tyrosines then serve as docking sites for Stat proteins. All Stats have a tyrosine residue near their SH2 domain that is used as a substrate for phosphorylation. As such, Stat proteins are activated after specific binding of Stat SH2 domains and receptor phosphotyrosine residues. Stat proteins can homodimerize or heterodimerize after being phosphorylated and are released from the receptor. The dimerized Stats are rapidly translocated from the cytoplasm to

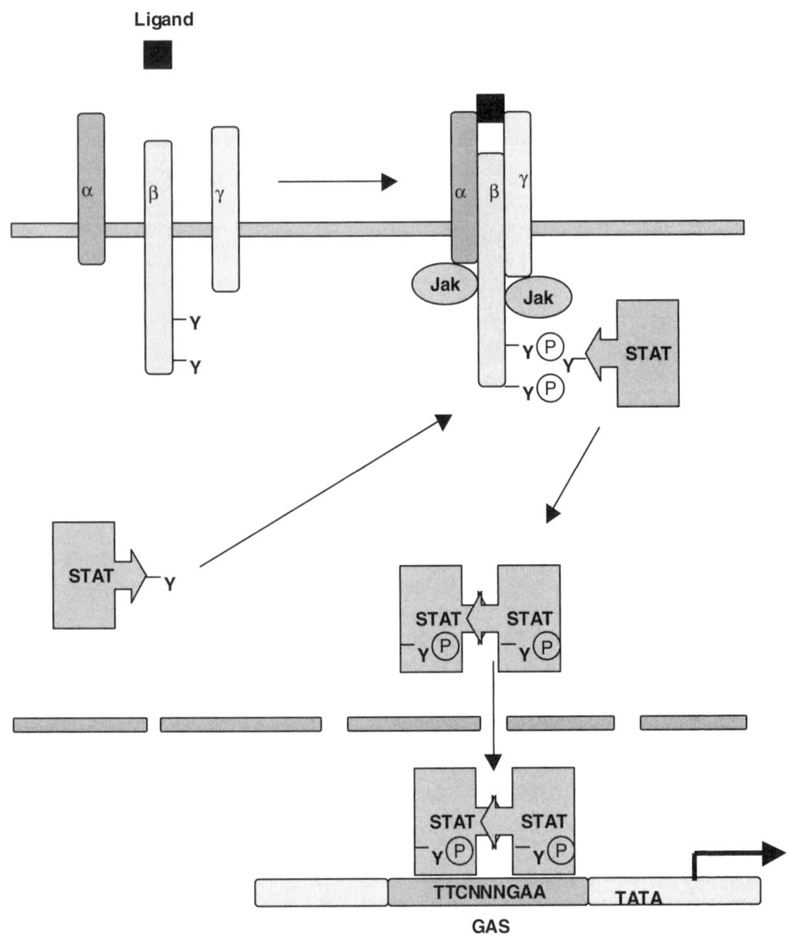

Figure 11. The JAK/STAT signaling pathway.
A ligand binds to the receptor resulting in the activation of receptor-bound Jaks. The activated Jaks then promote phosphorylation of tyrosine residues on the receptor which serve as signals for the recruitment of Stats. These Stats also become phosphorylated and are released from the receptor. They then dimerize and are translocated into the nucleus where they subsequently bind to the GAS family of enhancers and regulate gene expression. GAS=γ-activated site; Jak=Janus Kinase; P=phosphorylated residues; STAT=signal transducers and activators of transcription; TATA=TATA box; Y=tyrosine residues.

the nucleus where they bind to specific sequence elements (usually γ-activated sequence enhancers) on DNA and modulate the expression of target genes (see Figure 11) (References 162–165).

Besides cytokine receptors, non-cytokine receptors like GPCRs and RTKs are able to activate signal transducer and activator of transcription proteins. For example, through RTKs and GPCRs (such as the angiotensin II receptor) EGF and PDGF activate the Janus family tyrosine kinase/signal transducer and activator of transcription signaling pathway. Also, the Janus family tyrosine kinase/signal transducer and activator of transcription signaling pathways can be regulated by different intrinsic and environmental stimuli, protein tyrosine phosphatases, or protein inhibitors. The suppressor of cytokine signaling proteins that bind directly to Jaks and inactivate the kinases, and the protein inhibitors of activated Stats, which prevent DNA recognition by binding to phosphorylated Stat dimers, are two examples of Janus family tyrosine kinase/signal transducer and activator of transcription signaling pathway protein inhibitors.

The association of the Janus family tyrosine kinase/signal transducer and activator of transcription signaling pathway with cardiac dysfunction and its important role in the pathogenesis of myocardial ischemia have been demonstrated in a rat model. Treatment of hearts with tyrphostin AG490 (a Jak protein inhibitor) resulted in the recovery of cardiac function showing that Jak activation is involved in ischemia-induced dysfunction of the heart. The Janus family tyrosine kinase/signal transducer and activator of transcription pathway also may be implicated in various other diseases of inflammatory or hematopoeitic dysregulation such as asthma, immunodeficiency, and cancer (References 168–170).

Summary

Molecular and cellular biology not only serve as the foundations of biological science, but are dynamic disciplines evolving in ways that result in technological and pharmacological advancements in the diagnosis and management of patients with a spectrum of clinical diseases. By understanding cellular structure and function, gene processing and regulation, and cellular signaling, practitioners begin to narrow the gap between the basic and clinical sciences. With the advancement of molecular-based drug therapies through genomics research, the clinician will be called upon to translate approaches to patient care from the scientific bench to the patient's bedside. A functional understanding of molecular and cellular biology principles is imperative in order to identify new drug targets, optimize currently available therapies, and improve patient outcomes.

References

1.   Newport JW, Forbes DJ. The nucleus: structure, function, and dynamics. Annu Rev Biochem 1987;56:535–65.

2.   Pante N, Aebi U. The nuclear pore complex. J Cell Biol 1993;122(5):977–84.

3.   Davis LI. The nuclear pore complex. Annu Rev Biochem 1995;64:865–96.

4.   Forbes DJ. Structure and function of the nuclear pore complex. Annu Rev Cell Biol 1992;8:495–527.

5.   Scheer U, Hock R. Structure and function of the nucleolus. Curr Opin Cell Biol 1999;11(3):385–90.

6.   Doudna JA, Rath VL. Structure and function of the eukaryotic ribosome: the next frontier. Cell 2002;109(2):153–6.

7.   Hill WE, Dahlberg A, Garrett RA, Moore PB, Schlessinger D, Warner JR. The Ribosome: Structure, Function, and Evolution. Washington, D.C.: American Society for Microbiology, 1990.

8.   Noller HF. Ribosomal RNA and translation. Annu Rev Biochem 1991;60:191–227.

9.   Cooper GM. Protein sorting and transport. In: Cooper GM, ed. The Cell: A Molecular Approach. Sunderland: Sinauer Associates, Inc., 1997:347–87.

10. Wolfe SL. Protein Sorting, Distribution, Secretion, and Endocytosis: Introduction to Cell and Molecular Biology. Belmont: Wadsworth Publishing Company, 1995:571–604.

11. Keenan RJ, Freymann DM, Stroud RM, Walter P. The signal recognition particle. Annu Rev Biochem 2001;70:755–75.

12. Pahl HL. Signal transduction from the endoplasmic reticulum to the cell nucleus. Physiol Rev 1999;79(3):683–701.

13. Abeijon C, Hirschberg CB. Topography of glycosylation reactions in the endoplasmic reticulum. Trends Biochem Sci 1992;17(1):32–6.

14. High S, Greenfield JJ, Meacock SL, Oliver JD. Membrane-protein biosynthesis at the endoplasmic reticulum. Biochem Soc Trans 1999;27(6):883–8.

15. Batt AM, Magdalou J, Vincent-Viry M, et al. Drug metabolizing enzymes related to laboratory medicine: cytochromes P-450 and UDP-glucuronosyltransferases. Clin Chim Acta 1994;226(2):171–90.

16. Griffing LR. Comparisons of Golgi structure and dynamics in plant and animal cells. J Electron Microsc Tech 1991;17(2):179–99.

17. Rothman JE, Orci L. Movement of proteins through the Golgi stack: a molecular dissection of vesicular transport. Faseb J 1990;4(5):1460–8.

18. Hirschberg CB, Snider MD. Topography of glycosylation in the rough endoplasmic reticulum and Golgi apparatus. Annu Rev Biochem 1987;56:63–87.

19. Munro S, Pelham HR. A C-terminal signal prevents secretion of luminal ER proteins. Cell 1987;48(5):899–907.

20. Pelham HR. The retention signal for soluble proteins of the endoplasmic reticulum. Trends Biochem Sci 1990;15(12):483–6.

21. Teasdale RD, Jackson MR. Signal-mediated sorting of membrane proteins between the endoplasmic reticulum and the Golgi apparatus. Annu Rev Cell Dev Biol 1996;12:27–54.

22. Burgess TL, Kelly RB. Constitutive and regulated secretion of proteins. Annu Rev Cell Biol 1987;3:243–93.

23. Sherratt HS. Mitochondria: structure and function. Rev Neurol 1991;147(6-7):417–30.

24. Cooper GM. Bioenergetics and metabolism. In: Cooper GM, ed. The Cell: A Molecular Approach. Sunderland: Sinauer Associates, Inc., 1997:389–421.

25. Wolfe SL. Cellular Oxidations and the Mitochondrion: Introduction to Cell and Molecular Biology. Belmont: Wadsworth Publishing Company, 1997:207–45.

26. Cooper GM. Replication, maintenance, and rearrangements of genomic DNA. In: Cooper GM, ed. The Cell: A Molecular Approach. Sunderland: Sinauer Associates, Inc., 1997:175–224.

27. Stillman B. Cell cycle control of DNA replication. Science 1996;274(5293):1659–64.

28. Dutta A, Bell SP. Initiation of DNA replication in eukaryotic cells. Annu Rev Cell Dev Biol 1997;13:293–332.

29. Ogawa T, Okazaki T. Discontinuous DNA replication. Annu Rev Biochem 1980;49:421–57.

30. Wang JC. DNA topoisomerases. Annu Rev Biochem 1996;65:635–92.

31. Pulleyblank DE. Of topo and Maxwell's dream. Science 1997;277(5326):648–9.

32. Bambara RA, Murante RS, Henricksen LA. Enzymes and reactions at the eukaryotic DNA replication fork. J Biol Chem 1997;272(8):4647–50.

33. Wold MS. Replication protein A: a heterotrimeric, single-stranded DNA-binding protein required for eukaryotic DNA metabolism. Annu Rev Biochem 1997;66:61–92.

34. Waga S, Stillman B. The DNA replication fork in eukaryotic cells. Annu Rev Biochem 1998;67:721–51.

35. Hubscher U, Maga G, Spadari S. Eukaryotic DNA polymerases. Annu Rev Biochem 2002;71:133–63.

36. Takemura M. Evolution and degeneration of eukaryotic DNA replication system. Biosystems 2002;65(2-3):139–45.

37. Livneh Z. DNA damage control by novel DNA polymerases: translesion replication and mutagenesis. J Biol Chem 2001;276(28):25639–42.

38. Washington MT, Johnson RE, Prakash L, Prakash S. Accuracy of lesion bypass by yeast and human DNA polymerase eta. Proc Natl Acad Sci U S A 2001;98(15):8355–60.

39. Yavuz S, Yavuz AS, Kraemer KH, Lipsky PE. The Role of Polymerase eta in Somatic Hypermutation Determined by Analysis of Mutations in a Patient with Xeroderma Pigmentosum Variant. J Immunol 2002;169(7):3825–30.

40. Tanaka K, Wood RD. Xeroderma pigmentosum and nucleotide excision repair of DNA. Trends Biochem Sci 1994;19(2):83–6.

41. Twyman RM, Wisden W. Replication: Advanced Molecular Biology: A Concise Reference. New York: Bios Scientific Publishers Limited, 1998:389–409.

42. Stillman B. Smart machines at the DNA replication fork. Cell 1994;78(5):725–8.

43. Baker TA, Bell SP: Polymerases and the replisome: machines within machines. Cell 1998;92(3):295–305.

44. Yuzhakov A, Turner J, O'Donnell M. Replisome assembly reveals the basis for asymmetric function in leading and lagging strand replication. Cell 1996;86(6):877–86.

45. Tjian R. Molecular machines that control genes. Sci Am 1995;272(2):54–61.

46. Conaway JW, Shilatifard A, Dvir A, Conaway RC. Control of elongation by RNA polymerase II. Trends Biochem Sci 2000;25(8):375–80.

47. Myer VE, Young RA. RNA polymerase II holoenzymes and subcomplexes. J Biol Chem 1998;273(43):27757–60.

48. Asturias FJ, Kornberg RD. Protein crystallization on lipid layers and structure determination of the RNA polymerase II transcription initiation complex. J Biol Chem 1999;274(11):6813–6.

49. Young RA. RNA polymerase II. Annu Rev Biochem 1991;60:689–715.

50. Wu J, Parkhurst KM, Powell RM, Brenowitz M, Parkhurst LJ. DNA bends in TATA-binding protein-TATA complexes in solution are DNA sequence-dependent. J Biol Chem 2001;276(18):14614–22.

51. Nikolov DB, Chen H, Halay ED, Hoffman A, Roeder RG, Burley SK. Crystal structure of a human TATA box-binding protein/TATA element complex. Proc Natl Acad Sci U S A 1996;93(10):4862–7.

52. Roeder RG. The role of general initiation factors in transcription by RNA polymerase II. Trends Biochem Sci 1996;21(9):327–35.

53. Werner T. Models for prediction and recognition of eukaryotic promoters. Mamm Genome 1999;10(2):168–75.

54. Dvir A, Conaway JW, Conaway RC. Mechanism of transcription initiation and promoter escape by RNA polymerase II. Curr Opin Genet Dev 2001;11(2):209–14.

55. Buratowski S. The basics of basal transcription by RNA polymerase II. Cell 1994;77(1):1–3.

56. Bentley D. The mRNA assembly line: transcription and processing machines in the same factory. Curr Opin Cell Biol 2002;14(3):336–42.

57. Lodish H, Berk A, Zipursky SL, Matsudaria P, Baltimore D, Darnell J. RNA Processing, Nuclear Transport, and Post-transcription Control: Molecular Cell Biology. New York: W.H. Freeman and Company, 2000:404–94.

58. Cooper GM. RNA synthesis and processing. In: Cooper GM, ed. The Cell: A Molecular Approach. Sunderland: Sinauer Associates, Inc., 1997:255–72.

59. Zawel L, Reinberg D. Common themes in assembly and function of eukaryotic transcription complexes. Annu Rev Biochem 1995;64:533–61.

60. Korzheva N, Mustaev A. Transcription elongation complex: structure and function. Curr Opin Microbiol 2001;4(2):119–25.

61. Burley SK, Roeder RG. Biochemistry and structural biology of transcription factor IID (TFIID). Annu Rev Biochem 1996;65:769–99.

62. McKeown M. Alternative mRNA splicing. Annu Rev Cell Biol 1992;8:133–55.

63. Herbert A, Rich A. RNA processing and the evolution of eukaryotes. Nat Genet 1999;21(3):265–9.

64. Rosenthal N. Regulation of gene expression. N Engl J Med 1994;331(14):931–3.

65. Sharp PA. Split genes and RNA splicing. Cell 1994;77(6):805–15.

66. Divoky V, Bisse E, Wilson JB, et al. Heterozygosity for the IVS-I-5 (G→C) mutation with a G→A change at codon 18 (Val→Met; Hb Baden) in cis and a T→G mutation at codon 126 (Val→Gly; Hb Dhonburi) in trans resulting in a thalassemia intermedia. Biochim Biophys Acta 1992;1180(2):173–9.

67. Latchman DS. Transcription-factor mutations and disease. N Engl J Med 1996;334(1):28–33.

68. Kornberg RD. Eukaryotic transcriptional control. Trends Cell Biol 1999;9(12):M46–9.

69. Hanna-Rose W, Hansen U. Active repression mechanisms of eukaryotic transcription repressors. Trends Genet 1996;12(6):229–34.

70. Cowell IG. Repression versus activation in the control of gene transcription. Trends Biochem Sci 1994;19(1):38–42.

71. Harrison SC. A structural taxonomy of DNA-binding domains. Nature 1991;353(6346):715–9.

72. Wolfe SA, Nekludova L, Pabo CO. DNA recognition by Cys2His2 zinc finger proteins. Annu Rev Biophys Biomol Struct 2000;29:183–212.

73. Harrison SC, Aggarwal AK. DNA recognition by proteins with the helix-turn-helix motif. Annu Rev Biochem 1990;59:933–69.

74. McKnight SL. Molecular zippers in gene regulation. Sci Am 1991;264(4):54–64.

75. Burgess-Beusse B, Farrell C, Gaszner M, et al. The insulation of genes from external enhancers and silencing chromatin. Proc Natl Acad Sci U S A 2002;1:1.

76. Khorasanizadeh S, Rastinejad F. Nuclear-receptor interactions on DNA-response elements. Trends Biochem Sci 2001;26(6):384–90.

77. Torchia J, Glass C, Rosenfeld MG. Co-activators and co-repressors in the integration of transcriptional responses. Curr Opin Cell Biol 1998;10(3):373–83.

78. Funder JW. Glucocorticoid and mineralocorticoid receptors: biology and clinical relevance. Annu Rev Med 1997;48:231–40.

79. Tenbaum S, Baniahmad A. Nuclear receptors: structure, function and involvement in disease. Int J Biochem Cell Biol 1997;29(12):1325–41.

80. Issa LL, Leong GM, Eisman JA. Molecular mechanism of vitamin D receptor action. Inflamm Res 1998;47(12):451–75.

81. Singal R, Ginder GD. DNA methylation. Blood 1999;93(12):4059–70.

82. Kouzarides T. Acetylation: a regulatory modification to rival phosphorylation? Embo J 2000;19(6):1176–9.

83. Cress WD, Seto E. Histone deacetylases, transcriptional control, and cancer. J Cell Physiol 2000;184(1):1–16.

84. Bjorklund S, Almouzni G, Davidson I, Nightingale KP, Weiss K. Global transcription regulators of eukaryotes. Cell 1999;96(6):759–67.

85. Sterner DE, Berger SL. Acetylation of histones and transcription-related factors. Microbiol Mol Biol Rev 2000;64(2):435–59.

86. Marks PA, Richon VM, Breslow R, Rifkind RA. Histone deacetylase inhibitors as new cancer drugs. Curr Opin Oncol 2001;13(6):477–83.

87. Murata T, Kurokawa R, Krones A, et al. Defect of histone acetyltransferase activity of the nuclear transcriptional coactivator CBP in Rubinstein-Taybi syndrome. Hum Mol Genet 2001;10(10):1071–6.

88. De Silva B. What syndrome is this? Rubenstein-Taybi syndrome. Pediatr Dermatol 2002;19(2):177–9.

89. Cooper GM. Protein synthesis, processing, and regulation. In: Cooper GM, ed. The Cell: A Molecular Approach. Sunderland: Sinauer Associates, Inc., 1997:273–311.

90. Bolsover SR, Hyams JS, Jones S, Shephard EA, White HA. Translation and Protein Targeting: From Genes to Cells. New York: John Wiley and Sons, Inc., 1997:189–208.

91. Arnez JG, Moras D. Structural and functional considerations of the aminoacylation reaction. Trends Biochem Sci 1997;22(6):211–6.

92. Sachs AB, Sarnow P, Hentze MW. Starting at the beginning, middle, and end: translation initiation in eukaryotes. Cell 1997;89(6):831–8.

93. Kozak M. Recognition of AUG and alternative initiator codons is augmented by G in position +4 but is not generally affected by the nucleotides in positions +5 and +6. Embo J 1997;16(9):2482–92.

94. Thach RE. Cap recap: the involvement of eIF-4F in regulating gene expression. Cell 1992;68(2):177–80.

95. Chaudhuri J, Si K, Maitra U. Function of eukaryotic translation initiation factor 1A (eIF1A) (formerly called eIF-4C) in initiation of protein synthesis. J Biol Chem 1997;272(12):7883–91.

96. Lee JH, Choi SK, Roll-Mecak A, Burley SK, Dever TE. Universal conservation in translation initiation revealed by human and archaeal homologs of bacterial translation initiation factor IF2. Proc Natl Acad Sci U S A 1999;96(8):4342–7.

97. Pestova TV, Lomakin IB, Lee JH, Choi SK, Dever TE, Hellen CU. The joining of ribosomal subunits in eukaryotes requires eIF5B. Nature 2000;403(6767):332–5.

98. Pestova TV, Borukhov SI, Hellen CU. Eukaryotic ribosomes require initiation factors 1 and 1A to locate initiation codons. Nature 1998;394(6696):854–9.

99. Rodnina MV, Wintermeyer W. Ribosome fidelity: tRNA discrimination, proofreading and induced fit. Trends Biochem Sci 2001;26(2):124–30.

100. Nakamura Y, Ito K, Isaksson LA. Emerging understanding of translation termination. Cell 1996;87(2):147–50.

101. Heurgue-Hamard V, Karimi R, Mora L, et al. Ribosome release factor RF4 and termination factor RF3 are involved in dissociation of peptidyl-tRNA from the ribosome. Embo J 1998;17(3):808–16.

102. Goessling LS, Daniels-McQueen S, Bhattacharyya-Pakrasi M, Lin JJ, Thach RE. Enhanced degradation of the ferritin repressor protein during induction of ferritin messenger RNA translation. Science 1992;256(5057):670–3.

103. Kozak M. Regulation of translation in eukaryotic systems. Annu Rev Cell Biol 1992;8:197–225.

104. Cocito C, Di Giambattista M, Nyssen E, Vannuffel P. Inhibition of protein synthesis by streptogramins and related antibiotics. J Antimicrob Chemother 1997;39 Suppl A:7–13.

105. Jacobson A, Peltz SW. Interrelationships of the pathways of mRNA decay and translation in eukaryotic cells. Annu Rev Biochem 1996;65:693–739.

106. Decker CJ, Parker R. Mechanisms of mRNA degradation in eukaryotes. Trends Biochem Sci 1994;19(8):336–40.

107. Hartl FU. Molecular chaperones in cellular protein folding. Nature 1996;381(6583):571–9.

108. Craig EA. Chaperones: helpers along the pathways to protein folding. Science 1993;260(5116):1902–3.

109. Agard DA. To fold or not to fold. Science 1993;260(5116):1903–4.

110. Taubes G. Misfolding the way to disease. Science 1996;271(5255):1493–5.

111. Jentsch S. When proteins receive deadly messages at birth. Science 1996;271(5251):955–6.

112. Gereben B, Goncalves C, Harney JW, Larsen PR, Bianco AC. Selective proteolysis of human type 2 deiodinase: a novel ubiquitin- proteasomal mediated mechanism for regulation of hormone activation. Mol Endocrinol 2000;14(11):1697–708.

113. Jentsch S, Schlenker S. Selective protein degradation: a journey's end within the proteasome. Cell 1995;82(6):881–4.

114. Miranda FF, Teigen K, Thorolfsson M, et al. Phosphorylation and mutations of Ser16 in human phenylalanine hydroxylase. Kinetic and structural effects. J Biol Chem 2002;15:15.

115. Bjorklof K, Lundstrom K, Abuin L, Greasley PJ, Cotecchia S. Co- and posttranslational modification of the alpha(1B)-adrenergic receptor: effects on receptor expression and function. Biochemistry 2002;41(13):4281–91.

116. Zitzmann N, Mehta AS, Carrouee S, et al. Imino sugars inhibit the formation and secretion of bovine viral diarrhea virus, a pestivirus model of hepatitis C virus: implications for the development of broad spectrum anti-hepatitis virus agents. Proc Natl Acad Sci U S A 1999;96(21):11878–82.

117. Spiro RG. Protein glycosylation: nature, distribution, enzymatic formation, and disease implications of glycopeptide bonds. Glycobiology 2002;12(4):43R–56R.

118. Huby RD, Dearman RJ, Kimber I. Why are some proteins allergens? Toxicol Sci 2000;55(2):235–46.

119. Liu F, Zaidi T, Iqbal K, Grundke-Iqbal I, Merkle RK, Gong CX. Role of glycosylation in hyperphosphorylation of tau in Alzheimer's disease. FEBS Lett 2002;512(1-3):101–6.

120. Mehta A, Carrouee S, Conyers B, et al. Inhibition of hepatitis B virus DNA replication by imino sugars without the inhibition of the DNA polymerase: therapeutic implications. Hepatology 2001;33(6):1488–95.

121. Beato M, Klug J. Steroid hormone receptors: an update. Hum Reprod Update 2000;6(3):225–36.

122. Ignarro LJ. Endothelium-derived nitric oxide: pharmacology and relationship to the actions of organic nitrate esters. Pharm Res 1989;6(8):651–9.

123. Goldstein SA. Ion channels: structural basis for function and disease. Semin Perinatol 1996;20(6):520–30.

124. Sherwood L. Neuronal physiology. In: Sherwood L. ed. Human Physiology. St. Paul: West Publishing Company, 1993:79–103.

125. Bockaert J, Pin JP. Molecular tinkering of G protein-coupled receptors: an evolutionary success. Embo J 1999;18(7):1723–9.

126. Northup JK, Smigel MD, Sternweis PC, Gilman AG. The subunits of the stimulatory regulatory component of adenylate cyclase. Resolution of the activated 45,000-dalton (alpha) subunit. J Biol Chem 1983;258(18):11369–76.

127. Shorr RG, Lefkowitz RJ, Caron MG. Purification of the beta-adrenergic receptor. Identification of the hormone binding subunit. J Biol Chem 1981;256(11):5820–6.

128. Hur EM, Kim KT. G protein-coupled receptor signalling and cross-talk: achieving rapidity and specificity. Cell Signal 2002;14(5).397–405.

129. Attwood TK, Findlay JB. Fingerprinting G protein-coupled receptors. Protein Eng 1994;7(2):195–203.

130. Schertler GF, Villa C, Henderson R. Projection structure of rhodopsin. Nature 1993;362(6422):770–2.

131. Neer EJ. Heterotrimeric G proteins: organizers of transmembrane signals. Cell 1995;80(2):249–57.

132. Coleman DE, Sprang SR. How G proteins work: a continuing story. Trends Biochem Sci 1996;21(2):41–4.

133. Neves SR, Ram PT, Iyengar R. G protein pathways. Science 2002;296(5573):1636–9.

134. Hamm HE. The many faces of G protein signaling. J Biol Chem 1998;273(2):669–72.

135. Vaughan M. Signaling by heterotrimeric G proteins minireview series. J Biol Chem 1998;273(2):667–8.

136. Gilman AG. G proteins: transducers of receptor-generated signals. Annu Rev Biochem 1987;56:615–49.

137. Clapham DE, Neer EJ. New roles for G-protein beta gamma-dimers in transmembrane signalling. Nature 1993;365(6445):403–6.

138. Neer EJ. G proteins: critical control points for transmembrane signals. Protein Sci 1994;3(1):3–14.

139. Wong SK, Ross EM. Chimeric muscarinic cholinergic:beta-adrenergic receptors that are functionally promiscuous among G proteins. J Biol Chem 1994;269(29):18968–76.

140. Carty DJ, Padrell E, Codina J, Birnbaumer L, Hildebrandt JD, Iyengar R. Distinct guanine nucleotide binding and release properties of the three Gi proteins. J Biol Chem 1990;265(11):6268–73.

141. Arshavsky V, Bownds MD. Regulation of deactivation of photoreceptor G protein by its target enzyme and cGMP. Nature 1992;357(6377):416–7.

142. Brady AE, Limbird LE. G protein-coupled receptor interacting proteins: emerging roles in localization and signal transduction. Cell Signal 2002;14(4):297–309.

143. Roush W. Regulating G protein signaling. Science 1996;271(5252):1056–8.

144. Berman DM, Wilkie TM, Gilman AG. GAIP and RGS4 are GTPase-activating proteins for the Gi subfamily of G protein alpha subunits. Cell 1996;86(3):445–52.

145. Zhong H, Neubig RR. Regulator of G protein signaling proteins: novel multifunctional drug targets. J Pharmacol Exp Ther 2001;297(3):837–45.

146. Farfel Z, Bourne HR, Iiri T. The expanding spectrum of G protein diseases. N Engl J Med 1999;340(13):1012–20.

147. Bockaert J, Claeysen S, Becamel C, Pinloche S, Dumuis A. G protein-coupled receptors: dominant players in cell-cell communication. Int Rev Cytol 2002;212:63–132.

148. Bergsma DJ, Ellis C, Kumar C, et al. Cloning and characterization of a human angiotensin II type 1 receptor. Biochem Biophys Res Commun 1992;183(3):989–95.

149. O'Dowd BF, Heiber M, Chan A, et al. A human gene that shows identity with the gene encoding the angiotensin receptor is located on chromosome 11. Gene 1993;136(1-2):355–60.

150. Stadel JM, Wilson S, Bergsma DJ. Orphan G protein-coupled receptors: a neglected opportunity for pioneer drug discovery. Trends Pharmacol Sci 1997;18(11):430–7.

151. Schlessinger J. Cell signaling by receptor tyrosine kinases. Cell 2000;103(2):211–25.

152. Hubbard SR, Till JH. Protein tyrosine kinase structure and function. Annu Rev Biochem 2000;69:373–98.

153. Ullrich A, Schlessinger J. Signal transduction by receptors with tyrosine kinase activity. Cell 1990;61(2):203–12.

154. Heldin CH. Dimerization of cell surface receptors in signal transduction. Cell 1995;80(2):213–23.

155. Schlessinger J. SH2/SH3 signaling proteins. Curr Opin Genet Dev 1994;4(1):25–30.

156. Pawson T. Protein modules and signalling networks. Nature 1995;373(6515):573–80.

157. Lowes VL, Ip NY, Wong YH. Integration of signals from receptor tyrosine kinases and G protein-coupled receptors. Neurosignals 2002;11(1):5–19.

158. Robertson SC, Tynan J, Donoghue DJ. RTK mutations and human syndromes: when good receptors turn bad. Trends Genet 2000;16(8):368.

159. Zwick E, Bange J, Ullrich A. Receptor tyrosine kinase signalling as a target for cancer intervention strategies. Endocr Relat Cancer 2001;8(3):161–73.

160. Hao D, Rowinsky EK. Inhibiting signal transduction: recent advances in the development of receptor tyrosine kinase and Ras inhibitors. Cancer Invest 2002;20(3):387–404.

161. Slamon DJ, Godolphin W, Jones LA, et al. Studies of the HER-2/neu proto-oncogene in human breast and ovarian cancer. Science 1989;244(4905):707–12.

162. Gelb MH. Protein prenylation, et cetera: signal transduction in two dimensions. Science 1997;275(5307):1750–1.

163. O'Shea JJ, Gadina M, Schreiber RD. Cytokine signaling in 2002: new surprises in the Jak/Stat pathway. Cell 2002;109 Suppl:S121–31.

164. Kisseleva T, Bhattacharya S, Braunstein J, Schindler CW. Signaling through the JAK/STAT pathway, recent advances and future challenges. Gene 2002;285(1-2):1–24.

165. Leonard WJ, O'Shea JJ. Jaks and STATs: biological implications. Annu Rev Immunol 1998;16:293–322.

166. Leonard WJ, Lin JX. Cytokine receptor signaling pathways. J Allergy Clin Immunol 2000;105(5):877–88.

167. Darnell JE, Jr., Kerr IM, Stark GR. Jak STAT pathways and transcriptional activation in response to IFNs and other extracellular signaling proteins. Science 1994;264(5164):1415–21.

168. Aaronson DS, Horvath CM. A road map for those who know JAK-STAT. Science 2002;296(5573):1653–5.

169. Mascareno E, El-Shafei M, Maulik N, et al. JAK/STAT signaling is associated with cardiac dysfunction during ischemia and reperfusion. Circulation 2001;104(3):325–9.

170. Xuan YT, Guo Y, Han H, Zhu Y, Bolli R. An essential role of the JAK-STAT pathway in ischemic preconditioning. Proc Natl Acad Sci U S A 2001;98(16):9050–5.

Self-Assessment Questions

1. It was discovered that a certain mitochondrial enzyme found in high concentrations in normal myocardium is depleted in patients with heart failure. You hypothesize that supplementation with this enzyme may improve clinical outcomes in patients hospitalized for worsening heart failure. After conducting a small study, you find that patients who received enzyme supplementation were 2 times less likely to be rehospitalized in the proceeding 12 months than those who did not receive supplementation. Which one of the following is the most plausible molecular mechanism to explain the apparent benefit?

    A. Increased efficiency of protein sorting and vesicular transport.
    B. Modulation of electron and proton transfer during oxidative phosphorylation.
    C. Phosphodiesterase III inhibition and increased intracellular calcium concentrations.
    D. Enhanced binding of transcription factors to the promoter region of the β_1-adrenergic receptor.

2. The activity of which one of the following organelles is specifically mediated through an acidic pH?

    A. Endoplasmic reticulum.
    B. Golgi apparatus.
    C. Lysosomes.
    D. Mitochondria.

3. You have cloned the deoxyribonucleic acid (DNA) for the gene that encodes Antiselin, a protein that is a potent suppressor of prostate tissue growth. Before developing this compound for the treatment of benign prostatic hypertrophy, you decide you need a better understanding of Antiselin's transcriptional regulation. Which one of the following is the best first step in the process of elucidating Antiselin transcriptional regulation?

    A. Identify common genetic sequence variations in 50 individuals.
    B. Isolate the promoter sequence of the Antiselin gene.
    C. Characterize the transcription factor binding domains.
    D. Identify what *cis* elements are required for Antiselin transcription.

4. Which one of the following statements is true for promoters in eukaryotic messenger RNA (mRNA) synthesis?

    A. Promoters are the upstream regions of DNA to which DNA polymerase binds to initiate transcription.

B. Promoters are found approximately 10 to 100 bps upstream from the first intron of the gene.
C. Promoters are necessary for second messenger-mediated cell signaling.
D. Promoters usually contain a TATA box that is important in recognition by transcription proteins.

5. Which one of the following schematics best represents the sequence of events in the processing of eukaryotic mRNAs?

A. DNA→pre-mRNA→3' polyadenylation→mRNA splicing→ 5' capping→export to cytoplasm.
B. pre-mRNA→mRNA splicing→5' capping→3' polyadenylation→ DNA→export to cytoplasm.
C. DNA→pre-mRNA→5' capping→3' polyadenylation→mRNA splicing→export to cytoplasm.
D. DNA→pre-mRNA→mRNA splicing→5' capping→3' poly-adenylation→export to cytoplasm.

6. In translation of mRNA, which one of the following statements best describes the function of transfer RNA (tRNA)?

A. Transports specific amino acids to ribosomes where they are aligned along the mRNA template.
B. Catalyzes the synthesis of amino acids used in protein synthesis.
C. Transports nucleotides to ribosomes for protein synthesis.
D. Serves as a template for amino acid alignment and protein synthesis.

7. You have decided to investigate whether genetic variations in the estrogen receptor gene modify the effects of estrogen replacement therapy on low-density lipoprotein cholesterol in post-menopausal women. Which one of the following gene mutations is least likely to influence estrogen replacement therapy effects on low-density lipoprotein?

A. A mutation in an intron.
B. A mutation in an exon.
C. A mutation in the promoter region.
D. A mutation in a splice site.

8. Angiotensin-converting enzyme inhibitors exert their antihypertensive effects by blocking the activity of angiotensin-converting enzyme. You identify an enhancer sequence upstream from the promoter region of the angiotensin-converting enzyme gene found in 10 percent of patients with hypertension. Which one of the following would you expect the comparative blood pressure lowering with angiotensin-converting

enzyme inhibitors to be in patients with the mutation versus patients without the mutation?

A. Smaller relative blood pressure reduction.
B. Larger relative blood pressure reduction.
C. No difference in blood pressure reduction between groups.
D. The difference is irrelevant since the mutation only occurs in 10 percent of patients.

Questions 9 and 10 pertain to the following case.
You are conducting mutagenesis studies on a GPCR found on the surface of cardiac myocytes with the purpose of better characterizing the in vitro activity of the receptor. You decide to introduce two mutations in the receptor. The first is a mutation in the extracellular amino terminus of the receptor. The second is in the cytoplasmic tail in a highly conserved region proximal to the seventh transmembrane spanning domain.

9. Which one of the following is the most likely result of introducing the mutation in the extracellular tail of the receptor?

    A. Altered receptor trafficking as either upregulation or downregulation.
    B. Altered G protein-coupling.
    C. Increased sensitivity to agonist-induced apoptosis.
    D. The mutation is not likely to have any effects on cell signaling.

10. Which one of the following is the most likely result of introducing the mutation in the intracellular tail of the receptor?

    A. Altered receptor trafficking as either upregulation or downregulation.
    B. Altered G protein-coupling.
    C. Increased sensitivity to agonist-induced apoptosis.
    D. The mutation is not likely to have any effects on cell signaling.

Analysis of the Human Genome and Proteome

H. Trent Spencer, Ph.D.

Key Words

Genome, proteome, pharmacogenomics, polymerase chain reaction, polymorphisms, deoxyribonucleic acid sequence analysis, expressed sequence tags, microarray analysis, and gene therapy.

Abstract

Technical advancements in analytical or procedural methodologies have driven the development of novel approaches for studying biological processes and the subsequent translation of biological information to clinical practice. This is especially true for the analysis of nucleic acid sequences that comprise the human genome and the analysis of interactions among the proteins that compose the human proteome. Pharmacogenomic studies focus on describing the interaction of specific nucleic acid sequences and drug action. Only by identifying differences at the molecular level among individuals can clinicians understand how specific drugs function in a heterogeneous population. The technologies that have been driving recent genome- and proteome-based discoveries are discussed in this chapter. Applications based on the sequencing of individual genes, simultaneous analysis of thousands of expressed genes, analysis of protein-protein interactions, and strategies used to manipulate the human genome using gene therapy approaches are all discussed to provide a comprehensive understanding of the paradigm shifts now taking place in molecular medicine.

Outline

Learning Objectives

1. Understand the technology and methodology driving nucleic acid- and protein-based discoveries and understand the potential impact of these discoveries on drug therapy.
2. Understand the technologies driving advances in the field of gene therapy.
3. Appropriately apply new deoxyribonucleic acid-based methodology to the analysis of specific disease states.
4. Understand the realized versus potential benefits of genome and proteome analysis.

Abbreviations in this Chapter

2-D	Two dimensional
AAV	Adeno-associated virus
BRCA1	Breast cancer susceptibility gene
cDNA	Complementary deoxyribonucleic acid
Cy3	Cyanine 3
Cy5	Cyanine 5
dATP	Deoxyadenosine triphosphate
dCTP	Deoxycytidine triphosphate
ddATP	Dideoxyadenosine triphosphate

ddNTP	2',3'-Dideoxynucleotide triphosphate
dGTP	Deoxyguanine triphosphate
DNA	Deoxyribonucleic acid
dNTP	Deoxynucleotide triphosphate
dTTP	Deoxythymidine triphosphate
DOPE	Dioleoyl L-α-phosphatidylethanolamine
EDTA	Ethylenediamine tetraacetic acid
EST	Expressed sequence tag
LTR	Long-terminal-repeat
MALDI-TOF	Matrix-assisted laser desorption coupled MS with ionization time-of-flight mass spectrometry
mRNA	Messenger ribonucleic acid
MSI	Microsatellite instability
MSI-H	High-frequency microsatellite instability
MSI-L	Low-frequency microsatellite instability
MSS	Microsatellite stable
NHGRI	National Human Genome Research Institute
NIEHS	National Institute of Environmental Health Sciences
NIGMS	National Institute of General Medical Sciences
PCR	Polymerase chain reaction
RFLP	Restriction fragment length polymorphism
RNA	Ribonucleic acid
SDS-PAGE	Sodium dodecyl sulfate-polyacrylamide gel electrophoresis
SNP	Single nucleotide polymorphism
SSCP	Single-strand conformational polymorphism
TDT	Terminal deoxynucleotidyl transferase
UV	Ultraviolet

Historical Perspectives

Past generations are remembered for the remarkable accomplishments of their time. One of the legacies of the present generation likely will be the sequencing of the entire human genome, and subsequently the development of molecular medicine. Sequencing the human genome was certainly a colossal endeavor, but the less publicized accomplishments of creating methods to sequence millions of base pairs are equally impressive. Identifying mutations and genetic markers in known regions of the human genome is no longer an arduous task. It is now possible to screen large regions of the genome using a variety of techniques, such as analysis of single nucleotide polymorphisms (SNPs), and methods for screening the entire genome are now being developed. This chapter and the Bioinformatics chapter describe how human genes are sequenced, how polymorphisms within the population are identified, and how the vast amount of information being generated from the human genome project is being analyzed.

During the past four decades, biological sciences have witnessed a revolution. It is becoming increasingly clear that the achievements of molecular biology, cell biology, and analytical chemistry have provided great potential for advancing medical research and the practice of medicine. Since the initial confirmation that genetic alterations can cause defined disease states, the pervasive outlook has been that the future for genetic medicine is promising. However, applying the potential information stored in the genetic code has been problematic. Obtaining the valuable information initially required thousands of work-hours to sequence a single gene, whereas today laboratories dedicated to genome analysis can sequence thousands of base pairs daily, and high school students working on summer research projects can be required to sequence and clone specific deoxyribonucleic acid (DNA) sequences. With respect to the field of clinical pharmacology, sufficient examples exist to believe that the impact of genetic analysis has already been significant and that genetic analysis will continue to play a major role in the future of diagnostic testing. But it has yet to be realized if these advancements will truly define a fundamental change in the potential for human health.

Historically, "first-generation" methods for detecting disease were available several hundred years ago and relied on observation or growth of specific microorganisms. Advancements in novel testing methodologies were driven by improvements in microscopy. "Second-generation" methods were substantially more rapid than methods that depended on particular growth characteristics, and relied on measuring specific cellular components unique to a diseased state. A major force driving the development of these methods was the production of monoclonal antibodies. Current technologies, or "third-generation" methodologies, are nucleic acid-based and detect genetic sequences specific to the disease state. These technologies often make use of hybridization protocols. Hybridization (or annealing) is the process of complementary base pairing between two single-stranded molecules of DNA or of DNA and ribonucleic acid (RNA). Nucleic acid-based tests are divided into two major categories: one in which the target sequence is directly analyzed, and a second in which the target sequence is amplified. The predominant amplification method, called the polymerase chain reaction (PCR) logarithmically amplifies specific target sequences. Because of the ease of amplifying specific nucleic acid sequences, methods based on the PCR have become commonplace.

Technologies Driving DNA-based Discoveries

Analysis of the Human Genome by PCR Amplification

Many PCR techniques have been developed and validated for clinical applications, and PCR has become a fundamental tool for genetic research and genome analysis. Because of its simplicity, sensitivity, and reliability, PCR amplification of DNA is now the foundation of many techniques designed to detect differences in DNA sequences among individuals. In 1985, Dr. Kary Mullins and colleagues invented PCR while working at the Cetus Corporation and received the Nobel Prize for this achievement about 10 years later. It cannot be overstated how important the PCR is to the analysis of human genes, and how a major foundation of pharmacogenomics relies on PCR methodology.

To amplify a known sequence of DNA using the PCR, the basic protocol requires two primers (Figure 1). One primer is designed to specifically anneal upstream of the target sequence on the 3'→5' strand of DNA, and the second is designed to anneal to the 5'→3' strand downstream of the target

Polymerase Chain Reaction

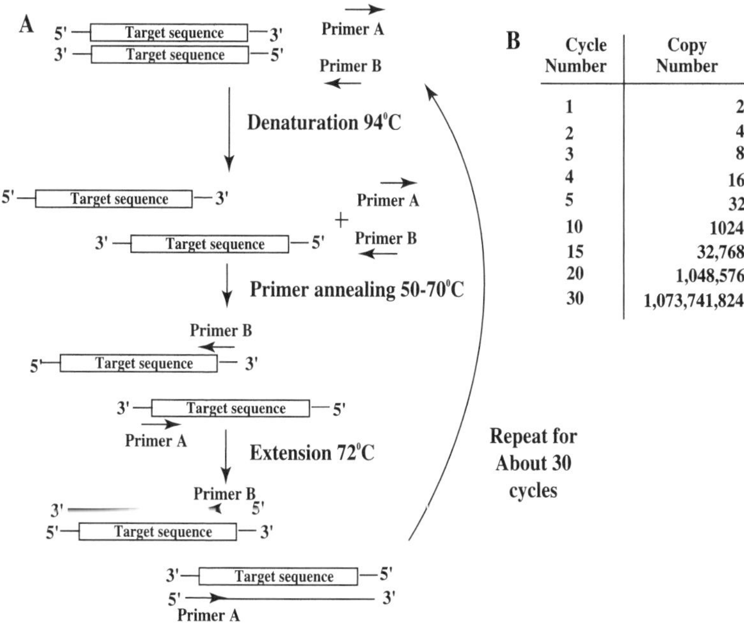

Figure 1. A) Schematic of the polymerase chain reaction. B) Theoretical amplification of copy number after each cycle of the polymerase chain reaction.

sequence, which is used to synthesize the complementary strand. Also included in the reaction are a thermostable DNA polymerase and the four nucleotides, adenine (A), guanine (G), thymidine (T), and cytosine (C). As shown in Figure 1, isolated DNA and the primers are mixed and the hydrogen bonds holding the two strands of DNA together are broken by heating the sample to around 95°C using a thermal cycler. The reaction is then rapidly cooled to the optimum temperature for hybridizing (or annealing) the primers to their target sequences on the DNA (typically 50–65°C, but annealing temperatures depend on each specific primer pair). The annealing temperature is critical for specific annealing of the primers to unique sites of the template DNA, thus ensuring the fidelity of the PCR amplification. Once the primers are annealed, the reaction is heated to 72°C, which is the optimum temperature for DNA polymerase. Deoxyribonucleic acid polymerase is the enzyme that adds incoming deoxyribonucleoside triphosphates (dNTPs) to the annealed primers. Because DNA polymerase requires double-stranded DNA to initiate DNA synthesis, the double-stranded region generated by primer annealing allows the polymerase to synthesize DNA beginning at a single site in the genome. After primer extension, the first denaturation → annealing → synthesis cycle is completed. Deoxyribonucleic acid is amplified by repeating this cycle about 30 times. A typical cycle includes denaturation at 94°C for 30 seconds, annealing at 60°C for 30 seconds, then synthesis at 72°C for 1 minute. After the second cycle, synthesized DNA becomes the template for the next round of amplification. Because amplification of DNA is exponential (Figure 1B), large amounts of a specific DNA sequence can be generated even though relatively few copies of the target sequence are initially available.

As can be imagined, the efficiency of a DNA amplification depends on how well the primers are designed, selection of the annealing temperature, and the accuracy of the DNA polymerase. Guidelines for choosing primers typically include the following:

i) Primers are typically 21–24 nucleotides long.
ii) Primers should be designed with an overall G + C content of 40–60 percent.
iii) A primer pair should have relatively equal G + C content.
iv) Repeats of a single base within a primer or complementary sequence between primers should be avoided.
v) At least one and preferably both primers should anneal to unique sequences in the template DNA.

Although following these general guidelines usually results in successful amplification reactions, programs are available that aid in selecting primer pairs. For example, the Whitehead Institute for Biomedical Research offers a freely shared program at *http://wwwgenome.wi.mit.edu/ftp/distribution/software/primer.0.5/.*

Accuracy of the DNA polymerase is extremely critical. Because the synthesized DNA becomes the template for later reactions if incorrect bases are incorporated into the newly synthesized segments of DNA, especially within the first few cycles of amplification, some of the final amplified product will not accurately represent the original DNA sequence. A major advance in PCR technology was the characterization of thermostable DNA polymerases. Because the synthesis reactions are performed at high temperatures and because many enzymes are denatured at temperatures above 37°C, thermostable DNA polymerases allow many cycles to be performed without the need to replenish the enzyme. The first characterized thermostable DNA was isolated from Thermus aquaticus in the mid 1970s. This enzyme has a temperature maximum between 70 and 80°C. A second polymerase, named Taq polymerase and isolated in the mid 1980s from the same organism, catalyzes DNA synthesis at an optimum temperature of 75–80°C. Several additional polymerases that function at high temperatures are now available.

An important feature of some DNA polymerases is their ability to proofread which bases are incorporated into the growing DNA strand. For example, Pfu DNA polymerase has a 3'→5' exonuclease activity that allows it to remove bases that are incorrectly added, a feature that Taq polymerase lacks. Error rates are as low as one in 1 million misincorporated bases for Pfu DNA polymerase to as high as one in 100,000 for Taq DNA polymerase. Using Taq DNA polymerase, 40 percent of products from an amplification of a 1000 base pair target sequence can have in vitro generated mutations. Although accuracy may not be a concern for qualitative analysis, such as cases of paternal determinations, greater accuracy is required for studies involving the genotyping of individuals, which is commonly needed in pharmacogenomic studies, or cloning DNA for functional studies.

After the amplification reaction is completed, the product is typically characterized by agarose gel electrophoresis. Gels are easily prepared by dissolving agarose in a Tris/acetate or borate/ethylenediamine tetraacetic acid (EDTA) buffer at a concentration of 0.6 percent (for larger DNA products such as 10,000 base pairs) to 1.5 percent (for smaller DNA products such as 200 base pairs). A DNA-intercalating dye, such as ethidium bromide, typically is added to the agarose because it allows visualization of DNA bands under ultraviolet (UV) light. Deoxyribonucleic acid markers of known size are run alongside the amplified product for accurate size determinations. Figure 2 shows the amplification of variant β-tubulin genes that confer resistance to paclitaxel. After amplification of specific DNA sequences, PCR products can be isolated directly from agarose gels or by gel filtration using size exclusion columns. The isolated products can then be analyzed using a variety of techniques.

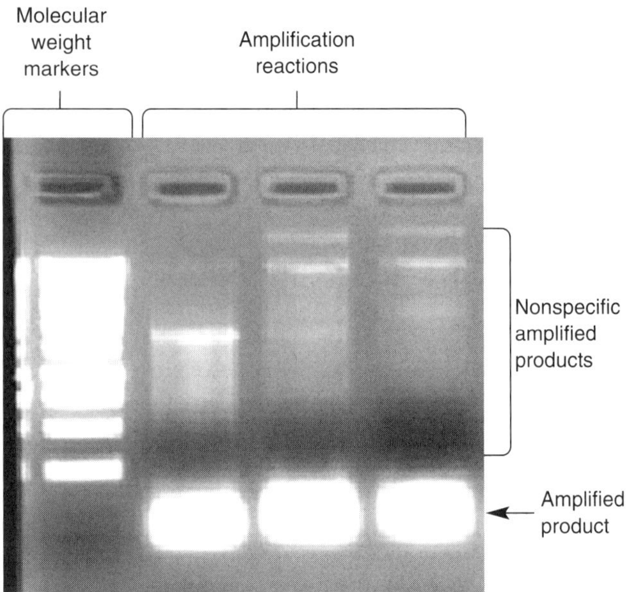

Figure 2. Amplification of a specific region of the Ψ-tubulin deoxyribonucleic acid (DNA) sequence. Tumor cells were grown in culture with increasing concentrations of paclitaxel. Because paclitaxel is known to bind to β-tubulin, polymerase chain reaction (PCR) primers were designed to amplify a specific region of the β-tubulin DNA. Deoxyribonucleic acid was extracted from drug resistance cells and a 400 base pair region was amplified. The amplified product was then submitted for DNA sequencing to determine if mutations in the β-tubulin sequence correlated with drug resistance.

Direct DNA Sequencing

When the human genome project was initiated, it quickly became obvious that faster and automated sequencing methods would be required to handle the volume of samples needed for a timely completion of the project. The field of pharmacogenomics is now benefiting from the advancements achieved in high throughput DNA sequencing. Variations of the Sanger method for DNA sequencing are uniformly used for high throughput and accurate determinations of DNA sequences. The Sanger method relies on the use of 2',3'-dideoxynucleotide triphosphates (ddNTPs) which differ from deoxynucleotides by having a hydrogen atom at the 3' carbon position rather than a 3'-hydroxyl group as in deoxynucleotides. Deoxyribonucleic acid synthesis is terminated when these molecules are introduced into a strand of DNA because the phosphodiester bond linking the bases cannot be formed.

The sequencing reaction is initiated by annealing a specific primer to the strand of DNA to be sequenced (Figure 3). Also included are a DNA polymerase, the four deoxynucleotides (deoxyadenosine triphosphate

[dATP], deoxycytidine triphosphate [dCTP], deoxyguanine triphosphate [dGTP], and deoxythymidine triphosphate [dTTP]) and a particular dideoxynucleotide, such as dideoxyadenosine triphosphate (ddATP), at about 1 percent of the concentration of the corresponding deoxynucleotide. The dideoxynucleotide is randomly incorporated at various sites in the growing strand, producing a series of DNA strands with various sizes (Figure 3). This reaction is performed using the four different dideoxynucleotides, then applied to a 6 percent denaturing polyacrylamide gel and electrophoresed to separate the various lengths of DNA. The shortest DNA fragments migrate the farthest, whereas the mobility of the larger fragments is hindered so that their migration distance is shorter (Figure 3).

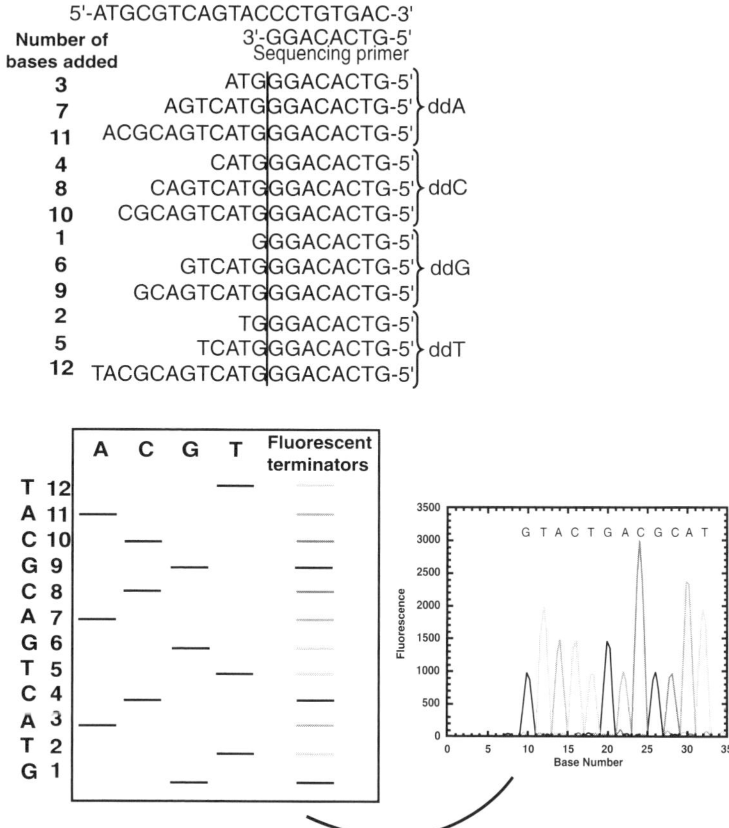

Figure 3. Schematic showing the process of deoxyribonucleic acid (DNA) sequencing using both radiolabeled and fluorescently labeled probes.

Initially, radiolabeled primers or radiolabeled deoxynucleotides were used to detect the DNA fragments. Although radiolabeled nucleotides were used extensively in sequencing reactions, during the 1990s the field moved toward the use of fluorescent labels. Nonradioactive fluorescent labels have allowed for the development of high throughput and extremely sensitive sequencing procedures. For example, the ABI Prism dRhodamine terminator cycle sequencing kit uses dideoxynucleotides conjugated to fluorescent dyes. Each nucleotide is conjugated to analogs of dichlororhodamine creating the dRhodamine dye terminators, the structures of these compounds are shown in Figure 4. These dyes have narrow emission spectra which decrease spectral overlap among the dyes. Using a thermal cycler programmed for 25 denaturation, annealing, and synthesis cycles, the target DNA is amplified and terminators are randomly introduced into the sequence, generating various length products ending in specific Rhodamine conjugated bases. Because a single primer is used for sequencing, product accumulation is linear instead of exponential as in PCR reactions. The signal to noise ratio is low for the four dye terminators and because each dye has a unique fluorescence property, the labeled products can be separated by running the entire reaction in a single lane of a polyacrylamide gel or by

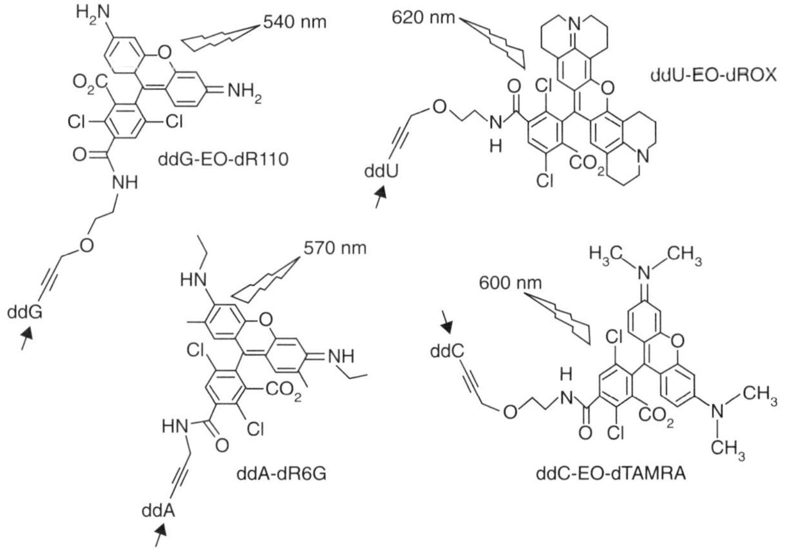

540 nm
ddG-EO-dR110
ddG
620 nm
ddU-EO-dROX
ddU
570 nm
ddA-dR6G
ddA
600 nm
ddC
ddC-EO-dTAMRA

Figure 4. Structures of fluorescent dyes used in high throughput deoxyribonucleic acid (DNA) sequencing. Development of these dyes greatly enhanced the efficiency of nucleic acid sequencing.
C = Carbon; Cl = Chlorine; ddA = Dideoxyandenosine; ddC = Dideoxycytidine; ddG = Dideoxyguanine; ddU = Dideoxyuridine; H = Hydrogen; N = Nitrogen; O = Oxygen.

capillary electrophoresis. Using equipment specifically designed to scan the individual lanes of a sequencing gel (such as the ABI Prism 377 DNA Sequencer) or record data from samples separated by capillary electrophoresis (such as the ABI Prism 310 DNA Sequencer), an electropheragram is generated (as shown in Figure 3). Sequences can be stored digitally and incorporated into downstream processes as discussed in the Bioinformatics chapter.

Expressed Sequence Tags
The Gene-to-Function-to-Potential Drug Paradigm

Advances in the technologies allowing for rapid genetic sequencing transformed many of the processes used to identify new molecular targets for drug discovery. Although the field of pharmacogenomics is particularly focused on the contribution of multiple genes to the variability of drug response, it is important to recognize how new drug targets are being identified and the need to understand the biochemical processes regulated by these newly discovered targets. Defining biochemical pathways traditionally has driven the identification of molecular targets for drug discovery. Typically, an enzyme or receptor is identified in a specific pathway and is then isolated and characterized. It is hoped that the gene can then be cloned and activity studies of the recombinant protein are used to confirm the protein's function. Rational drug design or high throughput compound screening is then used to develop modifiers of the protein's activity. Although the time involved in this "function-to-gene paradigm" is costly, a well-defined target can be identified. This paradigm is in the process of changing. High throughput sequencing can rapidly identify thousands of genes of unknown function (Reference 3). The paradigm shift, referred to as "from gene-to-screen" is now occurring where drug discovery teams are identifying genes that encode proteins that are attractive therapeutic targets.

About 100,000 genes are expressed from the entirety of the human genome. Therefore, expressed genes constitute only about 5 percent of the 3 billion nucleotides of the genome. Current technology does not allow prediction of which 5 percent of the genome encodes functional proteins. To quickly identify expressed sequences, a method now referred to as "expressed sequence tagging" was developed. Expressed sequence tags (ESTs) are generated by first isolating messenger ribonucleic acid (mRNA) from selected tissues. Because mRNA is transcribed from only genes expressed in the specific tissue, converting mRNA into DNA using the enzyme reverse transcriptase generates complementary deoxyribonucleic acid (cDNA) that represents the expressed genes of the tissue (Figure 5). The cDNA sequences can then be cloned into plasmids from which cDNA libraries can be constructed. Using automated sequencing techniques short stretches of DNA can then be sequenced from individual clones. Theoretically, it is possible that every expressed gene in a given tissue can be *partially* sequenced using this approach. Expressed sequence tag

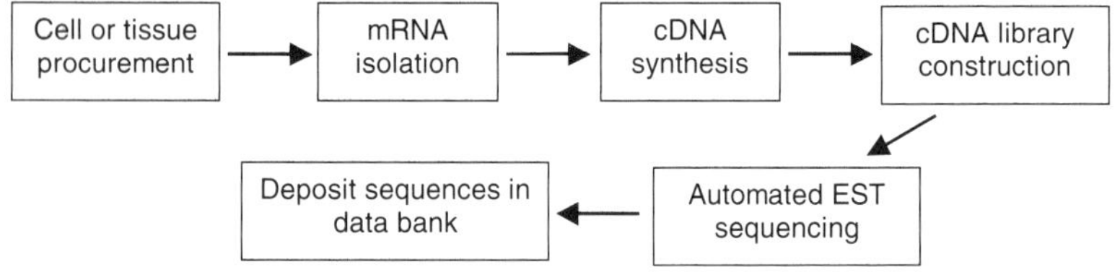

Figure 5. Schematic showing the process by which expressed sequence tags are generated. cDNA = complementrary deoxyribonucleic acid; EST = expressed sequence tag; mRNA = messenger ribonucleic acid.

sequences often are sufficiently long to provide enough sequence data to predict the molecular function of the gene product through homology searches. Millions of cDNAs have been sequenced, and the ESTs have been deposited in several sites for easy access. These sites include The Institute for Genomics Research Web site at *http://www.tigr.org/* and the National Institutes of Health Web site *http://www.ncbi.nlm.nih.gov/dbEST/*.

Deriving Drug Targets by EST Analysis: Discovery of Cathepsin K

Because thousands of genes are expressed in any given cell type, once EST sequences have been determined and deposited in data banks, a practical problem becomes how to identify which sequences are involved in disease progression and how can the sequences be translated into valid drug targets. SmithKline Beecham Pharmaceuticals developed a process by which more than 500 cDNA libraries were constructed, and thousands of ESTs were sequenced from these libraries.

To target the specific disease of osteoporosis, it was predicted that ESTs generated from osteoclasts, the cells responsible for bone resorption during bone remodeling, would provide unique targets for drug discovery. However, because osteoclasts are not easily isolated, researchers generated cDNA libraries from osteoclastoma tumors. Of the hundreds of ESTs sequenced, about 4 percent encoded a novel cysteine protease. Subsequent studies demonstrated that expression of the novel protein, which was later called cathepsin K, was not only restricted to osteoclasts but restricted to sites of bone resorption. Based on these preliminary observations, a detailed study on the biochemical analysis of the protein was initiated. It was determined that cathepsin K is a member of the papain family of cysteine proteases and can cleave bone proteins, such as type I collagen, osteopontin, and osteonectin. Mutations of the gene encoding cathepsin K result in pycnodysostosis, an autosomal recessive condition where osteoclasts from affected individuals demineralize normally but do not degrade the bone protein matrix, resulting in osteoporosis and increased bone fragility. Because additional studies suggested that inhibition of cathepsin K should result in a reduction of osteoclast-mediated bone resorption, inhibitors of cathepsin K were developed.

These studies demonstrate that 1) ESTs can be generated from target cells, 2) ESTs contain enormous amounts of information regarding gene expression, 3) new targets for drug discovery can be identified using rational genetic approaches, and 4) new treatments for disease, such as osteoporosis, can be targeted using sophisticated genetic methodologies.

Identification of DNA Sequence Variations, SNPs

A major focus of pharmacogenomics is determining why individuals respond differently to specific drugs. This focus is especially pertinent in light of many recent studies that clearly show individuals with certain DNA sequence variation metabolize specific drugs differently. Polymorphic markers have been used for decades to distinguish individuals within a given population. As discussed in the Principles of Genetic Medicine chapter, numerous studies have shown the relationship between DNA sequence (or genotype) and biology (or phenotype). Through detailed genetic studies it is becoming increasingly clear how genotypic alterations effect phenotypic responses. In addition, the influence of an individual's environment at the level of DNA sequence and the effect genetic changes (i.e., acquired mutations) have on biological processes can now be studied using polymorphic marker analysis.

Early polymorphic marker studies focused on identifying differences of blood groups or serum proteins. Polymorphic marker development depended on the discovery of proteins, or gene products, and not directly on the analysis of the gene. However, in the late 1970s it was shown that variations in DNA sequence occur not only in regions coding for proteins, but in noncoding regions as well. These results were extremely significant because they showed that not only are regions encoding protein products important, but also noncoding regions can contain valuable information. By the early 1980s it was well established that DNA polymorphisms could be used as a basis for defining molecular markers and that markers within arbitrary sequences of DNA could be as valuable as markers within gene-coding regions.

Several methods for rapidly detecting genetic polymorphic regions were subsequently developed. After the discovery of PCR, most genetic marker studies now rely on PCR amplification of specific DNA sequences followed by downstream analysis of the PCR product. Four major classes of DNA polymorphisms are routinely used as genetic markers, including:

i)   Single nucleotide polymorphisms (representing single base pair substitutions, insertions, and deletions).

ii) Restriction fragment length polymorphisms (RFLPs) (representing nucleoside changes that can be analyzed using restriction endonucleases).

iii) Variable number of tandemly repeated sequences (representing small portions of DNA sequences repeated variable number of times).

iv) Randomly amplified polymorphic DNAs (representing random sequences of DNA amplified by variable amounts).

Identification of SNPs by Sequence Analysis, Detection of DNA Polymorphisms

Deoxyribonucleic acid sequence analysis using high throughput and automated technology is being used to identify and genotype polymorphisms in hundreds of human candidate genes (References 6, 11). Candidate genes currently are being sequenced across a panel of 90 individuals representative of United States populations. This sequencing effort is designed to identify common sequence variations that ultimately will be used for functional analysis and population-based studies. Homozygote and heterozygote polymorphisms can be identified using high quality sequence data. Hundreds of genes are being targeted for SNP analysis including genes involved in DNA repair, cell cycle control, cell signaling, cell division, homeostasis and various metabolic pathways. Additional information on the National Institute of Environmental Health Sciences (NIEHS)-SNPs program and SNP databases can be found at *http://egp.gs.washington.edu/welcome.html, http://www.genome.utah.edu/ genesnps/,* or *http://wwwgenome.wi.mit.edu/snp/human/.* Also, the National Human Genome Research Institute (NHGRI), in collaboration with the National Institute of General Medical Sciences (NIGMS) and its Human Genetic Cell Repository, is developing a resource of cell lines and DNA samples from 450 unrelated individuals that reflect the diversity in the human population for the purpose of investigating DNA sequence polymorphisms. General information regarding the repository can be found at *http://locus.umdnj.edu/nigms/.*

In addition to identifying polymorphic markers, the NIEHS has developed an Environmental Genome Project that is focused on examining the relationships between environmental exposures and interindividual sequence variation in human genes and disease risk in United States populations. The NIEHS SNPs program is targeting the systematic identification and genotyping of SNPs in environmental response genes. Initially, efforts are focused on finding common sequence variation (SNPs) in human genes involved in DNA repair and cell cycle pathways. The ultimate goal of the project is to provide a dense genetic map of human genes that can be used to evaluate human disease risk with environmental exposures.

Detection of DNA Polymorphisms by Single-strand Conformational Polymorphism Analysis

Single-strand conformational polymorphism (SSCP) analysis is a convenient method for identifying differences among known and variant DNA sequences and is relatively straightforward. Single-strand conformational polymorphism analysis is used to screen PCR products from test samples for single base-pair changes relative to control DNA (Reference 9). Unlike SNP analysis, because this method does not initially rely on DNA sequencing, rapid screening of large numbers of samples for polymorphic differences is possible. As shown in Figure 6, SSCP analysis is based on the principle that the two strands (5'→3' and 3'→5') of a PCR product can be separated, and under the appropriate conditions can independently reanneal. The conformation each strand assumes after independent reannealing is sequence dependent. The individual strands can then be separated on a nondenaturing polyacrylamide gel. Strand migration rates depend on the conformation of each strand. Polymerase chain reaction products derived from samples with sequences variant from the control sample can be identified by their different migration properties. The major advantages of this technique are 1) the rapid screening of many samples and 2) sequencing efforts can be focused on the most important samples. However, as can be imagined, because all mutations do not induce differential conformational changes, false-negative rates can be as high as 10 percent, indicating all mutations are not identified by this method. Also, because analysis of PCR products of around 200 base pairs is most accurate, only small stretches of DNA are typically analyzed by SSCP analysis.

Detection of DNA Sequence Polymorphisms by RFLP

Compared to SSCP analysis, specific polymorphisms in longer stretches of DNA can be quickly assayed by RFLP analysis, which is based on the use of restriction endonucleases. These enzymes recognize and cleave double-stranded DNA of specific sequence. As shown in Figure 7A, the sites recognized by these enzymes are typically 4–8 nucleotides in length. The sites also are palindromic, meaning they have a 2-fold symmetry where the sequence read 5'→3' is the same for both strands. Because these enzymes are so highly specific for precise DNA sequences, if a polymorphism occurs

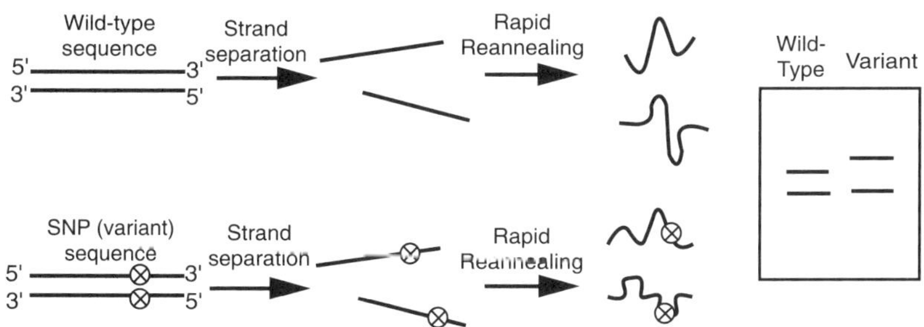

Figure 6. Schematic showing the basis for differences observed between wild-type and variant deoxyribonucleic acid (DNA) sequences when using single-stranded conformational polymorphism analysis.
SNP = single nucleotide polymorphism.

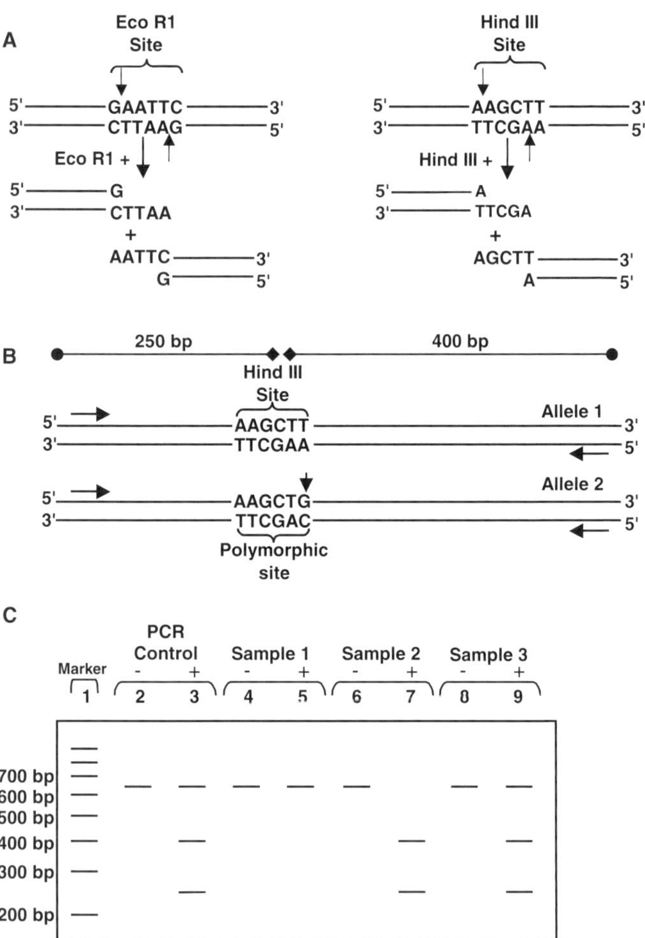

Figure 7. Schematic showing the basis for differences observed between control samples and test samples when using RFLP analysis. Panel A shows the recognition site of two restriction enzymes, Eco R1 and Hind III. Panel B shows a hypothetical restriction site and the size of products obtained after enzymatic digestion with Hind III, a 250 and a 400 bp product. If a single nucleotide polymorphic site is present in the Hind III site, Hind III will not cleave the DNA sequence and a 650 base pair product is observed. Panel C shows three possible RFLP results, the control sample contains a mixed population of DNA without addition of Hind III (650 bp band, lane 2), and with Hind III (lane 3, the 650 bp band represents polymorphic DNA sequences, and the 250 and 400 bp bands represent DNA sequences containing the Hind III site). Deoxyribonucleic acid from sample 1 is from an individual with the polymorphic site at both alleles (lanes 4 and 5), whereas DNA from sample 2 is from an individual without the polymorphic sequence (lanes 6 and 7), and sample 3 is from an individual with both alleles (lanes 8 and 9).

bp = base pair; DNA = deoxyribonucleic acid; PCR = polymerase chain reaction; RFLP = restriction fragment length polymorphism.

within the recognition site of a restriction enzyme, the site is not recognized by the enzyme. Alternatively, the polymorphism may create a new recognition site. Once a polymorphic restriction site is identified, many samples can be analyzed rapidly and accurately.

When introduced in 1978, RFLP analysis was labor-intensive and, because of poor detection limits of the time, required several days to weeks before a result was obtained. However, by combining the use of PCR to rapidly amplify regions of genomic DNA and specific restriction endonucleases, a powerful tool for detecting polymorphisms was established. Current technology allows for DNA isolation to polymorphism detection in as little as an afternoon. An RFLP analysis begins with the isolation of genomic DNA from a patient or laboratory sample. Specific primers are used for PCR amplification of a targeted region of DNA. After amplification and purification of the PCR product, a restriction endonuclease is added and the digested products are separated by agarose gel electrophoresis (Figure 7 B and C). If the PCR product is digested, then the restriction site is present; if the PCR product is not digested, the target site contains an altered DNA sequence at the enzyme recognition site.

Obviously, the major drawback of this method is the requirement of first knowing which region(s) of DNA contain useful polymorphic restriction sites. This information is obtained either by trial and error or by sequencing a limited number of samples to identify possible polymorphic regions. But once the polymorphic region is identified, large numbers of samples are quickly and easily screened.

Detection of DNA Sequence Polymorphisms by Microsatellite Analysis

Microsatellites are repetitive sequences of DNA composed of one to five base pair units, and they are one of the most abundant classes of intergenetic repetitive sequences dispersed on the human genome. These repeat sequences have become the most important markers for gene mapping and linkage analysis studies, and comprehensive human genetic linkage maps have been generated based on microsatellite data. The most common microsatellites used for the analysis of polymorphisms are dinucleotide, trinucleotide, and tetranucleotide repeats, where dinucleotide repeats are common in the human genome, particularly the dinucleotide sequence C-A (cytidine-adenosine). The most common method available to detect microsatellites is PCR amplification using two primers that flank the repeat. After PCR amplification, the products are separated by gel electrophoresis. For example, if a dinucleotide repeat differs from the population by a single repeat unit, the PCR product differs in size by two base pairs, which is easily resolved by acrylamide gel electrophoresis.

Although detection of microsatellites within populations appears relatively straightforward, several technical details inhibit unambiguous interpretations (Reference 8). For example, the Taq polymerases used in PCR amplifications have a confounding property of being able to add bases indiscriminately to the ends of PCR products. This terminal deoxynucleotidyl transferase (TDT) activity results in PCR products that can vary in size by one or two base pairs. If the microsatellite polymorphism being studied is only a two base pair addition, the TDT activity of Taq polymerase can be problematic. In addition, Taq polymerases can "slip" during a PCR amplification. Slippage occurs when the polymerase mistakenly replicates a stretch of DNA repeatedly or, because of possible secondary structures of DNA, skips a stretch of DNA. Because of slippage, various sizes of PCR products can be amplified, especially in a region of repetitive sequence. Although it is difficult to control for polymerase slippage, compensation for TDT activity can be achieved using the 3' exonuclease activity of T4 DNA polymerase, which removes the additional nucleotides added by Taq polymerase.

Because microsatellite polymorphisms appear to be stable within individuals they have been ideal markers for linkage analysis studies. However, in the early 1990s it was reported that one class of microsatellites with dinucleotide repeats was unstable in some human cancers, meaning the number of repeats of a specific microsatellite sequence was different when comparing tumor samples to normal tissue. Since the initial finding, microsatellite instability has been observed in many cases of sporadic cancers and numerous studies documenting microsatellite differences have been reported for a wide variety of human cancers. It was later found that the differences in microsatellite sequences, termed microsatellite instability, were the result of defects in DNA-mismatch-repair processes. In general, enzymes involved in DNA-mismatch-repair remove nucleotides that loop out from a strand created by slippage of the replicational polymerases, which can occur on repetitive sequences during DNA replication. Deoxyribonucleic acid-mismatch-repair mechanisms also are crucial for the removal of nucleotides mispaired by DNA polymerases during cell division. Inactivation of the DNA-mismatch-repair system leads to a hypermutable state where repetitive sequences of DNA are unstable during DNA replication. Microsatellite instability can, therefore, be an efficient method for detecting defective DNA-mismatch-repair and has been implicated in about 15 percent of sporadic colorectal cancers.

The ability to incorporate fluorescent tags into PCR products, using technologies similar to those described for automated sequencing of DNA, has helped standardize microsatellite analysis. For the purpose of detecting microsatellite instability in cancer samples, specific microsatellite sequences can be amplified from genomic DNA isolated from cancer tissue and noncancerous tissue. Several different dyes are available for DNA labeling during PCR amplification. One dye can be incorporated into the PCR product generated from the cancer sample and a second into the PCR product generated from a noncancerous sample. After T4 DNA polymerase treatment to compensate for TDT activity, the two amplified products can be mixed and separated by electrophoresis. Because two different dyes are used, both samples can be applied to a single lane, which minimizes migration errors. If a shift is observed in the size of products amplified from the tumor sample, as shown in Figure 8, then microsatellite instability at the particular loci is present.

An ultimate goal of microsatellite analyses is to assess the risk for cancer in a given individual. However, because different sets of microsatellite markers initially were used by various laboratories, it was impossible to compare results from independent investigators. To achieve the goal of using microsatellite instability as markers for cancer risk, the National Cancer Institute sponsored an international workshop focused on microsatellite instability and cancer detection. Several definitions and guidelines were derived from the meeting, including:

> "(a) The form of genomic instability associated with defective DNA-mismatch-repair in tumors is to be called microsatellite instability (MSI). (b) A panel of five microsatellites has been validated and is recommended as a reference panel for future research in the field. Tumors may be characterized on the basis of: high-frequency microsatellite

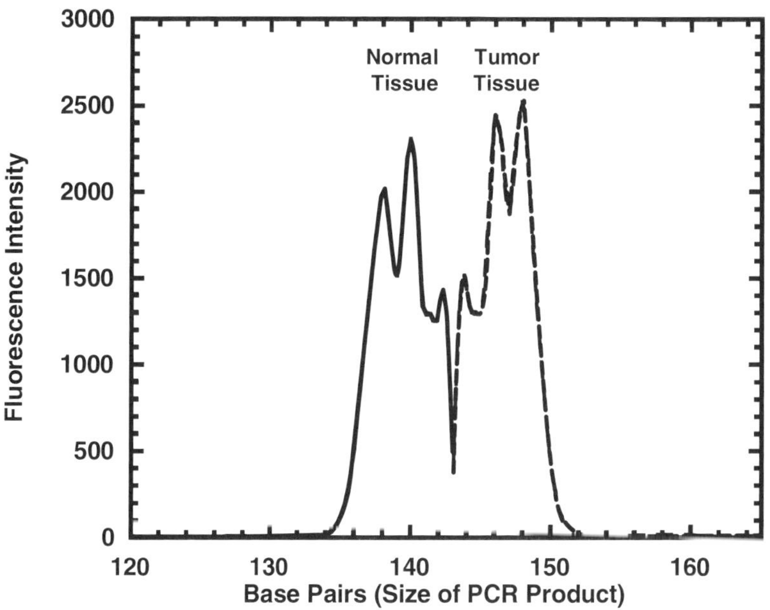

Figure 8. Microsatellite analysis of deoxyribonucleic acid (DNA) amplified from normal tissue compared with DNA amplified from tumor tissue.
PCR = polymerase chain reaction.

instability (MSI-H), if two or more of the five markers show instability (i.e., have insertion/deletion mutations), and low-frequency microsatellite instability (MSI-L), if only one of the five markers shows instability. The distinction between microsatellite stable (MSS) and MSI-L can only be accomplished if a greater number of markers is used. (c) A unique clinical and pathological phenotype is identified for the MSI-H tumors, which comprise about 15 percent of colorectal cancers, whereas MSI-L and MSS tumors appear to be phenotypically similar. The MSI-H colorectal tumors are found predominantly in the proximal colon, have unique histopathological features, and are associated with a less aggressive clinical course than are stage-matched MSI-L or MSS tumors. Preclinical models suggest the possibility that these tumors may be resistant to the cytotoxicity induced by certain chemotherapeutic agents. The implications for MSI-L are not yet clear. (d) MSI can be measured in fresh or fixed tumor specimens equally well; microdissection of pathological specimens is recommended to enrich for neoplastic tissue; and normal tissue is required to document the presence of MSI. (e) The "Bethesda guidelines", which were developed in 1996 to assist in the selection of tumors for microsatellite analysis, are endorsed. (f) The spectrum of microsatellite alterations in noncolonic tumors was reviewed, and it was concluded that the above recommendations apply only to colorectal neoplasms." (Reference 1).

In addition to their potential applications to cancer diagnosis, polymorphisms of nucleotide repeats have been implicated in affecting nervous system function. Nucleotide repeats within a gene are normal and typically do not confer disease phenotypes. However, through a variety of possible mechanisms, regions of nucleotide repeats can be amplified during DNA replication to such an extent that a disease phenotype develops. For example, Huntington's disease occurs when the C-A-G (cytidine-adenosine-guanosine) repeat located in the IT15 gene, which encodes the huntingtin protein, expands to an abnormal range of between 36 and 120 repeats (Figure 9). Because CAG is the codon for glutamine, the resulting huntingtin protein has a polyglutamine insertion that can

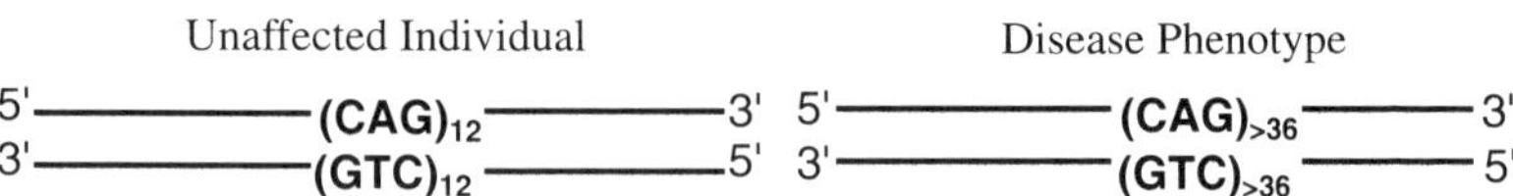

Figure 9. The huntingtin protein is encoded by the IT15 gene. If a C-A-G region of the gene is amplified Huntington's disease occurs.

alter interactions between huntingtin and other proteins. The altered protein-protein interactions are believed to activate cell-death mechanisms. Identification of the expanded CAG repeats can easily be identified by PCR amplification using primers flanking the CAG repeat sequence.

Gene Expression Profiling

Expression Profiling by Microarray Analysis

Specific changes in gene expression are believed to be the initiating factor for many or all human diseases. This hypothesis has generated tremendous commercial interest in gene expression profiling at the whole genome level. For the majority of genes, it is believed that the steady state mRNA levels in a cell approximate the levels of protein translated by their mRNA. Although this assumption is being critically evaluated, determination of mRNA levels can provide important information regarding changes in gene expression. The development of techniques for generating fluorescent probes from mRNA and the ease by which these probes can be analyzed by hybridization-based assays has driven many of the advancements in genome-based research. As shown in Figure 10, an

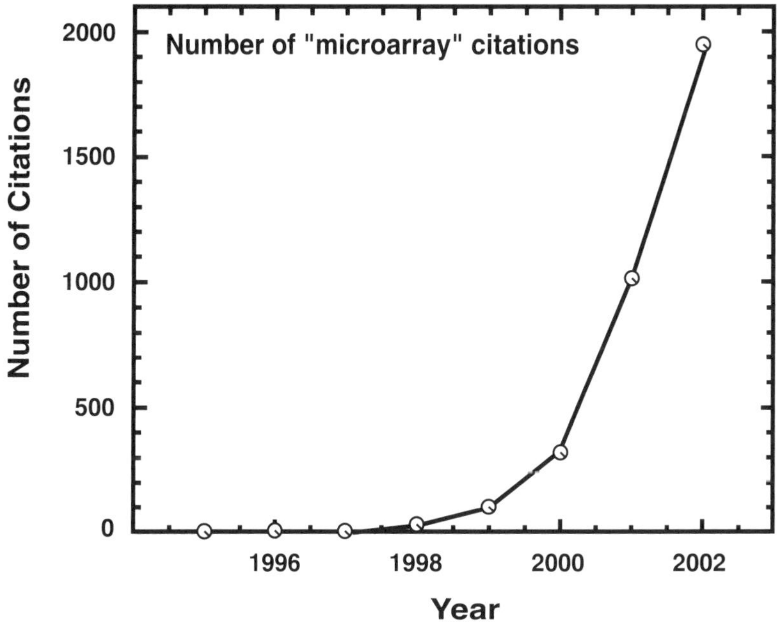

Figure 10. Graph showing the exponential growth in citations using microarray technology.

explosion of literature citing microarray applications has appeared within the past 3 years. The explosion of applications using microarray analysis makes it virtually impossible to cover all aspects of array technology. The goal of this section is to provide essential information regarding the basis of microarray technology and to provide sufficient examples to demonstrate the potential power of microarray analysis. Although it should be emphasized that techniques using microarray analysis have not been fully optimized for any individual target, based on the popularity of the method it is only a matter of time before standardized protocols are developed.

In general, microarray experiments are based on hybridization of nucleic acid samples, either DNA or RNA, with cDNA sequences that are immobilized to a solid substrate. Extremely precise methods have been developed for immobilizing DNA sequences to solid supports, producing the microarray. Numerous methods have been developed to use these arrays including: 1) quantitating differential gene expression, 2) screening and cloning differentially expressed genes, 3) detecting SNPs, 4) identifying drug targets, 5) profiling diseases, 6) subdividing diseases into drug sensitive or nonresponding disease, 7) determining drug actions and/or toxicities, or 8) determining gene expression differences during metabolically distinct states (Reference 7). For some applications, the solid substrate is a simple microscope slide (Figures 11 and 12) and for others specific microchips have been designed. Major advancements in DNA microarray technology have been in the development of methods to generate slides with thousands of immobilized oligonucleotide or cDNA sequences.

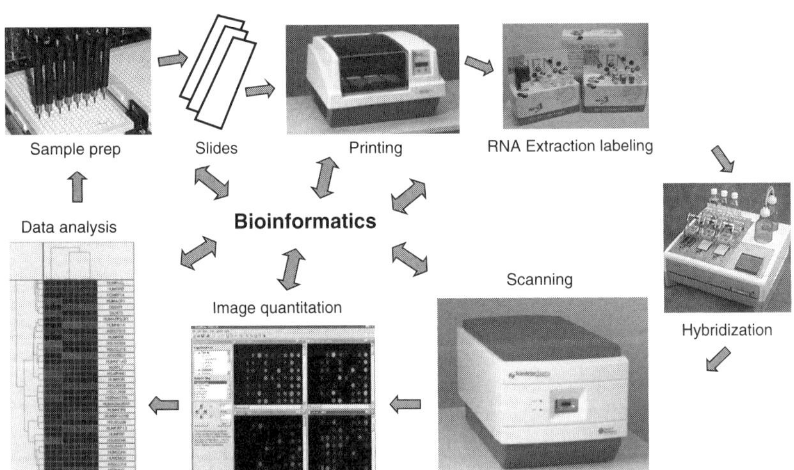

Figure 11. Schematic showing the processes of microarray techniques from the printing of DNA onto slides to the impact of bioinformatics on the entire microarray process (Variation of figure printed with permission from PerkinElmer Life Sciences).
RNA = ribonucleic acid.

Slides are made using robotic "arrayers" that use capillary printing tips (Figure 11). Recent technologies enable the printing of more than 25,000 individual elements on a single slide, which allows for the simultaneous analysis of thousands of gene products. The immobilized elements printed on the slides can be PCR products, DNA fragments from individual DNA library clones such as from ESTs, or chemically synthesized DNA sequences. Many companies now offer a variety of pre-arrayed slides with immobilized DNA from a wide variety of sources.

A typical microarray experiment is initiated by isolating mRNA from a test sample (Figure 11 and 12). The mRNA can be isolated using an oligo-dT resin (i.e., a series of thynidine bases linked by phosphodiester bonds that hybridize to the poladenosine tail at the 3' end of mRNAs) and then reverse transcribed (conversion of RNA to cDNA) using the enzyme reverse transcriptase. Although oligo-dT resin is used to isolate a pure mRNA sample, methods have been developed that use total RNA which in many cases is easier to isolate but consists of not only mRNA but also ribosomal RNA. Dye-labeled nucleotides are incorporated into the newly synthesized cDNA molecules during the reverse transcriptase reaction. In experiments designed to compare the relative expression of genes from two

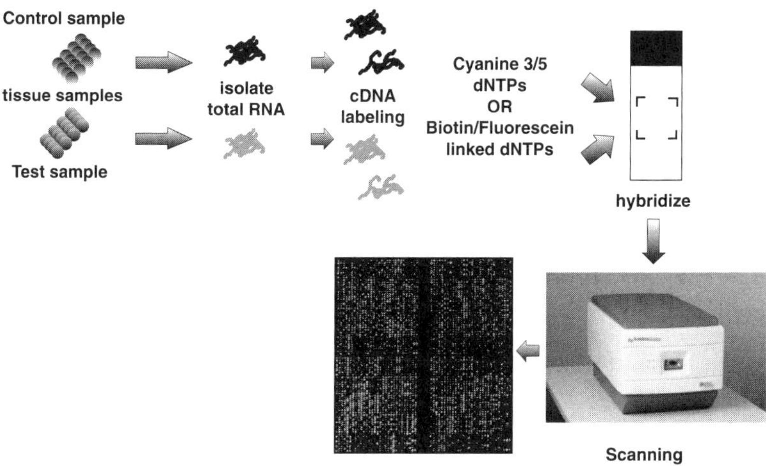

Figure 12. Several procedures are available to perform microarray experiments. This figure shows a general schematic depicting the isolation of ribonucleic acid (RNA) from control and test samples, converting RNA to complementary deoxyribonucleic acid (DNA) and labeling the synthesized DNA with either cyanine 3 and 5 or biotin, hybridizing the samples to a prepared microscope slide that contains thousands of immobilized DNA gene sequences, and detecting differential gene expression using a microarray scanner (Variation of figure printed with permission from PerkinElmer Life Sciences).
cDNA = complementary deoxyribonucleic acid; dNTPs = Deoxynucleotide triophosphates; RNA = ribonucleic acid

separate samples, for instance, samples isolated from cancer cells compared to normal tissue, the two samples are labeled with different fluorescent dyes. Typically, one dye is Cyanine 3 (Cy3) and the other Cyanine 5 (Cy5). The labeled samples are then mixed and hybridized to the microarray slide. After hybridization and washing, the microarray slide is inserted into a microarray scanner. Scanners have an excitation energy source, such as lasers of defined wavelength, that are focused onto the microarray slide. The fluorescent dyes are excited and the fluorescence energy emitted by the dyes is collected and focused onto a detector that converts the fluorescent signal into an electrical signal. The scanner must be able to measure low-level fluorescence from specific microscopic areas on the microarray slide. As can be imagined, if more than 20,000 genes are represented on a single slide, the area occupied by each is exceedingly small. The relative expression of individual genes is determined by comparing the fluorescence intensities of the two dyes. For example, if the fluorescence of Cy3 and Cy5 are about equal then the expression of the specific gene is equivalent in the two samples. If Cy3 fluorescence is greater, then expression of the specific gene is greater in the Cy3 labeled sample.

Alternatively, instead of comparing samples from a single individual, it is possible to compare gene expression in samples obtained from different patients diagnosed with similar diseases. Direct comparison of samples is not informative because expression comparisons are not relative to a common standard. To compensate for this problem, RNA extracts from an individual patient can be prepared and RNA expression can be compared to a standard RNA sample isolated from a reference source. The reference source can be a specific cell line or other suitable control. Although the reference source is one of the most critical aspects of microarray analysis, there currently is no general consensus as to what is the best reference. After the arrays have been processed, a major challenge for the investigator using microarrays is what to do with the vast amount of data generated from a single microarray experiment, and how to compare data generated from different experiments. An evolving subspecialty of the field of bioinformatics is dedicated to this type of analysis, which is covered more fully in the next chapter.

As an example, it has been well established that women with breast cancer diagnosed with the same stage of disease can have markedly different treatment outcomes. To determine if gene expression profiling can predict clinical outcomes of breast cancer patients, RNA was extracted from 98 primary breast cancers (Reference 14). From the 98 samples, a reference sample was prepared by mixing RNA from a subset of patients who developed sporadic metastatic disease. Each RNA sample from the 98 patients was then compared to the reference control. The microarray data from this study can be viewed at the Web site *http://www.rii.com/publications/default.htm.* It was shown that gene expression profiling does indeed allow for the prediction of clinical outcomes by identifying an expression signature that strongly predicted a short interval to metastatic lesions. In addition, an expression signature for breast cancer susceptibility gene (BRCA1) carriers was defined that can possibly be used to improve the diagnosis for hereditary breast cancer. Signatures also were identified that provided a strategy for stratifying patients who are most likely to benefit from adjuvant therapy compared to patients where adjuvant therapy may not necessarily be beneficial.

Microarray technology also has been coupled with recent advances in tissue preparation. When tissue is harvested from patient samples, it is virtually always a heterogeneous population of cells. For example, cancer cell biopsies contain endothelial cells, stromal cells, as well as cancerous cells. Ribonucleic acid isolated from a heterogeneous cell mass represents an average of all cells present in the sample. To more specifically identify differences in only cells of interest, the method of *laser capture microdissection* was developed. To capture cells from tissue samples, a section of the sample is mounted on a slide and viewed under an inverted microscope. A transparent cap loaded with a transfer film is placed directly above the tissue slice. Cells of interest are then harvested by triggering a laser beam. The laser beam activates an adhesive material that is applied to the transparent cap. Cells in the path of the laser beam become focally attached to the cap and can be lifted off for processing. A detailed description of laser capture can be found at *http://www.arctur.com*. The isolated cells can then be processed for microarray analysis or other postharvest processing, such as genomic PCR analysis.

Microarray Analysis of Nonhuman Genomes: Host-Microbe Interactions

Although a high proportion of genomic studies focus on understanding the intricacies of the human genome, many investigators have focused on identifying genetic characteristics of nonhuman genomes. The genomes of many microbes have been completely sequenced using high throughput sequencing techniques. Similar to the rate of sequence information obtained from the human genome project, sequence information for nonhuman genomes has accelerated at a similar rate. The Web site *http://www.tigr.org/tdb/mdb/mdbcomplete.html* contains links to the genome sequences of more than 60 microbial genomes with more than a dozen from human pathogens. New strategies for studying host-pathogen interactions can now be contemplated that include analysis of the entire pathogen genome. Using sequence similarities, the function of uncharacterized genes can be predicted, and by monitoring microbial gene expression, the effects of novel drugs can be precisely tested. For example, the sequence of the deadly human malarial parasite, *Plasmodium falciparum*, recently was completed, so researchers now have available the genome sequence of the parasite, the mosquito carrier, and the human host (References 4, 5). Together, the complexities of an infection that affects more than 500 million people can be better defined. In addition, growth patterns of many microbes allow several generations to be studied in a relatively short time. Because errors in microarray data collection often require analysis of duplicate samples, this can be accomplished easily with many microbial systems.

With respect to direct applications in pharmacogenomics, microarrays are being used to analyze polymorphisms of pathogenic microbes that confer drug-resistance phenotypes. For instance, microarray analysis of gene expression in *Mycobacterium tuberculosis* has identified targets for new antituberculosis drugs. Also, because microarrays can be used to simultaneously measure expression levels of thousands of genes, it is possible to determine how a specific drug affects cellular metabolism and genetic regulation on a genomic scale. In addition, DNA microarrays have been generated that contain every expressed gene of the *Saccharomyces cerevisiae* genome and have been used to identify changes in gene expression induced by various metabolic challenges. Although proof-of-concept has been well established for applying microarray technology for identifying and validating new drug targets, novel agents have yet to be developed based on these studies. However, it should be emphasized that this technology has only recently been introduced, especially to the field of pharmacogenomics, and it is typically expected that given time new agents will be introduced through this technology.

Methods for Analyzing the Human Proteome

In contrast to genomic studies that identify polymorphisms in nucleic acid sequences or relative changes in RNA expression, studies of the human proteome focus directly on identifying changes in protein expression. Although proteomic studies have been active for decades, the term "proteomic" was only introduced in the mid 1990s. The increase in attention to proteomic studies can be partially linked not only to the advancements in genomic studies but also to notable advancements in techniques for protein analysis.

It has been estimated that the human genome contains about 100,000 genes, which is an estimate that continues to fluctuate because of the lack of understanding of gene structure and function. But it is well understood that for every eukaryotic gene a single protein is translated. However, because of extensive post-translational modifications, every transcribed gene can generate as many as 10 differently processed proteins, making the number of functional proteins in a given cell at a given time much more difficult to estimate than the number of genes in the genome. As discussed in the Applied Molecular and Cellular Biology chapter, differential processing of proteins can lead to differential protein activity, differential protein stability, or altered selectivity of proteins for specific ligands. The field of proteomics focuses on the large-scale analysis of differential protein expression in the context of the whole cell.

Two-dimensional (2-D) gel electrophoresis was introduced in the early 1970s and is the classical method for separating complex mixtures of proteins. Although the techniques of 2-D gel electrophoresis are relatively straightforward, the methods for analyzing 2-D gels can be extremely complex. Tissue or cell samples are processed by first separating cellular protein components from cellular membrane components. The mixture of soluble proteins are then separated by gel electrophoresis based on their charge characteristics, a technique termed isoelectric focusing. Using commercially available gel strips, it is possible to separate proteins that have relatively small differences in charge. However, because of the large number of proteins in a cell, isoelectric focusing alone does not sufficiently separate each protein. After isoelectric focusing, proteins are further separated by sodium dodecyl sulfate-polyacrylamide gel electrophoresis (SDS-PAGE). This second dimension separates proteins based on their size (i.e., molecular weights). Once separated, individual proteins imbedded in the polyacrylamide gel can be visualized by Coomassie Blue staining, CYPRO Ruby fluorostaining, copper staining, or silver staining (Figure 13). Because of the ease and sensitivity of Coomassie-Blue and silver staining, these approaches are often used.

Combining isoelectric focusing and SDS-PAGE is an excellent method for separating complex mixtures of proteins, and computer programs are being created to analyze differences in protein spots separated by 2-D gel electrophoresis. But in many cases this technique may not be sufficient to separate and identify the enormous diversity of cellular proteins (Reference 13). For example, the most abundant protein in many cell types

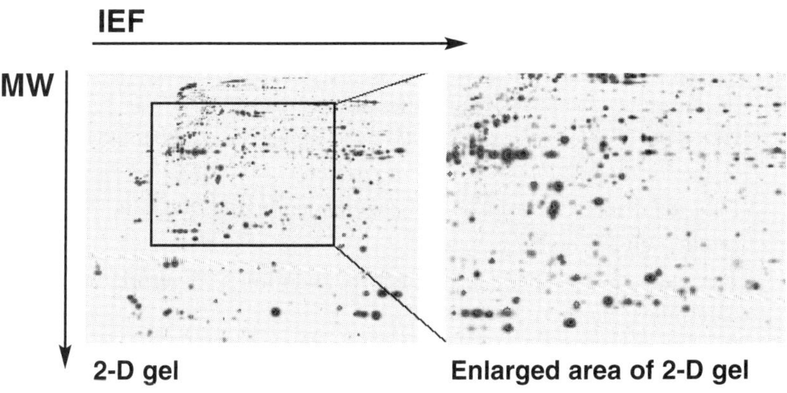

Figure 13. Using polyacrylamide gel electrophoresis, proteins are separated in the first dimension by charge (i.e., isoelectric point) and in the second dimension by their mw. 2-D = two dimensional; IEF = isoelectric focusing; MW = molecular weight.

is actin, and it is estimated that there can be as many as 100 million molecules of actin in a given cell. On the other hand, some cellular receptors or proteins involved in signal transduction pathways are only present at 100 molecules/cell. Standard 2-D gel electrophoresis techniques are not capable of handling this huge difference in protein abundance.

Newer and extremely more sensitive methods for identifying proteins from complex mixtures rely on coupling 2-D gel electrophoresis with various additional techniques, such as mass spectrometry (Reference 10). For example, in the late 1980s matrix-assisted laser desorption coupled with ionization time-of-flight mass spectrometry (MALDI-TOF MS) was introduced which increased the sensitivity of mass spectrometry and allowed analysis of samples with large masses. By enzymatically digesting proteins into smaller peptides, protein samples can be analyzed by MALDI-TOF MS. These innovations allowed mass spectrometry to become a major tool in biological research. Several underlining reasons for the growing use of MALDI-TOF MS in proteomic studies include: 1) its high sensitivity, 2) relatively rapid data collection, 3) extreme accuracy, 4) versatility, and 5) high informational content contained in a mass spectrometry spectra.

Using current technologies, a representative proteomic study can be described as:

- Protein is isolated from the sample(s) of interest.
- The complex mixture of proteins is crudely separated using a variety of methods, such as ammonium sulfate precipitation or by chromatographic techniques, which decreases the complexity of the sample used in downstream processing.
- Individual proteins are then separated by 2-D gel electrophoresis and visualized by Coomassie blue staining.
- Gel spots of interest are identified by computer-assisted comparison of two or more 2-D gels.
- Individual spots are excised and enzymatically digested with trypsin or other endoproteinase.
- The mass of each peptide product (peptide mass fingerprinting) is determined by MALDI-TOF MS.
- Based on peptide mass determinations, proteins are identified by matching the peptide mass fingerprint to databases containing known proteins, such as the SWISS-2DPAGE (*http://us.expasy.org/ch2d/*) or University of California at San Francisco (*http://prospector.ucsf.edu/*) proteomic Web sites.

Methods for Transferring Specific Genetic Sequences—Gene Therapy Techniques and Applications

It is anticipated that a better understanding of the human genome will allow more rational approaches for the design of treatments based on genetic manipulations. Currently, major efforts are focused on developing methods to treat human diseases using gene transfer techniques (i.e., gene therapy). Currently, the major limitations facing gene therapy investigators are the inability to genetically modify sufficient numbers of target cells and the inability to express the transferred gene(s) over prolonged periods. In many respects, the fundamental cause of these hurdles is not different than those faced by pioneers of other treatments, which is mainly a lack of understanding of the biological systems being manipulated. Even so, great strides have been achieved with respect to the transfer of nucleic acid sequences, expression of the transferred gene, and the clinical practice of gene therapy.

Initially, it was proposed that gene therapy could be used to cure the vast array of inherited disorders. However, there currently are more than 600 gene therapy clinical trials registered worldwide and 60 percent of these are focused on cancer as the target illness (*http://www.wiley.co.uk/ genetherapy/clinical*) (Figure 14). Obviously, the techniques of gene transfer are more versatile than originally envisioned. The versatility is partially because of the various methods used to transfer specific gene sequences. Several methods can be used to genetically engineer target cells, the majority of which can be divided into either nonviral (i.e., transfection) or viral (i.e., transduction) gene transfer procedures. Nonviral techniques are attractive because the components of the gene transfer system can be chemically synthesized. A formulation that can be well regulated is certainly more appealing when it comes to Food and Drug Administration approval compared

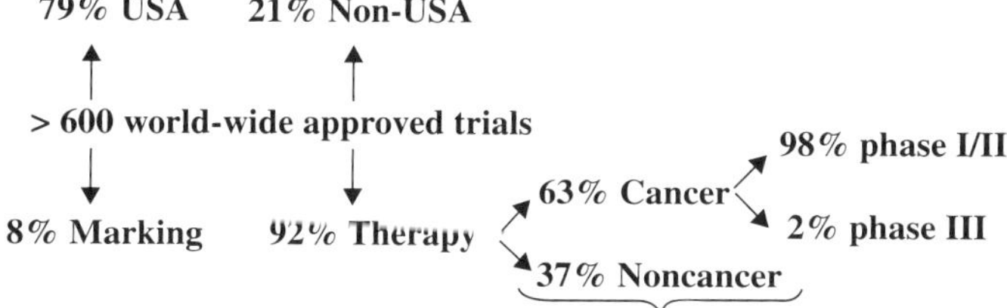

Figure 14. Summary of gene therapy clinical trials.

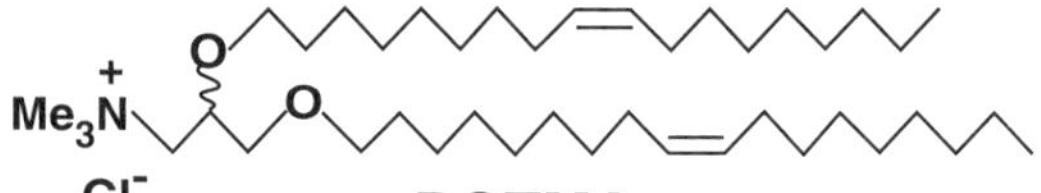

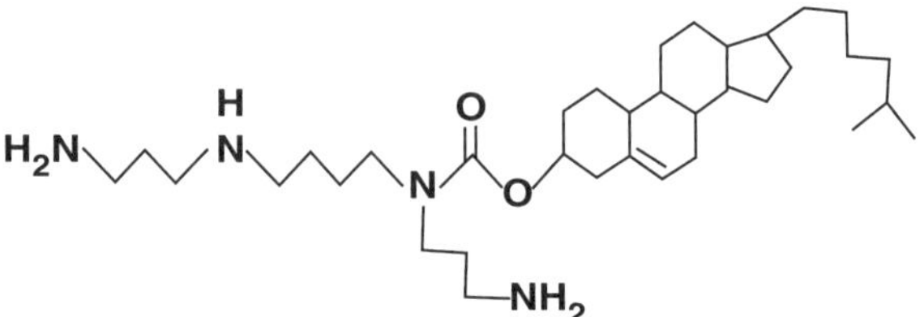

Me₃N⁺

Cl⁻ **DOTMA**

H₂N **GL 67** NH₂

Figure 15. Structures of two compounds used in nonviral gene transfer applications. Cl = Chlorine; DOTMA = N-[1-(2,3-dioleoyloxy)-propyl]-N, N, N-trimethyl-ammonium chloride; H = hydrogen; Me = methyl; N = nitrogen; O = oxygen.

to viral transfer systems that require a myriad of nonstandardized components. Although newer formulations used in nonviral gene transfer systems are excellent at achieving high transfection efficiencies, compared to viral transfer methods, nonviral systems are ineffective at maintaining gene expression over prolonged periods.

Nonviral gene transfer is typically accomplished by mixing DNA with a synthetic cationic amphiphile such as DOTMA or GL67 (Figure 15) and a neutral lipid, such as dioleoyl L-α-phosphatidylethanolamine (DOPE). Plasmid DNA is typically transferred and expression of the transferred gene is often under the control of a constitutive or lineage specific promoter. The efficiency of gene transfer varies based on cell type and the molar ratios of DNA and liposomal components (Reference 2). Once ratios are optimized, extremely high gene transfer efficiencies can be achieved. Cationic polymers and various peptide complexes such as poly-L-lysine also are used to deliver plasmid DNA. Because extremely high transfer efficiencies can be achieved, if conditions require short-term gene expression, nonviral transfer systems are ideal.

Viral gene transfer systems are used if high transduction efficiencies and long-term gene expression are needed. The basic concept for producing recombinant viruses is the use of a packaging cell line. Packaging cells are derived by generating cell lines that have controlled expression of wild-type viral sequences. As shown in Figure 16, the genome of a wild-type murine leukemia retrovirus contains two long-terminal-repeat (LTR) regions, the 5' and 3' LTRs. The 5'-LTR contains a promoter that drives the expression of the viral RNA transcript as well as enhancer sequences that increase the efficiency of gene expression. The proteins necessary for assembly of an infectious viral particle are translated from the gag, pol, and env sequences. The matrix, capsid, and nucleic acid-binding protein are translated by the gag gene, which encodes a single polyprotein that subsequently is cleaved into the three viral components. The reverse transcriptase and integrase proteins are encoded by the pol gene. Of key importance, the preprocessed RNA transcript is packaged into the viral particle by recognition of the Psi (Ψ) region as the viral particle is assembled. The resulting packaged genome of the viral particle contains the full length RNA transcript. Envelope proteins are encoded by the env gene and dictate to which cells the virus can attach. After adhesion to target cells, the viral RNA transcript is "injected", and the RNA transcript is reverse transcribed into DNA and incorporated into the genome of the target cell. Once the viral genome is incorporated into the cell's genome, additional virus is generated and the cycle is repeated. Because the viral sequence integrates into the genome of the target cell, the viral sequence is replicated when the infected cell divides.

Generation of recombinant viruses for gene therapy applications is based on the biology of wild-type viral replication. To generate cell lines that produce recombinant replication incompetent virus (i.e., viruses that infect target cells but do not contain the necessary elements needed to generate

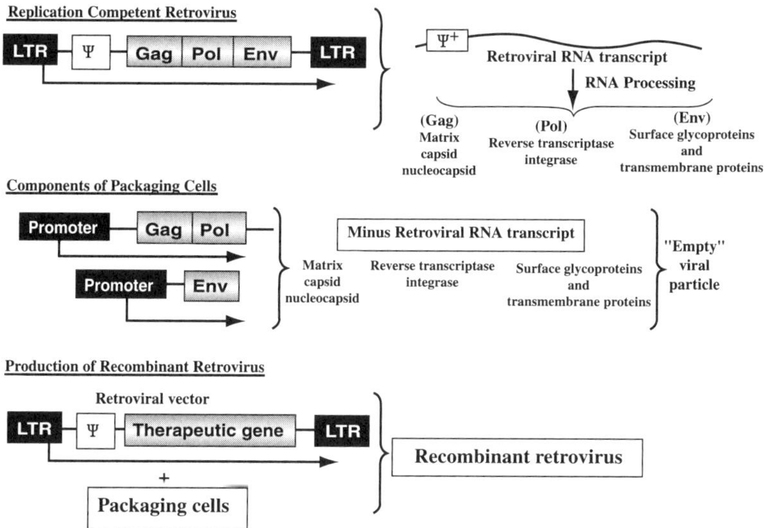

Figure 16.   Schematics showing 1) replication competent retroviruses and the proteins necessary to produce a viable virus, 2) components of packaging cells that generate the necessary proteins to form a virus particle but lack a retroviral RNA transcript for packaging, and 3) retroviral vectors used in combination with packaging cells to produce recombinant retroviruses.
LTR = long-terminal-repeat; RNA = ribonucleic acid.

more virus), the viral genome of wild-type viruses are cloned into expression plasmids and transferred into tissue culture cell lines (Figure 16). In general, packaging cells are derived by expressing the gag and pol genes from one plasmid and the env gene from a second plasmid. Cells genetically modified to express these genes can function as retroviral producer cell lines. However, the Ψ region is deleted from these expression constructs, so although viral particles can be generated, no viral RNA is packaged into the viral particle (Figure 16).

Recombinant retroviral vectors are created which contain intact Ψ regions and are used to generate recombinant retrovirus. Retroviral vectors contain 5' and 3' LTRs, the intact Ψ regions, and the nucleic acid sequence required to encode the therapeutic protein of interest (Figure 16). On transfection of the retroviral vector into a packaging cell line, synthesis of the retroviral vector RNA is driven by the 5' LTR. Because the recombinant retroviral RNA transcript contains a proper Ψ region, the RNA sequence is recognized by the viral particle and a recombinant virus is produced (Figure 16). The supernatant of the producer cells contains the recombinant virus and can be collected and used to infect target cells. Of importance, only the therapeutic nucleic acid sequence is transferred. Because no wild-type virus gene sequences are transferred to the target cell, infectious virus is not produced by the genetically modified cell. Using this basic method, noncompetent recombinant retroviruses can be used to safely introduce specific gene sequences into target cells.

Although the majority of gene therapy clinical trials are based on recombinant retrovirus gene transfer systems, more sophisticated and complex viral transfer systems are being created. Deoxyribonucleic acid virus vectors, such as adenovirus, adeno-associated virus (AAV), and herpes simplex virus, are finding their own niches in the field of gene therapy. Recombinant adenovirus is used extensively in preclinical and clinical cancer gene therapy applications (Reference 15), and several companies have been established that can provide preclinical grade recombinant adenovirus. The genome of the adenovirus is a single, double-stranded DNA molecule of about 36,000 base pairs. If prolonged expression is required, a weakness of using recombinant adenovirus is adenoviral DNA does not integrate into the cell's genome but replicates in an extra-chromosomal state and is, therefore, eventually degraded by intracellular DNAase. Also, initial administration of recombinant adenovirus generates immune responses that limit the effectiveness of subsequent virus administrations. These immune responses can be severe and possibly fatal if uncontrolled. Adeno-associated virus is particularly interesting because recombinant AAV can be engineered to integrate specifically into the long arm of human chromosome 19, unlike retroviruses that integrate randomly into the genome (Reference 12). The ability to isolate purified recombinant AAV has increased the feasibility of using AAV derived vectors in gene therapy applications.

Using gene transfer techniques, the manipulation of the human genome is certainly possible, and there are many systems available that can be used to efficiently genetically engineer target cells. Although about 50 percent of patients in clinical trials are being treated with recombinant retroviruses and an additional 18 percent of patients receive recombinant adenovirus (*http://www.wiley.co.uk/genetherapy/clinical*), because of limitations of each system it is impossible to predict which gene transfer system(s) will ultimately prevail. A likely scenario is that each system will gain its own niche and based on the specific requirement of the transferred gene sequence (e.g., high expression over short time periods or moderate expression over prolonged periods) a specific transfer system will be available.

Conclusions and Future Directions

Clearly, there are many methods available for analyzing the human genome and proteome. As limitations to each method are identified, more sophisticated techniques are continually being introduced. The information obtained from sequencing studies is only the first step toward understanding the complexity of the human genome. In addition to genetic analysis, recent advancements in the field of gene therapy allow for the genetic manipulation of genomes by introducing specific nucleic acid sequences. Although more than 95 percent of the human genome has been sequenced, putting the finishing touches on the entire sequence is not simple and tremendous efforts are being directed at resolving the final sequence. Determining where genes are located and how each is regulated is the next major hurdle facing genetic researchers. In addition, the derived sequence will be representative of only a small number of individuals. Genetic variations occurring throughout the human population can only be determined by high throughput sequencing endeavors, which are currently under way. It must then be determined to what degree each polymorphism effects various phenotypes, such as different disease states, changes in drug sensitivity and metabolism, aging, and others. Although scientists have available a tremendous amount of information, they are still fairly ignorant in understanding how genomic variability influences the human condition, especially with respect to issues important to the field of pharmacogenomics. However, researchers have the tools to proceed and to answer many of the intriguing questions generated by analysis of the humane genome.

Summary of Referenced Web Sites

Polymerase chain reaction primer design
1. *http://www-genome.wi.mit.edu/ftp/distribution/software/primer.0.5/*

Expressed sequence tag databases
2. *http://www.tigr.org/*
3. *http://www.ncbi.nlm.nih.gov/dbEST/*
Single nucleotide polymorphism databases
4. *http://egp.gs.washington.edu/welcome.html*
5. *http://www.genome.utah.edu/genesnps/*
6. *http://www.genome.wi.mit.edu/snp/human/*
7. *http://locus.umdnj.edu/nigms/*
Results of microarray analysis of breast cancer tissue
8. *http://www.rii.com/publications/default.htm*
Laser capture methodology
9. *http://www.arctur.com*
Links to microbial genomes
10. *http://www.tigr.org/tdb/mdb/mdbcomplete.html*
Proteomic Web sites
11. *http://us.expasy.org/ch2d/*
12. *http://prospector.ucsf.edu/*
Gene therapy clinical trials
13. *http://www.wiley.co.uk/genetherapy/clinical*

References

1. Boland C, Thibodeau S, Hamilton S, et al. A National Cancer Institute Workshop on Microsatellite Instability for cancer detection and familial predisposition: development of international criteria for the determination of microsatellite instability in colorectal cancer. Cancer Res 1998;58:5248–57. Review.

2. Chesnoy S, Huang L. Structure and function of lipid-DNA complexes for gene therapy. Annu Rev Biophys Biomol Struct 2000;29:27–47.

3. Debouck C, Metcalf B. The impact of genomics on drug discovery. Annu Rev Pharmacol Toxicol 2000;40:193–207. Review.

4. Gardner MJ, Hall N, Fung E, et al. Genome sequence of the human malaria parasite *Plasmodium falciparum*. Nature 2002;419:498–511.

5. Holt R. The genome sequence of the malaria mosquito *Anopheles gambiae*. Science 2002;298:129–49.

6. Kruglyak L, Nickerson D. Variation is the spice of life. Nat Genet 2001;27:234–6.

7. Marton M, Derisi J, Bennett H, et al. Drug target validation and indentification of secondary drug target effects using DNA microarrays. Nat Med 1998;4:1293–301.

8. Maehara Y, Oda S, Keizo S. The instability within: problems in current analyses of microsatellite instability. Mutat Res 2001;461:249–63.

9. Orita M, Iwahana H, Kanazawa H, Hayashi K, Sekiya T. Hayashi Detection of polymorphisms of human DNA by gel electrophoresis as single-strand conformation polymorphisms. Proc Natl Acad Sci 1989;86:2766–70.

10. Rabilloud T. Two-dimensional gel electrophoresis in proteomics: old, old fashioned, but it still climbs up the mountains. Proteomics 2002;2:3–10.

11. Rieder M, Taylor S, Clark A, Nickerson D. Sequence variation in the human angiotensin converting enzyme. Nat Genet 1999;22:59–62.

12. Srivastara, A. Gene transfer with adeno-associated vectors. In: Cid-Arregui A, Garcia-Carranca A, eds. Viral Vectors Basic Science and Gene Therapy. Westborough, MA: Eaton Publishing, Co., 2000:11-26.

13. Toda T. Proteome and proteomics for the research on protein alterations in aging. Ann N Y Acad Sci 2001;928:71–8.

14. van't Veer I, Dai H, Van de Vijver M. Expression profiling predicts clinical outcome of breast cancer. Nature 2002;415:530–6.

15. Zhang WW. Development and application of adenoviral vectors for gene therapy of cancer. Cancer Gene Therapy 1999;6:113–38.

Self-Assessment Questions

1. Deoxyribonucleic acid (DNA) microarrays are least likely to be used for which one of the following?

    A. Determining differential gene expression.
    B. Determining gene function.
    C. Identifying new drug targets.
    D. Classifying diseases into subgroups.

2. Which one of the following steps of a polymerase chain reaction (PCR) amplification is performed at 72°C?

    A. Strand denaturation.
    B. Annealling.
    C. Elongation.
    D. Hybridization.

3. The search for single nucleotide polymorphisms (SNPs) throughout the genome will do which one of the following?

    A. Identify the complete repertoire of expressed genes.
    B. Allow for the rapid parallel analysis of thousands of genes.
    C. Target regulatory sequences involved in drug metabolism.
    D. Enable the development of individualized drug therapy.

4. Which one of the following DNA methods requires restriction endonucleases?

    A. Single-strand conformational polymorphism.
    B. Single nucleotide polymorphism.
    C. Restriction fragment length polymorphism.
    D. Sanger sequencing.

5. Which one of the following pieces of information can be obtained from proteomic analysis using two-dimensional gel electrophoresis that cannot be obtained from genomic analysis?

    A   Post-translational modifications.
    B. Relative expression of gene sequences.
    C. Protein structure.
    D. Protein-DNA interactions.

6. Which one of the following would not be used to screen for cytochrome P450 2D6 allelic variations?

    A. Single-strand conformational polymorphism.
    B. Expressed sequence tag.

C. Restriction fragment length polymorphism.
D. Direct deoxyribonucleic acid sequencing.

7. Which one of the following regions of the viral genome is deleted to generate retroviral producer cells?

A. Env.
B. Gag.
C. Pol.
D. Psi (Ψ).

8. For which one of the following reasons is it difficult to use PCR amplification to determine microsatellite instability?

A. Polymerase chain reaction products from microsatellite regions are not stable.
B. Taq polymerases nonspecifically add bases to the ends of PCR products.
C. Taq polymerases nonspecifically cleave bases from the ends of PCR products.
D. Polymerase chain reaction amplification does not efficiently amplify small regions of genomic DNA.

9. Use of fluorescent dyes in DNA sequencing reactions aids in which one of the following?

A. Detection of labeled fragments.
B. Lowering sequencing error rates because DNA polymerases have higher affinities for the modified bases.
C. Polymerase chain reaction-based sequencing.
D. Sequencing of multiple repeated stretches of DNA.

10. The advantage of using Pfu polymerase over Taq polymerase for PCR amplifications is which one of the following?

A. Pfu is less expensive.
B. Taq polymerase has a $5'\rightarrow3'$ proofreading activity that lowers its efficiency.
C. Pfu has a $3'\rightarrow5'$ exonuclease activity.
D. Pfu has terminal deoxynucleotidyl transferase activity.

Bioinformatics

Austin L. Hughes, Ph.D.

Key Words

Bioinformatics, homology search, microarray data, phylogenetic analysis, secondary structure prediction, sequence alignment, sequence analysis, and sequence databases.

Abstract

Bioinformatics involves the use of computational methods to analyze the sequence structures and expression of biological macromolecules. The application of these methods now plays an essential role in virtually every aspect of the biological sciences. Important database resources for bioinformatics include the sequence and structural databases maintained by the National Center for Biotechnology Information. Widely used computer programs implement methods for sequence homology search, sequence alignment, estimation of the patterns of nucleotide substitution in deoxyribonucleic acid (DNA) sequences, protein structure prediction, and phylogenetic reconstruction. An increasingly important area of bioinformatics applications is the analysis of gene expression data from microarray studies. This chapter provides an introduction to the principles behind these methods so that readers will be able to apply widely used bioinformatics databases and software and be able to assess literature that makes use of these methods.

Outline

Learning Objectives

1. Recognize the major resources and methods in bioinformatics.
2. Recognize the kinds of questions that can be addressed by bioinformatics studies.
3. Explain how bioinformatics studies apply to pharmacogenomics.
4. Explain how bioinformatics studies apply to pharmacology in general.
5. Analyze studies that apply basic bioinformatics techinques.

Abbreviations in this Chapter

BLAST   Basic Local Alignment Search Tool
CDD   Condensed Domain Database

CLL	Chronic lymphocytic leukemia
DNA	Deoxyribonucleic acid
EMBL	European Molecular Biology Laboratory
GCG	Genetics Computer Group
IL	Interleukin
ME	Minimum evolution
MHC	Major histocompatibility complex
ML	Maximum likelihood
MMDB	Molecular Modeling Database
MP	Maximum parsimony
mRNA	Messenger ribonucleic acid
NCBI	National Center for Biotechnology Information
NJ	Neighbor-joining
NMR	Nuclear magnetic resonance
OMIM	Online Mendelian Inheritance in Man
PAM	Percent Accepted Mutation
PAUP	Phylogenetic Analysis Using Parsimony
PIR	Protein Information Resource
RNA	Ribonucleic acid
SNP	Single nucleotide polymorphism
UPGMA	Unweighted pair-group means using arithmetic averages

Introduction

What is Bioinformatics?

The name bioinformatics suggests an interaction of the biological or biomedical sciences (as indicated by the prefix "bio-") with the information or computational sciences ("informatics"). Of course, the uses of computational methods cover a broad spectrum in biology and medicine today. The computational methods range from the use of computer models of population growth in ecology to the computational problems associated with the storage and retrieval of patient records in clinical medical practice. The Office of Extramural Research at the National Institutes of Health provides a broad definition of "bioinformatics": "Research, development, or application of computational tools and approaches for expanding the use of biological, medical, behavioral or health data, including those to acquire, store, organize, archive, analyze, or visualize such data." (See *http://grants.nih/gov/grants/bistic/bistic.cfm.*) However, those people active in the field of bioinformatics typically use a more restricted definition. For example, Baxevanis and Ouellette see bioinformatics as "loosely defined at the intersection of molecular and computational biology" (Reference 2). Mount's recent textbook Bioinformatics (Reference 10) is subtitled "sequence and genome analysis." In this chapter, a definition that reflects these authors' ideas is used: bioinformatics is the use of computational methods to analyze the sequences, structures, and expression of biological macromolecules.

The pharmaceutical industry has invested heavily in bioinformatics in recent years, and this trend is likely to continue. The main reason for increased interest in bioinformatics is that, given the large amounts of data now being made available by genomic sequencing projects and gene expression studies, there is an "informational bottleneck" in the process of drug discovery and development. If analysis of sequence information can provide a path to guide drug discovery studies through all of this information, it can considerably accelerate the process of identifying possible new drug targets. Computational methods that can uncover patterns in molecular biological data have thus become important tools in the arsenal of pharmacology, as well as in many other branches of both basic and applied biomedical science.

This chapter provides an overview of the database resources and analytical tools for bioinformatics and introduces some of the key ideas and approaches in this rapidly growing field. Readers who are interested in acquiring a hands-on familiarity with computational resources for bioinformatics are encouraged to visit the Web sites providing such resources, many of which are identified in this chapter.

Historical Background

The rise of bioinformatics was made possible by the availability of techniques for determining the amino acid sequences of polypeptides and the three-dimensional structures of proteins. The key paper that launched bioinformatics as a separate discipline was Zuckerkandl and Pauling's discussion of the potential for comparative study of protein sequences (Reference 16). Although the two did not use computers, the discussion showed that protein sequences can be aligned and that studying the differences among sequences at aligned positions can yield important biological information. In subsequent years, the number of available protein sequences expanded greatly, and Margaret Dayhoff had the foresight to realize the need for accumulating these sequences in a database that would be updated periodically. So was born the first sequence database, maintained by Dayhoff and colleagues at the National Biomedical Research Foundation; these database later became known as the Protein Information Resource (PIR), which is available at *http://www-nbrf.georgetown.edu/pir*.

With the advent of rapid methods for sequencing deoxyribonucleic acid (DNA), the number of available nucleotide sequences and predicted protein translations skyrocketed. The first DNA sequence database in North America was the Genbank database, originally maintained at Los Alamos National Laboratory in New Mexico, but subsequently moved to the National Center for Biotechnology Information (NCBI) under auspices of the National Library of Medicine in Bethesda, MD. A European database was founded at the European Molecular Biology Laboratory (EMBL) in

Heidelberg, Germany, and a Japanese database, the DNA Data Bank of Japan in Mishima. All three databases now exchange data continually; so that sequences submitted to any one of the three automatically appears in the other two.

As database resources were being developed in the 1970s and 1980s, the earliest computational methods for analyzing sequences were likewise being developed. Dayhoff played a pioneering role in this new area by developing models of amino acid sequence evolution based on the comparison of closely related and highly conserved sets of proteins. Gibbs and McIntyre in 1970 introduced the dot matrix method of sequence comparison, a tool still widely used to detect regions of sequence similarity. Alignment of nucleotide and amino acid sequences depends on the algorithm developed by Needleman and Wunsch in 1981, which, in aligning two sequences, compares all possible alignments and finds the one that is optimal according to preselected scoring criteria. Finally, Fitch in 1971 introduced the use of phylogenetic methods in reconstructing the evolutionary relationships among sequences in developing the theoretical basis for the method of phylogenetic reconstruction now known as maximum parsimony.

Theoretical Foundations
The discipline of bioinformatics depends on evolutionary reasoning. Aligning molecular sequences and examining the differences among them only make sense if researchers assume that these sequences are descended from a common ancestor and have changed as a result of mutations accumulated throughout time. The theoretical understanding of the mechanisms of sequence change over evolutionary time is based on the work of the great Japanese population geneticist Motoo Kimura. Kimura is best known for developing the so-called Neutral Theory of Molecular Evolution (Reference 8). The neutral theory provides a mathematical formulation of the processes by which the frequency of allelic variants within populations changes over time. This theory is important to bioinformatics analysis because every observable difference between related sequences ultimately originated as a mutation within a population.

The eventual fate of such a mutation—whether it eventually disappears from the population or whether, alternatively, it becomes fixed (i.e., reaches 100 percent frequency)—depends on the interaction of many factors. One obvious factor is natural selection. A new mutation may be selectively disadvantageous or selectively advantageous; selectively advantageous mutations are more likely to increase in frequency in populations than those that are disadvantageous. Even when a new mutation is selectively neutral (i.e., neither advantageous nor disadvantageous), there is some probability that it can increase in frequency in a population and even reach fixation by the random process known as genetic drift.

Kimura was able to obtain elegant mathematical formulations for the probabilities of fixation of mutations under a variety of conditions. Kimura also made the prediction that genetic drift, rather than natural selection, is the predominant factor in evolution at the molecular level. The most widespread form of natural selection is predicted to be selection against deleterious new mutations. This form of natural selection is often called "conservative" or "purifying" natural selection. However, Kimura predicted that cases where natural selection actively favors a new mutation are quite rare at the molecular level. This idea was intensely controversial when Kimura first proposed it in the late 1960s; by now, due to the success of the neutral theory in explaining sequence evolution, Kimura's ideas have gained wide acceptance among biologists.

The mathematics used in formulating the neutral theory is quite advanced, but a few simple expressions can be derived from the theory. Perhaps the most important consequence of the neutral theory, at least for bioinformatics, is expressed in the following simple equation:

$$K = u_T f_0$$

(Equation 1)

where K is the rate of fixation of selectively neutral mutants per generation; u_T is the total mutation rate per generation; and f_0 is the fraction of mutations that are neutral. This equation can be used to predict differences among nucleotide or amino acid sites with respect to the rate of evolutionary change. Assuming a constant mutation rate across sites, the rate of evolutionary change is highest at sites or amino acid sites where f_0 is high. Conversely, the rate of evolutionary change is low at sites where f_0 is low. In most cases, the frequency of selectively advantageous mutants is so low as to be negligible. Thus, most non-neutral mutations are selectively disadvantageous. This means, in turn, that the rate of molecular evolution is high at sites that are not functionally important; most mutations are neutral at these sites because changes make no difference to the fitness of the organism. However, equation 1 predicts that the rate of evolution is low at functionally important sites.

Equation 1 provides the theoretical basis for a wide variety of bioinformatics analyses. For example, one expects that protein-coding regions of a genome evolve more slowly than noncoding regions. This information can be used in gene-finding. Likewise, equation 1 predicts that slowly evolving regions of a protein are likely to be functionally important. Biologists make use of this prediction whenever they align amino acid sequences and look for conserved regions as a tool for predicting protein function.

Database Resources

Introduction to NCBI

The most important Internet source for bioinformatics data and other resources is the Web site maintained by the NCBI (*http://www.ncbi.nlm.nih.gov/*) (Reference 15). This Web site provides access to the Genbank database of DNA sequence data, as well as protein sequence and structure databases. This Web site provides links to related databases such as the Online Mendelian Inheritance in Man (OMIM) database, which provides information regarding the function of mapped human genes, with emphasis on their role in disease. The PubMed database of literature published in all major biomedical research journals can be searched from the same site; each sequence data file is linked to a PubMed file, which includes the complete citation and abstract of the paper in which the sequence was reported. The NCBI site also provides many bioinformatics tools, the most important of which are the Basic Local Alignment Search Tool (BLAST) programs used to conduct homology searches of nucleotide and protein sequence databases (see "Homology Searches").

Types of Databases

Molecular biology databases can be either *factual* databases or *knowledge* databases (Reference 7). Factual databases include databases of nucleotide sequences, amino acid sequences, or three-dimensional protein structures. Factual databases are the results of experimental studies, compiled in the form of a database. Knowledge databases, on the other hand, have the capacity to generate new knowledge from stored knowledge. An example is the Conserved Domain Database (CDD) of conserved protein domain alignments, which not only has grouped protein domains into families, but also includes tools that can be used to predict domains in other protein sequences that are not themselves part of the database.

Factual sequence and structure databases can be classified further as primary or secondary databases. A primary sequence database contains sequences as were submitted by the experimental laboratory that generated the sequence. A secondary database has been "curated" or annotated by the managers of the database. In curation of the data, database managers include additional information not present in the original sequence submission. This may include information on protein structure or information on differences among sequences of the same gene from different laboratories, which may correspond to polymorphisms in the population.

The Genbank Entry

Figure 1 shows an example of a Genbank file or individual entry in the Genbank sequence database. This is a sequence of the messenger ribonucleic acid (mRNA) for the human cytokine interleukin (IL)-10. The

```
LOCUS       HUMIL10                   1601 bp    mRNA    linear   PRI 07-
MAR-1995
DEFINITION  Human interleukin 10 (IL10) mRNA, complete cds.
ACCESSION   M57627
VERSION     M57627.1  GI:186270
KEYWORDS    cytokine synthesis inhibitory factor; interleukin 10.
SOURCE      Human T cell line B21, cDNA to mRNA, clone H15C.
  ORGANISM  Homo sapiens
            Eukaryota; Metazoa; Chordata; Craniata; Vertebrata;
Euteleostomi;
            Mammalia; Eutheria; Primates; Catarrhini; Hominidae; Homo.
REFERENCE   1  (bases 1 to 1601)
  AUTHORS   Vieira,P., de Waal-Malefyt,R., Dang,M.N., Johnson,K.E.,
            Kastelein,R., Fiorentino,D.F., deVries,J.E., Roncarolo,M.G.,
            Mosmann,T.R. and Moore,K.W.
  TITLE     Isolation and expression of human cytokine synthesis inhibitory
            factor cDNA clones: homology to Epstein-Barr virus open reading
            frame BCRFI
  JOURNAL   Proc. Natl. Acad. Sci. U.S.A. 88 (4), 1172-1176 (1991)
  MEDLINE   91142134
   PUBMED   1847510
FEATURES             Location/Qualifiers
     source          1..1601
                     /organism="Homo sapiens"
                     /db_xref="taxon:9606"
                     /map="Unassigned"
                     /clone="H15C"
                     /cell_line="B21"
                     /cell_type="T cell"
     gene            1..1601
                     /gene="IL10"
     CDS             31..567
                     /gene="IL10"
                     /codon_start=1
                     /evidence=experimental
                     /product="interleukin 10"
                     /protein_id="AAA63207.1"
                     /db_xref="GI:186271"
                     /db_xref="GDB:G00-128-636"
                     /translation="MHSSALLCCLVLLTGVRASPGQGTQSENSCTHFPGNLPN-
MLRDL
                     RDAFSRVKTFFQMKDQLDNLLLKESLLEDFKGYLGCQALSEMIQFYLEEVM-
PQAENQD
                     PDIKAHVNSLGENLKTLRLRLRRCHRFLPCENKSKAVEQVKNAFN-
KLQEKGIYKAMSE
                     FDIFINYIEAYMTMKIRN"
     sig_peptide     31..84
                     /gene="IL10"
                     /note="G00-128-636"
     mat_peptide     85..564
                     /gene="IL10"
                     /product="interleukin 10"
                     /note="G00-128-636"
BASE COUNT      445 a     368 c      356 g      432 t
ORIGIN
        1 aaaccacaag acagacttgc aaaagaaggc atgcacagct cagcactgct ctgttgcctg
       61 gtcctcctga ctggggtgag ggccagccca ggccagggca cccagtctga gaacagctgc
      121 acccacttcc caggcaacct gcctaacatg cttcgagatc tccgagatgc cttcagcaga
     1501 tttaactaga atttattcaa ttcctctggg aatgttacat tgtttgtctg tcttcatagc
     1561 agattttaat tttgaataaa taaatgtatc ttattcacat c
```

Figure 1. Example of a Genbank file (locus name HUMIL10, accession number M57627). The file is cross-referenced to the bibliographic resources Medline and PubMed. The portion of the sequence that is coding is indicated under the heading CDS, and the protein translation is provided. The unique identifying numbers (GI numbers) are 186270 for the DNA sequence and 186271 for the amino acid sequence. (For reasons of space, a portion of the deoxyribonucleic acid sequence was eliminated from this figure.) Reprinted with permission from The National Center for Biotechnology Information (*http://www.ncbi.ndm.nih.gov/*).

sequence has been assigned a unique locus name HUMIL10 (Figure 1). As in this example, Genbank entries were formerly assigned locus names to reflect something of the gene's function. As the volume of entries has increased, this practice is no longer followed, and the locus name is now a meaningless string of letters and numbers identical to the accession number. In this example, the accession number is M57627. In addition, there is a number, the GI number, which is uniquely associated with each single version of each single sequence in Genbank and in all of the other database resources at NCBI. Thus, for the example in Figure 1, the GI number for the nucleotide sequence is 186270, whereas that for the protein sequence is 186271. The Genbank file also includes a citation of the original publication from which the sequence was derived. At the NCBI Web site, this reference is linked to PubMed (and its precursor Medline), the bibliographic database. By clicking on this link, one can access the abstract of the original paper.

Another important source of information in each Genbank file is the taxonomic information listed under the heading "Organism". The organism from which the sequence was derived is placed taxonomically, and clicking on the taxonomic categories leads to more information about these categories from NCBI's taxonomy resources. These links, in turn, lead to links to other species in the same taxonomic group from which sequences are available in the database. For example, these links can be used to find out about other primates besides humans for which there are sequences in Genbank.

SWISS-PROT and RefSeq

SWISS-PROT is an example of a secondary or curated database of amino acid sequences. Another example is PIR, which was previously discussed. Both of these databases are directly accessible from the NCBI Web site. SWISS-PROT is probably the more informative of these two databases, as illustrated here by the example of human IL-10 (Figure 2). In the SWISS-PROT file, the human IL-10 sequence has a "locus name" IL10_HUMAN and an accession number P22301 (Figure 2). It also includes a unique GI number, 124292 (Figure 2). Now that protein sequences are derived primarily from nucleotide sequences, researchers must be aware of the nucleotide sequences on which a given protein sequence is based. Thus, the SWISS-PROT file gives cross-references by GI number to all nucleotide sequences of the human IL-10 gene in the Genbank database and their predicted protein translations. In our example, there are 10 such cross-references (Figure 2), including reference to the mRNA sequence shown in Figure 1 and its translation.

Unlike the individual Genbank entry, the SWISS-PROT file lists numerous bibliographic references. There are a total of eight references cited in the IL10_HUMAN entry, which are not shown in Figure 2 to conserve space. These include not only references to papers reporting the sequence, but also references regarding the three-dimensional structure of the

RX   MEDLINE=3D91142134; PubMed=3D1847510; [NCBI, ExPASy, EBI, Israel, =
      Japan]
RA   Vieira P., de Waal-Malefyt R., Dang M.-N., Johnson K.E., Kastelein

CC   -!- FUNCTION: INHIBITS THE SYNTHESIS OF A NUMBER OF CYTOKINES,
CC   INCLUDING IFN-GAMMA, IL-2, IL-3, TNF AND GM-CSF PRODUCED BY
CC   ACTIVATED MACROPHAGES AND BY HELPER T CELLS.
CC   -!- SUBUNIT: HOMODIMER.
CC   -!- SUBCELLULAR LOCATION: Secreted.
CC   -!- TISSUE SPECIFICITY: PRODUCED BY A VARIETY OF CELL LINES, =
INCLUDING
CC   T CELLS, MACROPHAGES, MAST CELLS AND OTHER CELL TYPES.
CC   -!- SIMILARITY: BELONGS TO THE IL-10 FAMILY.
DR   EMBL; M57627; AAA63207.1; -. [EMBL / GenBank / DDBJ] =
[CoDingSequence]
DR   EMBL; AF418271; AAL06594.1; -. [EMBL / GenBank / DDBJ] =
[CoDingSequence]
DR   PIR; A38580; A38580.
DR   PDB; 1ILK; 10-JUL-95. [ExPASy / RCSB]
DR   PDB; 1INR; 14-OCT-96. [ExPASy / RCSB]
DR   MIM; 124092; -. [NCBI / EBI]
DR   GeneCards; IL10.
DR   Ensembl; P22301.
DR   SOURCE; IL10.
DR   InterPro; IPR000098; Interleukin_10.
DR   InterPro; Graphical view of domain structure.
DR   Pfam; PF00726; IL10; 1.
DR   PRINTS; PR01294; INTRLEUKIN10.
DR   ProDom; PD003687; Interleukin_10; 1.
DR   ProDom [Domain structure / List of seq. sharing at least 1 domain]
DR   SMART; SM00188; IL10; 1.
DR   PROSITE; PS00520; INTERLEUKIN_10; 1.
DR   BLOCKS; P22301.
DR   ProtoMap; P22301.
DR   PRESAGE; P22301.
DR   DIP; P22301.
DR   ModBase; P22301.
DR   SWISS-2DPAGE; GET REGION ON 2D PAGE.
KW   Cytokine; Glycoprotein; Signal; 3D-structure.
FT   SIGNAL   1   18   POTENTIAL.
FT   CHAIN   19   178   INTERLEUKIN-10.
FT   DISULFID   30   126   =20
FT   DISULFID   80   132   =20
FT   CARBOHYD   134   134   N-LINKED (GLCNAC...) (POTENTIAL).
SQ   SEQUENCE   178 AA; 20517 MW;   6825E9FA4337CDE4 CRC64;
      MHSSALLCCL VLLTGVRASP GQGTQSENSC THFPGNLPNM LRDLRDAFSR VKTFFQMKDQ

Figure 2. Example of a SWISS-PROT file (locus name IL10-HUMAN, accession number P22301). Brief descriptions of the function, quaternary structure, subcellular location, and tissue specificity are given, as well as structural features of the protein. (For reasons of space, references to the literature and all but the first line of the amino acid sequence have been eliminated from this figure.) Reprinted with permission from SWISS-PROT *http://www.expasy.org/cgi-bin/get-sprot-entry?P22301.*

IL-10 protein. When information on the function and expression of a protein is available, the SWISS-PROT file contains a brief summary of what is known. Information is provided regarding the basic biological function of the protein, its quaternary structure, its subcellular localization, and its tissue expression (Figure 2). Annotations on the sequence (listed under the heading "Features") include information about structurally and functionally distinct regions of the protein. In our example, the residues corresponding to the signal peptide (residues 1-18) are noted (Figure 2). The residues involved in two intra-chain disulfide bonds also are shown (Figure 2).

Recently, NCBI has begun creation of an additional secondary sequence database known as RefSeq.   Refseq provides standard, nonredundant reference sequence. It provides an entry for each known mRNA and protein for human and other organisms, particularly those whose complete genomes have been sequenced or are in the process of being sequenced. Refseq also includes entries for genomic DNA contigs. Figure 3 shows the Refseq entry for human IL-10 mRNA.

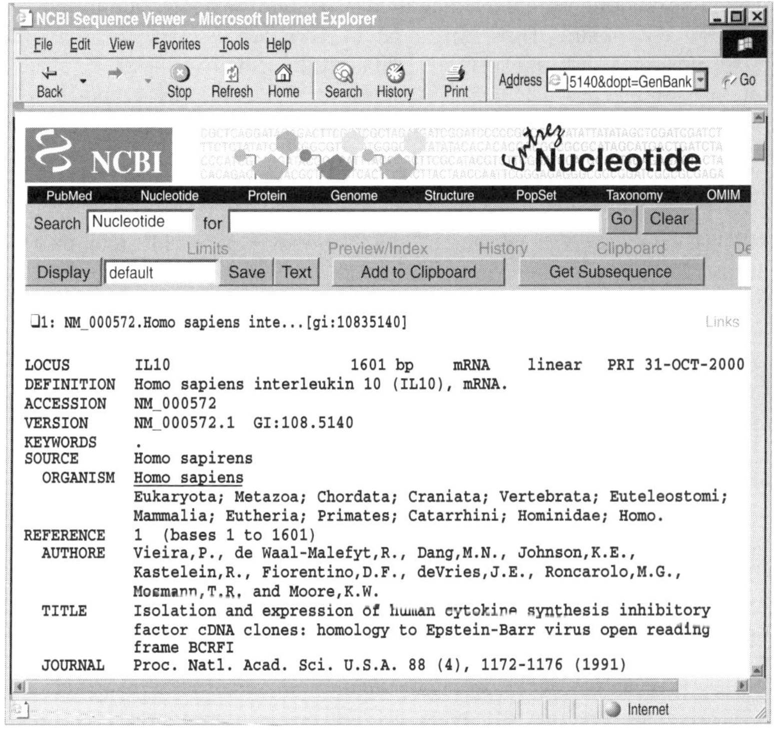

Figure 3. Example of a RefSeq file (accession number NM_000572) as it appears at the NCBI Web site. Reprinted with permission from National Center for Biotechnology Information (*http:/www.ncbi.ndm.nih.gov/*).

Genome Databases

In addition to NCBI, there are many other databases of relevance to bioinformatics. Among the most important are those associated with the genome sequencing projects. The Genome Sequencing Center at Washington University, St. Louis, Missouri, has a Web site with information regarding several of the genome projects, including the human genome (*http://genome.wustl.edu/gsc*). One of the best individual organism Web sites is PlasmoDB (*http://www.plasmodb.org/*), which is devoted to the genomes of malaria parasites (*genus Plasmodium*).

Single Nucleotide Polymorphism Databases

Deoxyribonucleic acid sequence analysis using high-throughput and automated technology is increasingly being used to identify genetic polymorphisms in human genes that are candidates for associations with genetic disease or other phenotypic traits of interest. Of particular interest are single nucleotide polymorphisms (SNPs) (Reference 4, 12). If a given segment of the genome is compared between two humans selected at random, on the average there is about one nucleotide difference per 1000 base pairs. Thus, this type of variation is widespread in the human genome, and one or more SNPs are expected in or close to most protein-coding genes. The dbSNP database at NCBI provides a repository of uncurated SNP data for both humans and other species, submitted directly by investigators (*http://www.ncbi.nlm.nih.gov/SNP/*). The GeneSNPs database provides data on SNPs at more than 500 human protein-coding loci classified by function (*http://www.genome.utah.edu/genesnps/*). The SNP500 database is a project of the National Cancer Institute to type previously known and new SNPs in a reference population of 102 individuals at about 500 loci with known or suspected associations with cancer (*http://snp500cancer.nci. nih.gov/home.cfm*).

Sequence Alignment

Sequence Homology

Two nucleotide sequences are said to be homologous if they are descended from a common ancestral sequence. Similarly, two amino acid sequences are said to be homologous if the nucleotide sequences that encode them are descended from a common ancestral sequence. Strictly speaking, homology is an "either-or" condition; two sequences are either homologous or they are not. Molecular biologists often speak of "percent homology" between two sequences; for example, in biological journals statements often appear such as: The two sequences are "75 percent homologous at the DNA level." Strictly speaking, statements of this kind are not correct. It would be more accurate to say, "The two sequences are 75 percent identical at the DNA level."

Similarly, statements often are made that amino acid sequences are "75 percent homologous" or the like. Again, this use of the term "homologous" should be discouraged. In the case of amino acid sequences, the *percent identity* is defined as the percentage of aligned sites at which the two sequences have identical amino acid residues. The *percent similarity* is defined as the percentage of aligned sites at which the two sequences have chemically similar amino acid residues.

Two sequences are said to be "orthologous" sequences (or orthologs) if they are descended from a common ancestor without gene duplication (Figure 4). However, two sequences are "paralogous" if one or more gene duplication event has intervened since their last common ancestor. Thus, two members of a multigene family are paralogous sequences or paralogs of each other. Both orthologs and paralogs are kinds of homolgous sequences, which can be aligned with one another and compared using the techniques outlined in this chapter.

Dot-matrix Comparisons

The simplest way of looking for evidence of sequence homology is a dot-matrix plot. In this technique, a grid is marked off in segments

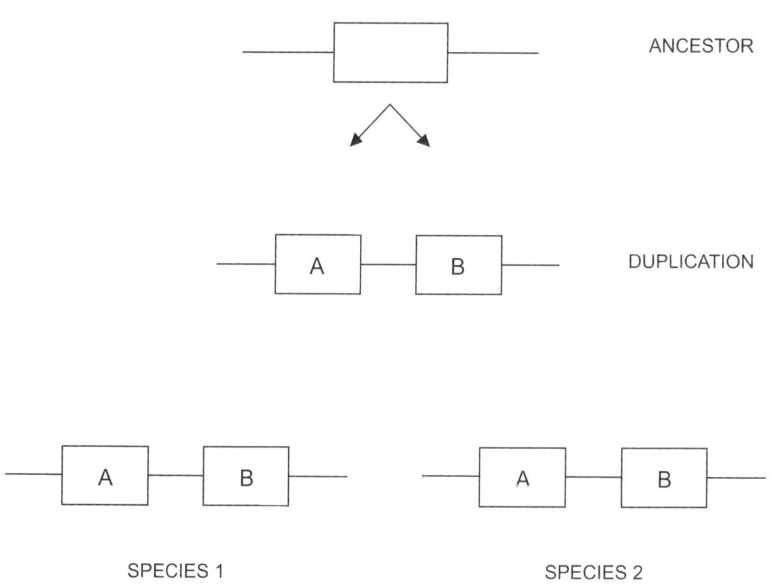

Figure 4. Evolutionary history of two related (homologous) genes (A and B) in two hypothetical species (1 and 2). Gene A in species 1 is orthologous to gene A in species 2, whereas gene B in species 1 is orthologous to gene B in species 2. Gene A is paralogous to gene B.

corresponding to each base in two nucleotide sequences being compared (or to each amino acid residue when two protein sequences are compared) (Figure 5). A dot is placed at every point in the grid where the two sequences are the same. A "diagonal" or line of such dots indicates a stretch of sequence homology (Figure 5). The example in Figure 5 is a comparison of rat and mouse tenascin-X genomic regions. The tenascin-X protein includes numerous fibronection type III repeats, each encoded by a separate exon. The cross-hatching pattern observed in the upper lefthand corner of Figure 5 shows the presence of these repeated exons; the numerous diagonal lines indicate the presence of repeated regions homologous to one another.

Pairwise Sequence Alignment

At the computational level, sequence alignment involves searching each of a pair of sequences for characters that are actually identical or are similar by some criterion (such as chemically similar amino acids) in both sequences. The two sequences are printed out in two rows in such a way that the identical or similar characters are aligned in columns (Figure 6). Nonidentical characters also may be aligned in the same column, or one may introduce a "gap" (a space with no character in it) in one of the sequences to correspond to a character in the other sequence (Figure 6).

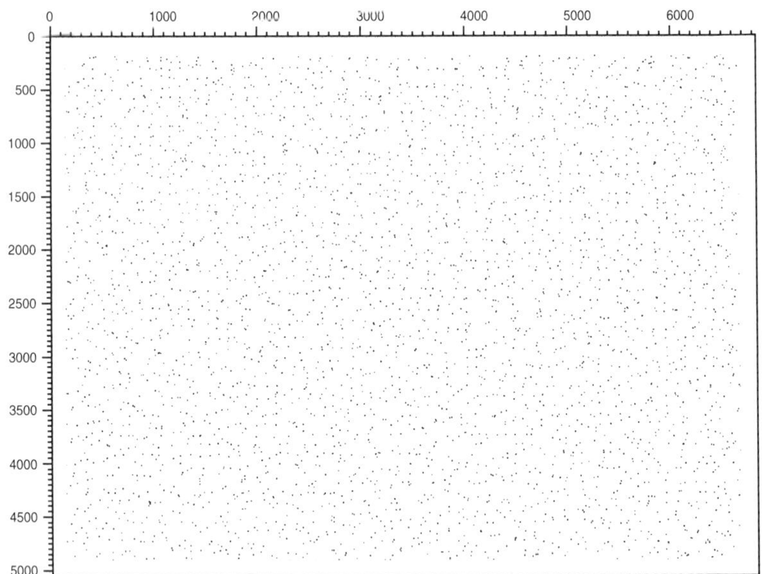

Figure 5. Dot-matrix plot of the genomic regions encoding the tenascin-X genes from mouse and rat.

Thus, at a purely computational level, alignment could be applied to any string of characters, whether biological or not. However, an alignment of nucleotide or amino acid sequences represents something more than the result of a computer algorithm that lines up similar characters. Rather, an alignment embodies an evolutionary hypothesis. Regarding sites at which the alignment shows a difference between the two aligned sequences, the alignment hypothesizes that an evolutionary change has taken place. In the case of nucleotide sequences, this change would involve substitution of one nucleotide for another. In the case of amino acid sequences, the change would involve one or more nucleotide substitutions at the DNA level that result in an amino acid change.

Regarding gaps, the alignment assumes that an insertion or deletion has occurred in one of the sequences since their common ancestor. Usually, it is unknown what the ancestor was like. Thus, it is unknown whether an insertion occurred in one of the sequences or a deletion occurred in the other sequence. Thus, use the term indel (meaning "insertion or deletion") to indicate such an event. Finally, where identical residues are aligned, the alignment assumes that this residue has been conserved over evolutionary time.

Alignment of two sequences may be *global* alignments (which align the sequences throughout their lengths) or *local* alignments (which concentrate on regions of high sequence similarity between the two sequences). For example, in the widely used Genetics Computer Group (GCG) package of bioinformatics computer programs, the GAP program provides a global alignment, whereas the BESTFIT program provides a local alignment.

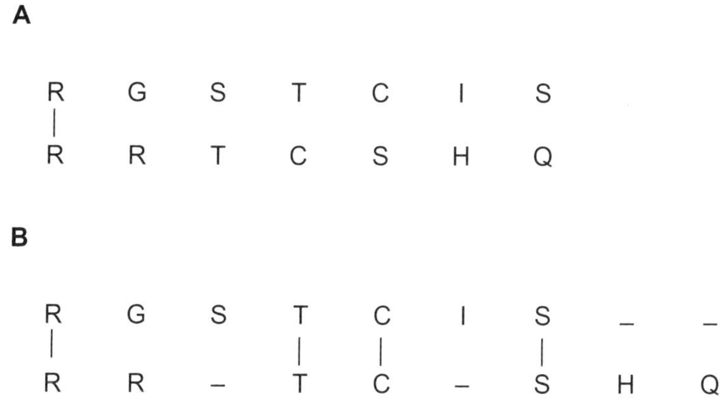

Figure 6. Possible alignments of two hypothetical amino acid sequences. In A, the number of gaps is minimized, but there is only one match of residues in the two sequences (indicated by vertical line). In B, the introduction of gaps increases the number of matches to four.

The usual approach to obtain a global alignment of two sequences uses dynamic programming. This approach is a computational technique that is guaranteed to find the alignment that optimizes a score reflecting the quality of the alignment. The score is based on a function that takes into account both mismatches and gaps. Because there is no straightforward way to develop a common currency for mismatches and gaps, a function (called a "gap penalty") must be defined to translate gaps into the same currency as mismatches. Different gap penalties may produce different results, and, in practice, it is often a good idea to try many different gap penalties to see how much difference the choice of gap penalty makes in the analysis of a given data set.

The simplest way to score mismatches is simply to tally the number of nonidentical residues. However, in the case of amino acid sequences, more sophisticated methods are available, based on the fact that certain amino acid replacements are more likely to occur in nature than others. The earliest attempt to incorporate information on the likelihood of particular amino acid replacements was the Percent Accepted Mutation (PAM) matrix, which was developed in the 1970s by Dayhoff. The PAM matrix was based on comparisons of closely related, highly conserved amino acid sequences for which the alignment was nonproblematic. In these comparisons, the frequency of amino acid replacements that have actually occurred in nature are counted. Such a replacement is said to be an "accepted mutation" because it has been "accepted" in the evolutionary process; in other words, it has not been eliminated by purifying selection. Another substitution matrix commonly used in alignments is the BLOSUM matrix. This matrix is based on observed amino acid differences in a sample of conserved amino patterns, called blocks.

Intuitively, one might predict that empirically derived matrices of amino acid substitution probabilities, such as PAM and BLOSUM, might not always accurately reflect the evolutionary process. These matrices are derived from conserved sequences, and evolution is not always conservative. When natural selection actually favors changes of function of proteins, nonconservative amino acid replacements often take place (Reference 6). However, in practice, such natural selection has little impact on alignments. First, as predicted by the neutral theory (Reference 8), evolution is mostly conservative. Second, the relatively small number of cases where natural selection acts to promote nonconservative changes typically only involves a small number of residues. A small number of nonconservative changes does not seem to have a marked effect on observed alignments.

In the case of DNA sequences, scoring matrices can be based on empirical comparisons of sequences or on a theoretical model of nucleotide substitution (see Nucleotide Sequence Comparisons). For example, in many nucleotide sequences, there is a higher rate of transition (mutation from one purine to another or from one pyrimidine to another) than of transversion (mutation from purine to pyrimidine or vice versa). Such a transitional bias can be readily accommodated on a scoring system for use in sequence alignment.

Multiple Sequence Alignment

The problem of simultaneously aligning more than two sequences using the criteria similar to those used in pairwise alignment is computationally difficult. Therefore, the usual approach taken to multiple sequence alignments starts with pairwise alignments and then, after using the scores of pairwise aligments to construct a phylogenetic tree (see the Phylogenetic Reconstruction Section), allows the phylogenetic tree to guide the sequential addition of sequences to the alignment. This approach was implemented in the widely used CLUSTALW program.

The alignment of mammalian IL-10 sequences shown in Figure 7 was produced by the CLUSTALW program. The program output marks with an asterisk sites conserved in all the sequences in the alignment. Examining such an alignment is a way of looking for sites that might be important for the function of the protein in question. In terms of equation 1, sites that are functionally important are expected to have a low f_0 and, thus, a low rate of

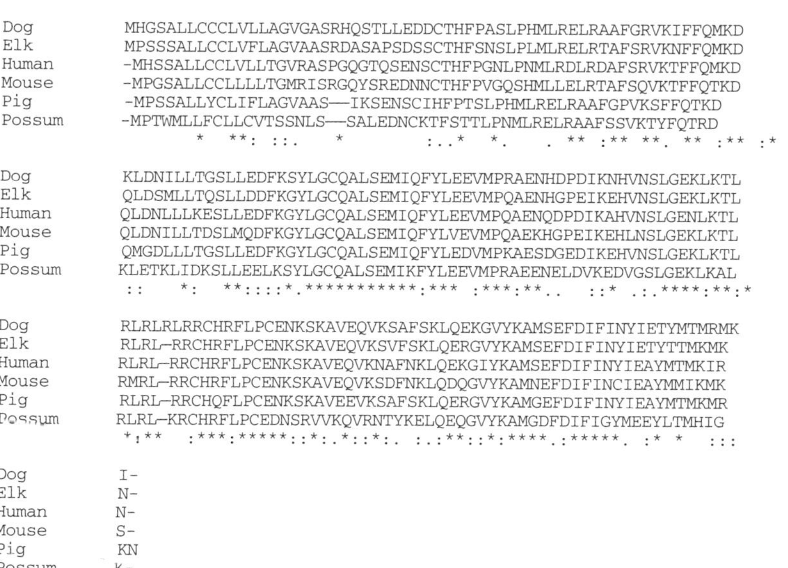

```
Dog      MHGSALLCCCLVLLAGVGASRHQSTLLEDDCTHFPASLPHMLRELRAAFGRVKIFFQMKD
Elk      MPSSSALLCCLVFLAGVAASRDASAPSDSSCTHFSNSLPLMLRELRTAFSRVKNFFQMKD
Human    -MHSSALLCCLVLLTGVRASPGQGTQSENSCTHFPGNLPNMLRDLRDAFSRVKTFFQMKD
Mouse    -MPGSALLCCLLLLTGMRISRGQYSREDNNCTHFPVGQSHMLLELRTAFSQVKTFFQTKD
Pig      -MPSSALLYCLIFLAGVAAS——IKSENSCIHFPTSLPHMLRELRAAFGPVKSFFQTKD
Possum   -MPTWMLLFCLLCVTSSNLS——SALEDNCKTFSTTLPNMLRELRAAFSSVKTYFQTRD
                  *   **:  ::.      *         :..*   *.     .  ** :** **. ** :** :*

Dog      KLDNILLTGSLLEDFKSYLGCQALSEMIQFYLEEVMPRAENHDPDIKNHVNSLGEKLKTL
Elk      QLDSMLLTQSLLDDFKGYLGCQALSEMIQFYLEEVMPQAENHGPEIKEHVNSLGEKLKTL
Human    QLDNLLLKESLLEDFKGYLGCQALSEMIQFYLEEVMPQAENQDPDIKAHVNSLGENLKTL
Mouse    QLDNILLTDSLMQDFKGYLGCQALSEMIQFYLVEVMPQAEKHGPEIKEHLNSLGEKLKTL
Pig      QMGDLLLTGSLLEDFKGYLGCQALSEMIQFYLEDVMPKAESDGEDIKEHVNSLGEKLKTL
Possum   KLETKLIDKSLLEELKSYLGCQALSEMIKFYLEEVMPRAEENELDVKEDVGSLGEKLKAL
          ::     *:   **:::.*.************.*** :***.**..   ::*  .:..****.**.*

Dog      RLRLRLRRCHRFLPCENKSKAVEQVKSAFSKLQEKGVYKAMSEFDIFINYIETYMTMRMK
Elk      RLRL—RRCHRFLPCENKSKAVEQVKSVFSKLQERGVYKAMSEFDIFINYIETYTTMKMK
Human    RLRL—RRCHRFLPCENKSKAVEQVKNAFNKLQEKGIYKAMSEFDIFINYIEAYMTMKIR
Mouse    RMRL—RRCHRFLPCENKSKAVEQVKSDFNKLQDQGVYKAMNEFDIFINCIEAYMMIKMK
Pig      RLRL—RRCHQFLPCENKSKAVEEVKSAFSKLQERGVYKAMGEFDIFINYIEAYMTMKMR
Possum   RLRL—KRCHRFLPCEDNSRVVKQVRNTYKELQEQGVYKAMGDFDIFIGYMEEYLTMHIG
          *,**   :***.*****::*:.*::*:.  :..:**::*:****.:*****. :*  *   :::

Dog      I-
Elk      N-
Human    N-
Mouse    S-
Pig      KN
Possum   K-
```

Figure 7. Alignment of amino acid sequences of interleukin-10 from selected mammals, produced by the CLUSTALW program. Underneath the sequences, '*' indicates a residue conserved in all sequences in the alignment; ':' indicates a position at which all residues have high similarity scores to one another; '.' indicates a position at which all residues have moderately high similarity scores to one another.

molecular evolution. Thus, by reasoning backward from evolutionary conservation, potentially important sites can be identified.

Homology Searches

One of the most important tools in biological research is a homology search, which involves taking a sequence of interest and searching a sequence database for possible homologs. The NCBI Web site provides free access to a family of tools for searching its nucleic acid and protein sequence databases. This is the BLAST family (Reference 1). These programs use a fast search strategy that involves searching for common sequence "words" or short stretches of sequence similarity between the query sequence and sequences in the database. The BLAST includes programs for searching both DNA and amino acid sequences. With coding sequences, it is typically preferable to search at the amino acid sequence level unless one is only interested in finding closely related sequences. Because of the higher rate of substitution at synonymous sites in coding regions than at nonsynonymous sites (see the Nucleotide Sequence Comparisons section), synonymous sites provide little evolutionary information for comparison of distantly related sequences.

Figure 8 illustrates the NCBI Web page for the BLASTP program, which is the ordinary method for conducting a homology search at the amino acid level. Input either a GI number for a protein sequence from any of the NCBI batabases or paste in the sequence itself using a word processor. The sequence that is pasted in should be in FASTA format (named for FASTA, another homology search program). In this format, the first line includes the character ">" followed by the name of the sequence (an arbitrary string of characters). The second and following lines include the sequence in the single-letter code for amino acids (either small or capital letters); the symbol "X" is used for undetermined amino acids.

As a default, BLAST searches all nonredundant sequences in the NCBI databases, both *primary* and *secondary*, (referred to as "nr" databases). Alternatively, the search can be limited to a given database (such as Swiss-Prot), to a group of organisms (such as primates or bacteria), or an individual species. The BLAST algorithm searches for the highest-scoring ungapped local alignment between the query sequence and the database in question and gives this alignment a score (S). The output of the BLASTP program lists potentially homologous sequences in order of decreasing S (Figure 9). In addition, a probability value called the "expect score" (E) is given. The E represents the probability of observing a score of the observed value S or higher in a search of the chosen database with the given query sequence by chance alone; in other words, E is the probability of a false-positive. Thus, the lower the E value, the stronger the evidence of homology.

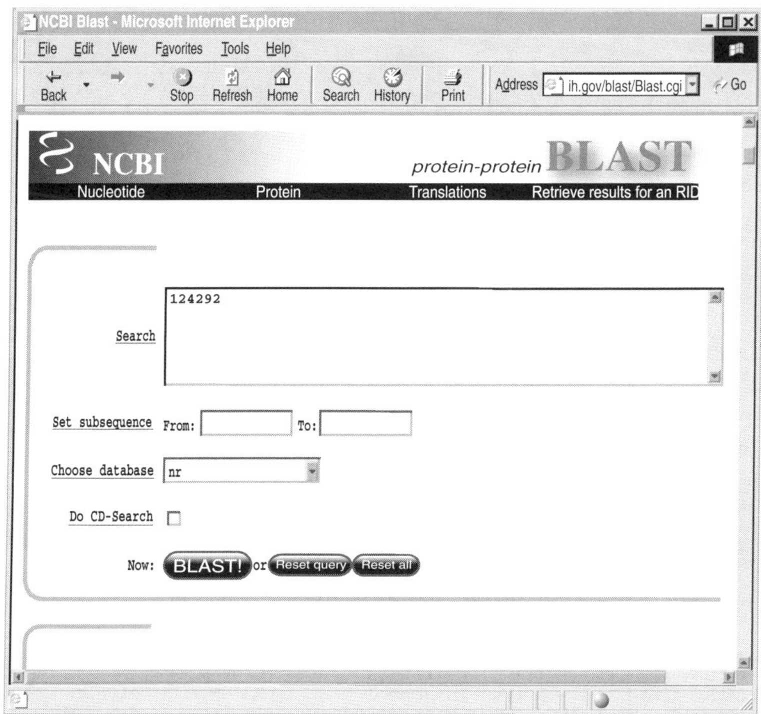

Figure 8. The Basic Local Alignment Search Tool (BLAST) homology search tool for proteins, showing the box in which one can type or paste a GI number corresponding to a query sequence (here 124292, the number for the human interleukin-10 sequence in Figure 2) or the query sequence itself. Reprinted with permission from National Center for Biotechnology Information (*http://www.ncbi.nlm.nih.gov/*).

Sequence Comparisons

Amino Acid Sequence Comparisons

Given an alignment between two sequences, the simplest way of characterizing the amount of difference between them is simply to compute the proportion of sequence identity. To compute this value, divide the number of identical sites by the number of aligned sites. For example, there are 178 aligned amino acid sites shared between human and mouse IL-10 (Figure 7), and there are differences between the two sequences at 48 of the sites. Thus, it can be said that the sites are 130/178 or 73 percent identical, or 27 percent different.

However, it is obvious that it is uncertain that, since the last common ancestor of human and mouse, only 48 amino acid changes have occurred in the two IL-10 proteins. Just because a site differs between the two proteins does not permit the statement to be made that only one change has occurred

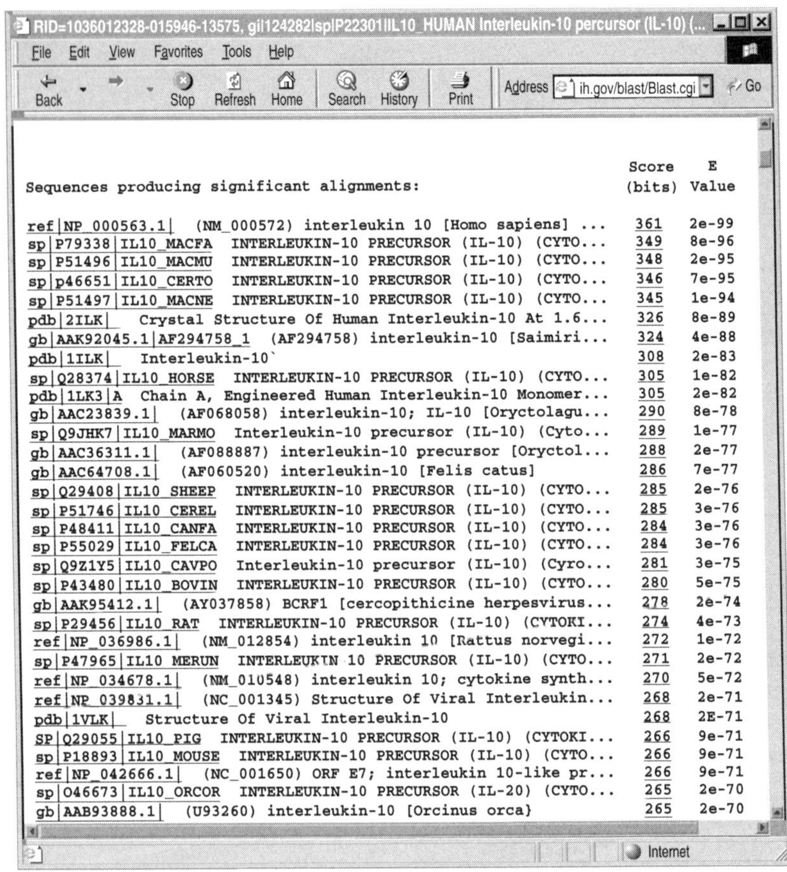

Figure 9. Output of the BLAST search initiated in Figure 8, showing the alignment scores (S) in decreasing order and the corresponding expect scores (E). Reprinted with permission from National Center for Biotechnology Information (*http://www.ncbi.nlm.nih.gov/*).

at that site since the last common ancestor. More than one change may have taken place. For this reason, biologists often use a statistical model to estimate the effects of unobserved changes that may have taken place in a sequence during the course of evolution.

For amino acid sequence, the simplest such model assumes that the number of amino acid replacements that have occurred at each site follows a Poisson distribution. Assuming this model yields a simple correction formula which can be used to estimate the number of animo acid replacements per site (d_{AA}) given the proportion of amino acid difference (p):

$$d_{AA} = -\ln(1-p)$$

(Equation 2)

The variance due to the error of estimation of d_{AA} is given by

$$V(d_{AA}) = p/[(1-p)n]$$

(Equation 3)

where n is the number of sites compared. In the case of the human and mouse IL-10 amino acid sequences (Figure 7), d_{AA} is estimated as 0.314 ± 0.43 (the standard error of estimation, or square root of the variance).

The Poisson correction formula makes some simplifying assumptions that are likely to be only about true under the best of circumstances. For example, it assumes that the rate of amino acid replacement is the same at all sites in the sequence. However, in most data sets, rates vary from site to site. Indeed, as previously discussed, the neutral theory predicts that sites that are functionally important evolve more slowly than sites of lesser importance to the protein's biological role. Because of the limitations of the Poisson model, some considerably more sophisticated ways of correcting statistically for unobserved changes in amino acid sequences have been developed.

One widely used method involves a so-called gamma correction. This method assumes that rates vary among sites, but that the variation among sites follows a kind of statistical distribution known as a gamma distribution. Other methods may use an empirically derived model of amino acid sequence evolution like the PAM matrix previously discussed.

Nucleotide Sequence Comparisons

As with amino acid sequences, DNA sequences can be compared simply by counting the percentage of identity or of difference. Between the DNA sequences for human and mouse IL-10 (data not shown), there are 101 differences at 534 sites; thus, the sequences are 18.9 percent different or 81.1 percent identical. Again, as with amino acid sequences, it may be desirable to correct the raw proportion of difference to take into account unobserved events in the past. The simplest correction formula is the Jukes-Cantor correction (Reference 11). This formula is based on the simplest possible model of DNA sequence evolution, which assumes that all four bases are used with equal frequency, and that there is a single substitution probability for all possible DNA substitutions. When this formula is applied to human and mouse IL-10, the number of nucleotide substitutions per site between the two sequences is estimated at 0.218 ± 0.023. For the details of the computation, see Reference 11.

More complex models assume that there are different probabilities for different types of substitution. For example, Kimura's two-parameter model assumes that there are different probabilities for transitions and transversions. A fully parameterized model for DNA sequences would assume 12 different substitution probabilities; that is, there would be a different substitution probability of each possible nucleotide substitution. In addition, a model can accommodate differences among sites with respect to the rate of substitution, for instance, by assuming that rates vary among sites following a gamma distribution. One problem with complex models is that, in comparing short sequences, there would not be enough information available to estimate every parameter accurately. Therefore, simpler substitution models are usually used in most applications, in spite of the fact that they make biologically questionable simplifying assumptions. However, when the level of difference between two sequences is small, model choice makes relatively little practical difference because all models yield similar results.

In the case of coding sequences, there is one important feature that is not captured by a simple model that assumes a constant rate of evolution at every site. In a protein-coding sequence, synonymous mutations (those that do not result in an amino acid change) can be distinguished from nonsynonymous mutations (those that do result in an amino acid change). In most protein-coding sequences, the rate of evolution at synonymous sites is much faster than that at nonsynonymous sites. That this should occur is a prediction of the neutral theory. Because synonymous mutations do not change the amino acid, they are all expected to be neutral or almost so. Thus, in the terminology of equation 1, f_0 is close to 1 at synonymous sites. At nonsynonymous sites, however, f_0 is expected to vary from site to site. It is expected to be much higher at sites which are not important to the protein's function than at sites which are important to the protein's function. But on average f_0 at nonsynonymous sites is expected to be much lower than f_0 at synonymous sites.

For this reason, it is often useful to estimate the number of synonymous nucleotide substitutions per synonymous site (symbolized d_S or K_S) separately from the number of nonsynonymous nucleotide substitutions per nonsynonymous site (symbolized d_N or K_a). For example, in the case of the human and mouse IL-10 sequences, d_S was estimated at 0.499 ± 0.087, whereas d_N was estimated at 0.156 ± 0.021. Thus, in this example, substitutions at synonymous sites are estimated to have accumulated more than 3 times as rapidly as substitutions at synonymous sites.

These estimates were produced by Nei and Gojobori's method, a widely used method of estimating numbers of synonymous and nonsynonymous substitution; for details of the computation, see Reference 11. This and some other methods of estimating numbers of synonymous and nonsynonymous substitution are available in the MEGA2 program (Reference 9), which is available at *http://www.megasoftware.net*.

Because of the higher rate of substitution at synonymous sites, synonymous sites eventually accumulate so many changes that no meaningful evolutionary information is present. Assuming the simplest model of DNA sequence evolution (with equal use of all four nucleotides), two DNA sequences are saturated with changes when they are 75 percent different (25 percent similar). At this point, the two sequences are no more similar to each other than two random sequences would be. If there is a bias in nucleotide content (for example, leading to a preference for G and C over A and T), the point of saturation will be reached at an even lower percentage of difference. In practice, given the rates of mutation that occur in eukaryotes, synonymous sites are at or near saturation when comparing sequences whose most recent common ancestor was about 200 million years ago.

Examining the pattern of synonymous and nonsynonymous nucleotide substitution can be a powerful tool for giving clues about protein function. Because synonymous mutations are largely selectively neutral, they accumulate over evolutionary time at a rate which is expected to be close to the mutation rate [equation 1]. Thus, in most cases, d_S is relatively similar across different regions of a gene. However, d_N varies from one region to another, depending on the strength of purifying selection.

For example, Table 1 shows estimates of d_S and d_N between the human and mouse platelet-derived growth factor receptor-α genes, computed separately for different regions of the gene. These gene regions correspond to structurally distinct region of this protein, which is a transmembrane receptor belonging to the immunoglobulin superfamily. The extracelluar portion of the molecule includes four immunoglobulin superfamily C-set domains (labeled C1-C4) and one immunoglobulin superfamily V-set domain (Table 1). The ratio of the highest d_S value (in C4) to the lowest (in the leader) is about 1.7. However, the ratio of the highest d_N value (in the leader) to the lowest (in the cytoplasmic domain) is about 22.4. Thus,

Table 1. Numbers of Synonymous Substitutions per Synonymous Site (d_S) and of Nonsynonymous Substitutions per Nonsynonymous Site (d_N), with Standard Errors, in the Comparison of Different Domains of Platelet-derived Growth Factor Receptor between Human and Mouse

Protein Domain	d_S	d_N
Leader	0.513 ± 0.221	0.179 ± 0.069
C1	0.614 ± 0.145	0.074 ± 0.019
C2	$0.752 + 0.179$	0.084 ± 0.022
C3	0.631 ± 0.139	0.073 ± 0.019
C4	0.851 ± 0.193	0.083 ± 0.020
V	0.617 ± 0.125	0.119 ± 0.023
Transmembrane	0.730 ± 0.278	0.049 ± 0.031
Cytoplasmic	0.715 ± 0.068	0.008 ± 0.003

there is a much greater variance from one domain to another in d_N values than there is in d_S values. The extremely low d_N value in the cytoplasmic domain suggests that this region is highly conserved evolutionarily, suggesting that it is likely to be functionally important. Note that d_S is not particularly low in the cytoplasmic domain; thus, low d_N in this domain cannot be attributed to a low mutation rate but must be the result of strong purifying selection on this domain, which in turn implies functional importance.

In a minority of genes, there is a reversal of the usual pattern, with higher rates of nonsynonymous than synonymous evolution. This unusual pattern is evidence that natural selection has acted to favor changes at the amino acid level. This type of selection is referred to as positive Darwinian selection, to distinguish it from the much more widespread negative or purifying selection. Perhaps the best-documented case of this sort involves the molecules of the vertebrate major histocompatibility complex (MHC), which present peptides to T cells. In the codons encoding peptide-binding region of the MHC molecule, d_N exceeds d_S, whereas in the rest of the gene d_S exceeds d_N as in most genes. This highly unusual pattern of nucleotide substitution indicates that natural selection has acted to diversify the amino acid sequences in the peptide-binding regions of MHC molecules, presumably because of the enhanced immune surveillance conferred on a host that is able to bind a diverse array of foreign peptides (Reference 6).

Phylogenetic Reconstruction

General Considerations

One way of thinking of a phylogenetic tree is as a picture or diagram that shows how similar the members of a set of sequences are to one another. However, biologists are accustomed to thinking of phylogenetic trees not simply as illustrations of sequence similarity but as actual representations of evolutionary history. Thus, the goal of phylogenetic reconstruction is not simply to cluster sequences that are similar but sequences that are closely related evolutionarily. Often, evolutionary biologists speak of the "true tree" as the ideal diagram that would represent the true relationships among the sequences, if they were known. What the researcher is trying to do in phylogenetic tree reconstruction is to find a good estimate or reconstruction of the true tree; but, in reality, researchers typically will not know whether this reconstruction faithfully reproduces the true tree. Thus, a phylogenetic tree is the expression of a hypothesis regarding the evolutionary relationships among the sequences used in reconstructing the tree.

It is useful to make a distinction between gene trees and species trees. A gene tree shows the relationship among a set of homologous genes, which may include orthologs, paralogs, or some mixture of orthologs and paralogs. A species tree shows the relationship among members of a set of species. In molecular evolutionary studies, it is customary to use a gene tree to estimate the species tree, but even if the gene tree is reconstructed with perfect accuracy, the researcher still may not have the true species tree.

There are two main biological reasons why a gene tree may not be the same as the species tree. First, to reconstruct the species tree from sequence data, be certain that all the genes used are orthologs rather than paralogs. However, in practice, it may be difficult to be certain that the genes are all orthologs. For instance, if there is no good knowledge of the genome of one of the species used, there may be a duplicate locus of which the researcher is unaware. In addition, if two or more speciation events occur in a short time window (1 or 2 million years or less), genetic polymorphism in the ancestral species may be apportioned to the descendent species in a way that does not reflect the species' actual relationships.

Reconstructing the true gene tree is problematic for many reasons. One reason is that there are many possible trees from which to choose. Phylogenetic trees are classified as rooted. In a rooted tree, there is one node known as the root, and a unique path leads from that node to any other nodes in such a way that the path corresponds to evolutionary time (Figure 10). The root, thus, corresponds to the most recent common ancestor of all the sequences in the tree. For n sequences, the number of possible bifurcating rooted trees is given by the formula:

$$N_R = (2n\text{-}3)! \, / \, 2^{\,n\text{-}2} \, (n\text{-}2)!$$
(Equation 4)

The number of possible bifurcating unrooted trees is given by the formula
$$N_U = (2n\text{-}5)! \, / \, 2^{\,n\text{-}3} \, (n\text{-}3)!$$
(Equation 5)

As can easily be seen by substituting values for n in these equations, the number of possible trees increases rapidly as *n* increases. For n = 4, there are three possible rooted trees and 15 possible unrooted trees. But for n = 14, there are more than 300 billion possible unrooted trees and almost 8 trillion possible rooted trees.

Many different methods have been proposed to help scientists decide among possible trees, and there has been considerable controversy among advocates of different methods. However, the most commonly used methods all share a similar set of assumptions: that the phylogeny that explains the observed data most simply is likely to be the true tree. In practice, three different criteria have been used to obtain this simplest phylogenetic hypothesis: 1) the maximum parsimony (MP) criterion, which seeks the tree that assumes the smallest number of mutational steps (character changes) among sequences; 2) the minimum evolution (ME) criterion, which starts from a matrix of pairwise distances among sequences and seeks the tree that

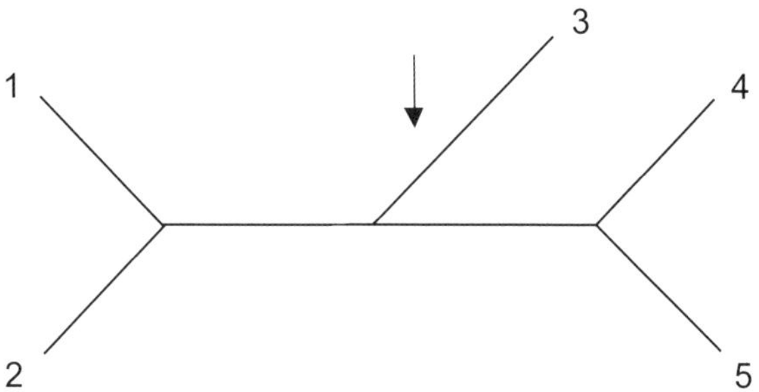

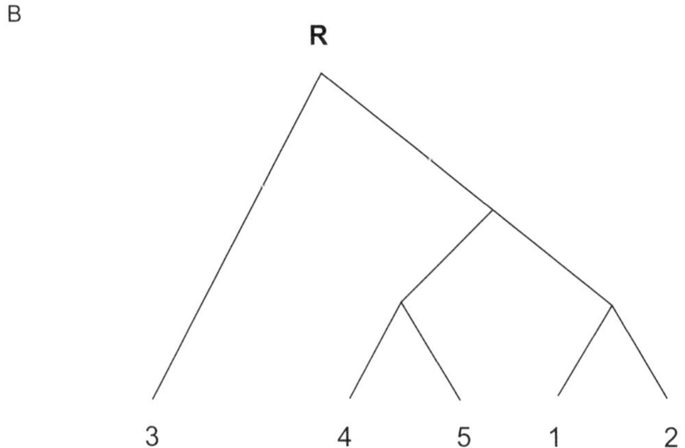

Figure 10. (A) An unrooted phylogenetic tree. (B) The same tree with the root placed as indicated by the arrow in (A).

assumes the minimum amount of evolutionary change; and 3) the maximum likelihood (ML) criterion, which assumes a model of sequence evolution, computes the likelihood of the observed sequence data and a given phylogenetic tree, and chooses the tree that gives the highest likelihood.

Maximum Parsimony

The MP criterion is the simplest. It is based on the concept of *informative sites*. An informative site is one that favors certain trees over others. The MP tree is the one that is supported by the most informative sites. This idea is easily illustrated in the case of four sequences (Figure 11A). Not all variable sites are informative sites. In this example, site 2 is an informative site because it supports one of the three possible unrooted trees over the others (Figure 11B). Site 2 supports tree I over trees II and III because, if tree I is true, only one mutational event at site 2 need be assumed, whereas two mutational events are required if assuming tree II or tree III (Figure 11B). By contrast, site 3 is not an informative site because one must assume two mutational events at this site under each of the three possible trees (Figure 11C).

The branch-and-bound computer algorithm is guaranteed to find the MP tree, but this algorithm can be time consuming when the number of sequences is large. For large numbers of sequences, there are heuristic search algorithms available, which are not guaranteed to find the MP tree, but typically come close. The Phylogenetic Analysis Using Parsimony (PAUP) program (Reference 14) is a widely used program that offers a variety of useful features for phylogenetic reconstruction, particularly using the MP method.

In some cases, there may be many different MP trees, all of which are equally parsimonious. However, these usually differ only in minor details. The PAUP and similar programs can compute the consensus tree of many equally parsimonious trees. A *strict consensus* tree includes only those branches which appear in all of the MP trees.

A *majority rule* consensus tree includes branches found in a majority of the MP trees.

Figure 12 shows the majority rule consensus tree of the mammalian IL-10 amino acid sequences from Figure 7. This is the consensus of four equally parsimonious trees, each assuming 187 amino acid replacements. The numbers on the branches indicate the percentage of the four trees in which the branch occurred. Ordinarily, the MP method produces an unrooted tree. However, the tree can be rooted based on biological knowledge. In the case of the IL-10 tree, the possum is the only marsupial in the set of species analyzed. Thus, it is reasonable to hypothesize that the possum IL-10 diverged before that of placental mammals. In this case, possum IL-10 is called an "outgroup" (i.e., a sequence that is known [or believed] to be more distantly related to the other sequences analyzed than the other sequences are to each other). The safest way to root an unrooted tree is with a known outgroup, although other methods for rooting trees in the absence of an outgroup have been proposed (Reference 11).

Minimum Evolution and Other Distance Methods

In using the ME criterion, start with a matrix of pairwise differences among sequences. These might simply be the uncorrected proportion of difference, or they might be corrected for multiple hits according to some statistical model (as previously discussed). The basic idea of the ME method

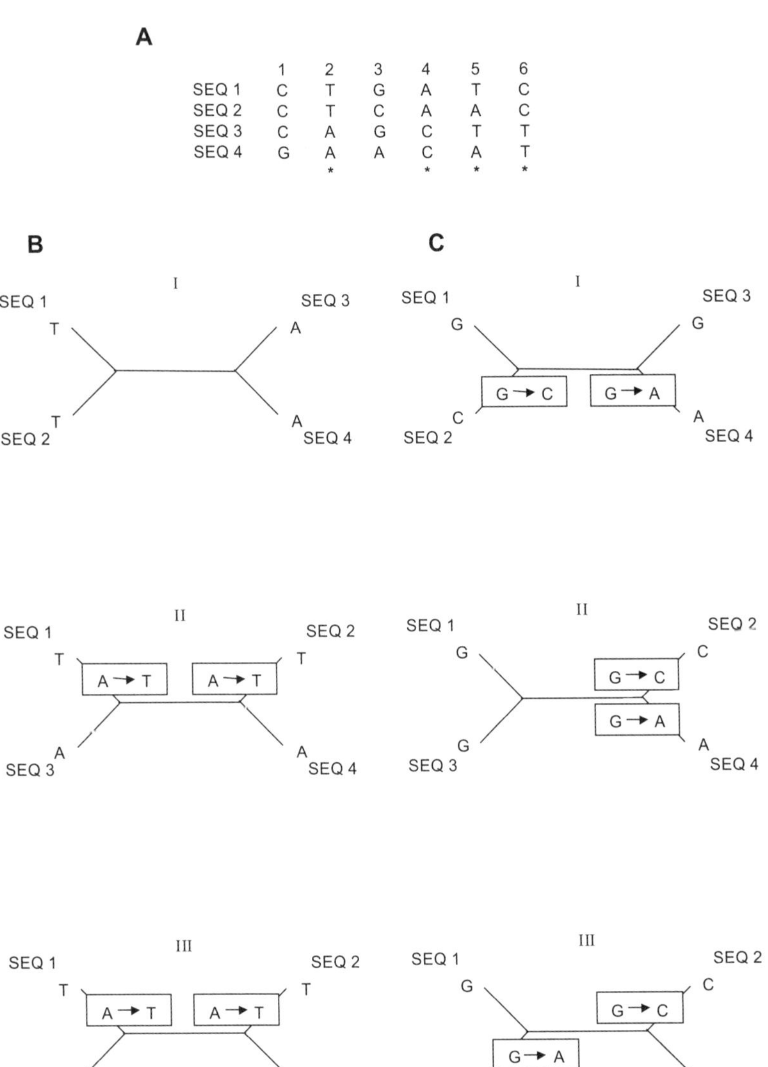

Figure 11. (A) Hypothetical sequences (SEQ1-SEQ4) illustrating the concept of phylogenetically informative sites. Asterisks indicate informative sites. (B) The pattern of evolutionary change that must be assumed at site 2 for each of the three possible unrooted trees (I, II, and III). Site 2 is an informative site because it favors tree I over trees II and III; that is, under tree I only one mutational change at site 2 need be assumed whereas under tree II or tree III two mutational changes must be assumed. (C) The pattern of evolutionary change that must be assumed at site 3 under the three possible unrooted trees. Site 3 is not an informative site because two mutational changes must be assumed under all three trees.

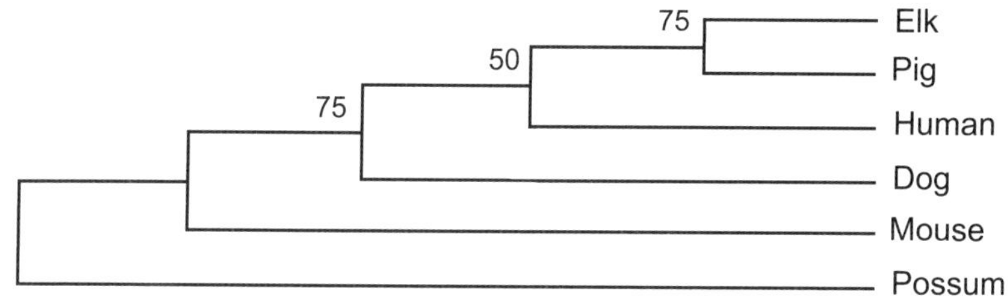

Figure 12. A majority rule consensus tree of four equally parsimonious trees based on the amino acid sequences is shown in A. Numbers on the branches correspond to the percentage of the four trees supporting the branch.

is that, given the distance matrix and a tree topology, a statistical method is used such as ordinary least squares to estimate the lengths of the branches in the tree that provide the best fit to the observed distances. If this is done for all possible trees, the ME tree is the one that provides the shortest total sum of the branch lengths for the whole tree.

In practice, unless the number of sequences is small, it is not possible to search all possible topologies to find the ME tree. Therefore, heuristic methods are used to find a tree that is at least close to the ME tree. One of the most widely used such heuristic methods is the neighbor-joining (NJ) method, which is a stepwise method based on minimizing the sum of the branch lengths in the tree as pairs of closely related sequences ("neighbors") are successively joined. The MEGA2 program (Reference 9) provides an easily accessible suite of methods for constructing NJ trees based on a variety of distance measures and for searching around the NJ tree for shorter trees.

Because NJ and ME are based on a distance matrix, they are sometimes classified as "distance methods." Another distance method is "unweighted pair-group means using arithmetic averages" (UPGMA). This method is now mainly of historical interest. The UPGMA method successively clusters sequences that have the lowest distances, but it is sensitive to unequal rates of evolution in different portions of the tree. Users of the GrowTree program in the popular GCG package should be aware of this and avoid the UPGMA option in most cases because most molecular data sets do not show a constant rate of evolution.

Maximum Likelihood

Maximum likelihood methods are time consuming computationally. For this reason, they are used less frequently than MP and NJ methods. However, as available computational power has increased, the tendency to use ML methods has increased also. In some respects, this is unfortunate because it is not clear that ML provides any advantages over simpler methods. Because ML is based on an explicit model of sequence evolution, the tendency is to use as complex a model as possible, in the belief that a more complex model is more likely to be biologically realistic. Yet it is unlikely that the same complex model holds true for every branch of a phylogenetic tree. Thus, a simple model often provides better results in practice, even if the simple model represents only an approximation of biological reality. However, if a simple model is used, it is unclear what is to be gained from using the complex and time-consuming ML algorithm, when much more rapid search methods (such as heuristic searches for MP or ME trees) are available for use with simple models.

Structure Prediction

The Brookhaven Protein Database (*http://www.pdb.bnl.gov*) maintains a database of protein structures obtained by crystallographic or nuclear magnetic resonance (NMR) methods. These structures also are available from NCBI's Molecular Modeling Database (MMDB). By using the BLAST tools, a new protein sequence can be used as a query to search for homologous proteins whose three-dimensional structures are known. If a query sequence has a close relative whose structure has been determined, this structure provides the best possible source of information for predicting the structure of the query sequence.

The prediction of the three-dimensional structure of proteins given only the amino acid sequence (primary structure) remains one of the great unsolved problems of biology. In the meantime, some progress has been made in predicting both secondary and tertiary structures of proteins by means of computers. However, none of the available methods is highly reliable, and there remains substantial room for improvement. Secondary structure prediction involves prediction of α helices and β strands. Available methods typically use a database of known secondary structures with which a query sequence is compared. A variety of methods for prediction of protein secondary and tertiary structure are available from the EMBLat *http://www.embl-heidelberg.de/predictprotein/doc/entry_intro.html*. Figure 13 shows the results of secondary structure prediction by the PHDsec program available at the EMBL site.

Gene Expression Data

Microarray Data

It is expected that gene expression studies using microarrays will play an increasingly important role in the future in all areas of both basic and applied biology (Reference 5, 3). Microarrays provide a way of measuring the abundance of mRNAs in cells under a variety of different conditions. Deoxyribonucleic acid samples on the microarray bind mRNA that has been fluorescently labeled, and thousands of such samples can be tested with a single microarray. Thus, the raw data of a microarray study are measures of the intensity of fluorescence of the spots on the array, which are correlated with the amount of mRNA present.

The analysis of microarray data are in its infancy. One important fact about these data to remember is that, as in any experimental system, there is expected to be substantial measurement error. Thus, if the same microarray is applied to analyze the same cell type on two different occasions, it is not likely the same results will be obtained. To estimate the extent of this experimental error and to account for it statistically, the ideal solution is to replicate the experiment many times. Unfortunately, given the cost of microarray runs, microarray studies are rarely replicated at the present time. For this reason, the power of this technique to address biological questions is somewhat muted due to the experimental error in the data.

The raw fluorescence intensities observed in a given microarray run are not directly comparable with those obtained by other studies using different equipment or different experimental conditions. Therefore, these data are typically standardized by comparison with some sort of control. These might be a set of control genes whose expression levels are known not to vary under the different conditions being examined in a given study. Alternatively, each ribonucleic acid (RNA) sample analyzed may have added to it an equal amount of some RNA standard. Thus, the relative level of expression of a given RNA can be expressed by an expression score which is the ratio of its observed fluorescence intensity to that of the control.

To provide a visual image of these expression scores, the fold deviation from the average expression score is color coded in a matrix of colored squares. The usual convention is to use red for genes with higher than average expression scores, green for those with lower than average scores, and black for average scores. Typically, the matrix of colored squares is arranged so that rows correspond to individual microarray elements (i.e., to the specific RNA bound by each such element) and columns correspond to different cell types or different experimental treatments. Although not all the colors are visible in the reproduction, Figure 14 provides an example of this approach. This

```
                  .   .   .   .   |   .   .   .   .   1   .   .   .   .   |   .   .   .   .   2
AA                M   P   S   Y   T   V   T   V   A   T   G   S   Q   W   F   A   G   T   D   D
PHD_sec                       E   E   E   E   E   E               E   E   E                   E
Rel_sec           *   *       *   *   *   *   *   *       *                       *   *

P_3_acc           b   e   e   b   e   b   e   b   b   b   b   b   e   b   b   b   b   e   e   e
Rel_acc                               *       *
```

Figure 13. Sample output from the PHDsec program. AA = the amino acid sequence analyzed. PHDsec: predicted secondary structure elements(E = extended; i.e., sheet).
Rel_sec: accuracy of the secondary structure prediction (* indicates strong prediction).
P_3_acc: predicted relative solvent accessibility (b = 0-9 percent, e = 36-100 percent). Rel_acc: accuracy of the solvent accessibility prediction (* indicates strong prediction).

figure summarizes data on the expression of 205 RNAs in 25 different B cell chronic lymphocytic leukemia (CLL) subtypes (Reference 13). The rows correspond to the 205 RNAs and the columns correspond to the 25 CLL subtypes.

Clustering Methods

Given expression data on a large number of genes, researchers often are interested in discovering similarities in expression pattern among genes. As an exploratory strategy for discovering and illustrating such similarities, researchers often use some form of hierarchical clustering. (This algorithm used for such clustering is actually identical to that used for the UPGMA method of phylogenetic tree construction as previously discussed.) In hierarchical clustering start with some measure of the similarity (or dissimilarity) among genes. When the same genes have been analyzed for different samples (such as the different CLL subtypes in Figure 14), the linear correlation (Pearson correlation coefficient) across samples is the most commonly used measure of similarity (Reference 3). Given a measure of similarity among any set of units, the hierarchical clustering algorithm sequentially groups units and clusters of units based on their average similarity.

In microarray studies, hierarchical clustering may be applied to genes to identify which genes have highly similar expression patterns. The "tree" or dendrogram on the left of Figure 14 provides an example of such clustering of genes. In addition, when multiple conditions or cell types are examined, hierarchical clustering can be used to highlight similarities among these as well. For example, the dendrogram at the top of Figure 14 illustrates clustering of CLL subtypes. This clustering shows a sharp distinction in gene expression pattern between immunoglobulin-mutated and unmutated CLL subtypes, which form two distinct clusters (Figure 14).

In addition to hierarchical clustering, microarray data are sometimes analyzed by k-means clustering, which clusters the data into a preassigned number (k) of clusters. In this case, each unit to be clustered is considered as a point in multidimensional space. The units to be clustered typically would be individual genes for which expression data has been obtained under many different conditions, and dimensionality of the space would correspond to the number of conditions examined. Clusters are established, and each gene is assigned to the cluster whose center in multidimensional space is closest to the point corresponding to that gene.

The Stanford Microarray Database (*http://genome-www5.Stanford.edu/MicroArray/SMD/*) provides a variety of computational tools for analyzing microarray data, including hierarchical clustering and k-means clustering. This database also stores the raw data from various microarray studies. Thus, it is possible to use these resources to reanalyze published microarray data using new perspectives.

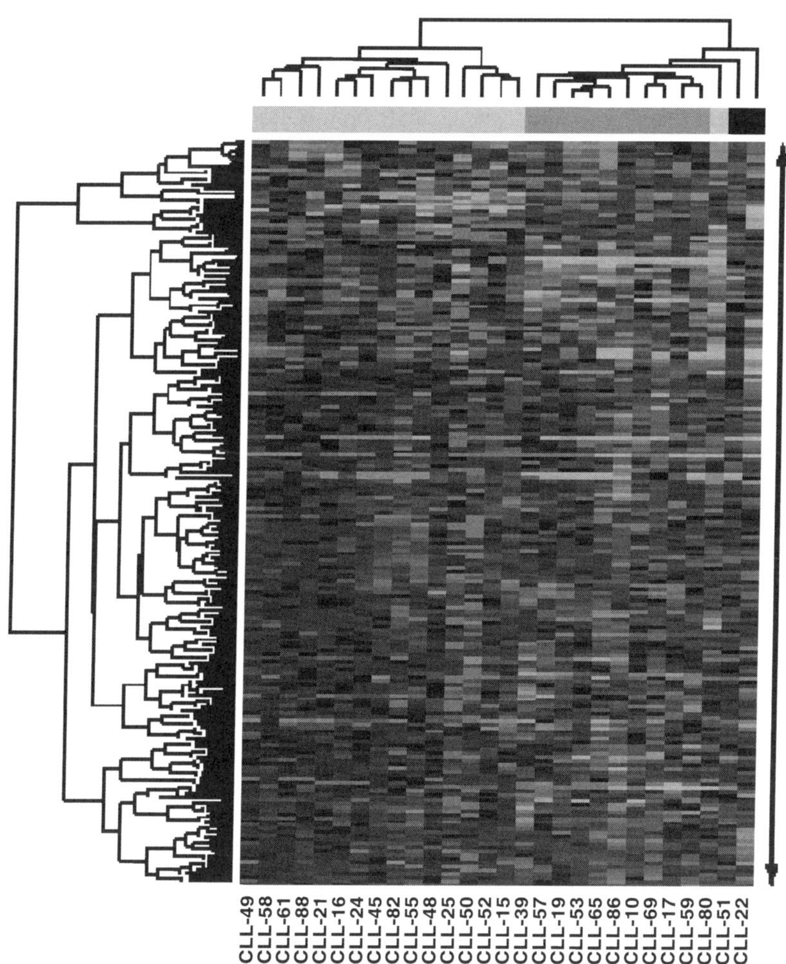

Figure 14. An example of a summary of microarray data. Rows correspond to 205 microarrays, and columns correspond to 25 B cell lymphocytic leukemia (CLL) subtypes. The tree to the left of the figure indicates clustering of ribonucleic acids, whereas the tree on the top of the figure indicates clustering of CLL subtypes. Reprinted with permission from Rosenwald A, Alizadeh AA, Widhopf G, et al. Reproduced from J Exp Med 2001;194:1639–47. Relation of gene expression phenotype to immunoglobulin mutation genotype in B cell chronic lymphotic leukemia.

Prospects for the Future

Microarray technology is a rapidly growing area, and technological advances are likely in the near future. In addition, it is likely that there will be improvements in the statistical methods for analyzing these data. For example, in the near future sequence and genomic databases will be linked to tools for the analysis of gene expression data. This link will make it straightforward to conduct studies that combine gene expression data with sequence-based information. For example, in some cases it may be of interest to compare gene expression patterns of genes mapping to different chromosomal regions and to look for differences between and within such regions. Software that combines information on the map location of genes with expression data will make such studies possible.

Likewise, it may be of interest to examine expression differences among members of a gene family or to compare expression patterns of different families. Such studies will be made possible by combining expression data with data on gene families established by sequence homology searches. Finally, gene expression data can be combined with the results of phylogenetic analyses to help scientists understand how expression patterns are correlated with evolutionary relationships among gene family members. Such linkages will be made possible by the creation of comprehensive knowledge databases for genomics, which provide software tools to integrate data at the levels of sequence, structure, and expression.

Web Sites of Interest

1. *http://lectures.molgen.mpg.de/.*

2. *http://www.angelfire.com/ga2/nestsite2/bioinform.html.*

References

1   Altschul SF, Gish W, Miller W, Myers EW, Lipman DJ. Basic local alignment search tool. J Mol Biol 1990;215:405–10.

2. Baxevanis AD, Ouellette BFF, eds. Bioinformatics: A Practical Guide to the Analysis of Genes and Proteins. New York: Wiley-Interscience, 1998.

3. Brazma A, Vilo J. Gene expression data analysis. FEBS Lett 2000;480:17–24.

4. Brookes AJ. The essence of SNPs. Gene 1999;234:177–86.

5. Clarke PA, te Poele R, Wooster R, Warkman P. Gene expression microarray analysis in cancer biology, pharmacology, and drug development: progress and potential. Biochem Pharmacol 2001;62:1311–36.

6. Hughes AL. Adaptive Evolution of Genes and Genomes. New York: Oxford University Press, 1999.

7. Kanehisa M. Post-genome Informatics. New York: Oxford University Press, 2000.

8.   Kimura M. The Neutral Theory of Molecular Evolution. Cambridge: Cambridge University Press, 1983.

9.   Kumar S, Tamura K, Jakobsen IB, Nei M. MEGA2: molecular evolutionary genetics analysis software. Bioinformatics 2001;17:1244–5.

10.   Mount DW. Bioinformatics: Sequence and Genome Analysis. Cold Spring Harbor, NY: Cold Spring Harbor Laboratory Press, 2001.

11.   Nei M, Kumar S. Molecular Evolution and Phylogenetics. New York: Oxford University Press, 2000.

12.   Riley JH, Allan CJ, Lai E, Roses A. The use of single nucleotide polymorphisms in the isolation of common disease genes. Pharmacogenomics 2000;1:39–47.

13.   Rosenwald A, Alizadeh AA, Widhopf G, et al. Relation of gene expression phenotype to immunoglobulin mutation genotype in B cell chronic lymphotic leukemia. J Exp Med 2001;194:1639–47.

14.   Swofford D. PAUP: Phylogenetic Analysis Using Parsimony (and other Methods). Software Version 4. Sunderland, MA: Sinauer, 2002.

15.   Wheeler DL, Church DM, Lash AE, et al. Database resources of the National Center for Biotechnology Information: 2002 update. Nucleic Acids Res 2002;30:13–16.

16.   Zuckerkandl E, Pauling L. Molecules as documents of evolutionary history. J Theor Biol 1965;8:357–62.

Self-Assessment Questions

1. Two genes are orthologous if they are which one of the following?

   A. Descended from a common ancestral gene without gene duplication.
   B. Descended from a common ancestral gene with gene duplication.
   C. At least 50 percent identical at the nucleotide level.
   D. At least 75 percent identical at the nucleotide level.

2. In trying to find bacterial homologues of a human gene, it is best to do which one of the following?

   A. Conduct a homology search at the nucleotide level.
   B. Conduct a homology search at the amino acid sequence level.
   C. Conduct a keyword search.
   D. Conduct an author search.

3. Derived databases in which sequences have been curated and annotated include which one of the following?

   A. Refseq.
   B. Genbank.
   C. European Molecular Biology Laboratory.
   D. The DNA Data Bank of Japan.

4. In basic local alignment search tool (BLAST) homology searches, the expect score (E) is a measure of which one of the following?

   A. The penalty for a mismatch.
   B. The penalty for a gap.
   C. The probability of a false-positive.
   D. The probability of a false-negative.

5. Hierarchical clustering cannot be used to do which one of the following?

   A. Look for similarities in expression patterns of different genes using microarray data.
   B. Look for similarities in the gene expression profile of different cell lines using microarray data.
   C. Look for similarities in the gene expression profile of cells subjected to different treatments using microarray data.
   D. Reconstruct the most parsimonious phylogenetic tree.

6. A phylogenetically informative site is which one of the following?

   A. A variable site.

B. An invariable site.
C. A site that favors some trees over others.
D. A site that supports the maximum parsimony tree.

7. If an amino acid residue is conserved in a set of aligned protein sequences, which one of the following is true?

    A. It may be functionally important because the rate of evolution is low at functionally important sites.
    B. It is unlikely to be functionally important because the rate of evolution is high at functionally important sites.
    C. It is subject to positive Darwinian selection.
    D. It is a synonymous site.

8. The most time-consuming of widely used methods of phylogenetic reconstruction is which one of the following?

    A. Maximum parsimony.
    B. Neighbor-joining.
    C. Unweighted pair-group means using arithmetic averages.
    D. Maximum likelihood.

9. The observed proportion of difference between two homologous sequences may not represent all of the change that has taken place since the last common ancestor of the two sequences because of which one of the following?

    A. The two sequences may not be related.
    B. The two sequences may be paralogous.
    C. The two sequences may be orthologous.
    D. More than one substitution may have taken place at a given site.

10. Synonymous and nonsynonymous sites in coding regions of most genes evolve at different rates because of which one of the following?

    A. Purifying selection is stronger at synonymous sites.
    B. Purifying selection is stronger at nonsynonymous sites.
    C. Positive Darwinian selection is common at synonymous sites.
    D. Positive Darwinian selection is common at nonsynonymous sites.

Applications of Genomics in Human Health and Complex Disease

Daren L. Knoell, Pharm.D., FCCP
Wolfgang Sadee, Ph.D.

Key Words

Quantitative trait loci, single nucleotide polymorphism (SNP), deoxyribonucleic acid (DNA) microsatellites, haplotype, association studies, and linkage disequilibrium (LD).

Abstract

The ability to interpret genome-based information will become an essential skill for understanding disease and optimizing drug therapy. Having prior knowledge of a patient's genetic composition will invariably change our approach to pharmacotherapy and the outcome of our patients. The purpose of this chapter is to provide a basic understanding of the terms and issues central to a genomic view of disease and therapy. This will permit the practitioner to follow the rapid developments in medical genetics and pharmacogenomics likely to impose profound changes in clinical practice over the coming decade. Examples have begun to emerge that demonstrate how genomics can provide new insight into the genetic basis of complex diseases. This chapter provides an overview of the polymorphisms that exist across the genome and discusses strategies that are currently used for determining the genetic identity and cause of complex disease in humans. This chapter also provides a framework that is complemented by contemporary examples that demonstrate how genomic information is being used to identify the mechanisms of common complex disorders, diagnose disease, and develop improved treatment strategies.

Outline

Learning Objectives

1. Distinguish how independently occurring polymorphisms could result in development of a complex disease.

2. Predict how individual patient genomic information will change the diagnosis, classification, and treatment of common diseases such as hypertension.
3. A healthy patient states that a genomic screen has predicted a 30 percent likelihood that he will develop a certain disease in his lifetime. Identify three major areas where pharmacists would be involved in using this information to help the patient.

Abbreviations in this Chapter

Apo	Apolipoprotein
CAD	Coronary artery disease
CETP	Cholesteryl ester transfer protein
cDNA	Complementary deoxyribonucleic acid
CFTR	Cystic fibrosis transmembrane conductance regulator
CIN	Chromosomal instability
cM	CentiMorgan
DNA	Deoxyribonucleic acid
HDL	High-density lipoprotein
HIV	Human immunodeficiency virus
HMG CoA	Hydroxymethyl glutaryl coenzyme A
HPLC	High pressure liquid chromatography
LD	Linkage disequilibrium
LDL	Low-density lipoprotein
LPL	Lipoprotein lipase
MDR	Multidrug resistance
MIN	Microsatellite instability
mRNA	Messenger ribonucleic acid
PCR	Polymerase chain reaction
QTL	Quantitative trait locus
RFLP	Restriction fragment length polymorphism
RNA	Ribonucleic acid
RT-PCR	Reverse transcriptase polymerase chain reaction
SNP	Single nucleotide polymorphism
STR	Simple tandem repeats
VNTR	Variable number tandem repeats

Introduction

Health care experts predict that at the time of birth every individual will receive a birth certificate and a personal "gene chip". The chip will contain the patient's "functional" genomic signature and will be used by pharmacists, physicians, and other health care professionals to determine disease susceptibility and how the patient will respond to the environment and drugs. Although such a prediction may appear fictitious, use of personal genetic information will inexorably change the way health care practitioners interact with patients. In particular, the ability to interpret genome-based information will become an essential skill for understanding disease and optimizing drug therapy for each patient (Figure 1) (Reference 1). Having prior knowledge of a patient's genetic composition will forever change the approach to pharmacotherapy and the outcomes of patients. The purpose of this chapter is to introduce the basic terms and issues central to the use of genomics to understand the pathogenesis of complex disease and the individualized response to therapy. After completing this chapter, the reader should be able to keep pace with discoveries in medical genomics that define the biological basis for complex diseases that, in turn, facilitate improved care for patients.

To begin, a fundamental distinction between single-gene diseases, with which most clinicians are familiar, and complex diseases, which occur more frequently but are less understood, must be made. Before the age of genomics, complex diseases were referred to as multifactorial. The terminology has changed to reflect the improved capability to determine the physiologic mechanisms responsible for disease. The principal difference that distinguishes a complex disease from a single-gene disease is that the former does not segregate. In other words, complex disease phenotype does not follow the classic Mendelian rules of inheritance. Although the multiple genes responsible for complex disease can segregate across families, the phenotype does not. In general, this is because complex diseases have multiple genes that specify multiple products that dynamically interact with the environment to produce a phenotype.

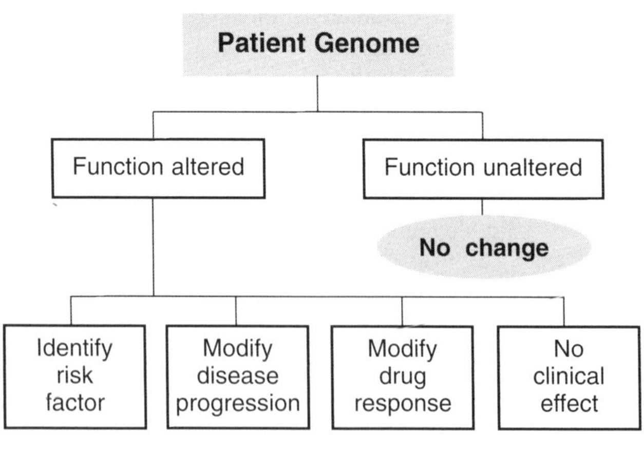

Figure 1.

To illustrate this point, if two individuals with the same genome and same predisposition to a complex disease were placed in two entirely different environments, one that favored disease occurrence and one that did not, only the individual in the disease favoring environment would manifest the disease. Of course, in reality the relationship among multiple genes, gene products, and the environment is difficult to determine, and at the present time only a partial view of just a few complex disorders exixts. Nevertheless, in the new era of genetics-genomics, the diagnosis of complex multigenic disease relies heavily on understanding the comprehensive genetic make up of the individual. As an example, in the clinic clinicians will no longer rely solely on recording a patient's blood pressure to derive a diagnosis of hypertension. Rather, a fingerprint of the genetic variations in multiple candidate genes will permit clinicians to establish the underlying causes of the disease and to stratify the patient into a discreet group of patients with hypertension who require a distinct therapy. At the present time, this is unachievable because complex diseases such as hypertension involve the dynamic interplay of multiple genes, their corresponding proteins, and the environment, which is not yet fully understood. The challenge of finding genes responsible for a complex disease is at the present time similar to having one individual read through an entire set of encyclopedias just to identify several misspelled words. Therefore, many obstacles remain to be resolved for genomic information to become clinically useful.

Examples have begun to emerge that demonstrate how genomics can provide new insight into the genetic causes of complex diseases (Reference 2, 3) and identify novel targets for drug discovery (Reference 4). Genome-wide scanning with genetic markers in association studies already has revealed quantitative trait loci (QTLs) and candidate genes that contribute to common complex diseases including type 1 and type 2 diabetes, multiple sclerosis, asthma, hypertension, atherosclerosis, and rheumatoid arthritis (Reference 5). Quantitative trait loci is a term used to define continuous traits that do not fall into discrete classes. When a population is analyzed for a continuous trait, a bell-shaped distribution is usually found. An example of a complex disease with a continuous trait is hypertension and blood pressure. Theoretically, when one individual with an extremely high blood pressure produces offspring with an individual who has low blood pressure, the blood pressure of their progeny may be intermediate to the two parents. If the blood pressures were examined over a larger population of family members, the readings would exhibit a bell-shaped distribution. Because continuous traits are often given a quantitative value, they are often referred to as *quantitative traits,* and the area of genetics that studies their mode of inheritance is called quantitative genetics. Furthermore, the genetic loci controlling these traits are called QTLs. These traits are controlled by multiple genes, each segregating according to Mendel's laws. As previously discussed, these traits also are affected by the environment to varying degrees.

Genome-wide scanning also is being used to identify host susceptibility toward infection and to characterize the virulence of pathogens (Reference 6). Although most health care practitioners do not immediately recognize a genetic basis for infection, there is considerable evidence that genotype can affect susceptibility to infection. It also is clear that the genotype of the pathogen should be taken into consideration. As an example, work is under way to fully characterize the genome of different human immunodeficiency virus (HIV) isolates taken from HIV-positive patients. The genetic sequence of each isolate is being determined and then compared in parallel with in vitro susceptibility testing against different antibiotics. The intent is to revolutionize anti-HIV therapy by developing individualized treatment strategies based purely on the pathogen's genetic signature. A major advantage to this strategy is that susceptibility to drugs could be determined in hours compared to the usual turnaround time of several days with conventional methods. Additional genome-based applications for infectious diseases will arise and may include improvements in diagnosis, determining antibiotic susceptibilities, determining host factor predisposition to allergy and drug response, and perhaps one day differentiate influenza from the common cold. The main challenge at this time is to identify all possible genetic variants, determine which genetic variants are biologically relevant, understand how the combined interactions contribute to disease, and determine the best outcome with therapy (Reference 2). The latter is encompassed in a field now termed pharmacogenetics or more broadly pharmacogenomics (Reference 7, 8).

This chapter provides an overview of the type of polymorphisms that exist across the genome and discusses strategies that currently are used for determining the genetic identity and cause of complex disease in humans. The field of applied genomics is still in its infancy and experiencing major breakthroughs on a daily basis. As a consequence, some of the content in this chapter is not yet established and subject to dynamic change. This chapter will provide a framework that is complemented by contemporary examples that demonstrate how genomic information is being used to identify the mechanisms of common complex disorders, diagnose disease and develop improved treatment strategies.

Genome Scanning Techniques

Genotyping

Initial association studies conducted in humans involved the identification of single nucleotide substitutions that resulted in the loss or acquisition of susceptibility to digestion by a restriction enzyme. Deoxyribonucleic acid (DNA) obtained from a patient was subjected to restriction enzyme digestion and then resolved on an agarose gel by electrophoresis. Changes in the number and mobility of the DNA fragments because of a single nucleotide polymorphism (SNP) could easily be detected and compared among patients. This type of polymorphism was, therefore, referred to as a restriction fragment length polymorphism (RFLP). An original map of all identifiable RFLPs constructed more than a decade ago included relatively few (about 400) landmarks across the entire human genome, therefore, severely limiting application to clinical practice.

There are many variations on genotyping methods for detecting SNPs, but most share several common features. The polymerase chain reaction (PCR) is currently the basis for most of the conventional methods used to rapidly amplify small starting quantities of DNA or ribonucleic acid (RNA). Detection of SNPs after DNA amplification is most commonly performed by hybridization of a probe with the wild-type or mutant allele, followed by a detection step (labeled primer extension, labeled hybridization probe, melting characteristics of the formed dimers, etc). Increasingly, use of microarrays with hundreds of thousands of oligonucleotide probes selective for either wild-type or mutant alleles permits the massive parallel analysis of literally thousands of SNPs on a single chip. Another strategy is to perform direct sequencing on the patient's amplified DNA.

Although the technology is rapidly advancing, the increased demand to determine a large number of SNPs in large patient populations still imposes a significant challenge using current techniques. With improvements in techniques and automation, it is anticipated that we will have the capability to derive all of the information necessary for patients from as little as one drop of blood. The DNA extracted from one drop of blood would be sufficient to permit rapid genome scanning for diagnostic purposes in a clinical setting. At the present time, reliance on amplification of the starting sample by PCR can be a rate-limiting step for genome-wide association studies because it requires 10,000–100,000 PCR reactions to span the genome of a single patient. Therefore, intense efforts are under way to develop novel techniques that are sufficiently sensitive and accommodate nanogram quantities of DNA without amplification by PCR.

Messenger Ribonucleic Acid Expression Analysis (Transcriptome)

Microarray expression analysis is a relatively new experimental technique that allows complete analysis of all expressed messenger ribonucleic acids (mRNAs) in a tissue of interest, which also is referred to as the transcriptome. This technique differs from conventional DNA-based sequencing techniques because it measures differences in gene expression between a test sample and a control tissue. Expression analysis needs to be complemented by analysis of relevant polymorphisms that could affect the level of mRNA expression or the function of the expressed protein. A patient's expression profile is acquired by dense spotting of many different complementary oligonucleotide or complementary deoxyribonucleic acid (cDNA) probes onto a slide. A sample of the patient's mRNA is then converted into a cDNA strand through a technique called reverse transcriptase polymerase chain reaction (RT-PCR). The patient's cDNA sample is then labeled with a fluorescent dye, applied to the "chip" containing oligonucleotide and cDNA probes, and hybridized. Typically, cDNA samples are generated from a disease tissue and compared with the normal control tissue, yielding expression ratios because most arrays cannot determine absolute expression values. This results in a quantitative estimate of the changes in mRNA expression between the two samples. Many variations on this theme are possible. Wholesale analysis of mRNA patterns has been applied to characterize and classify cancers, compare normal and diseased tissue with complex disease such as emphysema, and determine the effect of drugs on the target tissue. Searching for novel gene targets for drug discovery is one of the main goals in this area. At present, huge databases have emerged and are rapidly growing with diverse information on tissues, mRNA expression, drug effects, and phenotypes. These databases will become much more common and accessible in the public domain, such that all investigators will have these extraordinary tools available. The main challenge for clinicians is to prepare for this flood of new information, and make optimal use for understanding disease and optimizing therapy—an enormous task with great promise.

Protein Analysis (Proteome)

In general, genes, SNPs, and other polymorphisms are only relevant if they influence (or are linked to other genes that influence) the individual's phenotype (i.e., the pattern and function of all proteins in the cell). Moreover, each gene can give rise to numerous protein variants, either by differential splicing or post-translational modifications. Finally, proteins are sequestered into cellular compartments and interact with multiple partners, forming complex systems that determine a cell's behavior. Thus, proteomics (study of the sum of all proteins) has emerged as a new discipline, to help practitioners understand how protein networks function and what consequences arise from genetic variations or environmental stimuli. Use of microarrays for protein analysis, similar to those for DNA or RNA analysis, recently have emerged and add a new dimension to the available information, but they are technically much more challenging. Preliminary basic investigations exploring the proteome of single cell populations suggest that protein expression profiles and gene expression profiles do not match one to one. In other words, results taken from RNA expression may not be indicative of what is happening at the protein level. Therefore, to fully understand the mechanism of disease pathogenesis or treatment response we are obligated to explore both areas. Clearly, proper use and mining of these complex databases will be essential to exploit the vast potential for a new understanding of biology engendered by this novel approach.

Metabolite Analysis (Metabolome)

The comprehensive analysis of all small-molecular-weight solutes and metabolites in a given tissue also has risen to the forefront—a compelling extension to studies on the transcriptome and the proteome. Modern analytical techniques such as high pressure liquid chromatography (HPLC)-mass spectrometry permit wholesale analysis of thousands of solutes simultaneously, the requisite for comprehensive analysis. There are few examples as to how these diverse measurements have been integrated to obtain a better understanding of the cell's biology and the disease process. Yet, it is expected that this type of insight will emerge in the coming years.

Genetic Variability

The human genome consists of 3 billion base pairs in a double-strand DNA helix across 22 autosomes and the X and Y chromosomes. Although the nucleotide sequence has been revealed, the number of genes in the human genome remains to be accurately determined. Current estimates range from 30,000 to 50,000 functional genes underscoring the incomplete understanding of the principal components of the genome. Genes, including their introns and noncoding exons, cover about 10 percent of the genome, whereas the protein-coding regions within the genes make up only 2–3 percent. Moreover, the function of many genes remains unknown. Eric Lander of the Whitehead Institute, a pioneer in human genomics, remarked that the current position in functional genomics is similar to "having all of the parts to a 747 jet without having the instructions on how to put it together".

The genomic sequences among individuals are about 99.9 percent identical regardless of ethnic background. One important exception is that gender differences are quite substantial because of the presence of either XY or XX chromosomes, with transcription from one of the two X chromosomes largely inactivated at random in females. Therefore, it is necessary to ensure that clinical trials at all levels address gender as a factor in disease progression and treatment response. Despite the typically high level of similarity, 0.1 percent of each individual's genome is different and is predicted to account for most, if not all of the differences in phenotype, including susceptibility to disease and response to therapy. Based on this, substantial effort is now under way to identify all of the interindividual variation, or polymorphisms, within the human genome. Polymorphism is a popular term used to describe biological heterogeneity. Blood group antigens were among the first polymorphisms identified and studied in humans. Blood group antigen variation originally was predicted to arise from genetic diversity and, indeed, this turned out to be correct, thereby laying the foundation for the study of genetic diversity within humans. In general, a polymorphism arises in the genome every time a change in the nucleotide sequence occurs and gets transmitted through the germ cell lineages (Figure 2).

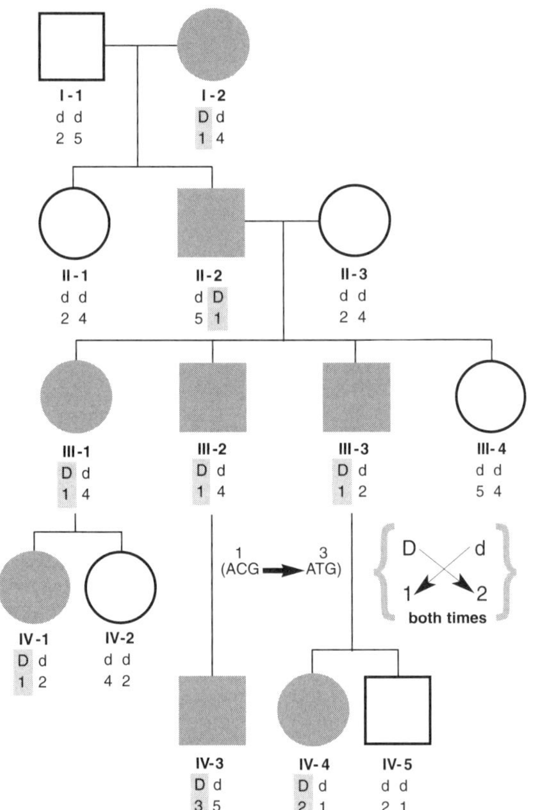

Figure 2.

On the other hand, somatic mutations or nongerm line mutations also occur throughout life, in some cases leading to disease or contributing to age-related changes. Although some polymorphisms directly alter gene function and influence disease or treatment response, most are biologically inert and do not account for phenotypic alterations in the individuals who harbor them. Nevertheless, it is clear that functionally silent polymorphisms can be used as "landmarks" in gene mapping and population-based studies. A rigorous effort is now under way to identify and geographically map all human polymorphisms that, in turn, will reveal the identity of candidate genes associated with complex disease. This information will reveal the biological basis for complex diseases and design optimal treatment strategies on an individual basis. Note that genetic polymorphisms are those occurring with an abundance of at least 1 percent; therefore, a more generic term is 'sequence variant', although usage of the term in the literature varies.

Identifying subtle changes in the human genome that account for disease, whether it is monogenic or complex, is a difficult task and requires a well-planned strategy. *Linkage disequilibrium* (LD) describes the nonrandom association of a particular allele at a given locus with a different allele (or mutation or polymorphism or variant, etc.) at a nearby unrelated locus among different families, as a result of shared ancestry. The *LD mapping* is a commonly used strategy but distinctly different from *linkage mapping* in that it exploits *across-family* associations. In this setting, one expects much more heterogeneity in the study population because of the large number of meiotic and recombination events in the genealogical links that connect individuals across families. As a result, LD mapping requires a dense map of markers because the size of the genetic distance between marker alleles that co-segregate with a disease allele across different families is usually small. Developing a map of all polymorphisms in the human genome will undoubtedly facilitate large scale "gene hunting" studies and improve the overall understanding of complex disease. A more detailed discussion of gene mapping strategies is provided in the Linking Genotype to Phenotype section of this chapter. An alternative strategy used to identify candidate genes associated with disease is *linkage mapping*. This strategy works by assessing the transmission and co-segregation of alleles at landmark spots on the genome with putative disease alleles *within* family members that manifest the disease. To work effectively, the marker alleles need to be in close proximity to the disease-causing alleles and be passed down through family members of the study population. However, recombinant events that allow alleles to cross over to different chromosomes during each generation can confound linkage mapping, particularly if the linkage marker is rather distant from the suspected disease locus. If successful, linkage analysis can help locate the approximate position of a locus harboring disease alleles relative to the position of the marker loci studied.

Single Nucleotide Polymorphisms

The vast majority of genetic variations in humans, about 80 percent, are accounted for by SNPs, that is the exchange of one nucleotide for another. Single nucleotide polymorphisms occur at a high frequency across the human genome. Estimates are that on average about one SNP occurs in every 300 base pairs. Human SNP databases have already collected more than 4 million human SNPs with more expected, but the error rate in these databases can be considerable. Even though there are four possible variants at each nucleotide position, an A, C, G, or T, commonly only two nucleotides are found at the same location, generating a biallelic SNP, as opposed to multiple alleles at the same position. As a convention, a single nucleotide change is a polymorphism when it occurs at a frequency of greater than 1 percent in the population. In contrast, single nucleotide changes occurring at lower frequencies are commonly referred to as genetic variants or mutations. Many of these rare variants are responsible for medically important monogenic disorders, such as sickle cell anemia, cystic fibrosis, and Marfan syndrome. Also, some of these mutations involve sequence variants other than SNPs.

For example, the most common mutation associated with cystic fibrosis (present in about 70 percent of all patients) involves a three base-pair deletion at position 508, referred to as the Δ 508 mutation. Nevertheless, most SNPs occur in intergenic regions, or in other words, regions of the genome where genes do not exist. This is not surprising because a low proportion of the human genome is composed of genes. Therefore, only a minority of SNPs are actually found within genes, which raises an important question. Should health care focus attention only on SNPs that exist within genes? The answer to this question is clearly no because SNPs that exist in intergenic locations can be used as important landmarks and may themselves confer changes in genomic functions. Single nucleotide polymorphisms found within a gene can occur either in the untranscribed promoter region or within the transcribed region. Within the transcribed region, a SNP may occur either in exons (which eventually become the mature RNA) or introns (which may contain regulatory sequences that are spliced out). Even if a SNP occurs in an exon, it may exist in untranslated 3' or 5' regions (which also have important regulatory functions), translated protein-coding regions that are processed out of the mature protein, or in a part of the gene which contributes directly to the sequence of a mature protein. The location where the SNP occurs in a gene is crucial because it can result in profound changes in the transcription and translation of the gene. As an example, SNPs located around intron-exon boundaries have the potential to affect mRNA splicing whereas SNPs that occur in promoter regions can influence the turning "on" or turning "off" of gene expression.

Finally, SNPs within regions that encode the actual protein can either be synonymous or nonsynonymous. Synonymous SNP is the common terminology used to identify SNPs that occur in the third (wobble) position of the codon and do not alter the protein sequence. Nonsynonymous SNPs result from nucleotide substitution at any location in the codon and generate either a missense codon that changes the encoded amino acid and could alter protein function, or a nonsense codon (e.g., a termination codon leading to protein truncation). It also is possible for a nonsynonymous SNP to not cause a change in protein function. An example is a nucleotide substitution in a codon that leads to incorporation of an aspartate instead of a glutamate, a similarly charged and sized amino acid that when substituted, leads to minimal or no functional alteration. Yet, nonsynonymous SNPs are most likely to affect the protein's function, although other SNP types can have multiple functional consequences (e.g., affecting the stability of mRNA). Nonsynonymous SNPs occur at considerably lower frequency than expected if mutations simply occurred at random, which is most likely the result of evolutionary selective pressure particularly in essential proteins.

Clinicians must understand the fundamental mechanisms by which SNPs influence the biologic function and overall phenotype of the patient. This knowledge is necessary to fully understand disease pathogenesis, incorporate this information into the diagnosis, and design the optimal therapeutic strategy. However, a basic understanding of SNP biology is not enough because it is impossible to predict the functional consequence of any given SNP. Rather, clinicians will need to understand how multiple SNPs interact dynamically and how these interactions, in turn, react with other genetic factors and with external factors, such as lifestyle, environment, age, and other clinical conditions. The next decade will likely produce a comprehensive listing of all known SNPs and other types of polymorphisms, and from this clinicians will eventually understand the dynamic interaction of different SNPs for a given patient and how they contribute to common complex diseases such as hypertension. Extensive information on SNPs is already available on the Web and it is highly recommended to visit the following sites: *http://dir.niehs.nih.gov/egsnp/status/, http://www.snps.com/, http://www.ncbi.nlm.nih.gov/LocusLink/, and http://www.ncbi.nlm.nih.gov/Omim/.*

Deoxyribonucleic Acid Microsatellite Variability

Another common type of polymorphism found in humans occurs when a strand of nucleotides is inserted or deleted in the genome. The most common type of insertion/deletion is referred to as tandem repeats. The size of the tandem repeats inserted or deleted can range from several hundred base pairs, referred to as variable number tandem repeats (VNTRs; minisatellites), to just two to four nucleotides repeated a variable number of times, referred to as microsatellites (or simple tandem repeats [STRs]). The genetic variation as a result of tandem repeats can lead to multiple alleles at a given locus, depending on the number of repeats present. Because tandem repeats are highly polymorphic, the chance that the exact same tandem repeat will randomly occur in two individuals is low so they are well suited as landmarks for association (linkage) studies.

Microsatellite Analysis of Altered Immune Function

The following provides a clinical example of how DNA microsatellite marking studies can be used to identify a candidate gene associated with disease. Recently, DNA microsatellite markers were used to identify a disease susceptibility gene responsible for disseminated mycobacterial infection (Reference 9). A family was identified that had a strong history of developing abnormal, lethal, disseminated mycobacterial infection. In this case, the infections only occurred in family members that originated from consanguineous marriages. Two affected family members were studied by genome-wide scanning using about 400 DNA satellite markers at 10 centiMorgan (cM) intervals across the genome. (One cM is the genetic distance between two loci with a 1 percent chance of a crossover event per generation. In physical terms, this is about 1 million base pairs, although the crossover frequency varies among different chromosomal segments.) The strategy was to look for regions of shared homozygosity because the family history predicted a recessive inheritance pattern. The investigators also took advantage of a detailed understanding of immune function in the affected individuals so that it would be easier to identify the key candidate gene within the mapped intervals. Indeed, their comparative analysis of both individuals revealed a mutation in the interferon-gamma 1 receptor. This mutation was subsequently proven to be responsible for the high susceptibility to mycobacteria. The mutation was a single nucleotide substitution that resulted in a stop codon and early truncation of the protein. The functional consequence was complete loss of interferon-gamma signaling through the type 1 receptor pathway that generated a major defect in early immune defense against the pathogen.

Since this initial discovery, additional rare mutations have been found in other gene family members involved in the type 1 cytokine response against pathogens. Although these variants are rare, they provide new leads that may be useful when looking at complex disorders involving type 1 immune dysfunction. This clinical study demonstrates a classic approach in which the investigators found microsatellite polymorphisms and used them for linkage analysis to identify a candidate region followed by identification of a specific nucleotide change.

Microsatellites and Chromosomal Instability in Cancer

In a majority of cancers, genetic instability plays a key role, leading to multiple mutations that eventually result in transformation of the cell to neoplastic behavior (Reference 14). Microsatellite instability (MIN), often resulting from mutation of a DNA mismatch repair gene, is considered to be a minor cause of cancer overall, but is seen at increased frequency in colon, endometrial, and gastric cancer and is a major factor in the autosomal dominant disorder hereditary nonpolyposis colon cancer. Most cancers are associated with chromosomal instability (CIN), which can arise from mutations in genes that play a role in chromosomal segregation during mitosis, or in maintaining chromosomal integrity. Changes include translocations between different chromosomes (e.g., the Philadelphia chromosome), duplications or deletions of chromosomal segments, or deletion or addition of entire chromosomes, leading to monosomy or trisomy. Loss of one or more chromosomes occurs frequently in cancers. This has the potential to exacerbate the impact of any mutations in genes that are retained on the remaining chromosomes. As an example, a mutant cancer-promoting gene (an oncogene) may be expressed but appear silent because expression of the corresponding wild-type gene in heterozygous normal cells dominates or overrides the cancer-causing gene. Loss of the entire chromosome carrying the wild-type gene leads to 'loss of heterozygocity' and sole expression of the mutated oncogene. Alternatively, chromosomal loss of a tumor suppressor gene, such as p53, could leave a single inactivated mutant tumor suppressor allele in the transforming cell. p53 mutations are implicated in almost half of all tumors. From these observations, it is clear that genetic and genomic changes have profound implications for oncogenesis even if at the present time the significance of most observed changes is uncertain.

Genomic variation undoubtedly has a major influence on the effectiveness of chemotherapy and is used to predict the host response. There are several ways by which genomic variation can be of influence and include alteration of the host response to various cancer treatments, induction of resistance as the tumor evolves dynamically under the pressure of cytotoxic agents, or provision of genetic landmarks to predict a patient's prognosis or optimal treatment regimen. Ultimate therapy failure is usually the result of highly resistant metastases that have evolved from the primary tumor. Several examples are listed here: 1) amplification of multidrug resistance (MDR) genes to clear chemotherapeutic drugs; 2) alteration of cell membrane channels and transporters or of metabolic machinery to exclude, inactivate, or fail to activate chemotherapeutic drugs; 3) escape from apoptosis through inactivation of p53 or other tumor suppressors; 4) presence or absence of specific receptors, such as estrogen and progesterone in breast cancer; 5) presence or absence of cell membrane antigens that can be targeted by monoclonal antibodies; 6) identification and targeting of novel fusion proteins unique to the cancer and arising from chromosomal rearrangements, as with the Philadelphia chromosome; 7) activation of oncogenes; 8) recently identified genetic variants predisposing to prostate cancer; and 9) the increased frequency of breast cancer among heterozygotes for ataxia telangiectasia, which might result from increased somatic mutation because of the DNA repair error in A•T, ultimately causing an accumulation of cancer-causing mutations.

Epigenetic Effects

Epigenetic effects refer to changes in gene activity that are unrelated to changes in the primary DNA sequence. An example is methylation of CpG islands, typically located in promoter regions, resulting in silencing of the adjacent gene. This mechanism is common for either permanently or temporarily shutting off expression of genes not required in a given cell at a given time. Another example is the inactivation of one of the two X chromosomes in females, although a few genes on the inactivated chromosome remain active. Presumably by similar mechanisms, hundreds of maternal and some paternal genes are imprinted (silenced) on autosomal chromosomes, leading to profound epigenetic changes that cannot be read from the primary sequence alone. Imprinting and X-inactivation are permanent events in all cells of a single individual, reversed only in germ cells during gametogenesis. Errors in imprinting and gene silencing have been implicated in several diseases, including mental illness and cancer, and there are now initial reports that suggest epigenetic influence may have a substantial role in drug response (e.g., of nitrosureas in cancer therapy). The ability to conduct genome-wide analysis for epigenetic changes is emerging but its potential impact in health care remains to be assessed and trails behind other leading areas such as SNP analysis.

Linkage Disequilibrium and Haplotypes

Linkage disequilibrium is the phenomenon whereby the presence of one allele on a chromosome suggests a high probability that a particular allele will be present at a neighboring site on the same chromosome (Figure 3) (Reference 10). The degree of LD is based on a scoring system that ranges from 0 (no linkage) to 1 (two alleles are always linked in a given population). In simple terms, if humans were all genetically identical and the genome never changed, the LD score for an associated marker and disease allele would always be 1. Of course, this is not the case. Finding candidate genes across families involved in the etiology of disease or treatment relies essentially on LD with a neighboring genetic marker that has been previously identified. Loss of LD between the marker gene and the

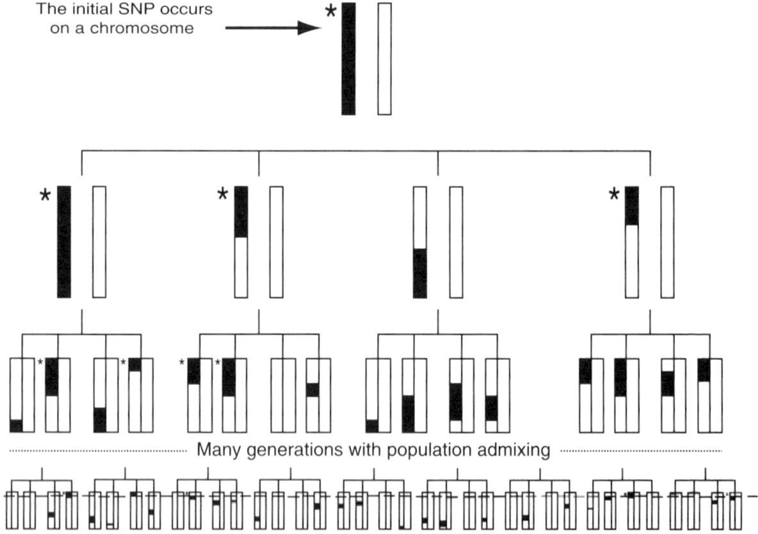

Figure 3.

functional gene locus can occur after meiotic recombination events among sister chromosomes with each generation. Such crossovers, or exchanging of DNA pieces between maternal and paternal chromosomes, occur in humans at a predicted frequency of about one per chromosome arm per meiosis. This occurrence translates into a 1 percent chance of losing LD between two loci that are about 1 million base pairs apart, a genetic distance defined as 1 cM. (Note: The definition of 1 cM is the genetic distance in which the likelihood of recombination in one generation is 1 percent; this translates into an average physical distance of 1 million base pairs; however, 1 million is not at all part of the definition. Therefore, the genetic distance [cMs] and physical distance [base pairs] are two entirely different units of measure. Applications that provide insight to family and population studies will be considered below).

By definition, multiple SNPs lined up on the same strand of DNA are in complete LD (i.e., LD=1). A specific pattern of alleles at several linked SNPs, arrayed together on one chromosome, represents phased SNPs and can be called a haplotype. Other polymorphic markers also can be included in a haplotype, and the markers are not limited just to SNPs. Given two adjacent bisallelic SNPs (1a,b and 2a,b), clinicians can expect 2 x 2 = 4 distinct haplotypes (1a-2a, 1a-2b, 1b-2a, 1b-2b). Because many genes contain multiple SNPs, the number of possible combinations (haplotypes) increases exponentially. For example, 10 linked SNPs theoretically can give rise to 2^{10}=1024 haplotypes. However, in any given population, only a few haplotypes actually account for a majority of the individuals. Hence, the potential complexity of haplotypes collapses into a manageable number of subgroups.

The haplotype of the individual, as opposed to a single SNP, will, in most cases, become the target to understand, diagnose, and treat disease. This emerges from two important aspects. Each gene associated with a given disease is likely to harbor several functional SNPs that may interact with each other when on the same haplotype. For example, the presence of one SNP may be identified on a receptor gene that conveys resistance to stimulation by an endogenous agonist, but this may be dominantly offset by an adjacent SNP on the gene that has an opposite effect. Therefore, only a consideration of both phased SNPs in combination would permit an accurate assessment of the encoded protein's function and the patient's response.

Equally important, haplotype frequencies often vary significantly in different ethnic groups. Therefore, haplotype analysis permits clinicians to stratify a patient population in the best genetic fashion. In other words, characteristic SNP allele patterns occur with different frequencies across ethnic populations, which improves study design if the haplotype is used to stratify study groups. This approach essentially considers the flow of chromosomal pieces through the human population over time (References 11, 12).

Here is a general example of how haplotype analysis can have a profound impact on the design of a genetic study. In founder populations (i.e., those which are descendent from relatively few individuals at a so-called genetic bottleneck), haplotype blocks with strong LD can extend over long genetic and generational distances. For example, in a Utah cohort derived from a relatively contained Northern European population about 800–1600 generations ago, LD may exceed 50 kilobase pairs (at a level of greater than 0.5), whereas in a less contained Nigerian population derived from a broader population about 4000 generations ago, 50 percent LD may be reached at less than 5 kilobase pairs (Reference 12). This infers that the Nigerian population studied is much more genetically diverse and significantly older because a higher number of recombination events have occurred through the generations. This example demonstrates how a genetic marker may be informative for a gene at considerable distance in some populations and at relatively shorter distances in others. The relevance of this finding is that the number of genetic markers required to perform a definitive diagnostic test would be substantially reduced in the northern European population. In contrast, with the more heterogeneous Nigerian population a significantly larger number of markers would be needed to conduct a meaningful genome-wide association study.

The potential value of haplotype analysis in genomics has only recently been fully recognized and there currently is an intense effort to catalogue the main haplotypes for each gene. Extensive haplotype information is being made available to the public at multiple Web sites (e.g., *http://genecanvas.idf.inserm.fr/*). Several examples of how the identification of polymorphisms is being applied to disease diagnosis and therapy are provided in the next section.

Asthma Haplotype Study

The Asthma Haplotype study first used SNP analysis of an index group of 77 normal adult patients consisting of 23 Caucasians, 19 African Americans, 20 Asians, and 15 Hispanic-Latinos (Reference 13). The β_2-adrenergic receptor, an intronless gene, was sequenced in each patient and 13 SNPs spanning the promotor and coding region were identified. Of the 2^{13} possible SNP combinations, only 12 haplotypes were found within the index group along with a strong divergence (up to 20-fold difference) in the frequency of certain haplotypes when the index group was stratified based on race. Moreover, only five haplotypes accounted for a majority of the patients. From this, each patient was assigned a genotype of the β_2-adrenergic receptor locus (i.e., the combination of two of the main haplotypes) with divergent frequencies of the genotypes across ethnic subgroups. This observation emphasizes a previous point that population-based studies involving SNP analysis require stratification of groups to account for different haplotype frequencies across ethnic backgrounds to achieve functionally meaningful results.

Next, the investigators applied the results of SNP analysis to identify a group of 121 adult Caucasian patients with asthma who harbored the five most common haplotype pairs (genotypes). After stratification based on genotype, each patient was tested for his or her bronchodilatory response to an inhaled β-agonist. In general, the response between the five genotype groups varied greater than 2-fold, and patient response was significantly related to the β_2-adrenergic receptor haplotype/genotype. The results suggested that the interactions of multiple SNPs, defined as a haplotype, influence the patient response to an inhaled β-agonist and that individual SNPs studied in isolation have poor predictive power. The investigators also compared normal patients to asthma patients to determine if the haplotype could be used to predict asthma. In this experimental setting, the haplotype was not a good predictor of asthma, perhaps suggesting that the β_2-adrenergic receptor plays a minor role in asthma pathogenesis but will be a predictor for response to β_2-adrenergic agonists.

Coronary Artery Disease and Genetic Predisposition

Ranked as the most prevalent cause of death in the United States, coronary artery disease (CAD) provides a key example for a complex multigenic disease. Aberrations in at least three main processes are thought to play a role in CAD (i.e., lipid metabolism, inflammation, and coagulation). More than 250 candidate genes have been identified as possibly contributing to cardiovascular diseases (Reference 5). It is understood but has yet to be proven that the spectrum of variant genes associated with cardiovascular diseases has a significant impact on an individual's risk and disease progression. Whereas the origin of CAD appears to be multigenic, rare mutations in single genes can cause the disease (e.g., mutations of the low-density lipoprotein [LDL] receptor). On the other hand, variant genes also can determine the outcome of drug therapy, a subject area of pharmacogenomics. Genetic variations that affect pharmacodynamics involve genes that either interact directly with the drug or contribute to the disease process per se (Reference 15, 16). For example, lipid-lowering drugs are important in the therapy of CAD. Specifically, hydroxylmethyl glutaryl coenzyme A (HMG CoA) reductase inhibitors which also are referred to as statins, are widely used but appear to be ineffective in one out of five patients to prevent disease progression.

Recently, numerous genetic variations predisposing to or associated with atherosclerosis and CAD have been proposed. Common genetic variations occur in genes encoding apolipoproteins, cholesteryl ester transfer protein (CETP), hepatic lipase, endothelial nitric oxide synthase, and others. Cholesteryl ester transfer protein activity is inversely related to high-density lipoprotein (HDL) levels (high HDL protects against CAD) and CETP polymorphisms thus may affect CAD. Of interest, the association between CETP genotype and HDL levels is abolished in smokers, indicating sensitivity to environmental factors.

Pharmacogenomics focuses on genetic variations affecting drug response. Recently, several hallmark papers have provided associations between genotype and CAD treatment. A recent study investigated the effect of CETP genotype on CAD progression and response to pravastatin, an HMG-CoA reductase inhibitor, in Caucasian males (Reference 15). Study results suggest that pravastatin efficacy correlates with CETP genotype. Whether smoking affects statin efficacy remains to be determined in the context of CETP genotype. Another study with pravastatin suggested an association between apolipoprotein (Apo) E alleles and therapeutic response, and outcome of intensive lipid-lowering therapy was associated with hepatic lipase gene variants (Reference 16). Moreover, a variant of lipoprotein lipase (LPL) was shown to modulate adverse metabolic effects of treatment with β-blockers. Genetic variations of CETP, Apo, and LPL also may determine part of the response to dietary intervention. Thus, multiple genetic markers have been implicated as possible predictors of CAD treatment.

Clinicians must investigate CETP polymorphisms to gain a better understanding whether and how such information can impact therapeutic decisions. Significant association between a common polymorphism in CETP and HDL levels may affect the progression of CAD. The CETP genotype B2/B2 is correlated with reduced CETP activity, which results in increased HDL levels—potentially protecting against atherosclerosis (Reference 15). However, the TaqIB polymorphism (presence or absence of a restriction site, alleles B1 and B2) is located within an intronic sequence of CETP, and, therefore, unlikely to affect CETP function. Rather, it is thought to serve as a marker for CETP or adjacent genes. Whereas there are known polymorphisms that abrogate CETP function (OMIM "118470) and might be in LD with the TaqIB polymorphism, these are too infrequent to account for this finding. Therefore, the functional significance of the TaqIB polymorphism is unclear. Single nucleotide polymorphisms can be in LD (on the same DNA strand) over extended distances (30–60 kilobases in 'bottleneck populations' [e.g., northern Europeans]) such that distant SNPs can be linked and informative. It is even possible that the TaqIB polymorphism is in LD with a functional variation in an adjacent gene (e.g., lipid transfer protein II).

To account for variations across the entire CETP gene and beyond, clinicians must determine all SNPs in this region, inferred from genomic databases (public and private) (about 80 percent accuracy of prediction), including large introns and about 60 kilobases on each side of CETP, to calculate haplotypes by statistical inference, or measure them by direct analysis of only one chromosomal strand of DNA. The main haplotypes of the CETP gene have already been published (*http://ifr69.vjf.inserm.fr/~canvas/*); however, the relationship between any given haplotype and disease progression or treatment outcome has yet to be clarified. It is anticipated that this type of association will become more reliable across different ethnic populations. Haplotypes could then serve as markers in clinical trials of pravastatin and other statins for CAD treatment. This has the potential to resolve the question whether genotyping can predict disease progression and therapeutic outcome, and under what conditions. It could have profound impact on CAD therapy.

Population admixture (race) is a main confounding factor for association studies with candidate genes and single polymorphisms that appear at different frequencies in ethnic groups. The haplotype analysis discussed for CETP is a more powerful approach to establish the distribution of functional blocks of DNA distributed over various patient populations. This serves to identify functional SNPs, or dynamic interactions among multiple SNPs. Considering haplotypes of multiple candidate genes adds another dimension to the power of genetic association analysis by defining subpopulations and gene-gene interactions, so that clinicians can expect such studies to emerge soon.

To summarize, a pharmacogenomics study focused on haplotype analysis of multiple candidate genes and applied to the therapy of CAD with statins has the potential to provide genetic information that is sufficiently accurate to predict disease progression and therapeutic response. In addition, single mutations with strong penetrance need to be considered, even if rare. Finally, drug metabolizing enzymes and transporters directly interacting with statins can play a significant role in drug efficacy and toxicity. Therefore, genetic variations must be considered in these corresponding genes as well. In combination, such an integrated approach significantly extends the scope of previous pharmacogenomics studies. Yet, it remains to be seen whether extensive use of complex genetic information indeed is capable of advancing clinical therapy for CAD. The main question remains whether the accuracy of predictions from genomic data is sufficient to influence a clinician's decision on how to treat an individual patient. During the coming decade, this crucial question will be intensely addressed not just for CAD, but many other multigenic complex diseases.

Linking Genotype to Phenotype

Monogenic Mendelian Disorders and Polygenic Diseases: Family Studies and Positional Cloning

The traditional genetic approach uses *linkage analysis* studies within families (Figure 4). This strategy is highly successful for monogenic diseases with a classic Mendelian pattern of inheritance studied over several generations within a large family. The basic assumption to this approach is that chromosomal segments containing the disease allele will bear other signature or marker alleles at nearby loci. By examining the pattern of co-segregation of marker locus alleles with the disease phenotype passed through generations in a single family, clinicians can estimate the chromosomal location of the candidate disease susceptibility gene and

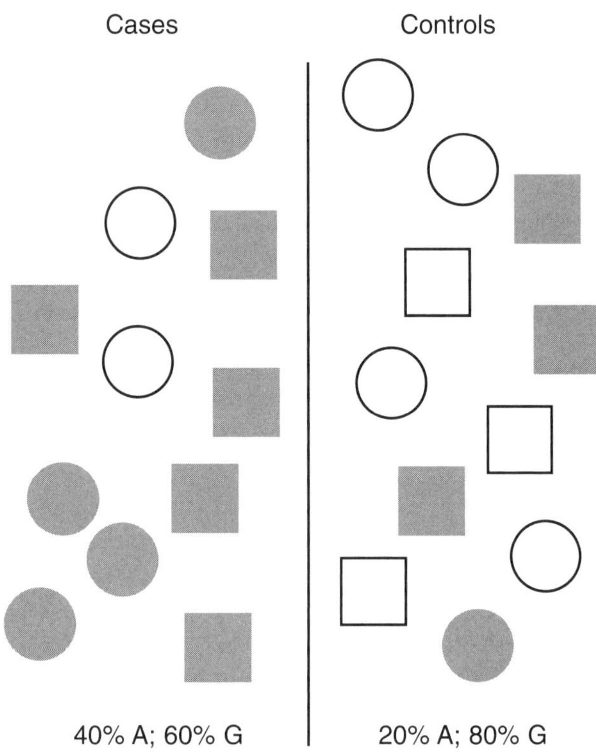

Figure 4.

determine the responsible allele. This gene detection strategy also is referred to as "positional cloning." Examples in clinical medicine where this has been useful to identify the genetic cause for a disease include cystic fibrosis, Duchenne muscular dystrophy, and Huntington's disease. Unfortunately, this approach cannot be readily applied to the study of common complex disorders such as hypertension, because there is usually more than one contributing gene and each one exerts a small to moderate effect on the disease (i.c., they have low penetrance). Attaining statistical significance of the gene-phenotype association could require the study of a large number of probands and families. To overcome this problem, attention has focused on

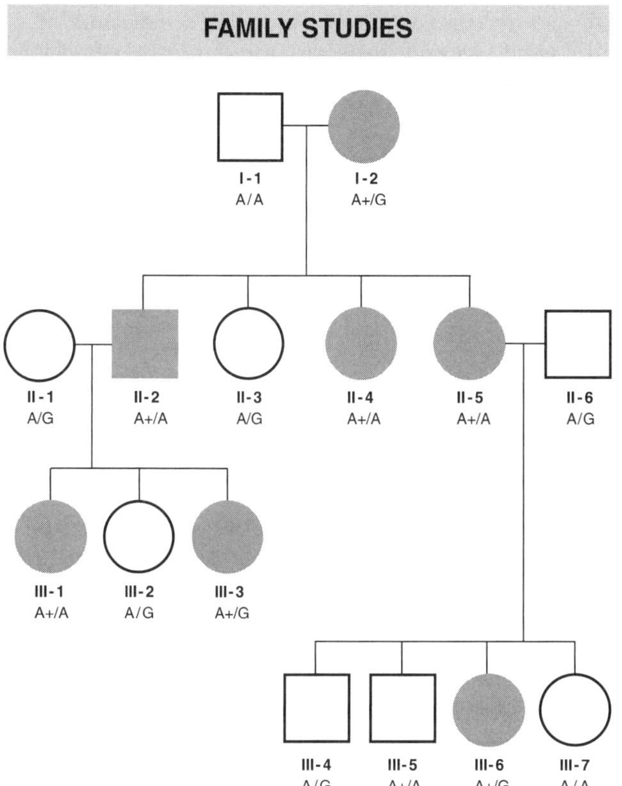

Figure 4. continued

the examination of multiple sets of polymorphisms (haplotypes) in several genes to better understand the factors leading to multifactorial disease.

Case-control Studies, Population Genetics

Historically, association analysis of genetic polymorphisms has been most often performed in a case-control setting, with unrelated affected subjects compared to unrelated unaffected subjects (Figure 4). Because many more recombinations have occurred in an unrelated outbred population, the regions of LD are considerably shorter when compared to those within members of a single family. Therefore, genetic markers have to be more closely spaced to serve as reliable indicators of a disease susceptibility locus. As previously discussed, the size of such haplotype blocks (i.e., regions in LD) can vary greatly among different ethnic populations. This has fostered interest in relatively homogeneous populations such as represented by the inhabitants of Iceland where considerably fewer genetic markers suffice for linkage analysis. Yet, a genetically diverse population may harbor many more diverse genotypes for the same phenotype that might be useful in understanding the genetic basis of disease. In practical terms, if a statistical association is observed between a marker allele and a phenotypic trait in a case-control study, then that location becomes a candidate region and it is studied further for the candidate gene(s) causing the disease or phenotype.

Several groups have shown that association studies in large populations can be a powerful approach for finding genetic determinants of complex disorders (Reference 17). The promise for case-control studies using LD to identify the cause of complex disorders is great but it also suffers from many challenges. If the cases include a heterogeneous collection of etiologies for a given disease, as most common complex disorders do, the power to detect a significant association will be reduced, requiring a large number of subjects. If the control groups include subjects that have not yet manifested a particular disease (e.g., high blood pressure) or have been misdiagnosed, the power also will decrease. The case-control association study design also is susceptible to spurious associations related to differences in population stratification between the case and control groups. Stratification can result from population admixing or differences in ethnicity between cases and controls. This can be a significant problem in areas where the population is diverse such as the United States.

Genome-wide Association Studies

Typically, association studies and positional cloning have been performed with the use of SNPs. A new approach includes the use of haplotypes with multiple phased SNPs (Reference 13, 18). This strategy provides several advantages because it reflects the true dissemination of chromosomal segments throughout the study population, it permits assessment of the combined functional effects of multiple phased SNPs, and it likely accounts for any bias arising from ethnic population admixture. The main haplotypes for most genes of interest will be available shortly on multiple Web sites. This represents a major advancement compared to early studies conducted in the 1980s that developed an RFLP map of the human genome. When completed, the map contained about 400 landmarks across the entire genome. For reasons previously discussed, the low density of RFLPs across the genome (about 1 RFLP per 7–10 megabases of DNA) severely limited the use of this map as a tool for identifying complex diseases. Under optimal conditions, the RFLP map was useful for linkage analysis in family studies.

Based on these limitations, investigators focused attention on polymorphisms found with higher frequency across the genome. Tandem repeats are well suited as landmarks for gene-mapping association studies because they are highly polymorphic and have a low probability for the same pattern occurring in two unrelated individuals. They also are found with a higher frequency in the genome compared to tested RFLPs. However, based on the relatively large number of SNPs that exist in the human genome, this type of polymorphism appears to hold the most promise for revealing the genetic cause of complex disease as well as the response to therapy.

Work is now under way to identify all human SNPs and to develop a dense map of SNPs and their distribution across the human genome (Reference 19). The SNP map is predicted to become the most useful tool in genome-wide association studies. In fact, the identification and cataloguing of all human SNPs has been identified as one of the next major steps taken from the human genome project. As previously discussed, SNPs occur with a relatively high frequency throughout the entire genome compared to other landmarks such as RFLPs or tandem repeats. Current estimates predict that more than 10 million SNPs will be identified such that one SNP will occur on average once every 200–300 bases. From the SNP map, clinicians will be able to establish haplotype information on the phasing of SNPs in genomic regions associated with disease. Despite the advantages previously discussed, the variable length of haplotype blocks in different populations will make it difficult to predict the needed density for finding any given disease susceptibility locus. It also remains to be determined how many haplotype markers will suffice for genome-wide scanning. Nevertheless, with the automation of rapid DNA sequencing and genotyping technology, genome-wide association studies have become feasible.

Summary

The conventional approach used to find the genetic basis of disease in humans has involved positional cloning strategies within family members possessing that disease. The positional cloning strategy typically begins by taking advantage of a sufficiently dense marker map around the suspected gene locus. The key to positional cloning is that it requires a good approximation of the specific chromosome segment where the disease gene(s) exist, and a strong pattern of inheritance between family members. If the initial estimate is off by a significant distance, the target gene will not be found. Until recently the "guess work" has been viewed as a major limitation to finding genes for complex disorders. Now that the entire human genome is known and many more markers are being revealed, the "guess work" will not be a determining factor for the successful identification of disease susceptibility genes. A sufficiently dense map of markers (SNPs) across the entire genome will allow genome-wide association studies that identify regions of LD around all disease susceptibility genes. This novel approach facilitated by technical advances in genotyping will be useful to study large populations with a high level of genetic diversity. It also will clearly open new avenues for understanding the genetic underpinning of complex disease without prior knowledge of chromosomal location or biochemical mechanisms.

References

1. Sadee, W. Pharmacogenomics. Interview by Clare Thompson. BMJ 1999;319(7220):1286.

2. Peltonen L, McKusick VA. Genomics and medicine. Dissecting human disease in the postgenomic era. Science 2001;291(5507):1224–9.

3. McKusick VA. Mendelian Inheritance in Man, 12 ed. Baltimore, MD: Johns Hopkins University Press, 1998.

4. Evans WE, Johnson JA. Pharmacogenomics: the inherited basis for interindividual differences in drug response. Annu Rev Genomics Hum Genet 2001;2:9–39.

5. Cambien F, Poirier O, Nicaud V, et al. Sequence diversity in 36 candidate genes for cardiovascular disorders. Am J Hum Genet 1999;65(1):183–91.

6. Hill AV. The genomics and genetics of human infectious disease susceptibility. Annu Rev Genomics Hum Genet 2001;2:373–400.

7. Mancinelli L, Cronin M, Sadee W. Pharmacogenomics: the promise of personalized medicine. AAPS PharmSci 2000;2(1):E4.

8. Evans WE, Relling MV. Pharmacogenomics: translating functional genomics into rational therapeutics. Science 1999;286(5439):487–91.

9. Newport MJ, Huxley CM, Huston S, et al. A mutation in the interferon-gamma-receptor gene and susceptibility to mycobacterial infection. N Engl J Med 1996;335(26):1941–9.

10. Schork NJ, Nath SK, Fallin D, Chakravarti A. Linkage disequilibrium analysis of biallelic DNA markers, human quantitative trait loci, and threshold-defined case and control subjects. Am J Hum Genet 2000;67(5):1208–18.

11. Patil N, Berno AJ, Hinds DA, et al. Blocks of limited haplotype diversity revealed by high-resolution scanning of human chromosome 21. Science 2001;294(5547):1719–23.

12. Reich DE, Cargill M, Bolk S, et al. Linkage disequilibrium in the human genome. Nature 2001;411(6834):199–204.

13. Drysdale CM, McGraw DW, Stack CB, et al. Complex promoter and coding region beta 2-adrenergic receptor haplotypes alter receptor expression and predict in vivo responsiveness. Proc Natl Acad Sci U S A 2000;97(19):10483–8.

14. Lengauer C, Kinzler KW, Vogelstein B. Genetic instabilities in human cancers. Nature 1998;396(6712):643–9.

15. Kuivenhoven JA, Jukema JW, Zwinderman AH, et al. The role of a common variant of the cholesteryl ester transfer protein gene in the progression of coronary atherosclerosis. The Regression Growth Evaluation Statin Study Group. N Engl J Med 1998;338(2):86–93.

16. Zambon A, Brown BG, Deeb SS, Brunzell JD. Hepatic lipase as a focal point for the development and treatment of coronary artery disease. J Investig Med 2001;49(1):112–8.

17. Sabatti C, Risch N. Homozygosity and linkage disequilibrium. Genetics 2002;160(4):1707–19.

18. Daly MJ, Rioux JD, Schaffner SF, Hudson TJ, Lander ES. High-resolution haplotype structure in the human genome. Nat Genet 2001;29(2):229–32.

19. Kruglyak L, Nickerson DA. Variation is the spice of life. Nat Genet 2001;27(3):234–6.

Self-Assessment Questions

1. Single nucleotide polymorphisms (SNPs) are commonly found in which of the following regions within chromosomes?

    A. Exons.
    B. Introns.
    C. Promotor regions.
    D. Exons, introns, and promotor regions.

Questions 2–5 pertain to the following case.

A comparative study was conducted in normal individuals and patients with cystic fibrosis homozygous for a common SNP mutation in the cystic fibrosis transmembrane conductance regulator gene and in normal individuals. The investigators analyzed each patient's genotype for a receptor protein associated with barrier defense in the lung in both groups. Patients homozygous for a normal functioning receptor were designated as A, whereas those homozygous for a genotype known to cause receptor dysfunction were designated as B. Several clinical end points, including pulmonary function, pneumonia susceptibility, and mortality, were followed more than 10 years. Some of the results are presented below.

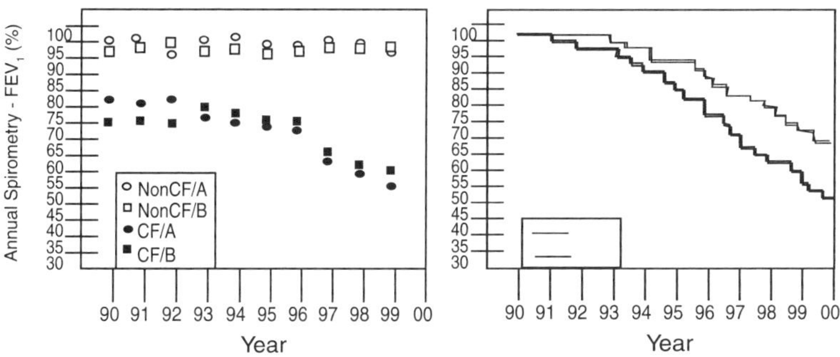

FEV_1 = forced expiratory volume in 1 second.

2. Which one of the following statements is most correct?

    A. The defective receptor is associated with pulmonary dysfunction in both normal and cystic fibrosis patients.
    B. The defective receptor does not appear to have any influence on pulmonary function in cystic fibrosis or normal patients.
    C. The defective receptor has a major impact on pulmonary function in patients with cystic fibrosis but not normal individuals.

D. The defective receptor has a major impact on pulmonary function in normal individuals but not patients with cystic fibrosis.

3. Which one of the following statements is most correct?

   A. The defective receptor does not influence survival in patients with cystic fibrosis.
   B. The defective receptor only has an impact on survival in normal individuals.
   C. The defective receptor appears to decrease survival in patients with cystic fibrosis.
   D. The defective receptor appears to increase survival in patients with cystic fibrosis.

4. Further analysis in patients with cystic fibrosis revealed that the higher level of mortality in patients with the B receptor correlated with a substantial increase in the number of *Pseudomonas* infections that patients experienced over the 10-year study period. Which one of the following conclusions can be drawn?

   A. That the B form of the receptor and defective cystic fibrosis transmembrane conductance regulator gene directly causes *Pseudomonas* pneumonia.
   B. That the B form of the receptor is directly responsible for *Pseudomonas* infections in patients with cystic fibrosis.
   C. The mechanism by which these genetic alterations result in a higher prevalence of *Pseudomonas* infections is unclear but they do correlate with a higher mortality.
   D. The higher incidence of *Pseudomonas* infections caused a further decrease in pulmonary infection function that ultimately resulted in mortality.

5. If the gene coding for the receptor protein is found on chromosome 1 and the cystic fibrosis transmembrane conductance regulator gene is found on chromosome 7, which one of the following statements is most accurate?

   A. Linkage disequilibrium is a valid strategy to find an association between defective receptor and cystic fibrosis alleles.
   B. Linkage analysis is a valid strategy to find an association between defective receptor and cystic fibrosis alleles.
   C. Genome-wide scanning that looks for multiple-phased SNP is the most effective method to find an association between defective receptor and cystic fibrosis alleles.
   D. A case-control study with relatively large numbers of patients is the most effective method to find an association between defective receptor and cystic fibrosis alleles.

Questions 6–8 pertain to the following case.

6. A patient comes to your clinic and indicates that she recently submitted a blood sample for deoxyribonucleic acid (DNA) SNP to determine her susceptibility to different forms of hypertension. She just received a preliminary report indicating that abnormalities were found but the doctor indicated that she should not be alarmed until the final report is provided. She asks for general advice on the worst-case and best-case scenarios. After carefully describing what an SNP is, which one of the following sets of answers are possible answers for this patient?

    i.   It is possible that one or more SNP could be found in areas on the chromosomes where genes do not exist but still contribute to significant changes that lead to hypertension.

    ii. It is possible that one or more SNP could be found in areas on the chromosomes where genes do exist but do not result in significant changes that cause hypertension.

    iii. It is possible that one or more SNP could be found in areas on the chromosomes where genes do exist and result in significant changes leading to hypertension.

    iv. It is possible that one or more SNP could be found in areas on the chromosomes where genes do not exist and do not result in significant changes leading to hypertension.

    A. i and ii.
    B. i, ii, and iii.
    C. i, ii, iii, and iv.
    D. ii, iii, and iv.

7. She comes back a month later, indicating that her physician predicted a high likelihood she will develop hypertension based on the DNA test. She is not terribly surprised because she has a strong family history, but remains confused. Her doctor indicated that some of the alterations found were simply used to help identify other alterations on the same chromosome that cause hypertension. Which one of the following responses best explains what the doctor meant?

    A. Hypertension is a common complex disease in which multiple genes interact with the individual's environment and contribute to high blood pressure.
    B. Segments on the chromosome that harbor the disease-causing gene stay in proximity to nondisease-causing genetic changes at neighboring locations. These nondisease-causing changes are passed down along with the disease-causing genes over generations and can, therefore, be used to locate the disease-causing genes.

C. Segments of chromosomes move around a lot from one chromosome to another as our cells divide. The nondisease-causing genetic alterations can, therefore, be used to locate the disease-causing genes because they are so hard to find.
D. Genetic tests such as these are only based on finding differences in disease-causing genes. Therefore, the information provided is inaccurate.

8. The patient now asks for advice about what to do next. Her doctor has said that her blood pressure is currently normal and that she does not require any drug. Which one of the following pieces of advice do you give her?

   A. Hypertension is the result of a dynamic interaction between a patient's genetic makeup and the environment that she lives in. Therefore, she can take many preventive measures, including but not limited to exercise, diet, weight control, and salt restriction.
   B. If she has children or other family members who could be affected, they should be tested so that they know their relative risk of developing hypertension and how to prevent it.
   C. Given her predisposition to hypertension, recommend ways to routinely monitor her blood pressure.
   D. All of the above are sound pieces of advice.

9. Which one of the following is not true regarding the strategy used in linkage disequilibrium studies?

   A. It requires a dense map of markers.
   B. It exploits within family studies.
   C. It relies on markers that occur close to disease alleles.
   D. It assumes that a marker has an indirect association with a given trait.

10. A case-control study is being conducted in a group of patients with congestive heart failure compared to normal individuals. The initial phase of the study was to determine the heterogeneity that exists for the angiotensin-converting enzyme gene between these two populations. In the group of 100 patients with congestive heart failure studied, a total of 15 different SNPs were found. The next phase was to determine if different haplotypes could be used to predict patient response to angiotensin-converting enzyme inhibitors. Which one of the following statements is correct regarding the number of possible haplotypes in this cohort?

   A. There are 2^{100} possible haplotypes.
   B. There are 2^{15} possible haplotypes.
   C. There are 200 possible haplotypes.
   D. There are 15,100 possible haplotypes.

Ethical, Legal, and Social Issues in Pharmacogenomics

William L. Allen, M.Div, J.D.

Key Words

Genetic discrimination, informed consent, confidentiality, eugenics.

Abstract

Understanding the ethical concerns about new genetic knowledge, such as pharmacogenomic information, requires an understanding of the history of racial, ethnic, and social discrimination that was reinforced by so-called "genetic knowledge," resulting in such public policy measures as involuntary eugenic sterilization and ethnically based immigration restrictions. In addition to the medical benefits of genetic information, the dynamics of predictive genetic information can have detrimental effects on patients, and must be considered and factored in to decisions to use genetic tests. In addition to the direct clinical issues, the potential nonmedical uses of probabilistic risk information from genetic testing, including pharmacogenomic profiles, will be of interest to third parties, such as insurers and employers who may use the information for genetic discrimination that is either unfair or unanticipated by the patient who receives such testing. Health care providers must understand these risks to appropriately preserve patient privacy and confidentiality, as well as explain the risks of genetic testing to potential candidates.

Outline

Learning Objectives

1. Understand the historical roots and dangers of genetic discrimination, which in part explain the anxiety associated with ethical issues arising from advances in genetic science and technology.
2. Understand how the traditional obligations of medical ethics, such as informed consent and confidentiality are applied in the context of clinical genetics.
3. Understand what new ethical, legal, and social challenges are posed by the development of functional genomics ensuing from the Human Genome Initiative.
4. Understand the risks of genetic discrimination.
5. Understand the scope and limitations of current regulatory protections against genetic discrimination and their professional obligation to inform patients of the risks of genetic discrimination that may result from submitting to a genetic test.

Abbreviations in this Chapter

ADA	Americans with Disabilities Act
ApoE	Apolipoprotein E
BNSF	Burlington Northern Santa Fe Railroad
EEOC	Equal Employment Opportunity Commission
ERISA	Employee Retirement Income Security Act
IRA	Immigration Restriction Act
HIPAA	Health Insurance Portability and Accountability Act
SNP	Single nucleotide polymorphism
TPMT	Thiopurine S-methyltransferase

Ethical, Legal, and Social Issues in

Pharmacogenomics

Historical Factors Coloring the Uses of Genetic Technology

In the contemporary period, advances in genetic technology have been associated with social and ethical concerns. At the beginning of the human genome era, such concern was manifest in a statement signed by a wide variety of clerics to the President warning of the dark possibilities that might accompany the dramatic technological advances being envisioned. Similar fears often accompany the prospect of rapid technological change, particularly when the technology affects such emotionally laden areas as human reproduction. Some prognosticators were so fearful of the ultimate consequences of genetic technology as to caution against research and discovery, not only on humans, but also on plants, animals, and microbes (Reference 1).

However, in the case of genetics, more is at work than the usual fear of technology. The history of genetic advances in the past century reveals some concrete reasons for concern. Much of the reason for the social and ethical concerns about advances in genetic knowledge and technology, including pharmacogenomics, has its roots in the history of social uses to which so called "genetic knowledge" and "genetic discoveries" have been put.

Eugenics was the term coined in late 19th century England for what its proponents advocated as a "science" of improving human stock by humanity taking control over its own evolution. Ensuring that "desirable" races and "strains of blood" prevailed and multiplied was called positive eugenics. Negative eugenics, by contrast, was conceived as a way of reducing or eliminating "bad genes" from the gene pool. This movement consisted primarily of people from the white middle and upper classes. Although laymen were involved, leadership from scientists, especially those who studied genetics, was crucial.

Eugenicists declared that they were concerned with preventing social degeneration, which they found glaring signs of in the social and behavioral discordances of urban industrial society—for example, crime, slums, and rampant disease—and the causes of which they attributed primarily to biology—to "blood," to use the term of inheritable essence common at the turn of the century (Reference 2).

They saw the new science of genetics as a way to accomplish social improvement. The key to reducing these chronic social ills was to identify, isolate, and prevent or discourage replication of the culprit deleterious genes. Negative eugenics entailed analysis of traits thought to be at the root of social burdens—traits of character, temperament, and behavior accounting for such problems as alcoholism, prostitution, criminality, and poverty.

The major early American leader of the eugenics movement was Charles B. Davenport, a Harvard professor, who held that various races and nationalities reflect biological differences manifesting distinct racial traits. He expected that the "great influx of blood from Southeastern Europe" would rapidly make the American population "darker in pigmentation, smaller in stature, more mercurial … more given to crimes of larceny, kidnapping, assault, murder, rape, and sex immorality" (Reference 2). There was virtually no research to support these claims, but they were expressed as if they were scientific truths. What little research did exist, such as a study of race mixing in Jamaica, was of no validity, already containing in its assumptions the "conclusion" that the results of race mixing in Jamaica demonstrated biological and social degeneration. Other such studies purported to show inheritance of such traits as "nomadism" and "shiftlessness." He claimed that "thalassophilia"—the love of the sea that he saw in naval officers—must be a sex-linked recessive trait, like color blindness, because it was manifest almost exclusively in males.

Another major problem held to be caused by genetics was mental deficiency—widely referred to as "feeblemindedness"—frequently demonstrated by intelligence tests. Feeblemindedness was used as an overarching genetic condition that was thought to lead to many varieties of socially undesirable behavior. Another eugenicist, Henry Goddard, speculated that this group was "a vigorous animal organism of low intellect but strong physique—the wild man of today." It was claimed that such specimens lacked the discretion to discern right from wrong, much less the self-control to restrain their primitive impulses. This explained their proclivity to become criminals, prostitutes, and paupers. The effects of these ideas were more than academic speculation. Public policies with profound results were implemented based on eugenic notions.

One of the most drastic attempts to eliminate problems perceived to be caused and perpetuated by unfettered reproduction of those deemed genetically inferior was involuntary sterilization. Of course, if one's goal were the efficient elimination of those with "inheritable feeblemindedness," the place to begin would be state entities where those deemed to be feebleminded were institutionalized.

By 1931, some 30 states had compulsory sterilization laws on their books, aimed mostly at the "insane" and "feebleminded." These categories were loosely defined to include many recent immigrants and others who were functionally illiterate or knew little or no English and who, therefore, did poorly on IQ tests. The laws also often were extended to so-called sexual perverts, drug fiends, drunkards, epileptics, and others deemed ill or degenerate (Reference 3).

In all, as many as 50, 000 individuals in the United States were subjected to this intervention. This measure was not implemented without some opposition, but ultimately the proponents prevailed in a case that was decided by the United States Supreme Court, Buck v. Bell, 274 US 200, 47 S.Ct. 584, 71L. Ed. 1000 (1927). At stake in this case was whether the State of Virginia had the right to assert a compelling state interest in carrying out involuntary sterilizations for eugenic purposes, or whether the state was prohibited from such measures by an individual's liberty interest as articulated in the United States Constitution. The state wanted to sterilize Carrie Buck, whom it deemed to be an imbecile due to inheritable transmission of feeblemindedness. The court upheld the state's right to carry out this sterilization, memorialized in a now infamous line from Justice Oliver Wendell Holmes that "...three generations of imbeciles is enough."

Many years later, Carrie Buck would be located and found to be mentally competent and regretful that she had never been able to bear children (Reference 4).

In Germany, the Nazis borrowed programs and rationales originated by eugenicists in Britain and the United States and implemented eugenic sterilization laws modeled on California's involuntary sterilization law, drafted in 1909, which required as a condition of release from a mental institution that patients undergo sterilization (Reference 5). In time, the German eugenic sterilization measures "were expanded to include Jews, homosexuals, Gypsies, Eastern European "Slavs," and other "inferior" types" (Reference 2). Eugenics was used to reinforce and provide "scientific" credence to Nazi racial hygiene ideology, leading ultimately to the extermination of millions in the Holocaust.

Involuntary sterilization was not the only manifestation of eugenics inspiring public policy measures. Davenport's warnings about the impact of immigration were augmented by others. Lewis Terman wrote:

The fecundity of the family stocks from which our most gifted children came appears to be definitely on the wane ... It has been figured that if the present differential birthrate continues 1000 Harvard graduates will at the end of 200 years, have but 56 descendants, while in the same period, 1000 South Italians will have multiplied to 100,000 (Reference 2).

Such fears eventually led to eugenically inspired immigration restrictions in the United States. In 1924, the United States enacted the Immigration Restriction Act (IRA), which set immigration levels by a formula designed to restrict immigration of southern Europeans to shift immigration to favor northern Europeans. These measures "prevented the immigration of countless Jews who were attempting to flee the Nazis, because they had been born in eastern Europe."

Application of these ideas on a grand scale by the Nazi regime ultimately cast eugenics in an unfavorable light. In the years after World War II, the eugenics movement's influence waned as the results of logical extension of racial hygiene ideas were eschewed. The ideas of its original proponents fell out of favor, not only because of its outcome in the holocaust, but also because later genetic researchers rejected the scientific inadequacies of the pioneers in favor of more rigorous methodologies and more cautious conclusions.

Of course, the social application of eugenics as a public health measure was fallacious from its inception because recessive genetic conditions are the result of carriers who do not manifest the condition. When carriers of one copy of a recessive allele reproduce, there is a 25 percent chance in each conception that the child will inherit two copies of the affected allele, one from each parent, thereby manifesting the condition. In light of the way recessive alleles function, targeting people who manifest real or perceived genetic conditions never made sense as a public health strategy because at best it could only address a small portion of those even with actual genetic maladies. The remarkable fact is that this knowledge was available, but provided no discouragement to the eugenics movement.

Although all this was known by 1908, before eugenic programs were instituted in the United States or in Germany, the old eugenic practices went on for several more decades, until changes in the political situation made them unacceptable.

The eclipse of eugenics was a welcome development, but it did not eliminate all controversy about the ethical acceptability of basing social distinctions on perceived disabilities believed to be inheritable. Even though such extreme policies as eugenic sterilization and eugenically based immigration quotas ended with the disfavor that overtook the eugenics movement, these historical moments have not lost their resonance in current discussions of genetic advances. Any current proposals for using applications of genetic analysis are inevitably seen against the background of the excesses of the eugenics movement. The emergence of genetic information, both real and perceived, is not neutral with respect to the social uses to which it may be put. An implicit burden of proof exists for those proposing genetic advances to demonstrate not only that the excesses of the past are not repeated, but also that more subtle and nuanced forms of unacceptable genetic discrimination do not emerge. By keeping in focus the egregious mistakes of the past as a cautionary tale of how subject genetic science has been to social mischief, perhaps such risks will be minimized.

Pharmacogenomics and the Principle of Nonmaleficence

This longstanding principle of health care ethics, originating in the Hippocratic tradition's maxim, "first, do no harm," also has been variously expressed as not only the duty to *do* no harm, but also the duty to remove harm and to prevent harm. One of the major reasons for pursuing pharmacogenomics has been the anticipation, already realized in some instances, of reducing adverse drug reactions. To the extent that pharmacogenomics can prevent a significant segment of such adverse drug reactions, pursuing this technology is ethically obligatory.

Before the ability to predict which patient would manifest an adverse reaction, the risk of death, even an adverse reaction resulting in death, is justifiable in some patients. Such risk can be justified because the anticipation of benefit dramatically exceeds the probability of harm or because the magnitude of harm without treatment, death, is equivalent to the magnitude of harm in the unlikely event of a fatal adverse reaction. Once there is a way to predict who is at risk from the treatment, it is obligatory under the principle of nonmaleficence to use such a means to prevent harm to those expected to be harmed.

Plausible arguments have been advanced that by using pharmacogenomic tests, people expected to have a substantial known risk of harm can be excluded from studies and that studies can prove effectiveness with smaller numbers of patients exposed to the harm of unknown risks as well. Targeting the protocol to include only those with pharmacogenetic indicators of expected efficacy would reduce the risks of harmful side effects for those who otherwise (as in conventional protocols) unknowingly incur risk without the likelihood of benefit. To the extent that a pharmacogenomic approach can reduce the numbers of research subjects exposed to reasonably anticipated harms in research, it is morally obligatory to make it available.

Pharmacogenomics and the Principle of Beneficence

The principle of beneficence exceeds the duty to avoid, remove, or prevent harm by enjoining the provider positively to promote the well-being and best interests of the patient. Thus, prevention of adverse drug reactions is not the only relevant ethical criterion for assessing pharmacogenomics. To the extent that efficacy can be improved by pharmacogenomic analysis and targeted therapeutic intervention, it would be morally obligatory to offer it.

In many, if not most contexts, beneficence cannot be considered in isolation from nonmaleficence because the prospect of potential for harm or even the necessity of some actual harm is entailed in an intervention expected to restore or improve the patient's overall well-being. In these cases, harm is tolerated as long as the expected benefits clearly outweigh the expected harms sufficiently to justify acceptance of the harm or risk of harm.

Of course, all of these reasons that pharmacogenomics might seem to be morally obligatory depend on projected scenarios in which the totality of positive outcomes greatly outweigh the bad outcomes. Any moral analysis that advocates pursuit of pharmacogenomics also is obligated to ensure that the prospect of unanticipated or unintended consequences that may accompany the anticipated benefits are prevented or mitigated as much as possible. A look at the issues that have arisen in the context of genetic testing in the past will help with that assessment.

Pharmacogenomics and the Principle of Autonomy

One of the primary rules of health care ethics stemming from autonomy is informed consent. Valid informed consent requires disclosure from providers and comprehension by patients of several elements necessary to medical decision making, including: 1) the potential risks and benefits of a recommended test or treatment option; 2) alternative potential diagnostic procedures or treatment options and their respective risks and benefits; and 3) the option of doing nothing, as well as the risks and benefits of no action.

One of the issues that must be determined in achieving informed consent is what degree of risk is too small or remote to require disclosure. In one of the classic cases articulating the standard of informed consent, the failure to disclose a 1 percent risk of paralysis after surgery was held to be sufficiently significant that a reasonable person might have refused the recommended surgery if the risk had been disclosed (Canterbury v. Spence, 464 F.2d 772, D.C. Circuit, Court of Appeals, [1972]). In the context of single nucleotide polymorphism (SNP) testing for drug responsiveness, it is interesting to note that the definition of a polymorphism is a genetic variation that occurs in at least 1 percent of the population. However, a 1 percent probability of harm is not an absolute threshold for assessing which risks warrant disclosure. Risk must be disclosed based not only on the basis of probability of harm, but magnitude of harm as well. Probabilities of harm substantially smaller than 1 percent may well be sufficient to influence the decisions of patients when the magnitude of harm is substantial. For example, azathioprine-induced profound myelosuppression secondary to thiopurine S-methyltransferase (TPMT) deficiency occurs in a subset of patients when using standard dosages of thiopurine. About 11 percent of Caucasians are heterozygous with one wild-type allele and one variant allele, resulting in intermediate enzyme levels, indicating susceptibility to early leukopenic episodes, who might be safely managed at reduced dosages. For the one in 300 Caucasians who inherit two variant alleles, resulting in no functional enzyme activity, however, severe myelosuppression can lead to serious morbidity and mortality. For a condition such as Crohn's disease, this risk may not be worthwhile because other therapeutic options exist. For acute lymphoblastic leukemia in children, however, the goal of prolonged remission may warrant use at lower dosages for those homozygous for the variant alleles. Although testing for genotype related to TMPT status currently is conducted at a few institutions, it has not yet become a clear standard of care. Nevertheless, when contemplating starting a patient on standard dosage of thiopurine without such testing, adequate informed consent must acknowledge not only the more common risk of leucopenia in the 11 percent of heterozygotes, but also the severe risks for the one in 300 homozygotes for the variant alleles. Even though the probability of serious harm is low for any given patient, the magnitude of harm can be fatal (Reference 6).

The ideal model of a pharmacogenetic test, in which identification of a particular SNP indicates a direct relationship between the drug and a harmful outcome with little or no benefit, the balance of harms and benefits may be fairly clear and straightforward, and disclosure necessary for valid informed consent is relatively straightforward as well. This pattern is likely to vary considerably, however, creating difficult choices for patients and providers about whether to have a test and how the result should influence care. In such complex scenarios, varying patient values and goals are crucial to the determination of whether to test and how clinical options are affected by testing. Informed consent in such scenarios is more difficult to achieve and requires considerable dialogue with patients to ensure adequate understanding for meaningful decision making.

Markers for certain drug responses for cardiovascular drugs, such as apolipoprotein (ApoE) for example, also may indicate an association with an increased likelihood of Alzheimer disease (Reference 7). Some patients may not want to know such probabilistic risk information, especially about a late-onset disease without clear measures of prevention or intervention. Consideration of whether to test for drug response in this situation must determine whether the patient would want to know other implications of the test results. If a patient does not want to know the predictive implications of a test result for a disease or condition, this factor must be balanced against the need to know the drug responsiveness. In some cases, even when there is a test available for drug responsiveness, but the burdens of empirical trial and error are not terrible, a patient may want to exhaust other treatment options or determine responsiveness empirically, without a genetic test, even if such an approach is more costly, labor intensive, and time-consuming.

One of the pervasive problems with the rise of molecular analysis and information is the tendency to what has been called geneticization (Reference 2). The term refers to an overly deterministic conception of the role of genes in phenotypic outcomes. The role of genes or of SNPs in phenotypic outcomes in some cases may be reasonably straightforward, but genetic heterogeneity, multiple interactions of genes or SNPs, and variable interactions of genes or SNPs with complex environmental factors complicate the inferences that can be drawn from associations between particular genes or SNPs and phenotypic outcomes (Reference 10).

This complexity undoubtedly complicates questions of access and informed consent. Although a single SNP may indicate a particular drug responsiveness outcome for some percentage of individuals, it is likely that other less frequent combinations of SNP(s) and/or environmental factors will lead to a similar outcome. In such cases, a positive test for a SNP may reliably indicate an adverse reaction to a particular drug, but a negative test for the same SNP will not necessarily mean there is no risk of the adverse reaction. Adequate patient understanding of the potential outcomes and meanings of such tests will be crucial for informed consent.

In a real sense, the professional role of genetic counselors has developed as a way of providing sufficient understanding of genetic testing and diagnosis to enable patients and their families to make informed decisions about whether the benefits of testing outweigh the risks in the context of their own personal values. One problem that has been identified with the advent and implementation of genetic tests is the projected inability to provide the equivalent of genetic counselors to meet the need for patient education and interpretation necessary to ensure that patients can make authentically informed decisions.

The role of pharmacists in ensuring the safe and effective use of drugs by patients has increased substantially, including drug therapy management service to physicians and patients managing problems such as anticoagulation, hyperlipidemia, diabetes, and asthma (Reference 11). In view of the increasing role of pharmacists in counseling and educating patients, pharmacists need to learn enough about pharmacogenetic analysis to educate and reinforce accurate understanding among the patients they serve. Because the deployment of pharmacogenomic analysis is likely to involve testing as well as prescribing, pharmacists need to understand the significance of tests and test results as well as outcomes and side effects of the prescribed drugs to be an informed resource for patients.

Among the issues that have become important in genetic counseling is the ethic of nondirectiveness. In general, the ethical commitment of genetics counselors has been to help patients understand the options they face and the meaning of the information relevant to those options, without directing the patients' choices of those options. Some questions have been raised as to whether it is possible to be completely neutral in counseling patients, but the ideal of nondirectiveness is important to ensuring that providers do not unduly influence patients' choices by imposing the providers' own values through recommendations that conflate personal choices with professional clinical judgment (Reference 12).

Issues in the Research Context

One of the issues that has been raised by genetic research in general is the changing paradigm of the banking of blood and tissue samples. Traditionally, leftover blood and tissue were thought of as disposable and insignificant from the source subject or patient's point of view. Because blood or tissue taken out of the subject's body were no longer useful, no one gave much thought to what else might be done with it or whether the source subject has any claims concerning it.

The increase in actual and potential information that can be extracted from extant tissue and blood samples about their original source by molecular genetic analysis makes such samples rich sources of information about any patient whose identity has remained linked to the sample. Not only is the sample a source of present information, but also a source of future information not yet analyzable, but potentially having profound impact on the source subject for years into the future, as long as the sample is linked to the source's identity.

The potential for as yet undetermined genetic testing, including pharmacogenomic analysis, raises a number of problems, not least of which is the complications it poses for valid informed consent. For example, if researchers who want to test blood or tissue samples already collected from a group of people with a particular disease to see whether there is a genetic marker for it, how do they obtain informed consent from the source donor subjects? Given the potential significance of what may be discovered, the original consent to obtain the sample cannot be deemed sufficient to imply that the donor has consented to whatever test anyone decides to do with it, especially as long as the sample retains identifiers. The simplest way to avoid some of these problems is to strip identifiers, but there are reasons the researchers may not want to do that. To answer some important questions, it might be necessary to acquire additional information about the donor's medical history, current condition, environmental factors, etc.

If identifiers are maintained to have access to such additional information, another thorny problem may arise. Although associations between certain genetic markers and physiological conditions may be suggested by research, such early data may not be sufficiently validated to be clinically useful, and disclosure to the donor may be more misleading than useful. In some cases, by contrast, findings may be such that the researchers may feel that the findings are sufficiently significant that the donor might want to know. Because individuals vary considerably in whether they want to know such information, the researchers have no way of knowing whether any particular donor would wish to learn the results. Because the donors could not have been informed of the genetic analysis and its potential meaning, benefits and harms before donating the sample, there is now no way to obtain informed consent after the findings have been made.

Of course, when contemplating the potential for genetic analysis of banked tissue when the tissue is collected, it is possible to obtain informed consent for specific genetic analysis that can be foreseen sufficiently to include the risks and benefits when the sample is donated. However, this is of limited help because numerous research possibilities will emerge from future genetic tests that have not yet been developed and which, therefore, cannot be sufficiently characterized to obtain informed consent at the time of donation. Therefore, it is impossible to obtain at the time of sample donation a blanket informed consent for any or all genetic research that may be desirable to conduct in the future on the same set of samples.

The remaining options are not ideal. One option is to return to the donor in each case for informed consent. This is labor intensive, and because of the difficulty in maintaining contact with subject donors, practically impossible in many cases. Another possibility is simply to have donors waive their right to informed consent for future research on their samples (Reference 13). If the samples can have identifiers completely eliminated, this is not so problematic, but eliminating the identifiers limits the additional data that can be acquired later. A middle possibility can be used in such cases. The identifiers can be maintained only in the file (medical record) of the subject's physician, and if a future researcher wants to conduct additional testing, the researcher can contact the subject's physician to approach the subject to see whether he or she is interested in participating in the new project based on the specific prospects of risks and benefits that may be anticipated.

Clinical Ethical Issues in Medical Genetics
Informed Consent

Another factor that complicates the informed consent, not only in the context of research, but also for clinical contexts, is the advent of multiplex testing. When multiple tests are available on a single computer chip that analyzes a blood sample for more than one test, which is more efficient than separate tests, the complexity of informed consent is magnified. A patient may legitimately want to know the results of one or more tests without knowing the results of others. Bundling tests together makes testing decisions more complicated.

Confidentiality

As with other medical information, genetic test results and their meanings are subject to confidentiality. More than other medical information, however, genetic information may have real or perceived implications not only for the test subject, but for his or her family as well. This means that a breach in confidentiality can be harmful not only to the patient, but also to family members, even though direct inferences about family members may not be accurate.

By the same token, the possibility of inheritable genetic traits means that some genetic information about an individual may raise concerns that could affect other family members. Some controversies have arisen among family members in which the test results of one individual were deemed by family members to be relevant to themselves and which led them to claim the results should be disclosed to potentially affected family members. In general, the better policy is to regard individual test results as the confidential information of the tested individual, not to be disclosed to other parties, even family members, without the consent of the tested individual. Although more often than not, tested patients are willing to share potentially relevant information with family members that may be affected, there are reasons that lead some to decide not to disclose such information to anyone. Refusal to disclose genetic test results to family has especially been the case where genetic test results leads to recognition of false paternity. When there is a risk of disclosure, mothers aware of the risk may choose not to have test results disclosed to family members.

Another ambiguity that has arisen around the issue of disclosure of genetic information is whether the provider has a duty to warn potentially at-risk family members, especially the individual's children, who may be at risk of inheriting the genetic condition. Two recent court cases on this issue have reflected somewhat divergent rulings. In Pate v. Threlkel, 661 So. 2d 278 (1995), the plaintiff sued her mother's physician for failure to tell the plaintiff's mother, his patient, that her medullary thyroid carcinoma was a genetically inheritable disease, which would have enabled the plaintiff's mother to warn her daughter of the risk to her in time to be tested and, if necessary, to pursue early intervention. The Florida Supreme Court held that even though the physician did not have a physician-patient relation with the daughter, he did have a duty to warn his patient that her daughter could inherit the condition, and that the daughter could sue her mother's physician for his failure to give that warning, so that the mother could pass it along to the daughter. However, the court went on to clarify that the physician's duty did not extend to a duty to warn the daughter directly because he would be prohibited from disclosure of his patient's condition without her permission. Thus, under Florida law, the physician's duty to disclose genetic information relevant to family members is limited to disclosure to the patient, and if the patient fails to pass on the information, the physician cannot be held liable.

However, a New Jersey appellate court explicitly chose not to follow the Florida Supreme Court's reasoning entirely. In Safer v. Pack, 677 A. 2d 1188 (1996), a woman sued her father's physician for failure to warn that her father's multiple polyposis of the colon was inheritable and which, left untreated, lead to metastatic colorectal cancer. The Appellate Division of the New Jersey Superior Court held that the physician had a duty to warn not only the patient himself, but also the members of the immediate family of the patient who may be affected.

Nonmedical Uses of Genetic Information and Genetic Discrimination

Insurance and Genetic Probabilistic Risk Profiles

The rationale for funding and pursuing the Human Genome Initiative was to provide a basis for improving medical understanding of human disease and the development of new therapies, both conventional and molecular interventions. Although the primary purpose of advances in predictive genetic information was to benefit patients and public health, the predictive information that is generated could have a much wider impact on other aspects of a test subject's life. Insurers and employers have interest in the probabilistic information generated by genetic tests bearing on morbidity, disability, and mortality beyond its clinical medical usefulness in making health care decisions that remain in the context of the provider-patient relationship. A prediction that an applicant for insurance or a covered employee is at significant risk of future onset for a costly medical condition provides incentives for an employer or insurer to avoid or restrict coverage to minimize the cost of future claims.

Although a "pharmacogenomic test" may not be designed to predict genetic disease per se, a test result that determines that the subject would be a nonresponder to a drug that is the only effective treatment for a condition would be of just as much interest to the insurer because it predicts loss, as a predictor of a high probability of the condition itself. Tests predicting that an individual either will have an adverse reaction or will not respond to a cheaper drug, which will necessitate resorting to a substantially more expensive drug, also are of interest to those providing health coverage for that individual. In the end, it is not whether genetic information predicts disease, disability, or drug responsiveness that determines the potential interest of insurers and employers, but rather what the implications of that information are for health benefit claims costs.

There are several ways insurers might use genetic information in the underwriting process. The most drastic way is to require genetic testing of everyone who applies for coverage as part of the underwriting process, and base coverage decisions as well as risk rating and premium pricing on such results. This approach would most violate the traditional ethical perspectives on genetic testing that discourages their use when there is no clear health-related rationale and the primary reason is to segment populations for purposes of distribution of social benefits, such as insurance. Although in an ultimate sense people would remain free to refuse testing as long as they were willing to forego insurance coverage, such an arrangement is extremely coercive to the extent that insurance coverage is a crucial social institution for the financial consequences of catastrophic loss or essential goods and services like health care access.

Most insurers have stated that they are not interested in making genetic testing a required part of the underwriting process for all underwriting decisions (Reference 14). Yet, all insurers recognize that, even if they are reluctant to initiate genetic testing as a part of the underwriting process, they are extremely vulnerable to a competitive disadvantage if their competitor(s) implement genetic testing in underwriting. An insurer that does not screen for genetic risks in underwriting when competitor(s) do use genetic screening risks insuring a pool of covered insureds with a substantially higher than expected risk profile because a larger number of high-risk applicants who were rejected by the competitor on the basis of their genetic risk profiles would gravitate to the insurer that did not use genetic screening.

Even if no extant competitor were to require genetic risk profiling as a part of the underwriting process, new market entrants could emerge that might base their entire marketing plan on selecting risks on the basis of genetic tests. Such a strategy might attempt to segment the lowest genetic risk pool possible by offering low rates to those who were willing to submit voluntarily to a genetic risk profile. If this were to happen, existing insurers would face enormous pressure to follow suit in self-defense.

In general, insurers have been much more insistent that their interest is not in requiring genetic tests of all applicants, but rather that they need access to those test results that insurance applicants have secured on their own before applying for coverage. Their argument is that when applicants know more about their risk than the insurers, the insurers are placed at an unfair advantage because they make coverage and premium decisions that do not adequately reflect risk and will ultimately lead to claims that exceed losses projected on underestimated risk assessments.

Insurers also have argued that the absence of accurate assessment of genetic risks reflected in premiums is unfair to those people in the insurance pool who are at lower risk. Lower risk individuals are held to be "unfairly" subsidizing those at higher risk as long as genetic risk is not reflected in underwriting and rating decisions. Critics of this perspective point out that it is the nature of insurance to spread risk. Moreover, it is an inherent feature of risk pools that it is impossible to segment them to reflect all distinctions among degrees of risk. Critics of the insurers argue that it is unfair to discriminate against people by using genetic risk projections in coverage and premium decisions, especially because genetic risks, unlike risk factors such as smoking, are neither voluntary nor under the control of the individual.

A substantial number of states have placed some restrictions on the ability of insurers to use genetic testing in insurance underwriting (Reference 15). The scope of protection these laws offer varies considerably among states. Even the state laws that offer the broadest protections are substantially limited by the preemption of the federal Employee Retirement Income Security Act (ERISA). This act specifies that state insurance regulations apply only to insurance companies, but not to employers whose health benefit plans are self-insured. Therefore, if a company pays for employee medical benefits out of its own funds rather than purchasing such benefits from an insurance company, state insurance regulations, such as those restricting the use of genetic information in insurance coverage, do not apply to self-insured employers. Most large employers self-insure, so their employees are not protected by state insurance laws.

Federal legislation does provide protection in some circumstances against the use of genetic information to deny or restrict health benefits under the Health Insurance Portability and Accountability Act (HIPAA). Thus, genetic information about risk of future illness is considered among the preexisting conditions that cannot be used as a basis for restricting health benefit coverage for a person moving from one employer with health coverage to another employer that provides coverage. Although this dimension of protection is not insignificant, it remains insufficient to protect people in situations not covered by HIPAA. People moving from an employer with health benefits, for example, to an employer without benefits are not protected. Any possibility from layoff to leaving an employer to become self-employed entails the risk that a genetic test result might be used as a preexisting condition exclusion of coverage or increased premiums. Because the most dynamic part of the economy is the creation of new companies, most of which have a small number of employees, it is precisely this segment of the workforce at risk of denied or restricted health insurance coverage (i.e., when employees leave large companies for start-up opportunities). The HIPAA protections, although welcome, are not entirely adequate. The number of individuals uninsured or underinsured in the United States has grown since the mid-1990s. The prospect of using genetic testing in underwriting health benefits threatens to exacerbate this problem.

Of course, different views on insurance, types of insurance, and notions of fairness have a lot to do with whether the use of genetic testing in the underwriting process is viewed as unacceptable or appropriate. In the United States, most of the concern manifest over this issue has centered around health insurance, because it has such an important bearing on access to health care and the percentage of Americans without health coverage has been a major problem. In England, which has a national health service to provide universal access, the primary focus has been not on health insurance, but on life insurance, especially because life insurance is required as a precondition for a mortgage. Although life insurance has not been regarded by some commentators as having the importance of health insurance in the United States, others have pointed to the basic role of life insurance in maintaining solvency and even preventing poverty of families in which the primary breadwinner dies. It is probably this balance that led the Netherlands to prohibit the use of genetic tests in underwriting life insurance policies with a face value up to the approximate amount of the average price of a house. For policies with a larger face value, genetic information concerning risk is allowed in underwriting life insurance (Reference 16).

Other important forms of insurance may be affected by predictive genetic testing. Disability income insurance provides protection against loss of ability (short of death) to provide income. As with life insurance, it can be crucial to prevent catastrophic impoverishment for families in which primary source of income is ended by serious disability. In fact, many financial advisors regard it as a higher priority for families and individuals than life insurance. Another form of insurance of increasing importance that could be affected by genetic risk information is long-term care insurance. With as many as one in four older Americans predicted to have Alzheimer's disease, the ability of insurers to determine that they are not vulnerable to underestimated risk of losses from the expense of long-term care for people who require so much attention, long-term care insurers will be interested in molecular markers associated with increased risk of Alzheimer's disease.

Employment

Some have looked to the Americans with Disabilities Act (ADA) as a source of protection against genetic discrimination in the employment context. Although the ADA does not offer protection from traditional underwriting in the provision of benefits such as insurance, it does prevent discrimination in hiring, promotion, and firing decisions if those decisions are based on physical or mental impairments that affect a major life activity, as long as the employee can perform the job with reasonable accommodations from the employer. One problem with finding protection from genetic discrimination in the ADA is that predictive genetic information is about predisposition to future impairments rather than presently manifested impairments. Thus, it is not clear whether predisposition to a future impairment would be protected because it does not currently affect a major life activity.

Advocates of protecting those at genetic risk from the perception that they are currently disabled have expressed reluctance to argue that future risk status should be regarded as a disability to fall under the scope of protection currently described in the ADA. The Equal Employment

Opportunity Commission (EEOC), the federal entity charged with regulating and enforcing the ADA in the employment context, has interpreted the ADA as offering substantial protection against the misuse of genetic or other medical tests by employers (Reference 17). These regulations also solve the problem of how to protect probabilistic genetic information on predisposition to illness without labeling risk of future illness as a present disability. These regulations do so by expanding protection from simply having a disability to include having a record of a disability (even if one no longer has the disability) and to the perception that one has a disability (such as treating a genetic test result predicting increased risk of future disability as if it were a present certainty of disability).

In a recent instance of an employer using genetic information to exclude coverage to save money on claims, Burlington Northern Santa Fe Railroad (BNSF) collected blood from employees and tested it without employee consent. The purpose of the genetic tests performed on employee blood samples was to deny workers' compensation claims by claiming that employees claiming work-related injuries had genetic predispositions to congenital defects that were the real cause of the injuries (Leigh Strope [AP labor writer] 2002). If BNSF could show that the injuries were caused by congenital defects instead of work done in the scope of employment, they could evade workers' compensation claims.

The EEOC sued BNSF for an injunction to prohibit the use of employee genetic tests in this fashion. Recently, BNSF and the EEOC settled the case, resulting in a fine and a consent agreement that BNSF would no longer engage in genetic testing of employees.

However, the effectiveness of the EEOC regulations in preventing employer use of genetic tests, in spite of its effectiveness in the BNSF case, has been called into question by a recent United States Supreme Court case (Toyota Motor Manufacturing, Kentucky, Inc., Petitioner v. Ella Williams 534 US 184; 122 S. Ct. 681; 151 L. Ed. 2d 615; [2002] US Lexis 400). The court reasoned that congressional intent when limiting the scope of protection under the ADA to impairments that affect a major life activity must be narrowly interpreted. According to the court, the entire rationale for the ADA was to provide relief for the minority of people with disabilities whose interests might not otherwise be adequately recognized in contexts designed for the majority who were not substantially disabled.

Although the court did not specifically address the implications of its ruling for genetic testing in the employment context, the substantial narrowing of the ADA's scope of protection is likely to undermine the breadth with which the EEOC regulations had interpreted the ADA with regard to genetic testing. In interpreting the scope of legal protection in a statute such as the ADA, the court is not bound by the way a federal agency such as the EEOC has interpreted congressional intent in its regulations designed to enforce the statute. Thus, in spite of the EEOC's successful settlement with BNSF, the value of this case as a disincentive for other employers, as well as the validity of the EEOC regulations protecting employees from employer use of testing for genetic predisposition to disease, is uncertain.

Before the widespread advent of SNP-based testing for adverse drug reactions, it is difficult to predict exactly how the standard of care will develop. In some cases, a particular drug may not be offered unless the genetic test is used first to screen for safety or effectiveness. However, in other cases, a test may be a choice left up to patients and their physicians. In some such cases, offering the test without requiring it may become the standard of care, and failure to offer it could result in liability. In other cases, the benefits of such a test may not be sufficiently clear that it becomes the standard of care, even though some physicians will offer it and some patients will choose it. Nevertheless, based on precedents, it is clear that once a test is available that can reliably predict significant responsiveness either in terms of safety and effectiveness, failure to offer such a test in the case of a patient who has a variant that causes the problematic responsiveness could well result in malpractice liability.

Although health benefit plans may begin to cover some pharmacogenetic tests as they become more widely used in practice, there undoubtedly will be periods when some tests that may be of benefit will not be covered, and the process of coverage for new tests as they are developed will be gradual. In this context, practitioners often feel caught in an impossible tension between recommending a test that may benefit the patient, yet knowing the patient's health benefit plan will not pay for the test. Too often, practitioners fail to inform patients of tests that they know the patient's plan will not cover. The fact that the patient's plan will not cover a test does not mitigate the practitioner's ethical or legal duty to inform the patient of such a test.

Practitioners should inform the patient of such tests anyway. In some cases, patients may want to pay for such a test out of pocket. Even if a patient is unable to pay out of pocket or simply chooses not to pay for the test, the patient must be informed of its existence and potential benefits, so that the patient's choice or inability to pay is the source of the decision not to test, rather than the practitioner's failure to inform the patient of the option. A practitioner cannot be held liable for the patient's or the health plan's choice not to pay for a recommended test, but the practitioner can be held liable for failing to inform the patient of the option of testing and the reason the patient might want to consider it.

Litigation has already been undertaken on the basis of an alleged failure to screen recipients of a Lyme disease vaccine for a variation in human leukocyte-associated antigen-DR4, which some scientists cautioned could cause a reaction to the vaccine that results in autoimmune arthritis (Reference 19). Although this case is a product liability case against the manufacturers, the same rationale for liability could be used to argue liability on the part of a physician who failed to offer the test to a candidate for the vaccine. Because pharmacists have an independent duty to patients to provide accurate information and sound advice, it is conceivable that a pharmacist also could be subject to liability on the same grounds.

The approach to ethical, legal, and social issues raised by advances in molecular genetics in the era of the Human Genome Initiative has been to address these issues as the technology is developed rather than as an afterthought, when the damage from unanticipated consequences has already been done. The difficulty with this approach is that specific legal and policy frameworks have not evolved to the point that definitive answers can be given as the basis for practical advice on these issues. Nevertheless, several recommendations can be made on the basis of what is already known about plausible developments in the technology and cautious approaches to clinical ethical issues based on current trends in law and public policy.

As pharmacogenetic or pharmacogenomic analysis becomes available, practitioners should make patients aware of the options where they are clinically relevant. Informed consent must entail not only the existence of such diagnostic tests, but also the tests' risks, benefits, and alternatives, including conventional trial and error approaches. Informed consent should include in the benefits and risks, not only the direct clinical information and decisions likely to result from such tests, but also the social and psychological ramifications of such information and the risks of genetic discrimination by insurers, employers, and other third parties who might use the information or its perceived implications in ways adverse to the patient's interests.

An example may help illustrate the range of issues that might confront a physician or pharmacist engaged in the use of pharmacogenetic analysis in the care of a patient. In managing a patient's drug therapy for cardiovascular disease, consideration is given to analyzing serum for typing ApoE. Should the process of informing the patient about the meaning of the test result include the association of ApoE with increased risk of Alzheimer's disease? If the test result is positive, what should the patient be told about the chances of his children to inherit the molecular structure that correlates with the relevant drug response and the increased risk of Alzheimer's disease? How secure is the patient's access to health benefit coverage? Should the patient be advised to acquire access to life insurance, disability insurance, and long-term care insurance before the ApoE test to prevent the possibility that the test result could make such insurance unobtainable or unaffordable? In view of these questions, would the patient prefer to pay for the testing himself rather than submit claims for reimbursement to his insurer or employer health benefit plan?

Informed consent for testing must not only enable patients to consider the potential benefits and risks of the genetic information for the clinical question that initially prompts its consideration, but also the other clinical conditions for which the outcome may contain associations or inferences. Informed consent should include accurate information about confirmed risks of offspring inheriting significant genetic conditions or susceptibilities to disease or drug responses. Such disclosure should be made to the patient rather than to family members, unless the patient gives permission to disclose the results to family members. Patients should be told what protections of confidentiality are in place to prevent unauthorized disclosure to third parties and warned to be cautious in signing authorizations for third parties to gain access to their medical records.

References

1. Rifkin, J. Algeny. New York, NY: The Viking Press, 1983.

2. Kelves DJ. The Code of Codes: Out of Eugenics: The Historical Politics of the Human Genome: Cambridge, MA: Harvard University Press, 1993:5–9.

3. Hubbard R. Exploding the Gene Myth: Boston: Genetic Labeling and the Old Eugenics: Cambridge MA: Beacon Press, 1997:16–24.

4. Human reproduction and birth: In: Furrow BR, Greaney TL, Johnson SH, Jost TS, Schwartz RL, eds. Health Law: Cases, Materials and Problems 3rd ed: St. Paul, MN: West Group, 1997:928.

5. Reilly PR. Eugenics Sterilization in the United States, Genetics and the Law III. 1985:231–2.

6. Lennard L. TPMT in the treatment of Chrohn's disease with azathioprine. Gut 2002;51:143.

7. Tang MX, Maestre G, Tsai WY, et al. Relative risk of Alzheimer's disease and age-at-onset distributions, based on APO-E genotypes among elderly African American, Caucasians and Hispanics in New York City. Am J Hum Genet 1996;58:574–84.

8. Roses AD. Apolipoprotein E and Alzheimer's disease. The tip of the susceptibility iceberg. Ann NY Acad Sci 1998;855:738–43.

9. Farlow MR, Lahiri DK, Poirier J, Davignon J, Schneider L, Hui SL. Treatment outcome of tacrine therapy depends on apolipoprotein genotype and gender of the subjects with Alzheimer's disease. Neurology 1998;50(3):669–77.

10. Issa AM. Ethical considerations in clinical pharmacogenomics research. Trends Pharmacol Sci 2000;21(7):247–9.

11. Brushwood DB. The challenges of pharmacogenomics for pharmacy education, practice, and regulation. In: Rothstein M, ed. Pharmacogenomics: Social, Ethical and Clinical Dimensions. Hoboken, NJ: Wiley-Liss, Inc., 2003:4.

12. Andrews LB, Fullarton JE, Holtzman NA, Motulsky AG. Assessing Genetic Risks: Implications for Health and Social Policy. Washington, D.C.: National Academy Press, 1994:148–52.

13. Daly MB, Offit K, Li F, et. al. Participation in the cooperative family registry for breast cancer studies: issues of informed consent. J Natl Cancer Inst 2000;92:452–6.

14. Bier R, Payne J. Report of the ACLI-HIAA Task Force on Genetic Testing. The American Council of Life Insurance, 1991:5.

15. Hall MA. Restricting insurers' use of genetic information: a guide to public policy. North American Actuarial Journal 1999;3(1):36.

16. Moseley R, Allen WL. What does genetic technology have to do with ethics? North American Actuarial Journal 1999;3(1):110.

17. Pagnattaro A. Genetic discrimination and the workplace: employee's right to privacy V. American Business Law Journal Fall, 2001 39 Am. Bus. L.J. 139.

18. Ioannou-Bouckaert, Kathy. "Genetic testing of employees raises some legal questions." St. Charles County Business Record. April 25, 2002.

19. Weiss R. The promise of precision prescriptions: "pharmacogenomics" also raises issues of race. The Washington Post, June 24, 2000:A1.

247

Self-Assessment Questions

1. Which one of the following statements is true of assessments of legal liability for failure to disclose risks of harm from a Food and Drug Administration-labeled drug?

    A. Legal liability for failure to disclose risk is limited to risks of 1 percent or higher probability.
    B. Only those risks of less than 1 percent probability that are likely to cause death are subject to legal liability if not disclosed to the patient.
    C. Even a low probability of a high magnitude of harm must be disclosed to patients.
    D. Full disclosure of all risks of harm is required only for unapproved uses of Food and Drug Administration-labeled drugs.

2. Which one of the following statements must be true for researchers to use banked blood or tissue samples from identified patients in as yet unspecified future research involving genetic analysis?

    A. The donor must provide a blanket informed consent that is valid for unspecified research protocols that may be conceived in the indefinite future.
    B. The researcher should contact the donor's physician so that the physician may ask the patient whether he or she is interested in being contacted to participate in new research on her sample(s).
    C. Donors must have already died to use their samples for additional research beyond the scope of the original protocol.
    D. Only blood or tissue obtained from biopsies, surgically removed organs, or excess blood may be used in unspecified future research, since these sources would otherwise be discarded.

3. Which one of the following statements is true of pharmacogenomic tests?

    A. Pharmacogenomic tests are unlikely to be used as a risk rating factor by insurers because they will not predict future onset of genetic disease.
    B. Pharmacogenomic tests may be of concern to insurers in cases in which the drug responsiveness would be expected to have implications for higher claims costs.
    C. Pharmacogenomic tests may not be used in insurance risk rating decisions because such uses are uniformly prohibited by law.
    D. Pharmacogenomic tests may be used in insurance underwriting, as long as no state law prohibits such uses in the state where the applicant resides.

4. Which one of the following statements describes the status of self-insured employers, who underwrite their own health benefit plans?

A. They are subject to the insurance laws on genetic testing of the state in which they are incorporated.
B. They are exempt from state insurance laws on genetic testing.
C. They are not subject to federal restrictions on genetic testing in health benefit coverage decisions.
D. They are exempt from the Equal Employment Opportunity Commission's (EEOC) regulations on genetic testing under the Americans with Disabilities Act (ADA).

5. What is the primary purpose of genetic counseling?

A. To determine whether the subject should have children in view of her genetic profile.
B. To provide psychotherapy for subjects whose tests show profound genetic abnormalities.
C. To promote the use of genetic tests for aborting congenitally deformed fetuses.
D. To provide informed consent on the risks and benefits of genetic testing and to interpret the meaning of test results for those who elect to undergo testing.

6. Which one of the following statements is true of legal precedents on the confidentiality of disclosing the risk of genetic conditions?

A. They clarify that practitioners have a duty to inform patients of the risk that their offspring may inherit the condition.
B. They clearly hold that practitioners must disclose genetic risk information, not only to the patient, but the duty directly to inform the patient's children as well.
C. They hold that patient confidentiality does not apply to withholding genetic risk information from a patient's children, since children share their parents' genetic material.
D. They conclude that practitioners may override a patient's refusal to warn offspring of inheritable genetic conditions when the practitioner determines that the offspring needs a warning to achieve early intervention.

7. A patient would be most likely to accept a pharmacogenomic test under which one of the following circumstances?

A. When the result may have implications, in addition to drug responsiveness, for predicting susceptibility to a disease for which there is no intervention.

B. When an empirical trial and error approach to drug responsiveness is inconvenient, but not harmful, and the patient wants to prevent genetic discrimination.
C. When the test result might reveal false paternity.
D. When the test result will prevent dosages that might otherwise result in high morbidity or mortality.

8. Germany's involuntary eugenic sterilization law followed the model of which one of the following state's program?

A. Virginia.
B. New York.
C. Massachusetts.
D. California.

9. Which one of the following was the purpose of the Immigration Restriction Act of 1924?

A. To prevent the influx of cheap labor that would weaken labor unions.
B. To prevent additional Asian immigration to California.
C. To favor Northern European immigrants over those from Southern and Eastern Europe.
D. To prevent introduction of contagious diseases sweeping Europe.

10. Which one of the following reasons for confidentiality of genetic test results might you expect to be more important to some mothers than fathers?

A. Discovery of false paternity.
B. Sex-linked genetic disorders, such as color blindness.
C. Women are more sensitive to stigma than men.
D. Women talk more about health concerns than men.

Pharmacogenetics:
A Historical Perspective

Werner Kalow, M.D.

Key Words

Pharmacogenetics, history, drugs, drug metabolism, receptors, molecular genetics, gene expression.

Abstract

Although pharmacology and genetics are sciences with very old backgrounds, they combined into 'pharmacogenetics' only about 50 years ago, when a few variant genes were found to alter drug effects. The discovery of butyrylcholinesterase variation is described as one of these findings. Numerous other observations followed, of which the discovery of variability of cytochrome P450 2D6, metabolizing debrisoquine, had a particular impact. The introduction of molecular genetic methodologies changed many aspects of pharmacogenetics, particularly in respect to patient classification, structural definition of drug metabolizing enzymes and of receptors, and interpretation of the widespread interethnic differences of drug responses. Other major changes were brought about by the recognition that most pharmacogenetic differences were dependent on multiple genes, interacting with environmental factors. It currently is recognized that gene expression is variable, causing functional variation in the absence of mutation. Because drugs may alter gene expression, an antithesis of pharmacogenetics, which deals with genes affecting drug action, is being seen.

Outline

Learning Objectives

1. Recognize the historical background of pharmacogenetics.
2. Understand why some early observations created pharmacogenetics as a new science.
3. Understand how to relate "phenotypes" and "genotypes" (i.e., the visible properties of an organism and its genetic constitution).
4. Compare old and contemporary discoveries in pharmacogenetics.

Abbreviations in this Chapter

CYP	Cytochrome P450
DNA	Deoxyribonucleic acid
G6PD	Glucose-6-phosphate dehydrogenase
NAT	*N*-acetyltransferase
PTC	Phenylthiocarbamide
SNP	Single nucleotide polymorphism

Early History of Pharmacogenetics

Two Independent Old Sciences Found Each Other

Pharmacogenetics is a combination of two old disciplines, genetics and pharmacology. It is worth a brief look to see how they arose as independent sciences, and how they came together to form the new science of pharmacogenetics.

Genetics

An accurate account of the history of genetics was published in 1986 (Reference 1). Inherited differences between different human beings were observed in ancient times. The Athenian philosopher Anaxagoras (500–428 BC), and later Aristotle and Plato commented on such observations. Genetics as a science is said to have started during the 19th century.   The Austrian botanist Gregor Mendel described in 1865 his experiments in peas which demonstrated inheritance; however, it took 35 years for Mendel's work to be recognized as background for the science of genetics.   Galton showed how to measure genetic effects in humans.   A stepping stone at the beginning of the 20th century was the work on the genetics of the human ABO blood groups.   The discovery of the deoxyribonucleic acid (DNA) structure by Watson and Crick in 1953 (Reference 2) opened the door to modern genetics.   It is now known (Reference 3) that humans have a genome which contains about 3 million base pairs of nucleic acids, of which about one in 500 are variant in the form of single nucleotide polymorphisms (SNPs).

Pharmacology

Knowledge of the medicinal activity of certain plants has been around for a long time.   Evidence indicates that opiates were grown on Swiss lakeshores 4000 years ago (Reference 4), apparently for medicinal use.   A recent history of pharmacology was compiled in 1963 (Reference 5).   The ancient Greeks used the word *Pharmacon* to indicate magic charm, poison, or a drug.   The book Pharmacologia by Samuel Dale of London reintroduced the concept in 1693.   In the 19th century, knowledge of medicinally active plants was supplanted by knowledge of the active chemicals within them.   Sertürner reported in 1806 that opium contains a substance which he called morphine after Morpheus, the Greek god of dreams.   There are similar histories of cocaine, cannabis, quinine, and other drugs.   In Canada, pharmacology training was initiated in 1824 (Reference 6).   Besides the attempts to find new drugs, many scientific efforts of academic pharmacology concentrated on the questions of how drugs act and what the body is doing with drugs.

According to historical accounts (References 7, 8), a connection of genetics and pharmacology was first envisioned by geneticists.   In 1931, Sir Archibald Garrod anticipated the occurrence of individual differences in human reaction to drugs and environmental chemicals in his book Inborn Factors in Diseases.   J.B.S. Haldane studied biochemical individuality, and in 1949, also predicted the occurrence of unusual reactions to drugs.   By that time, a few genetic differences in drug response were seen.   The inheritance of a deficient ability to taste phenylthiocarbamide (PTC) was a pharmacological observation.   Vitamin D-resistant rickets in certain children and abnormal drug effects in porphyria, were discovered in 1937. A genetic lack of atropine esterase in some rabbits prohibited these animals from eating belladonna-containing plants or they died.

The Start of Pharmacogenetics

The insights of Garrod and Haldane were prophecies rather than factual statements.   The quoted cases were isolated observations without general impact.   It can be argued that pharmacogenetics started in the 1950s with several discoveries, which together, established it firmly as a new science.

One of these early discoveries is a personal story, which I recently summarized (Reference 9). In 1956, I found a genetically controlled alteration of plasma cholinesterase, now officially named butyrylcholinesterase. Plasma cholinesterase destroys succinylcholine, a drug which had two clinical uses. The first use was injection before anesthesia to facilitate artificial ventilation during an operation. The other use was in psychiatry. Because there was no effective drug for schizophrenia, the patients often received electroshock therapy, which helped but frequently caused a brief but excessive muscle contraction, sometimes strong enough to break a patient's weak bones. Succinylcholine prevented such contractions.

Succinylcholine was the preferred muscle relaxant because the resulting paralysis typically lasts for a couple of minutes because it is rapidly destroyed by plasma cholinesterase. However, in some patients, the paralysis would last for as long as an hour.

I did not know this in the 1950s, but chance intervened. I worked in pharmacology in Berlin. My supervisor suspected that the plasma concentration of cholinesterase was affected by food intake, and he asked me to investigate. Because the standard methods of measuring that enzyme were complex, I developed a new method. I succeeded by using ultraviolet light to measure the concentration of some substrates in aqueous solution. The enzyme activity decreased the substrate concentration, and the rate of decrease could be measured. I had thereby created a precise and easy-to-use method for measuring the esterase activity (Reference 9).

The existence of this plasma cholinesterase was discovered in 1943 at the University of Toronto in the Department of Biochemistry as an enzyme distinct from acetylcholinesterase (Reference 10). When I joined that university in 1951, some biochemists still had investigations of this esterase in process. I informed them that I had a much better method to measure this enzyme's activity than the cumbersome gasometric method they used. I was asked to prove the validity of my method by comparing data obtained with the two methods. I did so by studying many students, using both methods, and found that they agreed. The biochemists were not satisfied because my students were young healthy subjects with esterase activities not far from average. They advised me to also try it in people with low esterase activity (Reference 9). I succeeded in locating such a person. A government laboratory had tested a patient's cholinesterase on demand from a psychiatrist because the patient regularly had a prolonged reaction to succinylcholine when treated with electroshock for his schizophrenia.

When I tested this patient's plasma in my ultraviolet spectrophotometer, his cholinesterase behaved differently from all others that I had seen. His cholinesterase was not missing, but the substrate disappearance curve was not as straight as usual—it was bent in a peculiar way. I had learned enough about enzyme kinetics to realize that the curvature indicated a low binding capacity (affinity) of the enzyme for its substrate. I could quickly show that the low affinity was not caused by an enzyme inhibitor. The low affinity implied a structural difference of the enzyme from normal. I concluded that a change of enzyme structure can only be genetic, and I asked the physician for contact with the patient's parents. The plasma enzyme in these parents did not seem normal but not as abnormal as that of their son. I assumed that they were heterozygotes (carriers) of an abnormal gene while their son was homozygous. I worked for a year to develop a method that allowed detection of the abnormality and a clear distinction between normals, carriers and fully affected subjects. Addition to the enzyme of dibucaine as a suitable enzyme inhibitor worked as intended (Reference 9).

My finding led anesthetists and psychiatrists to learn that the esterase was not missing but acting slowly. They simply had to wait for the patient's recovery while providing artificial respiration. This information prevented several fatalities, often contributed to by desperate medical actions to rescue the paralyzed patient.

In the 1950s, few known cases of human genetic variation allowed a clear-cut discrimination between homozygotes and heterozygotes. Furthermore, I had observed an unexpected principle—a genetically modified enzyme affected the action of a drug. I thought of my finding as a major discovery. This raised my interest in the question whether there were other cases of genetic control of a drug effect, or whether my observation was an isolated instance. I searched the literature and found cases which added to my excitement.

As has been reported (Reference 11), isoniazid was synthesized as a chemical in 1912. Forty years later, it was found to be capable of dramatically reducing the mortality of tuberculosis. In 1953, various authors observed numbness, pain, and tingling in arms and legs of some tuberculous patients who took the drug. This toxicity was explained by the interaction of high drug doses with pyridoxine (vitamin B_6). In 1954, the peripheral neuropathies of the drug were found to be associated with poor degradation by acetylation, finally explained by genetic deficiency of N-acetyltransferase (NAT). By 1960, various investigators measured isoniazid acetylation in different populations. Large differences between the proportion of slow and fast acetylators were seen when comparing Japanese, Eskimos (Inuit), and Europeans (Reference 12).

Another reported interplay between genes and drugs was an important observation during World War II, (Reference 13, 14). Some African-American soldiers developed a hemolytic disease after intake of the generally safe antimalarial drug primaquine. After the war, scientists in Chicago investigated the incidences. In 1954, they found an abnormality in the red blood cells of such sufferers, and in 1956 identified the cause as the genetic lack of the enzyme glucose-6-phosphate dehydrogenase (G6PD). The comparatively frequent occurrence of G6PD deficiency particularly in African Americans was explained by the discovery that the deficiency of the gene product protected its carriers from malaria. This is the reason for the relatively high frequency of the deficiency in Africa and other tropical countries. In nonmalaria exposed populations, the gene tends to be eliminated by Darwinian selection (Reference 13, 14).

Physicians and scientists were stimulated by these reports. A committee of the American Medical Association invited a geneticist (Reference 15) to write a paper titled "Drug Reactions, Enzymes, and Biochemical Reactions" in 1957 (Figure 1). In the same year, I started to summarize all known cases in a book (Reference 12), which was published in 1962. In 1959, a geneticist in Germany coined the word "Pharmacogenetics" (Reference 16), making pharmacogenetics an established entity.

The Rise of Classical Pharmacogenetics

As time went on, more pharmacogenetic discoveries were made (References 7 and 17). In 1960 and 1962, there were reports of the occurrence of excessively high body temperatures (hyperpyrexia) and rigidity among various family members in response to a general anesthetic. More than two-thirds of the reported cases were fatal. This condition was called malignant hyperthermia. Another example was the Swiss observation of a genetic lack of catalase, a lack seen before only in Japan. In 1966, there were reports from Germany of genetic variation of alcohol dehydrogenase. Many more cases were reported in the following years and some of the older reports were extended. For instance, malignant hyperthermia was found in 1970 to represent a biochemical defect in skeletal muscle that caused the muscle to respond abnormally to some drugs.

The 1977 report of abnormal metabolism of, and response to debrisoquine, had a great impact on the development of pharmacogenetics (Reference 18). The unusual story of this finding was later told by the primary discoverer, R.L. Smith in England (Reference 19). Smith was well aware of the existence of pharmacogenetics and of intricacies in the fate of drugs. One of his early colleagues was the famous investigator of drug metabolism, Tecwyn Williams. Debrisoquine is a sympatholytic antihypertensive agent. Smith was interested in the metabolism of this drug. He and his colleagues took a relatively high dose. He was the only one who suffered a marked and prolonged drop in blood pressure and an intensive dizziness, which made him unable to stand. It turned out that he lacked the main metabolite of debrisoquine in his urine. This encouraged him to initiate an investigation into the drug's metabolism in 94 volunteers. There were two groups of people who were defined as "poor and extensive metabolizers." The written 1977 description of this polymorphism (Reference 18) was widely read. In 1975, M. Eichelbaum in Germany had written a doctoral thesis which described a case of deficiency of the oxidation of sparteine, an antiarrhythmic and oxytocic alkaloid. Few people read a thesis, but in 1977, the story was published as a research paper (Reference 20). Subsequently, investigators in different countries showed

COUNCIL ON DRUGS

Report to the Council

The Council has authorized publication of the following report.
H.D. Kautz, M.D., Secretary.

Because of the renewed awareness of genetics in relation to the cause of disease and be-cause of an increasing interest in this subject, the following article is most timely. The author has prepared this report at the invitation of the Subcommittee on Blood Dyscrasias of the Committee on Research.
Norman De Nosaquo, M.D., Secretary,
Committee on Research.

DRUG REACTIONS, ENZYMES, AND BIOCHEMICAL GENETICS

Arno G. Motulsky, M.D., Seattle

In discussions of drug idiosyncrasy, careful distinction should be made between toxic reactions caused by immunologic mechanisms (drug allergy) and abnormal reaction caused by exaggeration or diminution of the usual effect of a given dose.[1] Although some progress has been made in the study of mechanisms of drug allergy, little was known un-til recently about the pathogenesis of hypersuscep-tibility reactions and hyposusceptibility reactions. Data are available now which suggest that reactions of this type may be caused by otherwise innocuous genetic traits or enzyme deficiencies.

Hockwald and his co-workers[2] demonstrated that approximately 10% of American Negroes and a very small number of caucasians developed hemolytic anemia when given an average dose of primaquine or chemically related drugs. Beutler and associates[3] showed that red blood cells of susceptible individuals possessed decreased numbers of nonprotein, sulfhydryl groups. It has now been pointed out that primaquine sensitivity is related to activity.[4] Investigations of glucose-6-phosphate dehydrogenase the genetics of this trait, now in progress, suggest that the abnormality is caused by a sex-linked gene of intermediate dominance.[5] The red blood cell abnormality per se has no known deleterious effect on the individual or on red blood cell life span. Excessive d o s e s

From the Department of Medicine, University of Washington Medical School. Dr. Motulsky is a John and Mary R. Markle Scholar in Medical Science.

Figure 1. The start of pharmacogenetics.
Copy of the title page of the first paper on pharmacogenetics (14) which appeared in the Journal of the American Medical Association, with inclusion of remarks by the Council on Drugs of this Association.

the identity of the debrisoquine and sparteine metabolizing enzyme. The enzyme is now defined as cytochrome P450 (CYP) 2D6 in the human liver.

This discovery had great scientific impact (Reference 9) for several reasons. First, oxidation is an important and widespread metabolic reaction in the human liver. Second, the deficiency was not a rare defect but a polymorphism, or a quite frequently occurring genetic alteration. Third, the enzyme CYP2D6 metabolized more than one drug. It is now known to metabolize perhaps as many as 20 percent of all clinically useful drugs, including tricyclic antidepressants and neuroleptic agents. Fourth, the medical consequences were not uniform. The enzyme deficiency caused many drugs to accumulate in the body, and thereby, produce an overresponse or toxicity. However, an underresponse, or lack of response, also could occur. For example, the debrisoquine-metabolizing enzyme converts codeine into morphine, thereby giving codeine its analgesic potency. When CYP2D6 is lacking, codeine does not relieve pain (Reference 21).

The scientific impact of this discovery is illustrated in several ways. A year after the initial publication of the deficiencies of debrisoquine and sparteine metabolism, 55 laboratories were exploring the topic (Reference 19). Current Internet data site about 2000 publications on CYP2D6. The pharmaceutical industry incorporated pharmacogenetics into programs of drug discovery and development. In Britain and the United States, drug regulatory bodies recommended an inclusion of pharmacogenetic information in physician's desk reference books. The study of genetic variation of the metabolism of drugs became a widespread effort in academia.

Nevertheless, the interest of medical practitioners in the topic remained small. A physician prescribing a drug for a patient does not always know anything about the fate of a drug in the patient unless that physician specifically demands pertinent biochemical information. Why should the physician care about a patient's biochemistry as long as the patient is alright? Thus, the medical impact of pharmacogenetics has remained small.

The quoted pharmacogenetic observations, including those of debrisoquine and sparteine, were based on clinical and biochemical measurements in individuals and their families, or on phenotype determinations. "Phenotype" indicates visible properties of an organism that are produced by the interaction of genes and the environment.

The Impact of Molecular Genetics on Pharmacogenetics

General Aspects of Molecular Pharmacogenetics

The gradual development of molecular genetics (Reference 22) changed pharmacogenetics from a phenotypic science into one which recognizes genes and gene alterations. The first studies of genes were done by using restriction endonucleases which served as DNA markers. As time went on, the DNA structure of genes was used more and more to ascertain genotype.

The clinical utility of DNA measurements depends on the fundamental fact that the nuclei of cells contain genes, although many of these genes are not active in all cells. Thus, each nucleated white cell in human blood, or in a hair root, contains all human genes, which can be tested in principle. However, to test a particular gene, the clinician has to know its normal DNA structure to be able to distinguish it from other genes in the cell, and to recognize any mutation.

Molecular biology has changed the outlook at genetic variability, but it is not a stationary science. Its emphasis on the structure of genes is changing to an interest in the genome. Only about 6 percent of all the DNA sequences in the genome are protein-producing genes. The genome is a collection of all genes, sequences, interactions, and nonuniform functions. This starts to change pharmacogenetics into pharmacogenomics.

Separate Areas of Molecular Pharmacogenetics

The repercussions of the changes brought about by molecular biology are considered separately for different areas of pharmacogenetics. Most of these areas are independently described by various authors (Reference 23).

Patient Classification

The ability to measure DNA sequences has changed the standard means to determine the pharmacogenetic status of individual patients. For instance, if a clinician could not sample a patient's liver but wanted to know whether the patient has a reduced ability to metabolize debrisoquine, the clinician had to give a separate test drug to the patient and to measure its fate in the body by appropriate tests of blood or urine. Now clinicians can take a sample of blood, isolate some white blood cells, and use a standard procedure to see whether the CYP2D6 gene is of normal structure. The patient does not need to be exposed to the test drug.

No exposure to the test drug means no danger of intoxication from that drug. The finding of a mutation which inactivates CYP2D6 may lead the physician to avoid prescribing to that patient any drug metabolized by that enzyme. Alternatively, if the drug needs to be prescribed, it may be applied at a smaller dose.

Today, if an abnormal drug response has an unknown cause, it is still possible to look for a responsible DNA change. This process is helped if clinical or biochemical data point to the gene which deserves the molecular investigation. If a mutation in the gene is found, the genetic nature of the case is indicated, perhaps requiring statistical verification. Since the most common genetic variations are changes of single nucleotides, special methods to determine SNPs are now widely used (Reference 24). Otherwise, a search of the genome may be needed.

Drug Metabolism

The impact of the change is illustrated by considering debrisoquine. Molecular genetics revealed (Reference 9 and 25) that the lack of CYP2D6 activity can be the result of frameshift mutations, splicing defects, gene deletion, or presence of a stop codon, or many different kinds of gene alteration. Gene duplication increases enzyme activity.

There are 74 CYP2D6 alleles, most containing several mutations; of these, six are registered as having normal activity, six have reduced, 23 no activity. The rest were genetically but not biochemically defined (Reference 50).

Similar though less extensive studies of variants of the enzymes cholinesterase, G6PD, and NAT have been made. There are at least 17 genetic variants of butyrylcholinesterase, 12 of these without activity (Reference 26). There are almost 400 different variants of G6PD; thus, it is perhaps the most heterogenous enzyme (Reference 14). *N*-acetyltransferase consists of two different enzymes—the new NAT1 and NAT2, the traditionally most-studied transferase. There are 26 variants of NAT1 and 29 variants of NAT2 (Reference 27).

Genetic analysis revealed the presence of alleles or mutations in many drug-metabolizing enzymes. A recent report counted 42 genetically variable enzymes in humans (Reference 28), which include two esterases, 16 transferases, three reductases, nine oxidases, and 13 CYPs.

Drug Receptors

Perhaps the most important consequence of the availability of molecular methods for pharmacogenetics is the ability to study genetic variation of drug targets, such as receptors. Many drugs act in the brain or other organs, affecting one or other cellular protein. Many proteins are genetically variable, and some variations alter drug binding or pharmacological reactions (Reference 29, 30). At the same time, such variation rarely can be directly measured.

Thus, if a researcher wants to know whether a drug receptor in the brain is of normal structure, he or she has to know the DNA structure of the receptor's gene to recognize the gene in blood cells. If the gene is identified in a blood specimen, the researcher can look for DNA variations of the gene (Reference 31). Because a variation can either be silent or cause variation of a protein structure, it will require biological observations and statistical evaluations to find out whether the DNA change has any medical or pharmacogenetic significance. MEDLINE cites about 6000 quotations dealing with human receptor polymorphism, indicating the medical importance of that problem.

There are two kinds of drug receptors (Reference 30)—cell surface receptors and nuclear receptors. Cell surface receptors are proteins inserted into the cell surface. They span the membrane and account for the action of most drugs. Cell surface receptors are proteins embedded into the outer cell membrane; they serve as the targets for most drugs. Best known in pharmacology is the A_H receptor which responds to nicotine, enhancing the formation of some drug-metabolizing enzymes. Nuclear receptors are located within the cell nucleus where they produce their actions. They typically react to glucocorticoids, estrogens, progesterone, aldosterone, thyroid hormone, and vitamin D. Agents acting on nuclear receptors must be able to enter the cell, directly or through a transporter.

The technical difficulties of studies of receptor variation may explain the fact that most of present pharmacogenetics deals with drug metabolism (Reference 31). Traditionally, an alteration of drug metabolism is investigated by measuring drug or metabolite in blood or urine, using old standard methods of chemistry. Investigations with methods of biochemical genetics could follow. However, the overwhelming frequency of metabolic pharmacogenetics also has an evolutionary explanation. The presence, absence, or genetic change of a drug-metabolizing enzyme may be irrelevant when there is no drug. Most people with the lack of such an enzyme do not realize it and live a normal life. By contrast, a drug receptor in the brain has a normal function. A genetic alteration of that function will probably affect the carrier, and the forces of Darwinian selection may tend to eliminate such carriers from a population. In short, this kind of variant may become rare.

Interethnic Pharmacogenetics

Interethnic comparisons of drug response have become a major aspect of pharmacogenetics. Ethnic differences in the frequency of deficiency of NAT (Reference 10) and of G6PD (Reference 13) have been known for a long time. Absence of the nicotine-metabolizing CYP2A6 varies between populations. Because elevation of nicotine levels reduces the desire for smoking, cigarette consumption differs much between populations (Reference 32). Ethanol consumption is much less in China and other Asian countries than in Europe, mainly because of structural differences of aldehyde dehydrogenase. This enzyme, which destroys the toxic primary ethanol metabolite, is frequently absent in China and makes the consumption of ethanol unpleasant (Reference 33). Altogether, at least 28 of 42 drug-metabolizing enzymes show differences between ethnically defined populations (Reference 28).

Methods of molecular genetics are necessary to know the extent a population difference in drug response is genetic (Reference 28). Within an ethnic group, family studies can be done routinely, and similarities between family members may point to inheritance and thereby to genetics. Genetic population differences cannot be studied by such methods. Drug metabolism, or many drug effects, are altered by environmental factors, such as by foods, nutritional status, temperature, endocrine factors, cigarette smoking, or drug intake. The choice of foods often differs between ethnically defined populations. Thus, even if a variation of drug response within each of two populations is genetic, that does not prove that a difference between these populations is genetic. Deoxyribonucleic acid analysis is necessary before a genetic cause for an ethnic difference in drug action or metabolism can be assured, and the magnitude of environmental contributions assessed.

Some observations of ethnic difference of drug response were part of the earliest records, and assumed to be genetic. As long as pharmacogenetics depended on clinical observations and biochemical measurements, only countable differences were recorded, or differences in the frequency of some abnormal reaction. Only with the advent of molecular genetics came the realization that the kinds of mutants often differ between populations.

The genetic lack of the activity of CYP2D6 has been known for some time to occur in roughly 7 percent of Europeans and in about 1 percent of Asians and Africans. However, of the 45 known mutants, only one is found everywhere (i.e., in Africa, Europe, and Asia) suggesting that the mutation originated more than 150,000 years ago before humans left Africa (Reference 28). Thus, it is not only the frequency but also the kind of a mutation that may differ.

Particularly because mutants often differ among populations, not all variants of a drug-metabolizing enzyme affect all substrates in the same way. Some mutations change enzyme properties so that a reduction of activity does not apply equally to all of its substrates. For instance, the normal form of CYP2D6 metabolizes both debrisoquine and metropolol. In some people of an African population with normal debrisoquine metabolism, the metabolism of metropolol by CYP2D6 was decreased (Reference 34), indicating a particular alteration of the CYP2D6 gene. Thus, unless the test substrate is appropriate, the presence of a genetic enzyme variant is not revealed. Only molecular studies of gene alteration can prove such cases.

Multifactorial Pharmacogenetics

Multifactorial control of drug action is the common situation. The usual response variation in a population is illustrated by normality of the (Gaussian) distribution curve. It indicates an interplay between environmental factors and numerous genes. The science of pharmacogenomics, with new analytical methods, will reveal more of the variant genes which may contribute to the control of fate and action of drugs in the body. The problems of multifactorial drug action are remote from the problems of classical pharmacogenetics, which dealt almost exclusively with alterations caused by single genes.

Even if a drug effect is not dramatically different among patients, drug effects are seldom exactly alike in different individuals, whether people or animals. This situation was formalized in 1927 (Reference 35) by the introduction of the concept of a median lethal dose called LD_{50}, indicating the drug concentration sufficient to kill 50 percent of a population. Later, this concept was widened and became the median effective dose called ED_{50}, the drug concentration having an expected effect in half the members of a population. The fact that this kind of human variation often has a genetic component was later demonstrated with the help of twin studies (Reference 36), or by comparing the effects of a drug between pairs of identical and fraternal twins. If the two members of a fraternal twin pair differ on average more from each other than those of an identical twin pair, the size of the genetic component is large, mathematically expressed as high heritability.

An example can be used to illustrate the background of multifactorial pharmacogenetics, (e.g., the metabolism of a drug). As seen in classical pharmacogenetics, the metabolism may fail because the enzyme is genetically inactive or poorly active because of a structural alteration. However, alternatively, the enzyme may be sparsely present because of low expression of its gene, which could be caused by independent genes, hormones, epigenetic silencing, age, or nutritional factors. The enzyme protein may degrade too fast. The enzyme may be inhibited by hormones or other drugs. The drug may not reach the intracellular enzyme because of a failure of the drug transporter. Several of these factors may be present at the same time. Thus, even a single event such as drug metabolism may represent a complexity.

As discussed in the Drug Receptors section, the pharmacological response to a drug may vary because the drug receptor is genetically altered. It may not bind the drug, or bind it too much. However, a normally structured receptor also could have an impaired function. There could be an improper G-protein, an auxiliary factor. The drug may not reach the receptor because of failure of a transporter, or the drug concentration at the site of the receptor may be low for various reasons, including failure of drug absorption; drug distribution in body fat; drug binding to albumin or other proteins; fast drug elimination through kidney, bile, or gut; or insufficient blood flow to the receptor area. Each of these factors could be controlled or influenced by one or several genes. In practice, a drug action never depends on a single factor, although sometimes a single factor has a predominating influence.

It is important to know whether a multifactorial drug action is under genetic control, or whether it is much affected by environmental factors. The classical way to answer this question is to determine the heritability through twin studies. However, some years ago a simpler method was introduced—take a group of patients and give them the same dose at appropriate intervals. The within-person variation, or a different response when a drug is taken repeatedly by one person, is almost certainly environmental. The differences among people are because of a combination of genetic and environmental influences. A statistical comparison of the between-person and the within-person variations allows clinicians to calculate the magnitude of the genetic component. This procedure (Reference 37, 38), called repeated drug administration test, is useful in commercial drug testing. It provides missed information with a modest increase of cost. The procedure is also usable in bioequivalence studies.

If two populations show a different average of a multifactorial drug response, a comparison of these averages has limited meaning. Deviant drug responses are clinically more significant than average responses. Patients with a drug response that diverges from the average are recorded on the edges of the bell-shaped curves which typically symbolize drug responses of a population (Reference 39). A different average may have pharmacogenetic meaning only in so far as it indicates a difference between the rims or edges of the distribution curves. Researchers should be aware of this complication.

New Problems Arising

Since the time when pharmacogenetics appeared, it has been a changing science. There are some problems of genetics which will exist for years to come, these problems started recently and are affecting pharmacogenetics.

Variable Gene Expression
Gene expression is principally measured by the amount of ribonucleic acid formed by a gene. Ribonucleic acid formation determines the protein production, the building stones of body, which also control functions.

The fact that variable gene expression exists and can be measured (Reference 40, 41) impacts pharmacogenetics in two different ways. First, it reduces the biological importance of the search for gene mutations. For a long time, any alteration of function (e.g., in pharmacogenetics as an interindividual difference in metabolizing capacities for a drug) was seen as evidence for a difference in the genetic structure of the metabolizing enzyme. The recognition that differences of gene expression exist means that an interindividual metabolic difference does not indicate the presence of a mutation. Thus, the science of pharmacogenetics (or of genetics) has broadened its perspectives.

Second, the ability to measure gene expression is opening a new means to study gene function. By comparing gene expression between a healthy and a diseased tissue allows clinicians to determine which gene alterations may cause the disease or are altered by the disease (Reference 42). A similar comparison of tissues before and after drug exposure can tell which genes are directly or indirectly affected by the drug (Reference 43). Thus, gene expression studies are starting to change the science of pharmacogenetics.

Drugs Affect Genes
It has been assumed that a drug affects one or another protein. The study of gene expression reveals that a drug may produce its effect by influencing

a gene and its function. This is now known to explain drug-induced increase of drug metabolism. An example showing the potential importance of this factor is the fact that drug addiction may represent an effect of the addicting drug on a gene rather than on a protein (Reference 44). This also explains why the state of addiction lasts longer than the effect of any single drug exposure (Reference 45). This problem affects not only pharmacogenetics, but also all pharmacology.

Epigenetics

Another problem is epigenetics (Reference 46, 47). Epigenetics refers to cytosine methylation in the DNA gene which usually causes gene inactivation. The methylation can be permanent or temporary. Epigenetics is an important regulator of multicellular life. Each cell has all genes but the genes not important for the function of a given cell are inactivated; thus, liver cells are different from muscle or brain cells. Gene inactivation varies with development, maturation, and aging. There are epigenetic differences between the sexes. Thus, the physiological and pathological significance of epigenetics is clear. What does epigenetics mean for pharmacogenetics? When describing gene expression, an epigenetic protein change may be mistaken for a mutation. A frequently occurring methylation of the gene which forms CYP1A2, reduces the activity of that enzyme in many people.

Summary

The science of genetics started with simple observations of effects of single genes and alterations caused by gene mutation. Genetics currently is involved with several complex problems, for instance, caused by the multiple genes, interactions of genes and environmental factors, variability of gene expression, and epigenetics. The changes in genetics are changing pharmacogenetics. Fatal adverse reactions to drugs are now known to represent about the fifth leading cause of death in the United States (Reference 48).

References

1. Vogel F, Motulsky AG. Human Genetics. Problems and Approaches. Berlin, Heidelberg, New York, Tokyo: Springer-Verlag, 1986.

2. Watson JD, Crick FHC. The structure of DNA. Quant Biol 1953;18:123–32.

3. Pennisi E. A closer look at SNPs suggests difficulties. Science 1998;281(5385):1787–9.

4. Lewin L. Phantastica; Die betäubenden und erregenden Genussmittel. Berlin: Georg Stilke, 1927.

5. Holmstedt B, Liljestrand G. Readings in Pharmacology. New York, NY: The Macmillan Company, 1963.

6. Marks GS. The history of pharmacology in Canada. Trends Pharmacol Sci 1994;15(7):205–10.

7. Weber WW. Pharmacogenetics. New York, NY: Oxford University Press, Incorporated, 1997.

8. Kalow W. Pharmacogenetics, ecogenetics, and pharmacogenomics. In: King RA, Rotter JI, Motulsky AG, eds. The Genetic Basis of Common Diseases. New York, NY: Oxford University Press. 2002:1033–9.

9. Kalow W, Grant DM. Pharmacogenetics. In: Scriver CR, Beaudet AL, Sly WS, et al, eds: The Metabolic & Molecular Bases of Inherited Disease. New York, St. Louis, San Francisco, Auckland, Bogota: McGraw Hill, 2001:225–55.

10. Mendel B, Rudney H. Studies on cholinesterase; cholinesterase and pseudocholinesterase. Biochem J 1943;37:59.

11. Evans DAP. Genetic Factors in Drug Therapy: Clinical and Molecular Pharmacogenetics. Cambridge: Cambridge University Press, 1993.

12. Kalow, W. Pharmacogenetics: Heredity and the Response to Drugs. Philadelphia, London: W.B. Saunders Co., 1962.

13. Beutler E. Study of glucose-6-phosphate dehydrogenase: history and molecular biology. Am J Hematol 1993;44(3):215–6.

14. Luzzatto L, Mehta A, Vulliamy T. Glucose-6-phosphate dehydrogenase deficiency. In: Scriver CR, BeaudetAL, Sly WS, Valle D, eds. The Metabolic & Molecular Bases of Inherited Disease. New York, NY: McGraw Hill, 2001:4517–53.

15. Motulsky AG. Drug reactions, enzymes, and biochemical genetics. JAMA 1957;165:835–7.

16. Vogel F. Moderne Probleme der Humangenetik. Ergebnisse der inneren Medizin und Kinderheilkunde 1959;12:65–126.

17. Kalow W. Historical aspects of pharmacogenetics. In: Kalow W, Meyer UA, Tyndale RF, eds. Pharmacogenomics. New York, Basel: Marcel Dekker, Inc., 2001:1–9.

18. Mahgoub A, Dring LG, Idle JR, Lancaster R, Smith RL. Polymorphic hydroxylation of debrsoquine in man. Lancet 1977;2:584–6.

19. Smith RL. The discovery of the debrisoquine hydroxylation polymorphism: scientific and clinical impact and consequences. Toxicology 2001;168:11–9.

20. Dengler VHJ, Eichelbaum M. Polymorphismen und defekte des arzneimittelstoffwechsels als ursache toxischer reaktionen. Arzneimitt Forsch 1977;27:1836–44.

21. Dayer P, Desmeules J, Leemann T, Striberni R. Bioactivation of the narcotic drug codeine in human liver is mediated by the polymorphic monooxygenase catalyzing debrisoquine 4 hydroxylation. Biochm Biophys Res Commun 1988;152:411–6.

22. Lodish H, Berk A, Zipursky SL, Matsudaira P, Baltimore D, Darnell JE. Molecular Cell Biology. New York, NY: W.H. Freeman & Co., 2000.

23. Kalow W, Meyer UA, Tyndale RF, eds. Pharmacogenomics. New York, Basel: Marcel Dekker, Inc., 2001.

24. Grant DM, Phillips MS. Technologies for the analysis of single nucleotide polymorphisms: an overview. In: Kalow W, Meyer UA, Tyndale RF, eds. Pharmacogenomics. New York, Basel: Marcel Dekker, Inc., 2001:183–90.

25. Daly AK, Brockmoller J, Broly F, et al. Nomenclature for human CYP2D6 alleles. Pharmacogenetics 1996;6:193–201.

26. Primo Parmo SL, Bartels CF, Wiersema B, van der Spek AF, Innis JW, LaDu BN. Characterization of 12 silent alleles of the human butyrylcholinesterase (BCHE) gene. Am J Hum Genet 1996;58:52–64.

27. Butcher NJ, Boukouvala S, Sim E, Minchin RF. Pharmacogenetics of the arylamine *N*-acetyltransferases. Pharmacogenomics 2002;2:30–42.

28. Kalow W. Interethnic differences in drug response. In: Kalow W, Meyer UA, Tyndale, RF, eds. Pharmacogenomics. New York, Basel: Marcel Dekker, Inc., 2001:109–34.

29. Linder MW, Valdes R Jr. Genetic mechanisms for variability in drug response and toxicity. J Anal Toxicol 2001;25(5):405–13.

30. Weber WW. Pharmacogenetics - receptors. In: Kalow W, Meyer UA, Tyndale RF, eds. Pharmacogenomics. New York, Basel: Marcel Dekker Inc., 2001:51–80.

31. Weidenhammer EM, Kahl BF, Wang L, Duhon M, et al. Multiplexed, targeted gene expression profiling and genetic analysis on electronic microarrays. Clin Chem 2002;48(11):1873-82

32. Tyndale RF, Sellers EM. Genetic variation in CYP2A6-mediated nicotine metabolism alters smoking behavior. Ther Drug Monit 2002;24:163–71.

33. Vasiliou V, Pappa A. Polymorphisms of human aldehyde dehydrogenases. Concequences for drug metabolism and disease. Pharmacology 2000;61:192–8.

34. Wennerholm A, Dandara C, Sayi J, et al. The African-specific CYP2D617 allele encodes an enzyme with changed substrate specificity. Clin Pharmacol Ther 2002 Jan;71(1):77–88.

35. Trevan JW. The error of determination of toxicity. Royal Soc London, Proceedings 1 Series B 1927;101:483–514.

36. Vesell ES. Polygenic factors controlling drug response. Med Clin North Am 1974;58:951–63.

37. Kalow W, Endrenyi L, Tang BK. Repeat administration of drugs as a means to assess the genetic component in pharmacological variability. Pharmacology 1999;58:281–4.

38. Kalow W, Ozdemir V, Tang BK, Tothfalusi L, Endrenyi L. The science of pharmacological variability: an essay. Clin Pharmacol Ther 1999;66:445–7.

39. Kalow W. Perspectives in pharmacogenetics. Arch Pathol Lab Med 2001;125:77–80.

40. Walker J, Rigley K. Gene expression profiling in human peripheral blood mononuclear cells using high density filter nased cDNA microarrays. J Immunol Methods 2000;239(1–2):167–79.

41. Madden SL, Wang C, Landes G. Serial analysis of gene expression: transcriptional insights into functional biology. In: Kalow W, Meyer UA, Tyndale RF, eds. Pharmacogenomics. New York, Basel: Marcel Dekker, Inc., 2001:223–52.

42. Bals R, Jany B. Identification of disease genes by expression profiling. Eur Respir J 2001;18:882–9.

43. Steiner S, Anderson NL. Expression profiling in toxicology - potentials and limitations. Toxicol Lett 2000;112–113:467–71.

44. Torres G, Horowitz JM. Drugs of abuse and brain gene expression. Psychosom Med 1999;61(5):630–50.

45. Nestler EJ. Molecular basis of long-term plasticity underlying addiction. Nat Rev Neurosci 2001;2(2):119–28.

46. Wolffe AP, Matzke MA. Epigenetics: regulation through repression. Science 1999;15:481–6.

47. Petronis A. Human morbid genetics revisited: relevance of epigenetics. Trends Genet 2001;17:142–6.

48. Lazarou J, Pomeranz BH, Corey, PN. Incidence of adverse drug reactions in hospitalized patients: a meta-analysis of prospective studies. JAMA 1998;279:1200–5.

49. Human Cytochrome P450 (CYP) Allele Nomenclature Committee Web site. Available at *http://www.imm.ki.se/CYPalleles/*.

Self-Assessment Questions

1. Pharmacogenetics started with observations of abnormal drug responses. Which one of the following drugs was *not* involved?

   A. Succinylcholine.
   B. Primaquine.
   C. Isoniazid.
   D. Caffeine.

2. Which one of the following drugs produces a response that is critically controlled by genetic variation of a single enzyme?

   A. Insulin.
   B. Magnesium.
   C. Codeine.
   D. Acetaminophen.

3. Large pharmacogenetic differences between ethnically defined human populations have not been observed for which one of the following drugs?

   A. Debrisoquine.
   B. Nicotine.
   C. Ethanol.
   D. Tylenol.

4. Which one of the following is the most accurate definition of the term "phenotype"?

   A. The visible property produced by genetics plus environment.
   B. An indicator of the genetic constitution of a person.
   C. An old term used only before the time of deoxyribonucleic acid testing.
   D. An indicator of the existence of genetic variation.

5. If there is a different drug response between human populations, how can a researcher be sure that the cause is mostly genetic rather than environmental?

   A. Measure pharmacogenetic factors in each population.
   B. See whether a population's food can alter the drug response.
   C. Compare geographic and genetic features of populations.
   D. Compare the genes which control the drug response between populations.

6. Comparing the utility of genotyping to phenotyping, which one of the following statements is incorrect?

   A. If genotyping does not explain the cause of a difference, an environmental cause may have to be looked for.
   B. Genotyping means less discomfort for the test subject.
   C. Use of white blood cells because they contain all human genes.
   D. Genotyping is reliable under all circumstances.

7. Which one of the following answers best describes the concept of multifactorial pharmacogenetics?

   A. It is contributed to by numerous genes plus environment.
   B. It is less common than monogenic pharmacogenetics.
   C. Current analytical methods have eliminated most problems.
   D. Only twin studies can reveal its heritability.

8. Among the human cytochrome P450s, which one of the following has the largest number of mutations, as currently known?

   A. Cytochrome P450 2A6.
   B. Cytochrome P450 2C9.
   C. Cytochrome P450 2D6.
   D. Cytochrome P450 2E1.

9. Counting some of the earliest cases of pharmacogenetics, which one of the following did not belong in this class?

   A. Isoniazid metabolism.
   B. Prolonged succinylcholine action.
   C. Insulin receptor variation.
   D. Primaquine-caused hemolysis.

10. Different mutations of a gene which control a drug-metabolizing enzyme have been found to alter one or other of its functions. Which one of the following effects has not been found?

   A. Abolish the enzyme activity.
   B. Make the enzyme act faster.
   C. Perpetuate the enzyme activity.
   D. Alter the enzyme's activity toward only some of its substrates.

Pharmacogenetics of Oxidative Drug Metabolism and Its Clinical Applications

Reginald F. Frye, Pharm.D., Ph.D.

Key Words

Cytochrome P450, drug metabolism, pharmacogenetics, drug oxidation polymorphism, flavin-containing monooxygenase, phenotype, poor metabolizer, interindividual difference, and pharmacokinetics.

Abstract

Genetic variation in drug metabolizing enzymes can be associated with significant clinical consequences. This chapter reviews the pharmacogenetics of the most important oxidative drug metabolizing enzymes, the cytochrome P450 and flavin-containing monooxygenase enzyme families. It is now appreciated that the efficacy of a drug and the likelihood of an adverse reaction often depend on the activity of these enzymes. The clinical consequences of genetic variation are reviewed for each enzyme and clinical scenarios in which prospective genotyping may improve clinical therapy are discussed.

Outline

Learning Objectives

1. Understand the role of pharmacogenetic variability in oxidative drug metabolizing enzymes on drug disposition, efficacy, and toxicity.
2. Discuss approaches used to estimate the in vivo activity (phenotype) of drug metabolizing enzymes.
3. Describe the molecular basis for a genetic variation influencing the functional activity of oxidative drug metabolizing enzymes.
4. Identify the areas of current and future potential applications of oxidative drug metabolizing enzyme pharmacogenetics to tailor drug therapy.

Abbreviations in this Chapter

Ah	Aryl hydrocarbon
AUC	Area under the curve
CO_2H	Carboxyl
CYP	Cytochrome P450
ERMBT	Erythromycin breath test
FMO	Flavin-containing monooxygenase
INR	International normalized ratio
NH_2	Amino
NNK	4-(methylnitrosamino)-1-(3-pyridyl)-1-butanone
OH	Hydroxy
SH	Sulfhydryl
SNP	Single nucleotide polymorphisms

Oxidative Drug Metabolism

It is well recognized that individuals may respond quite differently to the same dose or even the same concentration of a drug. Drug metabolizing enzymes are an important contributor to the observed variability in drug response as the activity of these enzymes is of critical importance in determining the steady-state plasma concentrations of pharmacological agents that are metabolized.

Most drugs or foreign chemicals (i.e., xenobiotics) undergo chemical modifications in the body before elimination. This biotransformation process serves to render lipophilic drugs more hydrophilic, thereby facilitating elimination. Drug biotransformation reactions traditionally have been classified as Phase I or Phase II reactions (Reference 1). Phase I reactions are considered functionalization reactions involving hydrolysis, reduction, and oxidation. These reactions introduce a polar functional moiety, such as an amino (NH_2), hydroxy (OH), sulfhydryl (SH), or carboxyl (CO_2H) group, onto the substrate to increase hydrophilicity and excretion, or prepare a compound for subsequent Phase II metabolism. Although Phase I metabolism typically decreases the reactive nature or toxicity of compounds, it also may lead to the formation of more reactive (and possibly toxic) metabolites (Reference 1).

Phase II (conjugating) enzymes catalyze the addition of small endogenous molecules to a broad range of compounds to increase their water solubility and elimination from the body (Reference 1). The major Phase II pathways are glucuronidation, sulfation, glutathione conjugation, acetylation, methylation, and amino acid and fatty acid conjugation. Both parent drugs and/or metabolic products of oxidative reactions may be conjugated, thus enhancing water solubility and facilitating excretion.

There have been incredible advances in the understanding of how genetics contributes to variability in drug response over the past few years, fueled by sequencing of the human genome and many technological advances. Phase I drug metabolizing enzymes are important contributors to interindividual variability, and genetic variation in these enzymes is associated with significant clinical consequences. The most important oxidative drug metabolizing enzymes are the cytochrome P450 (CYP) and flavin-containing monooxygenase (FMO) enzyme families. The purpose of this chapter is to review the pharmacogenetics of oxidative drug metabolism.

Cytochromes P450

The CYPs are a superfamily of enzymes having a heme-carbon monoxide complex that shows an absorption spectrum with a maximum near 450 nm (Reference 2). The CYP enzyme superfamily is one of the most important drug metabolizing enzyme systems in humans and is responsible for the oxidative metabolism of a large number of xenobiotics, including many drugs. In addition, CYP enzymes mediate the metabolism of many endogenous compounds, such as steroids and arachidonic acid (Reference 3). Not unexpectedly, there is substantial variability among individuals in the activity of CYP enzymes. Indeed, a variety of factors regulate CYP enzyme activity, including genetic polymorphisms, age, sex, disease states, and such environmental influences as smoking or exposure to environmental chemicals.

Cytochrome P450 enzymes primarily are located in the liver, although some are distributed in other tissues, such as intestine, lung, kidney, and brain. A standard nomenclature system has been developed in which CYP enzymes are named by the root "CYP", followed by an Arabic number designating the enzyme family, which is defined as enzymes having 40 percent amino acid sequence homology, a letter to indicate the enzyme subfamily (55 percent sequence homology), and another number denoting the individual CYP enzyme (e.g., CYP2C19) (Reference 4). For each enzyme, the most common or "wild-type" allele is denoted as *1 and allelic variants (i.e., alleles having one or more single nucleotide polymorphisms or [SNPs]) are sequentially numbered as identified (i.e., *2 and *3).

A total of 270 CYP gene families have been described to date (Reference 3). The 18 gene families that exist in mammals encode for 57 individual CYP genes (Reference 3). Despite the large number of CYP genes and enzymes, it appears that only the CYP1, CYP2, and CYP3 families of enzymes have a major role in drug metabolism. The remaining CYP families all have essential roles in intermediary metabolism, such as the CYP4 family which is involved in the oxidation of fatty acids,

Table 1. CYP Enzymes: Hepatic Content and Contribution to Drug Metabolism

Enzyme	Estimated Contribution to Drug Metabolism (% of drugs metabolized)[a]	Relative % of Total Hepatic CYP Content
CYP1A2	3	13
CYP2A6	2[b]	5–10
CYP2B6	2[b]	6
CYP2C8	18[c]	< 1
CYP2C9	18[c]	20[d]
CYP2C19	18[c]	20[d]
CYP2D6	25	2–4
CYP2E1	1	7
CYP3A4/5	51	30

[a]Relative contribution of the major human CYP isoforms to drug metabolism.
[b]CYP2A6 and CYP2B6 together metabolize about 2 percent of drugs.
[c]CYP2C8, CYP2C9, and CYP2C19 together metabolize about 18 percent of drugs.
[d]CYP2C9 and 2C19 together represent about 20 percent of CYP enzymes expressed in liver.
CYP = cytochrome P450.

prostaglandins, and steroids (Reference 3). Characteristics of these major human drug metabolizing CYP isozymes, including hepatic content and an estimate of the percentage of those drugs primarily eliminated by CYP-mediated metabolism that are metabolized by a specific CYP isozyme, are presented in Table 1 (Reference 5). Table 2 provides a partial listing of selected drugs that are substrates for the important CYP enzymes and Table 3 provides a listing of selected inhibitors and inducers for each CYP enzyme. Comprehensive and current information

Table 2. Selected Substrates for Drug Metabolizing Enzymes

Enzyme	Selected Substrates
CYP1A2	amitriptyline, caffeine, clomipramine, clozapine, estradiol, fluvoxamine, haloperidol, imipramine, mexiletine, naproxen, olanzapine, ondansetron, propranolol, riluzole, ropivacaine, tacrine, theophylline, verapamil, R-warfarin, zileuton, zolmitriptan
CYP2A6	coumarin, disulfiram, methoxyflurane, nicotine, valproic acid
CYP2B6	bupropion, cyclophosphamide, efavirenz, ifosfamide, S-mephenytoin, methadone
CYP2C8	amiodarone, chloroquine, dapsone, paclitaxel, repaglinide, retinoic acid, rosiglitazone
CYP2C9	diclofenac, fluoxetine, flurbiprofen, fluvastatin, glipizide, glyburide, ibuprofen, losartan, naproxen, phenytoin, tamoxifen, tolbutamide, torsemide, S-warfarin
CYP2C19	citalopram, cyclophosphamide, diazepam, imipramine, lansoprazole, nelfinavir, omeprazole, pantoprazole, primidone, progesterone, proguanil, S-mephenytoin, voriconazole
CYP2D6	amitriptyline, carvedilol, codeine, desipramine, dexfenfluramine, dextromethorphan, encainide, flecainide, fluoxetine, fluvoxamine, haloperidol, metoprolol, mexiletine, nortriptyline, paroxetine, perphenazine, propafenone, risperidone, thioridazine, tolterodine, tramadol, venlafaxine
CYP2E1	acetaminophen, chlorzoxazone, enflurane, ethanol, halothane, isoflurane, methoxyflurane, sevoflurane
CYP3A4/5	alfentanyl, alprazolam, amlodipine, atorvastatin, buspirone, cisapride, clarithromycin, cortisol, cyclosporine, diltiazem, erythromycin (not 3A5), estradiol, felodipine, fentanyl, finasteride, haloperidol, hydrocortisone, imatinib, indinavir, irinotecan, lidocaine, lovastatin, methadone, midazolam, nelfinavir, nifedipine, nisoldipine, nitrendipine, ondansetron, paclitaxel, progesterone, quinidine, ritonavir, saquinavir, sildenafil, simvastatin, sirolimus, tacrolimus, tamoxifen, testosterone, triazolam, verapamil, vincristine, zaleplon, zolpidem
FMO3	caffeine, cimetidine, clozapine, S-nicotine, ranitidine

Reprinted from Scordo MG, et al. Influence of CYP2C9 and CYP2C19 genetic polymorphisms on warfarin maintenance dose and metabolic clearance. Clin Pharmacol Ther 2002;72(6):702–10, with permission from Elsevier.
CYP = cytochrome P450; FMO = flavin-containing monooxygenase.

Table 3. Selected Inhibitors and Inducers for Drug Metabolizing Enzymes

Enzyme	Selected Inhibitors
CYP1A2	amiodarone, fluoroquinolones, fluvoxamine , ticlopidine
CYP2B6	thiotepa, ticlopidine
CYP2C19	felbamate, fluoxetine, fluvoxamine, ketoconazole, lansoprazole, omeprazole, paroxetine, ticlopidine, topiramate
CYP2C8	trimethoprim, gemfibrozil
CYP2C9	amiodarone, fluconazole, fluvastatin, fluvoxamine, gemfibrozil, isoniazid, lovastatin, paroxetine, sertraline, sulfamethoxazole, zafirlukast
CYP2D6	fluoxetine, metoclopramide, methadone, paroxetine, quinidine
CYP2E1	disulfiram
CYP3A4/5	amiodarone, clarithromycin, delavirdine, diltiazem, erythromycin, grapefruit juice constituents (e.g., dihydroxybergamottin), indinavir, itraconazole, ketoconazole, nefazodone, nelfinavir, ritonavir, saquinavir, verapamil

Enzyme	Selected Inducers
CYP1A2	omeprazole, smoking
CYP2B6	phenobarbital, rifampin
CYP2C19	carbamazepine, prednisone, rifampin
CYP2C8	rifampin
CYP2C9	rifampin
CYP2D6[a]	dexamethasone, rifampin
CYP2E1	ethanol, isoniazid
CYP3A4/5	carbamazepine, efavirenz, nevirapine, phenobarbital, phenytoin, rifabutin, rifampin, St. John's wort

[a]Although CYP2D6 is considered a noninducible enzyme, the clearance of multiple drugs predominately metabolized by CYP2D6 is increased in the presence of these drugs. CYP = cytochrome P450.

regarding substrates, inhibitors, and inducers of CYP enzymes can be found at the Indiana University School of Medicine Web site at *http://medicine.iupui.edu/flockhart/*.

Genetic Variation and Phenotype Characterization

The phenotype is an observed characteristic, such as drug clearance or rate of metabolism. The phenotype is influenced not only by a person's genetic makeup (i.e., genotype), but also by other factors, including age, sex, disease state(s), smoking, alcohol, and diet. Initial observations suggesting the presence of polymorphic CYP-mediated oxidative metabolism were based on interindividual differences in an observed characteristic (i.e., phenotype). An exaggerated response to the antihypertensive drug debrisoquine or the discovery of defective N-oxidation of sparteine, an antiarrhythmic and oxytocic drug, was reported in a small number of subjects being treated with one of these drugs (Reference 6). Subsequent studies revealed the genetic basis for these observations as being a polymorphism in the *CYP2D6* gene. These drugs were used later in large population studies to classify subjects on the basis of function (i.e., enzyme activity) as being "poor metabolizers", "intermediate metabolizers", "extensive metabolizers", or "ultrarapid metabolizers". This is illustrated in Figure 1, which shows the population distribution of CYP2D6 activity as estimated by the debrisoquine metabolic ratio, which varies 1000-fold. Thus, in these studies, debrisoquine and sparteine served as "probe drugs" to characterize enzyme activity.

Probe Drugs and Measures of Enzyme Activity

An approach that has become standard in pharmacogenetics research is to estimate the activity of a single enzyme in humans through the administration of a "probe" compound. As the term "probe" implies, it is a drug or chemical to search into, so as thoroughly to explore, or to discover something, according to the Oxford English Dictionary. A drug that has

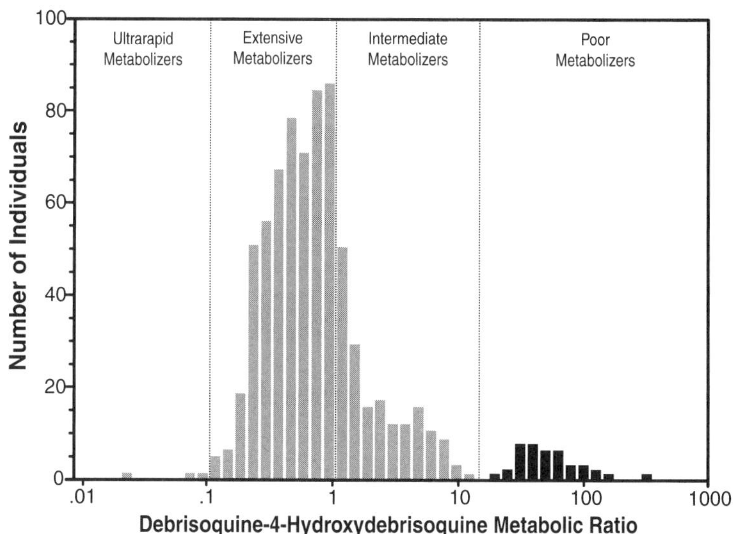

Figure 1. Population distribution of CYP2D6-mediated debrisoquine metabolism.
Distribution of the urinary debrisoquine-4-hydroxydebrisoquine metabolic ratio, which serves as an in vivo index of CYP2D6 activity, in 757 Swedish subjects. Breakpoints are used to classify individuals into ultrarapid, extensive, intermediate, and poor metabolizers on the basis of activity as shown. Note the apparent bimodal distribution, which was used in early studies to identify poor metabolizers. Reprinted from Steiner E, et al. Polymorphic debrisoquin hydroxylation in 757 Swedish subjects. Clin Pharmacol Ther 1988;44(4):431–5, with permission from Elsevier.
CYP = cytochrome P450.

been predominately or exclusively metabolized by an individual enzyme and is safe to administer can be considered for use as a probe drug. Information on the specific enzymes involved in the metabolism of a drug comes from in vitro studies using human liver microsomes or stably expressed human CYP enzymes. Although the relationship between in vitro observations and in vivo disposition often is not known, the in vitro data often provide the necessary justification for use of a particular drug to measure the activity of an individual enzyme.

After probe drug administration, a full pharmacokinetic study with extensive blood and/or urine collection is conducted to determine some measure of enzyme activity. The intrinsic clearance of a probe or of the metabolite(s) produced (formation clearance) is the best measure of enzyme activity (Reference 7). The formation clearance may be estimated by determining the amount of metabolite excreted in urine over time in reference to the area under the curve (AUC) of the parent compound over the same time period. However, in human studies, ethical and practical considerations often limit such an intensive approach because of blood volume, cost, or other considerations.

The goal of an intensive pharmacokinetic study with a candidate probe drug often is to develop a phenotypic trait measure, which represents a simplified method for estimating enzyme activity. A phenotypic trait measure is a parameter that best reflects the formation clearance, typically regarded as the gold standard, but is calculated from limited information and does not necessitate extensive sampling. Examples of trait measures include recovery ratios calculated from urinary recovery of parent compound and metabolite, a metabolic ratio using concentrations of parent drug and metabolite determined from a single plasma or urine sample, or total urinary recovery of a selected metabolite (Reference 8). Essentially a trait measure represents a noninvasive or less invasive means to estimate the activity of a particular enzyme after administration of a pharmacological probe and is a measure that can be more efficiently applied in large population studies.

Probe drugs and a suitable measure of enzyme activity have been used extensively in pharmacogenetics research. Initially, probe drugs were an essential tool used to identify subpopulations of subjects who would then be genotyped. More recently, probe drugs are being used to explore the clinical relevance of SNPs in drug metabolizing enzymes. Several probe drugs for specific CYP enzymes have been identified, and the advantages and disadvantages associated with each have been reviewed elsewhere (Reference 9). A partial listing of probe drugs and the enzyme evaluated is provided in Table 4.

Enzyme	Probe Drug
CYP1A2	caffeine, theophylline
CYP2A6	coumarin, nicotine
CYP2B6	bupropion (I), efavirenz (I), S-mephenytoin (I)
CYP2C8	paclitaxel (I)
CYP2C9	tolbutamide, flurbiprofen, warfarin
CYP2C19	S-mephenytoin, omeprazole
CYP2D6	dextromethorphan, debrisoquine, metoprolol, sparteine
CYP3A	cortisol, [^{14}C-N-methyl]erythromycin, midazolam
FMO3	S-nicotine (I), ranitidine

CYP = cytochrome P450; (I) = in vitro only; FMO = flavin-containing monooxygenase.

Genetic Variation in Oxidative Drug Metabolism

Overview

Genetic variation in drug metabolizing enzymes has been recognized as one of the major causes of interindividual variability in drug response. Cytochrome P450 enzymes are the most important enzymes involved in oxidative drug metabolism and they remain a major focus in pharmacogenetics research. Genetic variation has now been described for all of the major CYP enzymes that contribute to human drug and xenobiotic metabolism (Reference 10). A CYP nomenclature committee has been established and current information on genetic variants can be found at *http://www.imm.ki.se/CYPalleles*. For some enzymes (e.g., CYP2D6 and CYP2C19), allelic variants that have been identified are the result of SNPs that create an altered splice site, frameshift mutation, premature stop codon, gene deletion, or missense mutation, each of which produces "loss-of-function" alleles (i.e., nonfunctional alleles). Single nucleotide polymorphisms also may cause changes in the amino acid sequence, which often are associated with enzymes having catalytic activity altered compared to the fully functional *1 allele (e.g., CYP2C9*2) (Reference 11).

Pharmacogenetics of Specific Drug-metabolizing Enzymes

The *CYP1* Gene Family

The *CYP1* gene family is comprised of three genes, *CYP1A1*, *CYP1A2*, and *CYP1B1*. Cytochrome P450 1A1 and CYP1B1 appear to be of minor importance in drug metabolism, whereas CYP1A2 contributes to the metabolism of many drugs, including caffeine, clozapine, imipramine, and theophylline (Table 2).

Cytochrome P450 1A1 is distributed extrahepatically (e.g., lung) and is important in the bioactivation of environmental polycyclic aromatic hydrocarbons (Reference 10). The *CYP1A1* gene polymorphisms modify the risk of lung and prostate cancer (Reference 10). Cytochrome P450 1B1 expression is predominately extrahepatic with high expression in endometrial tissue (Reference 10). Cytochrome P450 1B1 is important in steroid metabolism, especially the 4'-hydroxylation of estradiol, and gene polymorphisms have been associated with higher risk for endometrial cancer and prostate cancer (References 12, 13). Genetic variation in *CYP1B1* also has been associated with primary congenital glaucoma (Reference 14).

Cytochrome P450 1A2

Cytochrome P450 1A2 is the major CYP1 enzyme and accounts for 13 percent of total hepatic CYP content. Cytochrome P450 1A2 demonstrates large interindividual variability in activity (up to 40-fold in vitro) and is well known as the enzyme induced by cigarette smoking. Cytochrome P450 1 gene family enzymes, such as CYP1A2, are induced by ligand binding at the aryl hydrocarbon (Ah) receptor. Compounds that are effective inducers include polycyclic aromatic hydrocarbons, such as those found in cigarette smoke (Reference 15). Thus, the clearance of many CYP1A2 substrates, including caffeine, clozapine, olanzapine, and theophylline, are increased in smokers compared to nonsmokers (Reference 15). Cytochrome P450 1A2 has been implicated in the bioactivation of heterocyclic amines, many of which are procarcinogens (References 3, 16). Polymorphisms in the coding region of CYP1A2 are rare; however, more common polymorphisms that may be functionally significant have been found in noncoding regions (Table 5). The most common *CYP1A2* polymorphisms, found in upstream sequences and in intron 1, are -2464T→delT (*CYP1A2*1D*) and -164A→C (*CYP1A2*1F*) (Reference 17).

In Vivo Activity. Caffeine has been extensively used as an in vivo probe of CYP1A2 activity since caffeine 3-demethylation was shown in vitro to be predominately mediated by this enzyme (Reference 18). Several phenotypic trait measures of CYP1A2 activity have been developed and include urinary caffeine metabolic ratios and plasma or saliva ratios (Reference 19). Caffeine is extensively metabolized, producing up to 14 metabolites in humans; CYP1A2 accounts for more than 90 percent of caffeine degradation in humans (Reference 20). The paraxanthine-caffeine plasma ratio appears to be the most robust measure of CYP1A2 activity (Reference 21).

Clinical Consequences of Genetic Variation. Cytochrome P450 1A2 activity, as measured using caffeine as an in vivo probe drug, exhibits wide interindividual variability. Caffeine metabolism is higher in smokers and initial evidence suggested that the

Table 5. Drug Metabolizing Enzymes: Common Alleles, Mutation(s), Functional Consequence, and Frequencies

Enzyme	Common Allelic Variant	Mutation/ Substitution	Consequence for Enzyme Function	Allele frequency (%)		
				Caucasians	African Americans	Asians
CYP1A2	CYP1A2*1D	5'flanking region	Unclear	5		42
	CYP1A2*1F	Intron 1	Increased inducibility	33		68
	CYP1A2*1K	Intron 1	Decreased	0.5		
CYP2A6	CYP2A6*1X2	Gene duplication	Increased	0.7		0–0.4
	CYP2A6*2	Leu160His	Decreased	3	0	< 1
	CYP2A6*4	Gene deletion	Nonfunctional	1		15–20
CYP2B6	CYP2B6*5	Arg487Cys	Unchanged	9–14		
	CYP2B6*6	Gln172His; Lys262Arg	Increased	16–26		16
	CYP2B6*7	Gln172His; Lys262Arg; Arg487Cys	Increased	13		0
CYP2C8	CYP2C8*2	Ile269Phe	Decreased	0.4	18	0
	CYP2C8*3	Arg139Lys; Lys399Arg	Decreased	2	13	0
CYP2C9	CYP2C9*2	Arg144Cys	Altered affinity	13–22	3	0
	CYP2C9*3	Ile359Leu	Decreased	4–5	1	3
	CYP2C9*5	Asp360Glu	Decreased	0	2	0
CYP2C19	CYP2C19*2	Splicing defect	Nonfunctional	15	17	30
	CYP2C19*3	Premature stop codon	Nonfunctional	0.04	0.4	5
CYP2D6	CYP2D6*2XN	Gene duplication	Increased	1–2		
	CYP2D6*3	Frameshift	Nonfunctional	1–2		< 1
	CYP2D6*4	Defective splicing	Nonfunctional	20	8	< 1
	CYP2D6*5	Gene deletion	Nonfunctional	4	6	4–6
	CYP2D6*6	Frameshift	Nonfunctional	1	< 1	< 1
	CYP2D6*10	Pro34Ser; Ser486Thr	Decreased	< 2	3	41
	CYP2D6*17	Thr107Ile; Arg296Cys; Ser486Thr	Decreased	< 1	22	
CYP2E1	CYP2E1*1D	5'-flanking region	Increased inducibility	2	13	20
	CYP2E1*2	Arg76His	Decreased	2.5		2.5
CYP3A4	CYP3A4*1B	5'flanking region	Unchanged	2–10	35–67	0
CYP3A5	CYP3A5*3	Splicing defect	Nonfunctional	85–95	27–45	70–75
	CYP3A5*6	Splicing defect	Nonfunctional	0	13–17	0
CYP3A7	CYP3A7*1C	Promoter polymorphism	Increased expression	3	6	
FMO3	FMO3*2	Glu158Lys; Glu308Gly	Decreased	17	3	14
	FMO3*3	Glu158Lys	Decreased	23	37	< 1
	FMO3*4	Val257Met	Decreased	7	7	20

CYP = cytochrome P450, FMO = flavin-containing monooxygenase.

-164A→C polymorphism (*CYP1A2*1F*) is associated with higher CYP1A2 inducibility by smoking (Reference 17). However, when evaluated in both smokers and nonsmokers, the *CYP1A2*1F* genotype had no impact on clozapine metabolism in patients with schizophrenia or on caffeine metabolism in pregnant women or patients with colorectal cancer (References 22–24). It is now known that the -164A→C polymorphism can be located in at least four different haplotypes and that it is important to consider the complete *CYP1A2* haplotype to assess the functional impact (References 25, 26). Individuals who were nonsmokers and heterozygous for *CYP1A2*1K* (-740G, -730T, -164A) haplotype had significantly lower CYP1A2 activity, as reflected by the caffeine metabolic ratio, when compared to nonsmoking subjects in other genotype groups (Reference 26). Also, there was no difference in enzyme activity observed between smokers or nonsmokers with *CYP1A2*1A/*1A* and *CYP1A2*1F/*F* genotypes. Finally, the *CYP1A2*1K* haplotype demonstrated 40 percent less induction in a cell-based reporter gene assay, but the impact of this haplotype on the magnitude of induction observed in vivo has not been evaluated.

CYP2 Gene Family

The *CYP2* gene family is the largest mammalian CYP family. It is comprised of 13 subfamilies, including CYP2A, CYP2B, CYP2C, CYP2D, and CYP2E, that encode for 16 CYP genes (Reference 3). Collectively, the CYP2 gene family enzymes contribute to the metabolism of nearly half of all drugs (Table 1).

Cytochrome P450 2A6

Cytochrome P450 2A6 predominantly is expressed in the liver, where it represents 5–10 percent of the total liver CYP content, and also is found in nasal mucosa and bronchial epithelial cells (Reference 27). Although CYP2A6 metabolizes a limited number of drugs (Table 2), it is the major enzyme that metabolizes nicotine, converting it to nicotine $\Delta^{1'(5')}$-iminium ion, which is further oxidized by aldehyde oxidase to cotinine (Reference 27). This is the rate-limiting step in nicotine metabolism and up to 80 percent of nicotine is metabolized to cotinine. Cytochrome P450 2A6 also is important in the activation of several procarcinogens present in tobacco smoke, including 4-(methylnitrosamino)-1-(3-pyridyl)-1-butanone (NNK) and *N*-nitrosodiethylamine (Reference 28).

Several functionally significant variant alleles have been identified and there are racial differences in their frequencies (Table 5). Several of the variant alleles that have been identified are associated with either loss of function or decreased activity. About 1 percent of Caucasians and up to 20 percent of Asians are poor metabolizers. The term "poor metabolizer" is used to describe an individual who lacks the capacity to metabolize a drug that is a substrate for the specific enzyme (e.g., coumarin and CYP2A6) as a result of inheriting two nonfunctional alleles; an "extensive metabolizer" is an individual having at least one functional allele (i.e., homozygous or heterozygous wild-type genotype). The most common variant allele in Asians is *CYP2A6*4*, which results in gene deletion. The most common variant allele in Caucasians is a point mutation, resulting in leucine to histidine conversion in codon 160 (*CYP2A6*2*), which yields an inactive protein and confers the poor metabolizer phenotype. Individuals having two copies of the wild-type gene (*CYP2A6*1/*1×2*) exhibit ultrarapid metabolism (Reference 28).

In Vivo Activity. Nicotine and coumarin have been used as in vivo probes of CYP2A6 activity (Table 4) (Reference 28). Phenotyping CYP2A6 activity with nicotine can be accomplished by having the subject chew a piece of nicotine gum and then collecting multiple plasma samples over time or a single plasma sample at 2 hours. A phenotypic trait measure that is used commonly is the cotinine to nicotine plasma concentration ratio. Coumarin is 7-hydroxylated by CYP2A6 and the amount of 7-hydroxycoumarin recovered in urine over a fixed time interval serves as an index of enzyme activity.

Clinical Consequences of Genetic Variation. The primary interest to date in CYP2A6 pharmacogenetics relates to its role in nicotine and procarcinogen metabolism. Cytochrome P450 2A6 activity, which is highly variable between individuals, may directly impact smoking behavior, risk of tobacco-related cancers, and treatment of nicotine addiction, as it is known that smokers regulate their smoking to maintain constant blood and brain nicotine concentrations (Reference 28). Individuals having one or more CYP2A6-null alleles are at lower risk to become smokers and will smoke fewer cigarettes (thereby reducing exposure to procarcinogens) if they are nicotine-dependent (Reference 29).

An interesting strategy to reduce cigarette smoking involves pharmacological inhibition of CYP2A6, which mimics genetically impaired metabolism (Reference 30). Methoxsalen (8-methoxypsoralen), which is used to treat psoriasis, is a potent inhibitor of CYP2A6. Consequently, methoxsalen decreases the first-pass metabolism and increases the bioavailability of nicotine and also prolongs nicotine exposure by decreasing systemic clearance. As a proof of concept, methoxsalen in combination with oral nicotine reduced smoking in a controlled setting, suggesting that this novel approach may be useful in treating tobacco dependence (References 30, 31).

Cytochrome P450 2B6

Cytochrome P450 2B6 was initially considered to be of minor significance because it was thought to constitute a small percentage of total hepatic CYP (and was not detected in all livers). However, it is now known that CYP2B6 represents about 6 percent of total hepatic CYP content (Reference 32, 33). Cytochrome P450 2B6 is expressed in liver and many extrahepatic tissues, including kidney and brain, and it plays an important role in the metabolism of drugs, such as cyclophosphamide, diazepam, efavirenz, and S-mephenytoin (*N*-demethylation) (Table 2). In addition, CYP2B6 has been implicated in the metabolism of procarcinogens including aflatoxin, 6-aminochrysene, and 7,12-dimethylbenz[a]anthracene (Reference 32).

Several polymorphisms have been identified in the *CYP2B6* gene (Table 5). Polymorphisms that result in a change in the amino acid sequence are termed nonsynonymous polymorphisms. Nonsynonymous polymorphisms in the *CYP2B6* gene that are functionally relevant include *CYP2B6*5* (Arg487Cys), *CYP2B6*6* (Gln172His; Lys262Arg), and *CYP2B6*7* (Gln172His; Lys262Arg; Arg487Cys) (References 34, 35).

In Vivo Activity. An in vivo probe for CYP2B6 activity has not been validated. However, bupropion and efavirenz have been used to characterize in vitro activity and one or both may prove to be useful for assessing in vivo activity (References 36, 37).

Clinical Consequences of Genetic Variation. It is likely that interindividual variability in CYP2B6 activity will contribute to clinically relevant differences in the systemic exposure of CYP2B6 substrates. The chemotherapeutic agent cyclophosphamide is a prodrug that must be 4-hydroxylated to its active metabolite. Cytochrome P450 2B6 has been shown in vitro to be an important enzyme in cyclophosphamide metabolism and greater catalytic activity was observed in *CYP2B6*6* carriers (Reference 38). A similar observation of higher intrinsic clearance values for the proteins CYP2B6.6 (*CYP2B6*6*) and CYP2B6.7 (*CYP2B6*7*) was shown in vitro with 7-Ethoxy-4-trifluoromethylcoumarin O-deethylation (Reference 39). Whether these in vitro observations are relevant in vivo is not known.

CYP2C Gene Subfamily

The CYP2C subfamily is of major importance to drug metabolism and is comprised primarily of CYP2C8, CYP2C9, and CYP2C19. These enzymes constitute about 20 percent of CYP protein content in human liver (Table 1), and contribute to the metabolism of numerous drugs, including losartan, nonsteroidal anti-inflammatory drugs (e.g., ibuprofen), phenytoin, proton-pump inhibitors (e.g., lansoprazole and omeprazole), and warfarin (Table 2).

Cytochrome P450 2C8. Cytochrome P450 2C8 primarily is distributed in the liver and is involved in the metabolism of paclitaxel, retinoic acid, and rosiglitazone (Reference 40). Cytochrome P450 2C8 also metabolizes arachidonic acid and retinoids (Table 2) (References 40, 41). Functionally relevant polymorphisms that have been identified in the *CYP2C8* gene include *CYP2C8*2* and *CYP2C8*3*. Allelic frequencies (percentage) have been estimated as 18 percent for *CYP2C8*2* in African Americans and 13 percent for *CYP2C8*3* in Caucasians (Table 5).

In Vivo Activity. An in vivo probe for CYP2C8 activity has not been established. Paclitaxel 6α-hydroxylation is used as an in vitro index reaction for CYP2C8 activity.

Clinical Consequences of Genetic Variation. The *CYP2C8*2* polymorphism encoding an Ile269Phe substitution is associated with a 2-fold lower intrinsic clearance of paclitaxel and a decreased affinity for 6α-hydroxypaclitaxel, a major metabolite of paclitaxel, whereas *CYP2C8*3*, which encodes Arg139Lys and Lys399Arg substitutions, is associated with decreased paclitaxel turnover (Reference 40, 41). However, the clinical relevance of these polymorphisms to the in vivo metabolism of CYP2C8 substrates, including paclitaxel, remains to be determined.

Cytochrome P450 2C9. Cytochrome P450 2C9 is the major CYP2C isoform found in human liver and it is involved in the metabolism of several clinically important drugs, including the narrow therapeutic index drugs phenytoin and warfarin. In addition, CYP2C9 metabolizes many nonsteroidal anti-inflammatory drugs (e.g., diclofenac, ibuprofen, piroxicam, and tenoxicam), losartan, several antidiabetic drugs (e.g., glipizide, glyburide, and tolbutamide), and torsemide (Table 2) (Reference 42, 43).

Genetic polymorphisms have been described in the *CYP2C9* gene and there are important interethnic differences in allele frequencies (Table 5). Single nucleotide polymorphisms within the coding region produce variant alleles *CYP2C9*2* and *CYP2C9*3*, which are found in up to 35 percent of Caucasians but are much less prevalent in African Americans and Asians (Reference 42). The *CYP2C9*5* allele encoding an Asp360Glu substitution is selectively found in African Americans (References 43, 44).

In Vivo Activity. Flurbiprofen, losartan, tolbutamide, and warfarin have been used as in vivo probes of CYP2C9 activity (Table 4) (References 43, 45). The CYP2C9 genotype-phenotype relationship has been extensively studied both in vitro and in vivo using S-warfarin as a probe. Clinical studies have shown that the unbound clearance of S-warfarin is significantly less in individuals carrying a variant allele (Figure 2). The formation clearance of 7-hydroxywarfarin serves as an in vivo index of CYP2C9 activity. Tolbutamide has been considered the standard probe for CYP2C9 activity and the cumulative urinary recovery of the tolbutamide metabolites 4'-hydroxytolbutamide and carboxytolbutamide or the molar ratio of these metabolites divided by tolbutamide recovery (i.e., metabolic ratio) are used as indexes of CYP2C9 activity (References 45, 46).

Clinical Consequences of Genetic Variation. The clinical relevance of *CYP2C9* polymorphisms relates primarily to its role in the metabolism of the narrow therapeutic index drugs phenytoin and warfarin, as the consequence of impaired metabolism of these drugs is great. The variant alleles that have been identified are associated with decreased enzyme activity, though the magnitude of effect varies. In fact, the magnitude of decrease in activity caused by expression of the CYP2C9 variant proteins may be substrate

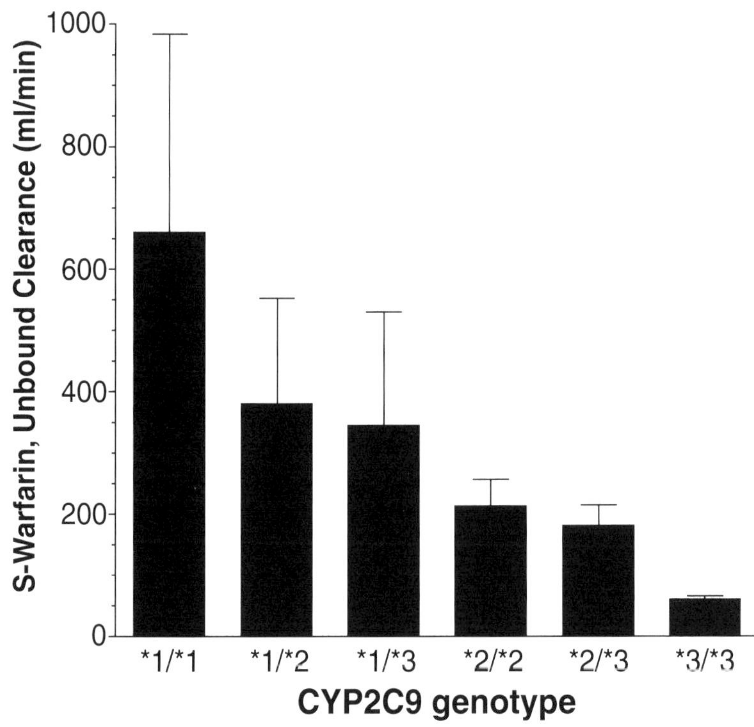

Figure 2. Effect of *CYP2C9* genotype on S-warfarin unbound clearance.
The relationship between phenotype and CYP2C9 genotype. The unbound clearance of S-warfarin is decreased in individuals carrying at least one copy of a variant allele. Data are from Scordo MG, et al. Influence of CYP2C9 and CYP2C19 genetic polymorphisms on warfarin maintenance dose and metabolic clearance. Clin Pharmacol Ther 2002;72(6):702–10.
CYP = cytochrome P450.

dependent. For example, the Ile359Leu substitution (*2C9*3*) produced a decrease in intrinsic clearance that ranged from 3-fold for diclofenac 4'-hydroxylation to 27-fold for piroxicam 5'-hydroxylation (Reference 47).

Warfarin is administered as a racemic mixture of R- and S-enantiomers. The enantiomers differ in potency with the S-enantiomer being 5-fold more potent than the R-enantiomer; it is estimated that the S-enantiomer is responsible for 60–70 percent of the anticoagulant effect with the R-enantiomer being responsible for the remaining 30–40 percent (Reference 48). The S-enantiomer is 7-hydroxylated predominantly by CYP2C9, whereas the R-enantiomer is 10-hydroxylated by CYP3A4 and 6- and 8-hydroxylated by CYP1A2 (Reference 48). As shown in Figure 2, there is a clear relationship between CYP2C9 genotype and the pharmacokinetics of the S-warfarin enantiomer; this pharmacokinetic difference directly affects the warfarin daily dose required to attain a target international normalized ratio. A summary of the gene dose effect across four studies totaling 794 Caucasian patients showed that the mean warfarin daily dose (target INR = 2.5) by genotype group was 5.28 mg, 4.59 mg, and 3.78 mg in the *1/*1, *1/*2, and *1/*3 genotypes groups, respectively (Reference 43). The single patient reported as having the *3/*3 genotype required only 0.5 mg/day. It also appears that the risk of major bleeding events, especially during the initiation of treatment, is greater in patients expressing one or more allelic variants (References 43, 48).

Phenytoin primarily is metabolized by CYP2C9 and to a lesser extent by CYP2C19. Due to toxicities associated with phenytoin use and its nonlinear pharmacokinetics, small changes in CYP2C9 activity likely are to be clinically relevant. A CYP2C9 gene-dose effect also has been observed for phenytoin with patients expressing at least one variant *CYP2C9* allele requiring a 30 percent lower phenytoin maintenance dose than patients with the *1/*1 genotype. Furthermore, the mean daily dose for patients with the *1/*1 genotype was 314 mg/day, whereas for the other genotype groups it ranged from 150 mg/day to 217 mg/day (Reference 43).

Thus, CYP2C9 genotype has clinically important implications for treatment with warfarin and phenytoin. The clearance of many other drugs also is impacted by the CYP2C9 genotype, but the clinical relevance remains unclear.

Cytochrome P450 2C19. Cytochrome P450 2C19 has been extensively evaluated over the past 20 years since it was one of the first enzymes recognized to exhibit genetic polymorphism. Cytochrome P450 2C19 is involved in the metabolism of many drugs, including citalopram, diazepam, imipramine, mephenytoin, and several proton-pump inhibitors (e.g., lansoprazole and omeprazole) (Table 2) (References 49, 50). Several allelic variants have been identified and there are marked interethnic differences in the allele frequencies. The most common allelic variants are *CYP2C19*2* and *CYP2C19*3* (Table 5). These nonfunctional variants are associated with the poor metabolizer phenotype, which occurs in 1–3 percent of Caucasians and 13–23 percent of Asians (References 49, 50).

In Vivo Activity. Mephenytoin and omeprazole have been used commonly as probes to estimate in vivo CYP2C19 activity (Reference 49). Mephenytoin is an anticonvulsant agent that is administered clinically as a racemic mixture; the S-enantiomer is rapidly hydroxylated by CYP2C19 to form 4'-hydroxymephenytoin, whereas the R-enantiomer is more slowly N-demethylated. An enantiomeric ratio of S-mephenytoin to R-mephenytoin in an 8-hour urine sample or the 8-hour cumulative recovery of 4'-hydroxymephenytoin are used to provide indexes of CYP2C19 in vivo activity. Mephenytoin was used in several large population studies to define the frequency of poor metabolizers; the genetic change was subsequently identified. The proton-pump inhibitor omeprazole is 5-hydroxylated by CYP2C19 and the plasma concentration ratio of omeprazole to 5-hydroxyomeprazole obtained 2–4 hours after drug administration has been used as an index of CYP2C19 activity (Reference 49).

Clinical Consequences of Genetic Variation. As would be expected, plasma drug concentrations of drugs predominately metabolized by CYP2C19 will be higher in CYP2C19 poor metabolizers. As a result, CYP2C19 poor metabolizers may experience more adverse effects. Indeed, the poor metabolizer phenotype was first recognized with a case of excess sedation after mephenytoin administration (Reference 49). However, CYP2C19 presents an interesting situation in that being a poor metabolizer may actually confer benefit rather than the more typical harm. The proton-pump inhibitors omeprazole and lansoprazole are predominately (more than 80 percent) metabolized by CYP2C19 and are used as part of dual or triple therapy for eradication of *Helicobacter pylori* infection (Reference 49). Several studies indicate that the cure rates of this treatment are higher in poor metabolizers (100 percent) as compared to heterozygous (60–90 percent) or homozygous (30–80 percent) extensive metabolizers (Reference 49, 50). This may be explained by the 5- to 10-fold higher omeprazole AUC in poor metabolizers, which results in a greater pharmacodynamic effect (i.e., increased gastric pH or serum gastrin concentration) but no greater incidence of adverse effects because of the wide safety margin of these drugs (Reference 49, 50). These data clearly demonstrate that CYP2C19 genotype affects the outcome of treatment with the proton-pump inhibitors.

Cytochrome P450 2DC

The pharmacogenetics of *CYP2D6* has been extensively studied since polymorphic hydroxylation of the well-known substrate debrisoquine was first reported more than 25 years ago. Although CYP2D6 is expressed at low levels, constituting only 2–4 percent of CYP protein content in human liver (Reference 51), it metabolizes 25–30 percent of all clinically used drugs, including antiarrhythmics, antidepressants (e.g., fluoxetine and nortriptyline), antipsychotics (e.g., haloperidol), β-blockers (e.g., carvedilol and metoprolol), codeine, and many other drugs (Tables 1 and 2) (Reference 5). *CYP2D6* has a high degree of genetic variability with more than 75 allelic variants identified to date (Reference 52). Although multiple nonfunctional alleles have been identified, four alleles, *CYP2D6*3*, *CYP2D6*4*, *CYP2D6*5*, and *CYP2D*6*, are predominately responsible for the poor metabolizer phenotype, with *CYP2D6*4* being the most common variant in Caucasians (Table 5). About 5–10 percent of Caucasians and 1 percent of Asians exhibit the poor metabolizer phenotype (References 10, 52). The poor metabolizer phenotype may result from being homozygous for one particular loss-of-function allele (e.g., *CYP2D6*4/*4*) or heterozygous for different defective alleles (e.g., *CYP2D6*4/*6*), which is termed compound heterozygosity. There are two allelic variants that have been associated with decreased catalytic activity—*CYP2D6*10*, which is common in Asians, and *CYP2D6*17*, which is found in African Americans. In addition to extensive metabolizers (i.e., individuals having at least one functional allele), up to 10 percent of Caucasians are classified as ultrarapid metabolizers, which is associated with duplication of the *CYP2D6* gene and greatly enhanced capacity for metabolism (Reference 10).

In Vivo Activity. Debrisoquine, dextromethorphan, metoprolol, and sparteine all have been used as in vivo probes of CYP2D6 activity, with dextromethorphan being the most commonly used probe because of issues relating to safety and availability (Reference 9).   Phenotyping with dextromethorphan typically involves oral administration of a 30-mg dose followed by collection of urine for up to 24 hours (though measurements in plasma or saliva may be more reliable) (Reference 53). Cytochrome P450 2D6 activity is estimated using the dextromethorphan metabolic ratio, which is calculated as the molar ratio of dextromethorphan to dextrorphan.

Clinical Consequences of Genetic Variation. Cytochrome P450 2D6 contributes to the metabolism of a broad range of substrates and the clinical importance of CYP2D6 pharmacogenetics has been demonstrated.   In general, the consequence of genetic variation is that compared with the majority of the population (i.e., extensive metabolizers), poor metabolizers will exhibit much higher plasma concentrations of a drug, whereas ultrarapid metabolizers will exhibit much lower plasma drug concentrations. The CYP2D6 poor metabolism genotype has been associated with lack of therapeutic efficacy and greater risk of adverse effects.   For example, codeine is metabolized to the active moiety morphine by CYP2D6, so poor metabolizers will not experience any therapeutic effect because of the absence of this conversion (Reference 10).   Adverse effects may be associated with the elevated plasma drug concentrations that are observed in poor metabolizers.   During metoprolol treatment, *CYP2D6* poor metabolizers had a 5-fold higher risk for developing adverse effects (e.g., symptomatic bradycardia) than extensive metabolizers (Reference 54). Extrapyramidal side effects (e.g., akathisia, Parkinsonism, and tardive dyskinesia) were much more common (45 percent vs. 14 percent) in poor metabolizers being treated with CYP2D6-metabolized antidepressants and/or antipsychotics than extensive metabolizers (Reference 55).   A gene-dose effect also was shown for haloperidol clearance and extrapyramidal symptoms (pseudoparkinsonism) (Reference 56).   At equivalent doses, poor metabolizers (80 percent) were much more likely to experience extrapyramidal symptoms than individuals expressing one or more functional alleles (16–20 percent) (Reference 56).

Cytochrome P450 2D6 activity may be lower in African Americans and Asians because of the higher frequency of alleles associated with decreased activity (i.e., *CYP2D6*17* and *CYP2D6*10*).   The enzyme CYP2D6.17 (*CYP2D6*17*) has decreased activity compared to the wild-type enzyme and also demonstrates unique substrate specificity. For example, the metabolism of debrisoquine and dextromethorphan is decreased in individuals with the *CYP2D6*17/*17* genotype compared to the *CYP2D6*1/*1* genotype, but the metabolism of codeine or metoprolol is not affected (Reference 57). The *CYP2D6*10* allele is associated with reduced activity, but the clinical importance, especially for heterozygotes, has not been shown consistently (References 58, 59).

Cytochrome P450 2E1

Cytochrome P450 2E1 is the only isozyme in the CYP2E subfamily and it constitutes about 7 percent of total hepatic CYP (Table 1). Although CYP2E1 has a limited role in drug metabolism, its toxicological significance is considerable because it is involved in the bioactivation of various protoxicant and procarcinogenic substrates, including halogenated anesthetics, alcohols, *N*-nitrosamines, and aromatic and halogenated hydrocarbons (Table 2) (Reference 60).

Several CYP2E1 allelic variants have been reported, with the most common being *CYP2E1*1D*, an insertion of a repeated nucleotide sequence in the 5'-flanking region, and *CYP2E1*2*, an Arg76His amino acid substitution (Table 5) (References 61, 62).

In Vivo Activity. Chlorzoxazone, a skeletal muscle relaxant, is the only validated probe drug for phenotyping CYP2E1 activity (Reference 63). Chlorzoxazone oral clearance or a plasma concentration ratio of 6-hydroxychlorzoxazone to chlorzoxazone in a single plasma sample obtained 2–4 hours after administering a 250-mg to 500-mg oral dose is used as an index of in vivo CYP2E1 activity.

Clinical Consequences of Genetic Variation. Although CYP2E1 has a minor role in drug metabolism, it metabolizes several organic solvents and several procarcinogens. Therefore, CYP2E1 pharmacogenetics may be most relevant in the evaluation of susceptibility to carcinogenic and/or toxicological effects of environmental exposures. Indeed, high CYP2E1 activity has been linked to increased susceptibility to chemical toxicity and cancer (Reference 60). Cytochrome P450 2E1 also may have a role in drug dependence because *CYP2E1*1D* has been linked to alcohol and nicotine dependence (Reference 64). Cytochrome 2E1 is induced by alcohol, obesity, and nicotine, and *CYP2E1*1D* has been associated with greater inducibility and higher CYP2E1 activity (Reference 62). The other common variant *CYP2E1*2* had less than 40 percent of the catalytic activity of the wild-type enzyme (Reference 61). Thus, these variants may be important contributors to interindividual variability in CYP2E1 activity.

CYP3 Gene Family

The *CYP3* gene family consists of four genes, *CYP3A4*, *CYP3A5*, *CYP3A7*, and *CYP3A43*. Cytochrome P450 3A enzymes are the most abundant in the liver and intestine and are considered the most important enzymes involved in drug metabolism. Cytochrome P450 3A enzymes constitute 30 percent and 70 percent of the CYP enzyme content in human liver and intestine, respectively, and are responsible for the metabolism of more than 50 percent of currently marketed drugs (Tables 1 and 2) (References 5, 65). Accordingly, CYP3A enzymes play a prominent role in the first-pass metabolism of drugs. Cytochrome P450 3A4 is considered the most abundant and clinically significant isozyme in human drug metabolism; it is expressed in human liver and intestine with intestinal protein concentrations averaging 10–50 percent of those found in liver. Cytochrome P450 3A5 is polymorphically expressed and typically displays decreased catalytic activity compared to CYP3A4. Cytochrome P450 3A7 originally was considered to exist only in fetal liver; however, recent evidence indicates that CYP3A7 messenger ribonucleic acid is highly expressed in both the liver and intestine of about 11 percent of adults (Reference 66). This suggests that CYP3A7 may contribute to interindividual variability observed in CYP3A-mediated metabolism. The relevance of CYP3A43 to drug disposition is not known.

There is intense interest in the pharmacogenetics of CYP3A enzymes given the prominent role these enzymes play in drug metabolism. Several allelic variants of *CYP3A4* have been identified, none of which are loss-of-function alleles. The most common variant that appears to have a modest functional consequence is *CYP3A4*1B*, which is an A-392G transition in the 5'-flanking region (Table 5) (Reference 67). Cytochrome P450 3A5 initially was considered less important than CYP3A4 because it was found in less than one-third of all livers and it appeared to metabolize far fewer substrates. However, an SNP in the third intron that creates an aberrant splice site and results in a truncated nonfunctional protein recently was identified (*CYP3A5*3*) (Reference 68). Identification of this SNP helped to explain variability in the expression of CYP3A5-only people who carry at least one copy of the *CYP3A5*1* allele express CYP3A5 and there is marked ethnic variation in the frequency of the variant alleles (Table 5). A mutation in the 5'-flanking region of *CYP3A7* consists of the replacement of 60 base pairs from the *CYP3A4* gene with the corresponding sequence from the CYP3A7 gene (*CYP3A7*1C*). Presence of this allele was associated with increased *CYP3A7* expression in both liver and intestine (Reference 66). It currently is not clear whether CYP3A7 expression contributes to higher CYP3A activity.

In Vivo Activity

Several drugs have been proposed as in vivo probes of CYP3A activity, including alprazolam, dapsone, dextromethorphan, erythromycin, midazolam, and nifedipine (References 9, 65). In addition, the 6β-hydroxylation of endogenous cortisol has been proposed as an index reaction for measuring CYP3A activity. Currently, midazolam and erythromycin are considered the gold standard probe drugs. An advantage of midazolam is that it can be given experimentally both orally and intravenously, thereby facilitating evaluation of intestinal and hepatic CYP3A activity. Midazolam clearance after oral or intravenous administration is used as a measure of CYP3A activity. In addition, these clearance values have been used to derive parameters reflecting hepatic and intestinal extraction (Reference 69). The erythromycin breath test (ERMBT) was one of the first selective in vivo CYP3A4 probe drugs validated for use in humans and involves intravenous administration of $[^{14}\text{C-N-methyl}]$erythromycin and collection of a breath sample at 20 minutes (Reference 65). Limitations of the ERMBT include the use of radioactivity and the fact that it does not provide information on intestinal metabolism. The urinary ratio of 6β-hydroxycortisol-cortisol is a useful and reliable marker of CYP3A enzyme induction (i.e., for within-subject comparisons) but it is not useful as a general index of enzyme activity (Reference 70).

Clinical Consequences of Genetic Variation

There is tremendous interindividual variability in CYP3A-mediated metabolism with the clearance of some substrate varying up to 20-fold. Thus, identification of any genetic determinants of enzyme activity would likely be of clinical importance. Although SNPs have been found in the coding region of *CYP3A4*, they are rare and appear to have limited impact on CYP3A4 activity (Reference 67). Although the *CYP3A4*1B* variant allele is associated with increased transcriptional activation in vitro, the in vivo data are not consistent and suggest only a modest effect (e.g., 30 percent difference in systemic midazolam clearance) (Reference 67).

Cytochrome P450 3A5 may be important with respect to interindividual variability in CYP3A-mediated metabolism. It is estimated that CYP3A5 may account for up to 50 percent of the total CYP3A content in people with at least one *CYP3A5*1* allele (Reference 68). A functional consequence of CYP3A5 expression was supported by the finding in vitro that midazolam hydroxylation was 2-fold higher in livers with at least one copy of the *CYP3A5*1* allele (Reference 68). It is likely that the impact of CYP3A5 genetic polymorphism will be drug-dependent to some extent because substrate specificity differs from CYP3A4. However, the clinical relevance of CYP3A5 pharmacogenetics as it pertains to drug clearance remains unclear. Indeed, there is some controversy regarding the contribution of CYP3A5 to hepatic drug metabolism, at least in Caucasians (Reference 71).

Cytochrome P450 3A5 is the primary extrahepatic CYP3A isoform and an interesting link recently was made between CYP3A5, the predominant CYP3A isoform in kidney, and blood pressure in African Americans (Reference 72). Cytochrome P450 3A5 protein content (8-fold) and catalytic activity (18-fold) were higher in renal microsomes from organ donors having the **1/*3* genotype compared to the **3/*3* genotype. In addition, the mean systolic blood pressure in homozygous carriers of *CYP3A5*1* was 19.3 mm Hg greater than that of homozygous carriers of *CYP3A5*3* in a population of 25 healthy African Americans, suggesting a possible link between CYP3A5 activity and the high prevalence of sodium-sensitive hypertension in African Americans (Reference 72). In addition to this observation, CYP3A5 may have other important physiological roles related to steroid metabolism (Reference 67).

Although multiple mutations have been identified in the *CYP3A* genes, the overall impact of genetic variation in concert with numerous nongenetic factors (e.g., enzyme induction and inhibition, and environmental factors) that affect activity must still be defined.

Oxidative Drug Metabolism—Other Enzymes
Flavin-containing Monooxygenase Gene Family

The FMOs are microsomal enzymes that catalyze the oxygenation of nucleophilic nitrogen-, sulfur-, phosphorus-, and other heteroatom-containing xenobiotics to their corresponding oxides. Flavin-containing monooxygenase-mediated metabolism typically increases water solubility and decreases toxic potential, though in some cases FMO can produce reactive metabolites. The nomenclature for these enzymes follows that *FMO* genes having 82 percent or more sequence homology are grouped within a family, which is designated by an Arabic numeral (i.e., 1, 2, or 3) (Reference 73). Flavin-containing monooxygenase-3 is the prominent form in adult human liver and also is found in brain (Reference 73). Flavin-containing monooxygenase-3 has a role in the metabolism of caffeine, cimetidine, clozapine, S-nicotine, and ranitidine (Table 2) (Reference 73). The physiological importance of FMO3 relates to its ability to N-oxygenate several endogenous and dietary amines, including biogenic amines (Reference 74).

Functionally significant allelic variants that have been discovered include missense, nonsense, and deletion or truncation mutants of human *FMO* (Table 5). The *FMO3* haplotype may be more relevant as the variants appear to be in linkage disequilibrium, which means that the variants occur in combination more often than expected based on the given frequency of each variant. The most common polymorphisms (Table 5) occur at sites 158 (Glu158Lys), 257 (Val257Met), and 308 (Glu308Gly) with the wild-type haplotype (Glu-Val-Glu) occurring in about 53 percent of Caucasians.

In Vivo Activity. There are few studies evaluating the in vivo activity of FMO3 using selective substrates. Drugs that have been used as probes to phenotype in vivo FMO3 activity include S-nicotine, caffeine, cimetidine, clozapine, and ranitidine (Reference 73). The metabolism of caffeine and clozapine was not associated with common FMO3 polymorphisms (Reference 75). However, a genotype-phenotype relationship has been observed with ranitidine N-oxidation in a Korean population (References 76, 77).

Clinical Consequences of Genetic Variation. The most clinically relevant consequence of genetic variation in FMO3 is associated with defective N-oxygenation of trimethylamine derived from choline-rich dietary sources. Excessive excretion of trimethylamine in urine (trimethylaminuria) and sweat causes individuals to emit an odor similar to rotting fish. Thus, this rare condition is known as fish-odor syndrome. Genetic polymorphisms in *FMO3* have been causally linked to trimethylaminuria (Reference 73). The impact of *FMO3* pharmacogenetics on the disposition or response to drugs is limited.

Approaches for Clinical Application of Oxidative Drug Metabolism Pharmacogenetics

Although multiple factors, including age, sex, disease, and environmental exposures, contribute to variability in drug response, it is clear that genetics plays a critical role in determining both the efficacy of a drug and the likelihood of an adverse reaction. Indeed, genetic variation in drug metabolizing enzymes, including CYP and FMO enzymes, is associated with significant clinical consequences. Although the pharmacogenetics of these enzymes continues to be unraveled, the incorporation of this knowledge into clinical practice is lagging behind. However, it is application of this knowledge that will help achieve the ultimate promise of pharmacogenomics, which is to provide "personalized medicine" or treatment that is tailored to individuals on the basis of their genetic makeup.

Integration into Therapy Selection Process

Current knowledge on the pharmacogenetics of drug metabolism supports the possibility that a suitable dosing regimen can be selected on the basis of a person's genotype. Although there is increasing evidence that this is feasible, it must be remembered that drug effects are not monogenic traits (i.e., involving single genes) but are determined by the interplay of several gene products. Inherited differences in both drug disposition genes (e.g., metabolizing enzymes and transporters) and drug target genes (e.g., receptors) will influence drug pharmacokinetics and pharmacodynamics, making polygenic determinants of drug effect essential. However, genotyping for variants of drug metabolizing enzymes may help guide successful treatment, such as through the development of dosing recommendations for different genetic subpopulations of patients.

Providing an example of how pharmacogenetics can be incorporated into clinical practice, starting dosing regimens for several antidepressants based on *CYP2D6* genotype have been developed (Reference 78). Cytochrome P450 2D6 pharmacogenetic implications are well documented, and *CYP2D6* genotype has been used to successfully predict drug clearance. For example, clearance of the CYP2D6 substrate nortriptyline, which is proportional to the number of functional CYP2D6 genes, is 80 percent lower in individuals carrying no functional genes compared to people with three functional genes (i.e., ultrarapid metabolizers) (Reference 79). Cytochrome P450 2D6 poor metabolizers exhibit supratherapeutic plasma concentrations and experience adverse drug reactions when receiving standard doses of the drug, whereas ultrarapid metabolizers often show evidence of therapeutic failure and may require up to 5 times the standard dose to achieve therapeutic plasma concentrations. The dose recommendations for nortriptyline are as follows: poor metabolizers should receive 50 percent, intermediate metabolizers 70 percent, extensive metabolizers 140 percent, and ultrarapid metabolizers up to 230 percent of the recommended starting dose of nortriptyline, which is 50 mg/day (Reference 78). Although this approach is attractive, prospective studies are still required to assess whether these genotype-based dosing guidelines will improve outcomes.

Other relevant examples in which prospective genotyping may improve clinical therapy include *CYP2C9* genotype and warfarin therapy and *CYP2C19* genotype and treatment for *H. pylori* infection. For example, the starting warfarin dose could be individualized based on the gene-dose relationship previously discussed (Reference 43). This approach may help to prevent bleeding complications during the initiation of therapy, as high-risk patients (e.g., *2C9*2/*3* or *2C9*3/*3* patients) would be started on treatment at lower doses.

Pharmacogenetics-oriented Therapeutic Drug Monitoring

The concept of drug therapy individualization is certainly not new. Therapeutic drug monitoring started in the early 1970s and is still commonly performed for selected drugs, such as aminoglycoside antibiotics. In the traditional sense, therapeutic drug monitoring is performed after the drug is administered by obtaining plasma concentration time data and applying appropriate mathematical interpretation and clinical judgment. Pharmacogenetics may permit proactive individualization of drug therapy, as pharmacogenetic information can be applied *a priori* for drug and dose selection (i.e., pharmacogenetics-oriented therapeutic drug monitoring) will make use of genotype data to individualize drug therapy (Reference 80). Drugs that are extensively and exclusively metabolized by a polymorphic enzyme (e.g., CYP2D6) have a narrow therapeutic index, and have a defined concentration response relationship are ideal candidates for early evaluations of this approach. Prospective clinical studies to assess outcomes and costs are needed to support implementation of this approach into clinical practice.

The ability to individualize or personalize drug treatment should improve as knowledge of genetic variations in proteins involved in drug disposition and response increases and more cost-effective testing methodology becomes available. The ultimate goal of pharmacogenomics is that on the basis of genetic makeup, the best drug and an individualized dosing regimen can be selected to attain maximal efficacy and minimal toxicity, thereby avoiding therapeutic misadventures and achieving optimal therapeutic outcomes.

References

1. Kumar GN, Surapaneni S. Role of drug metabolism in drug discovery and development. Med Res Rev 2001;21(5):397–411.

2. Omura T, Sato R. The carbon monoxide binding pigment of liver microsomes. I. Evidence for its hemoprotein nature. J Biol Chem 1964;239:2370–8.

3. Nebert DW, Russell DW. Clinical importance of the cytochromes P450. Lancet 2002;360(9340):1155–62.

4. Nelson DR, Koymans L, Kamataki T, et al. P450 superfamily: update on new sequences, gene mapping, accession numbers and nomenclature. Pharmacogenetics 1996;6(1):1–42.

5. Bertz RJ, Granneman GR. Use of in vitro and in vivo data to estimate the likelihood of metabolic pharmacokinetic interactions. Clin Pharmacokinet 1997;32(3):210–58.

6. Rusnak JM, Kisabeth RM, Herbert DP, McNeil DM. Pharmacogenomics: a clinician's primer on emerging technologies for improved patient care. Mayo Clin Proc 2001;76(3):299–309.

7. Wilkinson GR. Clearance approaches in pharmacology. Pharmacol Rev 1987;39:1–47.

8. Jackson PR, Tucker GT. Pharmacokinetic-pharmacogenetic modelling in the detection of polymorphisms in xenobiotic metabolism. Ann Occup Hyg 1990;34(6):653–62.

9. Streetman DS, Bertino JS Jr, Nafziger AN. Phenotyping of drug-metabolizing enzymes in adults: a review of in-vivo cytochrome P450 phenotyping probes. Pharmacogenetics 2000;10(3):187–216.

10. Daly AK. Pharmacogenetics of the major polymorphic metabolizing enzymes. Fundam Clin Pharmacol 2003;17(1):27–41.

11. Ingelman-Sundberg M, Oscarson M, McLellan RA. Polymorphic human cytochrome P450 enzymes: an opportunity for individualized drug treatment. Trends Pharmacol Sci 1999;20(8):342–9.

12. Sasaki M, Tanaka Y, Kaneuchi M, Sakuragi N, Dahiya R. CYP1B1 gene polymorphisms have higher risk for endometrial cancer, and positive

correlations with estrogen receptor alpha and estrogen receptor beta expressions. Cancer Res 2003;63(14):3913–8.

13. Tanaka Y, Sasaki M, Kaneuchi M, Shiina H, Igawa M, Dahiya R. Polymorphisms of the CYP1B1 gene have higher risk for prostate cancer. Biochem Biophys Res Commun 2002;296(4):820–6.

14. Stoilov I, Akarsu AN, Sarfarazi M. Identification of three different truncating mutations in cytochrome P4501B1 (CYP1B1) as the principal cause of primary congenital glaucoma (Buphthalmos) in families linked to the GLC3A locus on chromosome 2p21. Hum Mol Genet 1997;6(4):641–7.

15. Zevin S, Benowitz NL. Drug interactions with tobacco smoking. An update. Clin Pharmacokinet 1999;36(6):425–38.

16. Bartsch H, Nair U, Risch A, Rojas M, Wikman H, Alexandrov K. Genetic polymorphism of CYP genes, alone or in combination, as a risk modifier of tobacco-related cancers. Cancer Epidemiol Biomarkers Prev 2000;9(1):3–28.

17. Sachse C, Brockmoller J, Bauer S, Roots I. Functional significance of a C-->A polymorphism in intron 1 of the cytochrome P450 CYP1A2 gene tested with caffeine. Br J Clin Pharmacol 1999;47(4):445–9.

18. Tassaneeyakul W, Birkett DJ, McManus ME, et al. Caffeine metabolism by human hepatic cytochromes P450: contributions of 1A2, 2E1 and 3A isoforms. Biochem Pharmacol 1994;47(10):1767–76.

19. Fuhr U, Rost KL, Engelhardt R, et al. Evaluation of caffeine as a test drug for CYP1A2, NAT2 and CYP2E1 phenotyping in man by in vivo versus in vitro correlations. Pharmacogenetics 1996;6(2):159–76.

20. Berthou F, Flinois JP, Ratanasavanh D, Beaune P, Riche C, Guillouzo A. Evidence for the involvement of several cytochromes P-450 in the first steps of caffeine metabolism by human liver microsomes. Drug Metab Dispos 1991;19(3):561–7.

21. Fuhr U, Rost KL. Simple and reliable CYP1A2 phenotyping by the paraxanthine/caffeine ratio in plasma and saliva. Pharmacogenetics 1994;4:109–116.

22. Van Der Weide J, Steijns LS, Van Weelden MJ. The effect of smoking and cytochrome P450 CYP1A2 genetic polymorphism on clozapine clearance and dose requirement. Pharmacogenetics 2003;13(3):169–72.

23. Nordmark A, Lundgren S, Ask B, Granath F, Rane A. The effect of the CYP1A2*1F mutation on CYP1A2 inducibility in pregnant women. Br J Clin Pharmacol 2002;54(5):504–10.

24. Sachse C, Bhambra U, Smith G, et al. Polymorphisms in the cytochrome P450 CYP1A2 gene (CYP1A2) in colorectal cancer patients and controls: allele frequencies, linkage disequilibrium and influence on caffeine metabolism. Br J Clin Pharmacol 2003;55(1):68–76.

25. Han XM, Ouyang DS, Chen XP, et al. Inducibility of CYP1A2 by omeprazole in vivo related to the genetic polymorphism of CYP1A2. Br J Clin Pharmacol 2002;54(5):540–3.

26. Aklillu E, Carrillo JA, Makonnen E, et al. Genetic polymorphism of CYP1A2 in Ethiopians affecting induction and expression: characterization of novel

haplotypes with single-nucleotide polymorphisms in intron 1. Mol Pharmacol 2003;64(3):659–69.

27. Raunio H, Rautio A, Gullsten H, Pelkonen O. Polymorphisms of CYP2A6 and its practical consequences. Br J Clin Pharmacol 2001;52(4):357-63.

28. Xu C, Goodz S, Sellers EM, Tyndale RF. CYP2A6 genetic variation and potential consequences. Adv Drug Deliv Rev 2002;54(10):1245–56.

29. Pianezza ML, Sellers EM, Tyndale RF. Nicotine metabolism defect reduces smoking. Nature 1998;393(6687):750.

30. Sellers EM, Kaplan HL, Tyndale RF. Inhibition of cytochrome P450 2A6 increases nicotine's oral bioavailability and decreases smoking. Clin Pharmacol Ther 2000;68(1):35–43.

31. Sellers EM, Tyndale RF, Fernandes LC. Decreasing smoking behaviour and risk through CYP2A6 inhibition. Drug Discov Today 2003;8(11):487–93.

32. Ekins S, Wrighton SA. The role of CYP2B6 in human xenobiotic metabolism. Drug Metab Rev 1999;31(3):719–54.

33. Stresser DM, Kupfer D. Monospecific antipeptide antibody to cytochrome P-450 2B6. Drug Metab Dispos 1999;27(4):517–25.

34. Lang T, Klein K, Fischer J, et al. Extensive genetic polymorphism in the human CYP2B6 gene with impact on expression and function in human liver. Pharmacogenetics 2001;11(5):399–415.

35. Hiratsuka M, Takekuma Y, Endo N, et al. Allele and genotype frequencies of CYP2B6 and CYP3A5 in the Japanese population. Eur J Clin Pharmacol 2002;58(6):417–21.

36. Faucette SR, Hawke RL, Lecluyse EL, et al. Validation of bupropion hydroxylation as a selective marker of human cytochrome P450 2B6 catalytic activity. Drug Metab Dispos 2000;28(10):1222–30.

37. Ward BA, Gorski JC, Jones DR, Hall SD, Flockhart DA, Desta Z. The cytochrome P450 2B6 (CYP2B6) is the main catalyst of efavirenz primary and secondary metabolism: implication for HIV/AIDS therapy and utility of efavirenz as a substrate marker of CYP2B6 catalytic activity. J Pharmacol Exp Ther 2003;306(1):287–300.

38. Xie HJ, Yasar U, Lundgren S, et al. Role of polymorphic human CYP2B6 in cyclophosphamide bioactivation. Pharmacogenomics J 2003;3(1):53–61.

39. Jinno H, Tanaka-Kagawa T, Ohno A, et al. Functional characterization of cytochrome P450 2B6 allelic variants. Drug Metab Dispos 2003;31(4):398–403.

40. Bahadur N, Leathart JB, Mutch E, et al. CYP2C8 polymorphisms in Caucasians and their relationship with paclitaxel 6alpha-hydroxylase activity in human liver microsomes. Biochem Pharmacol 2002;64(11):1579–89.

41. Dai D, Zeldin DC, Blaisdell JA, et al. Polymorphisms in human CYP2C8 decrease metabolism of the anticancer drug paclitaxel and arachidonic acid. Pharmacogenetics 2001;11(7):597–607.

42. Goldstein JA. Clinical relevance of genetic polymorphisms in the human CYP2C subfamily. Br J Clin Pharmacol 2001;52(4):349–55.

43. Lee CR, Goldstein JA, Pieper JA. Cytochrome P450 2C9 polymorphisms: a comprehensive review of the in-vitro and human data. Pharmacogenetics 2002;12(3):251–63.

44. Dickmann LJ, Rettie AE, Kneller MB, et al. Identification and functional characterization of a new CYP2C9 variant (CYP2C9*5) expressed among African Americans. Mol Pharmacol 2001;60(2):382–7.

45. Lee CR, Pieper JA, Frye RF, Hinderliter AL, Blaisdell JA, Goldstein JA. Tolbutamide, flurbiprofen, and losartan as probes of CYP2C9 activity in humans. J Clin Pharmacol 2003;43(1):84–91.

46. Lee CR, Pieper JA, Hinderliter AL, Blaisdell JA, Goldstein JA. Evaluation of cytochrome P4502C9 metabolic activity with tolbutamide in CYP2C91 heterozygotes. Clin Pharmacol Ther 2002;72(5):562–71.

47. Takanashi K, Tainaka H, Kobayashi K, Yasumori T, Hosakawa M, Chiba K. CYP2C9 Ile359 and Leu359 variants: enzyme kinetic study with seven substrates. Pharmacogenetics 2000;10(2):95–104.

48. Daly AK, King BP. Pharmacogenetics of oral anticoagulants. Pharmacogenetics 2003;13(5):247–52.

49. Wedlund PJ. The CYP2C19 enzyme polymorphism. Pharmacology 2000;61(3):174–83.

50. Desta Z, Zhao X, Shin JG, Flockhart DA. Clinical significance of the cytochrome P450 2C19 genetic polymorphism. Clin Pharmacokinet 2002;41(12):913–58.

51. Shimada T, Yamazaki H, Mimura M, Inui Y, Guengerich FP. Interindividual variations in human liver cytochrome P-450 enzymes involved in the oxidation of drugs, carcinogens and toxic chemicals: studies with liver microsomes of 30 Japanese and 30 Caucasians. J Pharmacol Exp Ther 1994;270(1):414–23.

52. Bertilsson L, Dahl ML, Dalen P, Al-Shurbaji A. Molecular genetics of CYP2D6: clinical relevance with focus on psychotropic drugs. Br J Clin Pharmacol 2002;53(2):111–22.

53. Hu OY, Tang HS, Lane HY, Chang WH, Hu TM. Novel single-point plasma or saliva dextromethorphan method for determining CYP2D6 activity. J Pharmacol Exp Ther 1998;285(3):955–60.

54. Wuttke H, Rau T, Heide R, et al. Increased frequency of cytochrome P450 2D6 poor metabolizers among patients with metoprolol-associated adverse effects. Clin Pharmacol Ther 2002;72(4):429–37.

55. Vandel P, Haffen E, Vandel S, et al. Drug extrapyramidal side effects. CYP2D6 genotypes and phenotypes. Eur J Clin Pharmacol 1999;55(9):659–65.

56. Brockmoller J, Kirchheiner J, Schmider J, et al. The impact of the CYP2D6 polymorphism on haloperidol pharmacokinetics and on the outcome of haloperidol treatment. Clin Pharmacol Ther 2002;72(4):438–52.

57. Wennerholm A, Dandara C, Sayi J, et al. The African-specific CYP2D6*17 allele encodes an enzyme with changed substrate specificity. Clin Pharmacol Ther 2002;71(1):77–88.

58. Dalen P, Dahl ML, Roh HK, et al. Disposition of debrisoquine and nortriptyline in Korean subjects in relation to CYP2D6 genotypes, and comparison with Caucasians. Br J Clin Pharmacol 2003;55(6):630–4.

59. Mihara K, Kondo T, Yasui-Furukori N, et al. Effects of various CYP2D6 genotypes on the steady-state plasma concentrations of risperidone and its active metabolite, 9-hydroxyrisperidone, in Japanese patients with schizophrenia. Ther Drug Monit 2003;25(3):287–93.

60. Tanaka E, Terada M, Misawa S. Cytochrome P450 2E1: its clinical and toxicological role. J Clin Pharm Ther 2000;25(3):165–75.

61. Hu Y, Oscarson M, Johansson I, et al. Genetic polymorphism of human CYP2E1: characterization of two variant alleles. Mol Pharmacol 1997;51(3):370–6.

62. McCarver DG, Byun R, Hines RN, Hichme M, Wegenek W. A genetic polymorphism in the regulatory sequences of human CYP2E1: association with increased chlorzoxazone hydroxylation in the presence of obesity and ethanol intake. Toxicol Appl Pharmacol 1998;152(1):276–81.

63. Frye RF, Adedoyin A, Mauro K, Matzke GR, Branch RA. Use of chlorzoxazone as an in vivo probe of cytochrome P450 2E1: choice of dose and phenotypic trait measure. J Clin Pharmacol 1998;38(1):82–9.

64. Howard LA, Ahluwalia JS, Lin SK, Sellers EM, Tyndale RF. CYP2E1*1D regulatory polymorphism: association with alcohol and nicotine dependence. Pharmacogenetics 2003;13(6):321–8.

65. Thummel KE, Wilkinson GR. In vitro and in vivo drug interactions involving human CYP3A. Annu Rev Pharmacol Toxicol 1998;38:389–430.

66. Burk O, Tegude H, Koch I, et al. Molecular mechanisms of polymorphic CYP3A7 expression in adult human liver and intestine. J Biol Chem 2002;277(27):24280–8.

67. Lamba JK, Lin YS, Schuetz EG, Thummel KE. Genetic contribution to variable human CYP3A-mediated metabolism. Adv Drug Deliv Rev 2002;54(10):1271–94.

68. Kuehl P, Zhang J, Lin Y, et al. Sequence diversity in CYP3A promoters and characterization of the genetic basis of polymorphic CYP3A5 expression. Nat Genet 2001;27(4):383–91.

69. Lee JI, Chaves-Gnecco D, Amico JA, Kroboth PD, Wilson JW, Frye RF. Application of semisimultaneous midazolam administration for hepatic and intestinal cytochrome P450 3A phenotyping. Clin Pharmacol Ther 2002;72(6):718–28.

70. Tran JQ, Kovacs SJ, McIntosh TS, Davis HM, Martin DE. Morning spot and 24-hour urinary 6 beta-hydroxycortisol to cortisol ratios: intraindividual variability and correlation under basal conditions and conditions of CYP 3A4 induction. J Clin Pharmacol 1999;39(5):487–94.

71. Westlind-Johnsson A, Malmebo S, Johansson A, et al. Comparative analysis of CYP3A expression in human liver suggests only a minor role for CYP3A5 in drug metabolism. Drug Metab Dispos 2003;31(6):755–61.

72. Givens RC, Lin YS, Dowling AL, et al. CYP3A5 genotype predicts renal CYP3A activity and blood pressure in healthy adults. J Appl Physiol 2003;95(3):1297–300.

73. Cashman JR, Zhang J. Interindividual differences of human flavin-containing monooxygenase 3: genetic polymorphisms and functional variation. Drug Metab Dispos 2002;30(10):1043–52.

74. Cashman JR, Zhang J, Leushner J, Braun A. Population distribution of human flavin-containing monooxygenase form 3: gene polymorphisms. Drug Metab Dispos 2001;29(12):1629–37.

75. Sachse C, Ruschen S, Dettling M, et al. Flavin monooxygenase 3 (FMO3) polymorphism in a white population: allele frequencies, mutation linkage, and functional effects on clozapine and caffeine metabolism. Clin Pharmacol Ther 1999;66(4):431–8.

76. Kang JH, Chung WG, Lee KH, et al. Phenotypes of flavin-containing monooxygenase activity determined by ranitidine N-oxidation are positively correlated with genotypes of linked FMO3 gene mutations in a Korean population. Pharmacogenetics 2000;10(1):67–78.

77. Park CS, Kang JH, Chung WG, et al. Ethnic differences in allelic frequency of two flavin-containing monooxygenase 3 (FMO3) polymorphisms: linkage and effects on in vivo and in vitro FMO activities. Pharmacogenetics 2002;12(1):77–80.

78. Kirchheiner J, Brosen K, Dahl ML, et al. CYP2D6 and CYP2C19 genotype-based dose recommendations for antidepressants: a first step towards subpopulation-specific dosages. Acta Psychiatr Scand 2001;104(3):173–92.

79. Dalen P, Dahl ML, Ruiz ML, Nordin J, Bertilsson L. 10-Hydroxylation of nortriptyline in white persons with 0, 1, 2, 3, and 13 functional CYP2D6 genes. Clin Pharmacol Ther 1998;63(4):444–52.

80. Ensom MH, Chang TK, Patel P. Pharmacogenetics: the therapeutic drug monitoring of the future? Clin Pharmacokinet 2001;40(11):783–802.

81. Steiner E, Bertilsson L, Sawe J, Bertling I, Sjoqvist F. Polymorphic debrisoquin hydroxylation in 757 Swedish subjects. Clin Pharmacol Ther 1988;44(4):431–5.

82. Scordo MG, Pengo V, Spina E, Dahl ML, Gusella M, Padrini R. Influence of CYP2C9 and CYP2C19 genetic polymorphisms on warfarin maintenance dose and metabolic clearance. Clin Pharmacol Ther 2002;72(6):702–10.

Self-Assessment Questions

1. Which one of the following is the *least* likely explanation for an observation of a disparate genotype-phenotype relationship in the metabolism of a drug?

    A. The genotype study groups were not well defined.
    B. The enzyme of interest does not selectively metabolize the drug evaluated.
    C. The single nucleotide polymorphism(s) (SNP[s]) evaluated were not functionally significant.
    D. The drug is a substrate for the efflux transporter P-glycoprotein.

2. Which one of the following cytochrome P450 (CYP) enzymes plays the most prominent role in first-pass drug metabolism?

    A. CYP1A2.
    B. CYP2C9.
    C. CYP2D6.
    D. CYP3A4.

3. A patient who has been receiving codeine for pain after tooth extraction is not experiencing any therapeutic benefit (i.e., pain relief). If this patient's lack of response is because of an inability to metabolize codeine to the active moiety morphine, a homozygous genetic mutation in which one of the following genes is most likely responsible?

    A. *CYP2A6.*
    B. *CYP2C8.*
    C. *CYP2D6.*
    D. *CYP3A4.*

4. Which one of the following CYP enzymes has a genetic polymorphism in the promoter region that has been associated with altered inducibility?

    A. CYP1A2.
    B. CYP2C9.
    C. CYP2C19.
    D. CYP2D6.

5. There is evidence to support a role for genetically polymorphic CYP enzymes to influence the risk of drug dependence. Which one of the following enzymes has been linked to addictive behaviors, including smoking behavior?

    A. CYP1A2.

B. CYP2A6.
C. CYP2C19.
D. CYP3A4.

6. A patient who has been receiving nortriptyline to treat depression is not experiencing any therapeutic benefit as evidenced by a lack of change in the Hamilton Depression Rating Score. The patient was confirmed to be adherent to the treatment regimen, so plasma concentrations were assessed and were unexpectedly low. Genotyping determined that this patient has gene duplication, which is associated with which one of the following enzymes?

A. CYP1A2.
B. CYP2C19.
C. CYP2D6.
D. CYP3A4.

7. The utility of pharmacogenetics-oriented therapeutic drug monitoring for a drug that is oxidatively metabolized will *most* likely depend on which one of the following characteristics?

A. The drug does not have a narrow therapeutic index.
B. The polymorphic metabolic pathway is a major route of elimination for that drug.
C. The drug does not have pharmacologically active metabolite(s).
D. The variability in drug response cannot be easily determined clinically.

8. Proton-pump inhibitors (e.g., omeprazole and lansoprazole) are used as part of triple therapy for treating *Helicobacter pylori*-positive gastric ulcers. It has been noted that the cure rate is higher in CYP2C19 poor metabolizers. On average, which one of the following groups would you expect to have the higher response rate to triple therapy that includes omeprazole?

A. Caucasians.
B. African Americans.
C. Japanese.
D. European Caucasians.

9. Because of its important role in the metabolism of trimethylamine derived from dietary sources, which one of the following enzymes has genetic polymorphisms that have been associated with trimethylaminuria?

A. CYP1A2.
B. CYP2E1.
C. CYP3A4.

D. Flavin-containing monooxygenase-3.

10. A patient with deep vein thrombosis is being treated with warfarin at a standard dose of 5 mg/day. One week later, the patient presents with an intracerebral hemorrhage and the international normalized ratio is 11. The patient is genotyped and found to have a genetic mutation in the enzyme responsible for the metabolism of S-warfarin. The pharmacogenetics of which one of the following enzymes has been associated with adverse clinical outcomes (e.g., risk of bleeding complications) and warfarin maintenance dose requirements?

A. CYP1A2.
B. CYP2C9.
C. CYP2D6.
D. CYP3A4.

Drug Transporter Pharmacogenetics

Deanna L. Kroetz, Ph.D.
Tan D. Nguyen, Ph.D.c.

Key Words

Membrane transporters, multidrug resistance, nucleosides, organic anions, organic cations.

Abstract

Membrane transporters play an important role in the absorption, distribution, and elimination of numerous drugs. This chapter summarizes the current information on the localization and function of the multidrug resistance efflux transporters (MDR1) and multidrug resistance-associated proteins (MRPs) and solute carrier uptake transporters (organic cation, organic anion, and nucleoside transporters). Genetic variation in these membrane transporters and the functional significance of these variants in in vitro expression systems is reviewed. Finally, the clinical significance of genetic variation in membrane transporters is discussed. There has been much progress in recent years in understanding the importance of membrane transporters in drug response and toxicity. The field of membrane transporter pharmacogenetics is rapidly expanding and early studies suggest that genetic variation in drug transporters will need to be considered in determining optimal drug therapy.

Outline

Learning Objectives

1. Discuss the cellular and intracellular localization, substrate specificity, and proposed role of transporters in the absorption, distribution and elimination of drugs.
2. Describe clinical data supporting a role for efflux transporters in bioavailability, central nervous system exposure and tumor resistance.
3. Discuss the importance of neurotransmitter transporters as drug targets.
4. Describe the degree of genetic variation in drug transporters.
5. Discuss the functional implications of genetic variation in drug transporters and how this might affect the efficacy and safety of drugs.
6. Discuss the potential for prediction of altered drug response based on drug transporter genotypes.

Abbreviations in this Chapter

ABC	ATP-binding cassette
AMP	Adenosine monophosphate
ARA	Anthracycline resistance associated (protein)
ATP	Adenosine-5'-triphosphate
AUC	Area under the curve
BCRP	Breast cancer resistance protein
C_{max}	Maximum plasma concentration
cMOAT	Canalicular multispecific organic anion transporter
DNA	Deoxyribonucleic acid
$E_217\text{ß}G$	17β-estradiol glucuronide
GMP	Guanosine monophosphate

HIV	Human immunodeficiency virus
LTC_4	Leukotriene C_4
MDR1	Multidrug resistance gene
MPP^+	1-methyl-4-phenylpyridinium
mRNA	Messenger ribonucleic acid
MRP	Multidrug resistance-associated protein
MXR	Mitoxantrone resistance protein
NBD	Nucleotide-binding domain
Pgp	P-glycoprotein
PAH	*p*-Aminohippuric acid
PBMC	Peripheral blood mononuclear cells
PMEA	9-(2-phosphonylmethoxyethyl) adenine
PXE	Pseudoxanthoma elasticum
TEA	Tetraethylammonium
TMD	Transmembrane domain

Human Drug Transporters—Localization and Function

Efflux Transporters

The known human multidrug resistance transporters are efflux transporters and belong to three different gene subfamilies within the superfamily of adenosine-5'-triphosphate (ATP)-binding cassette (ABC) transporters (Reference 1). Multidrug resistance transporters typically contain two nucleotide-binding domains (NBDs) and at least two transmembrane domains (TMDs). The TMDs comprise 6-11 membrane-spanning α-helices and provide the substrate specificity for these transporters. The NBDs, which are highly conserved across species, each contain an ABC domain where ATP is used to drive the transport of substrates across the cell membrane. Characteristic motifs of ABC proteins are the Walker A and B sites, which are housed in the NBD. A signature C motif located upstream of the Walker B site distinguishes the ABC transporters from other ATP using proteins. The transporters of interest are multidrug resistance gene (*MDR1*), which encodes P-glycoprotein (Pgp), the multidrug resistance-associated proteins (MRPs), and the half transporter, mitoxantrone resistance protein (MXR). Their physiological roles and localization are discussed in more detail in the following sections.

MDR1 (ABCB1)

MDR1, which encodes Pgp, was the first cloned human ABC protein and is the most studied of the multidrug resistance transporters (Reference 2). P-glycoprotein was first characterized as an efflux transporter overexpressed in cancer cells, which is considered an important mechanism for resistance to many cancer chemotherapy agents. It is apically expressed in epithelial cells of the adrenal cortex, renal tubules, intestinal brush border membrane, and the canalicular membrane of the hepatocyte. P-glycoprotein also is localized to the capillary endothelial cells of the blood-brain and blood-testis barriers as well as various leukocyte lineages. P-glycoprotein is predicted to have two TMDs, each with 6 membrane-spanning regions. A wide range of hydrophobic cationic or neutral compounds are transported across membranes by Pgp. Substrates include anthracyclines, vinca alkaloids, paclitaxel, protease inhibitors, immunosuppressants, calcium channel blockers, opiates, digoxin, and numerous steroids. A wide variety of compounds also can inhibit the function of Pgp and they include the hormones tamoxifen and progesterone, the peptide cyclosporin A, and the antiarrhythmic quinidine.

Multidrug Resistance-associated Proteins
MRP1 (ABCC1)
MRP1 is sorted to the basolateral membrane in a variety of polarized cells (Reference 3). It is ubiquitously expressed throughout the body but has very low expression in the liver. Structurally, MRP1 is composed of three TMDs, compared to the two TMD structure of Pgp. It is predicted to have 17 membrane-spanning regions with the extra five transmembrane loops at the N-terminus. MRP1, like most MRPs, plays a role in organic anion transport. The substrate specificity of MRP1 is for amphiphilic organic anions that are conjugated with glutathione, glucuronide, or sulfates moieties. Experimentally, MRP1 has transported methotrexate, leukotriene C_4 (LTC$_4$), 17β-estradiol glucuronide (E$_2$17βG), and bile salt derivatives. The LTC$_4$ analog MK571, probenecid, sulfinpyrazone, and cyclosporin A inhibit MRP1.

MRP2 (ABCC2)
MRP2 was initially cloned from the liver and was named the canalicular multispecific organic anion transporter (cMOAT) (References 3, 4). MRP2 has three TMDs and is highly expressed at the canalicular membrane in the liver. It also is expressed at lower levels in the gut and kidney, and is the only member of the MRP family localized to the apical membrane of epithelial cells. The function of MRP2 is to extrude anionic conjugates from inside the cell for elimination. The most notable substrate is the heme metabolite bilirubin glucuronide, which is transported from within the hepatocyte into the bile canaliculi where it is eliminated. Substrate and inhibitor specificity is similar to MRP1 and only differs in substrate kinetics. Additional substrates for MRP2 are the chemotherapeutic agents vinblastine, methotrexate, and the glucuronide conjugate of SN-38, the active metabolite of irinotecan.

MRP3 (ABCC3)

MRP3, like MRP2, is expressed in the liver, intestine, and kidneys (References 3, 4). It also is found in the adrenal glands and the pancreas. MRP3 is localized to the basolateral membrane of polarized cells and has three TMDs. Substrate specificity overlaps with MRP1 and MRP2, with a higher preference for glucuronide conjugates. Because MRP3 is found in similar tissues as MRP2, it is believed that MRP3 plays a compensatory role. In the event that MRP2 no longer functions to transport substrates through the apical membrane, MRP3 can alleviate cellular accumulation of compounds by transporting through the basolateral membrane into the blood for renal elimination.

MRP4 (ABCC4)

MRP4 has a two-TMD structure similar to Pgp but its nucleotide sequence is more homologous to *MRP1* than *MDR1*. Recent studies have shown that MRP4 is highly expressed in the prostate and can be detected in the lung, testis, bladder, pancreas, and ovaries (Reference 5). MRP4 differs from the previously discussed MRPs in that it transports cyclic adenosine monophosphate (AMP) and cyclic guanosine monophosphate (GMP). Other substrates include cholestatic bile acids and dehydroepiandrostene sulfate. Overexpression of this transporter in mammalian cells has shown resistance to the antiretroviral nucleoside analog 9-(2-phosphonylmethoxyethyl) adenine (PMEA), and the anticancer agents 6-mercaptopurine and methotrexate (Reference 5).

MRP5 (ABCC5)

MRP5 is ubiquitously expressed with high levels in the brain, skeletal muscle, lung, and heart. It has a similar two-TMD structure as MRP4 and Pgp. MRP5 also transports nucleotide analogs as well as glutathione conjugates but does not transport typical MRP1-3 substrates such as LTC_4 or $E_2 17\beta G$ (Reference 5).

MRP6 (ABCC6)

MRP6 is localized to the basolateral membrane in the liver and kidneys (Reference 3). The topology of MRP6 resembles that of MRP1-3 and includes five additional transmembrane-spanning regions at the N-terminus. The biochemical and physiological function of MRP6 remains unclear and limited data suggest that it can transport glutathione conjugates, the cyclic pentapeptide BQ123 and some anticancer drugs. Of interest, the MRP6 gene lies close to MRP1 and the 3' end of the protein matches closely with the anthracycline resistance associated (ARA) protein.

MRP7 (ABCC7)

MRP7 can transport $E_2 17\beta G$ but has very low affinity toward LTC_4. The membrane topology of MRP7 is similar to MRP1. The tissue distribution and intracellular localization of MRP7 is not yet characterized (Reference 6).

Mitoxantrone Resistance Protein/Breast Cancer Resistance Protein (ABCG2)

Unlike the other ABC transporters, the MXR has only one NBD and one TMD and is, therefore, considered a half transporter (Reference 7). The single NBD is located at the N-terminus of the protein. MXR is predicted to dimerize to form a two-NBD, two-TMD protein typical of MDR transporters. MXR is able to confer resistance to mitoxantrone, and can transport anthracyclines, topotecan, and SN-38. One potent antagonist to MXR is fumitremorgin C, derived from *Aspergillus fumigatus* cultures. MXR has the highest expression in the placenta and liver, followed by the colon, small intestine, lung, kidney, and adrenal and sweat glands. Very low or no expression is found in the brain, heart, and stomach. MXR also is referred to as breast cancer resistance protein (BCRP).

Physiological Function of Multidrug Resistance Efflux Transporters

Multidrug resistance transporters modulate the disposition, metabolism, and elimination of numerous drugs. They interact with a myriad of large endogenous and exogenous compounds and are thought to play a protective role in the removal of toxic substances from tissues (References 2, 3, 8). In the gut, Pgp and possibly MRP2 mediate the efflux of drugs back into the lumen, thereby limiting their bioavailability. In the liver, Pgp and MRP2 mediate the elimination of drugs into the bile and renally expressed Pgp mediates urinary excretion of drugs. In regions such as the blood-brain and blood-testis barriers, the placenta, and the ovaries, they play a protective role in limiting toxins from entering these crucial organs. Studies in mice with genetic disruption of *mdr1* clearly reveal the importance of Pgp in limiting intracellular accumulation of drugs in the brain and the fetus. P-glycoprotein, MRP1, MRP4, and MRP5 have been implicated in multidrug resistance to anticancer and antiretroviral compounds and defects in MRP2 result in Dubin-Johnson syndrome (References 3–5, 8).

Uptake Transporters
Organic Cation Transporters

The human organic cation transporters consist of two distinct families, OCT and OCTN (Reference 9). All organic cation transporters have 12 putative transmembrane domains, with the exception of hOCTN1, which is predicted to have 11 transmembrane domains. They also share a large hydrophilic loop between transmembrane domains one and two that contains at least three potential sites for N-glycosylation and have multiple predicted sites for phosphorylation. Members of the OCTN family also contain a nucleotide-binding site sequence motif. Organic cation transporters interact with endogenous and xenobiotic organic cation compounds, including cimetidine, amantadine, pindolol, quinidine, and paraquat. The recent cloning of these transporters has led to an increased understanding of their role in the renal and hepatic transport of organic cations. The tissue distribution, localization, and functional properties of these transporters are summarized in the following sections.

OCT1 (SLC22A1)

hOCT1 is most highly expressed in the liver with lower levels found in the kidney, intestine, brain, and heart (References 9, 10). The intracellular localization has not been reported for hOCT1 but the rat orthologue is localized to the basolateral membrane of hepatocytes and renal tubular epithelial cells. Transport of the prototypical substrates tetraethylammonium (TEA) and 1-methyl-4-phenylpyridinium (MMP^+) is sensitive to membrane potential, consistent with the basolateral localization of this transporter. Choline, dopamine, epinephrine, 5-hydroxytryptamine, and norepinephrine are all transported by OCT1. Numerous cationic drugs, including procainamide, verapamil, quinidine, clonidine, acebutolol, quinine, and cimetidine, can inhibit OCT1 and are potential substrates.

OCT2 (SLC22A2)

hOCT2 is localized mostly to the kidney with only low levels found in the intestine and brain (References 9, 10). Within the kidney, hOCT2 is found on the brush border membrane where it may act as an organic cation:proton exchanger. The substrate and inhibitor profile is almost identical for hOCT1 and hOCT2, and, in general, most compounds have a higher affinity for the latter transporter.

OCT3 (SLC22A3)

The distribution of hOCT3 is distinct from the other two members of this family with high expression in the placenta, aorta, liver, prostate, salivary glands, adrenal glands, skeletal muscle, and fetal lungs (References 9, 10). The broad distribution of hOCT3 is in contrast to the relatively selective expression of mouse and rat OCT3 in the placenta and brain. Intracellular localization of OCT3 has not been reported in any species. In an oocyte expression system transport of prototypical substrates by OCT3 is membrane potential-dependent and proton-independent, consistent with the properties of a basolateral organic cation transporter. In addition to the substrates described for hOCT1 and hOCT2, corticosterone, desipramine, and histamine interact with hOCT3.

OCTN1 (SLC22A4)

hOCTN1 is broadly expressed with high levels detected in human adult kidney, trachea, and bone marrow, and in fetal liver, lung, and kidney (References 9, 10). Of interest, hOCTN1 is detected in numerous cancer cell lines. No members of the OCTN1 family have been localized intracellularly but transport of typical organic cations is stimulated by acidic pH, suggesting that transport is driven by a proton gradient. Proton-driven transport of organic cations is associated with a renal brush border membrane transport system. The substrate and inhibitor profile for hOCTN1 is similar to that reported for members of the OCT family.

OCTN2 (SLC22A5)

The second member of the OCTN family, hOCTN2, is highly expressed in both adult and fetal tissues (References 9, 10). hOCTN2 is found at highest levels in the fetal kidney and in the adult kidney, skeletal muscle, heart, brain, and placenta. hOCTN2 is unique among the organic cation transporters in that it does not transport the prototypical substrate TEA but can transport carnitine in a sodium-dependent manner. Carnitine transport is electrogenic and hOCTN2 cannot act as an organic cation:proton antiporter. Verapamil, valproic acid, and nicotine are among the drugs that have been shown to interact with hOCTN2.

Physiological Function of Organic Cation Transporters

The expression of organic cation transporters in the kidney and liver are consistent with their role in cellular uptake and renal secretion of drugs (Reference 11). Organic cation transporters on the basolateral membrane of renal epithelial cells mediate the uptake of organic cations from the blood into the tubule cells, the first step in the renal secretion of drugs. None of the human organic cation transporters have been definitively localized to the basolateral membrane but all three are sensitive to membrane potential, consistent with known transport mechanisms for organic compounds on the basolateral membrane. An organic cation:proton antiporter, possibly hOCTN1, mediates transport of organic cations across the brush border membrane of the kidney into the tubule lumen. Organic cation transporters also mediate the uptake of organic cations into the hepatocyte where they are exposed to drug metabolizing enzymes. The abundant expression of hOCT2 in the brain and its ability to transport monoamine neurotransmitters suggests a role for this transporter in dopamine transport within the brain.

Organic Anion Transporters

Transport systems for negatively charged organic molecules have been most extensively characterized for the intestine, liver, and kidney. Two distinct families of organic anion transporters, OAT and OATP (organic anion-transporting polypeptide), have been characterized (Reference 10). Members of the human OAT gene family encode 12 transmembrane domain transporters with up to five potential glycosylation sites in a large extracellular loop between the first two membrane-spanning regions. The structure of the organic anion transporters is very similar to that of the organic cation transporters, and they are all members of an amphiphilic solute facilitator family of transporters. The

OATP genes encode transporters with 8-12 transmembrane domains and share minimal sequence homology to organic anion transporters, thus comprising a distinct gene family. The tissue distribution, localization, and interactions with organic anions are discussed in the following sections for the known members of the human OAT and OATP gene families.

OAT1 (SLC22A6)

Human OAT1 is highly expressed in the kidney with much lower levels in the brain (References 10, 12). A variant of hOAT1 (hOAT1-1) has an additional 13 amino acids near the carboxy-terminus and two splice variants, hOAT1-3 and hOAT1-4, also have been identified. In the kidney, hOAT1 is localized to the basolateral membrane. *p*-Aminohippuric acid (PAH) is the prototype substrate for the organic anion transporters and transport of PAH by hOAT1 is sodium-independent and stimulated by an outwardly directed dicarboxylate gradient. Drug substrates of hOAT1 include adefovir and cidofovir. Numerous other anionic drugs inhibit PAH transport by hOAT1, including bumetanide, ibuprofen, indomethacin, furosemide, salicylates, probenecid, and losartan. Additional studies are needed to determine if these organic anions are actually transported by hOAT1.

OAT3 (SLC22A8)

The distribution of human OAT3 is similar to that of hOAT1, with high expression in kidney and much lower levels in the brain (References 10, 12). The subcellular localization and functional characteristics of hOAT3 have not been determined. The rat orthologue, rOAT3, mediates the uptake of PAH, estrone sulfate, cimetidine, and ochratoxin A. Inhibitors of rOAT3-mediated transport include bumetanide, zidovudine, penicillin G, probenecid, cefoperazone, furosemide, and methotrexate.

OAT4 (SLC22A11)

hOAT4 is highly expressed in the kidney and placenta but its subcellular localization is unknown (References 10, 12). *p*-Aminohippuric acid is not transported by hOAT4 but estrone sulfate, ochratoxin A, and dehydroepiandrosterone sulfate are substrates of hOAT4. Inhibition of hOAT4 transport is observed with many of the organic anions that interact with the other members of this gene family.

OATP1 (OATP-A, SLC21A3)

The OATP1 transporter was first cloned from the liver and is expressed in brain capillary endothelial cells and liver epithelial cells (References 10, 13). OATP1 messenger ribonucleic acid (mRNA) also has been detected in the kidney, lung, and testis. OATP1 mediates the uptake of bile salts such as cholate, taurocholate, and glycocholate, the peptide BQ123, and the anionic compound bromosulfophthalein. OATP1 also can transport prostaglandin E_2, fexofenadine, oubain, and some bulky organic cation compounds.

OATP-B (SLC21A9)

OATP-B was first cloned from the human brain, and mRNA levels have been detected in lung, kidney, ovary, heart, and brain (Reference 13). OATP-B is localized to the basolateral membrane in the liver and is believed to function as an uptake transporter to remove solutes from the blood. However, known substrates for the transporter are limited and include dehydroepiandrosterone sulfate, bromosulfophthalein, and benzylpenicillin. OATP-B also has been detected in the placenta where it is localized to the basal membrane facing the fetus.

OATP2 (OATP-C, LST1, SLC21A6)

hOATP2 is exclusively expressed in the basolateral membrane of the liver where it mediates the uptake of bile acids, eicosanoids, peptides, and anionic drugs from the sinusoidal membrane into the hepatocyte (References 10, 13). Pravastatin, an 3-hydroxy-3-methylglutaryl coenzyme A reductase inhibitor used to treat heart disease, is a substrate of OATP2 and other statins also may be transported by OATP2. In addition, bilirubin and its glucuronides are substrates for OATP2.

OATP-D (SLC21A11), OATP-E (SLC21A12) and OATP-F (SLC21A14)

Relatively little information is available about these members of the OATP family (Reference 13). OATP-D and OATP-E mRNA are ubiquitously expressed, although no protein has been detected. OATP-F protein has been found in the brain and testis. OATP-D transports benzylpenicillin, estrone-3-sulfate, and prostaglandin E_2. OATP-E can transport taurocholate, estrone-3-sulfate, $E_2$17ßG, and prostaglandin E_2.

OATP8 (SLC21A8)

OATP8 is similar to OATP2 in its amino acid identity and liver-specific localization (Reference 13). It transports similar substrates as OATP2 albeit with differing affinities. One exception is unconjugated bilirubin, which is not a substrate. OATP8 is the only member of the OATPs that transports digoxin.

Physiological Function of Organic Anion Transporters

Organic anion transporters mediate the cellular uptake of many bile acids, eicosanoids, and anionic drugs (References 9, 10, 12, 13). OAT1, and possibly OAT3 and OAT4, mediate transport across the basolateral membrane of renal tubular epithelial cells, thus facilitating the first step in organic anion secretion. Organic anion transporters in other tissues may aid in the uptake of essential compounds (References 10, 12). The uptake of bile acids into the liver by hOATP1, hOATP2 and hOATP8 helps maintain bile flow, whereas the transport of other drugs can be the initial step in hepatic metabolism. OATP transporters expressed on the sinusoidal membrane of hepatocytes mediate the first step in hepatic metabolism and may influence first pass bioavailability of these drugs (References 10, 13). OATP-B may be involved in the removal of natural substrates from the fetus into the mother's circulation.

Nucleoside Transporters

The cellular uptake of physiological purine and pyrimidine nucleosides and nucleoside drugs is mediated by nucleoside transporters of two major classes, the equilibrative and concentrative transporters (References 14, 15). The equilibrative transporters are facilitative transporters driven solely by the concentration gradient and concentrative transporters are driven by transmembrane sodium gradients. Equilibrative nucleoside transporters are expressed in most cells and have broad substrate selectivities. In contrast, concentrative nucleoside transporters have relatively narrow substrate selectivities and their expression is localized to specific cell types. The tissue distribution, subcellular localization, and substrate selectivity of the major equilibrative and concentrative nucleoside transporters are discussed in the following sections.

ENT1 (SLC29A1)

Human ENT1 was first cloned from placenta and encodes an 11 transmembrane domain protein with three potential N-linked glycosylation sites (Reference 14). hENT1 is widely expressed and most abundant in brain, colon, lung, placenta, liver, heart, spleen, testis, and many neoplastic tissues. Functional analysis suggests broad substrate selectivity for purine and pyrimidine nucleosides, including the nucleoside analogues cladribine, cytarabine, fludarabine, and gemcitabine.

ENT2 (SLC29A2)

hENT2 has a similar structure as hENT1 and also is widely distributed (Reference 14). It is particularly abundant in skeletal muscle and also highly expressed in brain, heart, prostate, kidney, pancreas, and placenta. The substrate selectivity for endogenous nucleoside analogues is similar to hENT1, although the affinity typically is less for hENT2. Xenobiotic substrates for hENT2 include zidovudine and didanosine and hENT2 also can transport the nucleobase hypoxanthine.

ENT3

hENT3 has a long hydrophilic N-terminal region preceding the first transmembrane domain which contains sequence motifs involved in the sorting of membrane proteins (Reference 14). Similarity of this sequence to a yeast ENT transporter suggests that hENT3 may be localized in some intracellular compartment. Expression of hENT3 is detected in kidney, placenta, breast, colon, testis, and numerous neoplastic tissues. Substrate selectivity is not yet characterized for hENT3.

CNT1 (SLC28A1)

hCNT1 was cloned from human kidney but its tissue distribution is still unclear (References 14, 16). Substrates for hCNT1 include zidovudine and gemcitabine, but not adenosine.

CNT2 (SLC28A2)

hCNT2 is expressed in the kidney, intestine, heart, liver, skeletal muscle, placenta, and brain (References 14, 16). Inosine, adenosine, guanosine, deoxyadenosine, didanosine, and 2-chloro-2'-deoxyadenosine are transported by hCNT2. Inhibitors of this transporter include 2',3'-dideoxyadenosine and 2',3'-dideoxyinosine.

CNT3 (SLC28A3)

The remaining member of the CNT family, hCNT3, is expressed in mammary gland, pancreas, bone marrow, liver, intestine, heart, and brain (Reference 17). hCNT3 transports physiological pyrimidine and purine nucleosides as well as antineoplastic and antiviral nucleoside drugs.

Physiological Function of Nucleoside Transporters

Nucleoside transporters mediate the cellular uptake of nucleoside analogs and, therefore, the pharmacological and/or toxicological response to these agents (References 14-16). The expression of hENT1 in numerous tumors suggests an important role for this transporter in the cellular uptake of nucleoside analogs used in cancer chemotherapy and hENT2 is predicted to be an important determinant of the cellular response to nucleoside analogs with antiretroviral properties (Reference 16). Hypoxanthine transport by hENT2 is important in the cellular uptake of this nucleobase into vascular endothelial cells and bone marrow where it serves as an important source of purines for salvage (Reference 16). The concentrative nucleoside transporters are thought to control the concentration of adenosine near purinergic receptors and may mediate the absorption of orally administered nucleosides or nucleoside analogs (Reference 15). Nucleoside transporters in tumor cells are likely to mediate the cellular uptake of cytotoxic nucleosides and nucleoside analogs and altered expression or function of these transporters could lead to resistance of the tumor cells to these drugs (References 15, 16). A similar role for these transporters is proposed for the cellular uptake of nucleosides and nucleoside analogs used to treat human immunodeficiency virus (HIV).

Genetic Variability in Drug Transporters

Genetic variation in membrane transporters is relatively uncharacterized compared to the extensive data available on drug metabolizing enzymes. A large scale effort to identify and characterize genetic variants of 24 membrane transporters provides interesting data about the degree and type of genetic variation in a group of proteins with similar structure (multiple transmembrane domains joined by alternating intracellular and extracellular loops) (Reference 18). Included in this analysis were four members of the ABC superfamily of transporters (including *MDR1*, *MRP1*, and *MRP2*) and 20 members of the solute carrier family of transporters (including *OCT1*, *OCT2*, *OCT3*, *ENT1*, *ENT2*, *CNT1*, and *CNT2*). A total of 680 variants was identified by screening exons and flanking intronic regions of these genes, and 155 of these variants caused an amino acid change. Amino acid diversity was significantly lower in transmembrane domains than in loop regions, consistent with an important functional role for the transmembrane domain. A comparison of two population genetic parameters, average heterozygosity, and the population mutation parameter, indicates that the genetic diversity in this group of membrane transporters is similar to that reported for other genes. Common genetic variants for important drug transporters are discussed below.

Efflux Transporters
MDR1

Genetic polymorphisms in *MDR1* have been well characterized. The most extensive characterization of *MDR1* genetic variation is in a group of almost 250 ethnically diverse individuals (Reference 19). Over a total of 9.8 kilobases of sequence, 48 variants were identified. Nineteen of the variants were in the coding region of *MDR1* and 13 were nonsynonymous changes leading to an amino acid change in Pgp. The most common nonsynonymous variants of *MDR1* and their allele frequencies are shown in Table 1. Haplotypes, the combination of genetic variants on a given chromosome, were statistically inferred for this same data set and two common haplotypes were identified out of a total of 64 haplotypes. The reference haplotype, *MDR1**1, is the most frequent in African Americans, whereas the most prevalent haplotype in Caucasians and Asian Americans, *MDR1**13, contains three intronic, two synonymous, and one nonsynonymous change relative to the reference haplotype and encodes for the Ala893Ser change in Pgp. A majority (60 percent) of the haplotypes encode for the reference Pgp, whereas 30 percent encode for the Ala893Ser variant. The remaining haplotypes encode additional amino acid changes and are all relatively rare. The six variants in *MDR1**13 are in tight linkage disequilibrium. Both unaltered and increased function have been associated with the Ala893Ser Pgp variant (References 19–21). No functional differences have been observed for the Asp21Asn, Ser400Asn, and Ala893Thr Pgp variants (Reference 21).

Multidrug Resistance-associated Protein
MRP1

MRP1 has the lowest degree of genetic variation of any of the ABC transporters characterized to date (Reference 18). An Arg433Ser variant in a predicted cytoplasmic loop of MRP1 has reduced function toward LTC_4 and oestrone sulphate (Reference 22). Cells expressing this variant MRP1 also show increased resistance to doxorubicin. An Arg1058Gln variant has been identified at a frequency of 7.3 percent in a Japanese population (Table 1) (Reference 23). Three additional nonsynonymous changes also were reported in the Japanese population at a 1 percent frequency. The functional significance of these variants is unknown.

Table 1. Common Nonsynonymous Variants of Membrane Transporters

Gene	AA Change	Function	Caucasian	African American	Asian	Reference
MDR1	Asn21Asp	↔	8%	0.5%	0%[a]	[19, 21]
	Ser400Asn	↔	2.5%	1.0%	0%[a]	[19, 21]
	Ala893Ser	↔,↑	46%	10%	45%[a]	[19-21]
	Ala893Thr	↔	3.6%	0.5%	6.7%[a]	[19, 21]
	Ser1141Thr	?	0%	11.1%	0%[a]	[19]
MRP1	Arg723Gln	?	ND	ND	7.3%[b]	[23]
MRP2	Val417Ile	?	ND	ND	12%[b]	[27]
OCT1	Arg61Cys	↓	9.1%	ND	ND	[30]
	Phe160Leu	↔	22%	ND	ND	[30]
	Gly401Ser	↓	3.2%	ND	ND	[30]
	Met408Val	?	60%	ND	ND	[30]
	Met420del	↔	16%	ND	ND	[30]
OCT2	Ala270Ser	↔	16%	11%	8.6%[a]	[31]
OATP-B	Ser486Phe	↓	ND	ND	31%[b]	[35]
OATP-C	Asn130Asp	↔	30%	74%	ND	[36]
	Pro155Thr	↔	16%	2.0%	ND	[36]
	Val174Ala	↓	14%	2.0%	ND	[36]
	Gly488Ala	↓	0%	9.0%	ND	[36]
	Glu667Gly	↔	2.0%	34%	ND	[36]

[a]Asian population had equal numbers of Chinese, Japanese, and Southeast Asians.
[b]Asian population was entirely of Japanese descent.
AA = amino acid

MRP2

The first characterized genetic variations in *MRP2* were identified in patients with Dubin-Johnson syndrome, a hereditary defect in bilirubin-glucuronide elimination leading to hyperbilirubinemia. A C2302T variant (Reference 24) is found in the signature C motif of the first nucleotide-binding domain and a 4175del6 variant (Reference 25) deletes two amino acids from the second nucleotide-binding domain. Both are believed to affect ATP-binding; however, functional characterization of the deletion variant shows impaired sorting of this mutant *MRP2* to the apical membrane (Reference 26). A C3196T variant (Reference 24) introduces a premature stop codon, leading to the loss of the second ABC. Additional mutations occur in the intronic regions of the mRNA and result in alternate splicing. Coding region variants in *MRP2* also have been identified in a healthy Japanese population and the location and frequency of the most common variants are shown in Table 1 (Reference 27). The functional significance of these variants is still unknown.

MRP6

Association of a region on chromosome 16p13.1 to the disease pseudoxanthoma elasticum (PXE) led to the identification of four variants of *MRP6* (Reference 28). C3421T and C3490T transitions both led to premature stop codons, a C4015T variant results in an Arg1339Cys change and a His632Gln change results from a C1896A transversion. The truncated proteins are predicted to result in an inactive protein but the significance of the other two variants is unknown. These variants have only been observed in patients with PXE and their allele frequency is expected to be low.

Mitoxantrone-resistance Protein

A genetic variant of *MXR* was identified in cell lines overexpressing this transporter and resulted in an Arg482Thr/Gly change in the transporter (Reference 29). Reference MXR was unable to transport rhodamine 123 or doxorubicin, whereas both the Arg482Thr and the Arg482Gly variant had significant activity with these prototypical substrates. Reference MXR and both variants can transport mitoxantrone. Additional variants have not yet been identified.

Uptake Transporters

Organic Cation Transporters

hOCT1

Twenty-five variants were identified in the promoter, exonic, and intronic regions of *hOCT1* in a panel of deoxyribonucleic acid (DNA) samples from 57 healthy Caucasians (Reference 30). The major nonsynonymous variants and their allele frequencies are noted in Table 1. The Arg61Cys variant showed reduced uptake of the prototypical substrate MPP^+, whereas the Cys88Arg and Gly401Ser variants were unable to transport this substrate.

Of interest, both Cys88Arg and Gly401Ser could transport TEA and serotonin, albeit at reduced levels.

hOCT2

Genetic variants of *hOCT2* have been identified in a collection of 247 individual DNA samples (Reference 31). Out of a total of 28 variant sites, eight nonsynonymous variants were identified that would alter the amino acid sequence of the transporter. The most common nonsynonymous variants are shown in Table 1. The K432Q *OCT1* variant has an increased affinity for MPP^+, and the A270S, R400C, and K432Q variants all have a lower K_i for tetrabutylammonium.

Organic Anion Transporters

OATP-A

A recent analysis in a Japanese population identified several variants in the 5'-flanking region of *OATP-A* but found no variants in the coding region (Reference 32). One regulatory region variant is in a putative hepatocyte nuclear factor 1α response element but its functional significance is unknown (Reference 33).

OATP-B

Two nonsynonymous variants have been reported in *OATP-B* and result in Thr392Ile and Ser486Phe changes in the protein sequence (Reference 34). The Thr392Ile variant was not found in a population of 267 Japanese individuals, whereas the C1457T variant leading to the Ser486Phe change was detected at a frequency of 31 percent (Reference 35). Functional characterization of this latter variant showed more than a 50 percent decrease in intrinsic transport activity relative to the reference protein.

OATP-C

Fourteen nonsynonymous variants have been reported for *OATP-C* and allele frequencies are highly dependent on ethnicity (Reference 36). The most common variants are included in Table 1. Haplotype analysis indicated that these variants were found in 16 haplotypes, five of which contained at least two nonsynonymous changes. Functional analysis of these variants using estrone sulfate and $E_2 17\beta G$ showed a significant loss of function with the following haplotypes: Phe73Leu, Val82Ala + Glu156Gly, Ile353Thr, Gly488Ala, Asp655Gly, Phe73Leu + Asp655Gly, and Val82Ala + Glu156Gly. In some cases, the altered transport was due to decreased plasma membrane expression of the transporters.

OATP8

Several polymorphisms in both the 5'-flanking and exonic regions of *OATP8* have been reported (References 13, 32). No significant differences in transport function have been reported for any of the exonic variants.

Clinical Consequences of Genetic Variability in Drug Transporters

Efflux Transporters

MDR1

The important role for Pgp in limiting drug absorption across the gastrointestinal tract, in preventing drug accumulation in the central nervous system, and in limiting intracellular levels of cancer chemotherapeutic agents has led to numerous studies to examine the effect of MDR1 genetic polymorphisms on Pgp function. The majority of the clinical studies have considered a single synonymous change in MDR1 at position 3435 (C3435T). The effect of the C3435T variant on digoxin bioavailability has been well studied but the outcomes are controversial. Comparison of digoxin area under the curve (AUC)0-4hour and/or maximum plasma concentration (C_{max}) values in individuals with the MDR1 3435TT and the 3435CC genotypes are consistent with increased, decreased, and unaltered Pgp function in those individuals homozygous for the variant allele (References 37-40). Additional consideration of the G2677T variant, which codes for an Ala893Ser change in Pgp led to similar discrepancies in studies with digoxin or fexofenadine (References 20, 41–44). The MDR1 3435TT genotype was associated with decreased trough levels of the protease inhibitor nelfinavir, consistent with increased intestinal Pgp function in individuals homozygous for this variant allele (Reference 45). MDR1 mRNA and Pgp levels measured in peripheral lymphocytes also were reduced in patients with HIV with the MDR1 3435TT genotype. Surprisingly, lower nelfinavir (and efavirenz, which is not a Pgp substrate) plasma concentrations in the 3435TT individuals were associated with increased antiviral response. The mechanism for this exaggerated response in the 3435TT individuals is not known.

The effect of *MDR1* genetic variation on expression also is controversial. P-glycoprotein function measured in peripheral blood mononuclear cells (PBMCs) is often used as a marker to reflect the systemic expression of this transporter. The 3435CC genotype is associated with increased Pgp function and MDR1 mRNA levels in PBMCs relative to the 3435TT individuals (References 44–46). However, in pure CD34$^+$ cells, transport of rhodamine is not affected by the *MDR1* genotype (Reference 47). In enterocytes, there is evidence for decreased MDR1 mRNA in 3435CC individuals relative to the 3435TT group, suggesting that the expression of lymphocyte and intestinal MDR1 mRNA are controlled by distinct mechanisms (Reference 48). Placental expression of Pgp also has been associated with *MDR1* genotype. In a study of 100 placentas from Japanese women, a maternal T-129C variant genotype was associated with increased Pgp levels (Reference 49). In the kidney, individuals homozygous for the

3435 reference allele had increased Pgp levels relative to the homozygous variant individuals (Reference 50). The lack of correlation between MDR1/Pgp expression and *MDR1* genotype across different tissues might reflect tissue-specific expression, but it also should be noted that most of these studies were done with only a small number of samples and definitive results will require that more samples are analyzed.

The influence of the *MDR1* genotypes for the three common coding region variants found in the *MDR1**13 haplotype, C1236T/G2677T/C3435T, on response to chemotherapeutic treatment of acute lymphoblastic leukemia recently was reported. Patients who were homozygous reference at all three of these sites had increased probability of relapse and decreased overall survival relative to patients who were homozygous for the variant allele at these sites (Reference 51). However, there was no gene dose response for this observation and the patients with the variant genotypes were more likely to have cytogenetic poor risk aberrations and decreased levels of MDR1 mRNA in peripheral blood mononuclear cells. Studies in a larger patient population will be necessary to fully understand the importance of these genotypes on response to acute lymphoblastic leukemia treatment. *MDR1* genetic variation also has been suggested to play a role in the development of renal cell carcinoma. The *MDR1* 3435TT genotype was overexpressed in both clear-cell and nonclear-cell renal cell carcinomas (odds ratio 3435TT vs. 3435CC genotype 1.7-2.5), suggesting that *MDR1* genotype influences an individual's predisposition to developing cancer (Reference 50). The possibility that a similar situation exists for other tumor types will need to be considered.

The prevention of neurotoxicity from exposure to numerous drugs is mediated at least in part by Pgp function on the blood-brain barrier. The tricyclic antidepressant nortriptyline is a modest Pgp substrate and is associated with postural hypotension. Patients homozygous for the *MDR1* 3435TT genotype have an increased risk of developing postural hypotension relative to 3435CC patients (odds ratio = 1.37), consistent with decreased Pgp function in these patients (Reference 52). Neurotoxicity also is a rate-limiting side effect of tacrolimus treatment. The *MDR1* G2677T/A variant genotype was a positive predictor of neurotoxicity, whereas the C3435T variant genotype was a negative predictor of neurotoxicity (Reference 53). Although these results suggest a potential role for *MDR1* genetic variation in determining an individual's susceptibility to neurotoxicity after tacrolimus treatment, the opposing effects of these two genotypes are not consistent with the tight linkage disequilibrium between the 2677 and 3435 variant sites. Of interest, in a relatively small sample set of 95 patients and 106 controls, the frequency of the *MDR1* 3435TT genotype was higher in patients with early-onset (36 percent) and late-onset (23 percent) Parkinson's disease relative to controls (19 percent) (Reference 54). These findings raise the interesting possibility that the *MDR1* C3435T variant, and/or other variants that are in tight linkage disequilibrium, might alter an individual's exposure to potential neurotoxins and, therefore, influence the development of neurodegenerative diseases such as Parkinson's disease.

MRP2

Dubin-Johnson syndrome is an autosomal recessive disorder characterized by a defect in elimination of anionic conjugates from the liver to the bile. This results in the accumulation of bilirubin glucuronide in the liver and a jaundice phenotype. The mechanistic basis for the development of Dubin-Johnson syndrome is the presence of *MRP2* variations that result in loss of transporter function (References 24-26). MRP2 is the primary transporter for conjugated bilirubin in the liver and absence of this transporter leads to accumulation of the MRP2 substrate bilirubin glucuronide. More common *MRP2* variants might result in altered elimination of numerous drugs and drug conjugates, including pravastatin and methotrexate.

MRP6

Pseudoxanthoma elasticum is an inborn disorder that causes a progressive calcification of elastic tissue in the skin, retina, and arterial walls. Variation in *MRP6* has been linked to PXE but there is no clear explanation for the role of this transporter in the disease (Reference 28). Individuals harboring the *MRP6* variants associated with PXE also have a significant increase in the prevalence of premature coronary artery disease (Reference 55).

Uptake Transporters
OCTN2

Primary carnitine deficiency is an autosomal recessive disease characterized by progressive cardiomyopathy, skeletal myopathy, hyperammonemia, and hypoglycemia. Studies in fibroblasts from patients with primary carnitine deficiency determined that the primary cause was a defect in transport in the plasmalemmal membrane. The transporter identified was OCTN2, and several mutations in *OCTN2* were found in patients with primary carnitine deficiency (Reference 56). The impact of these variants on the disposition of other compounds that interact with OCTN2, including valproic acid, verapamil, and nicotine, is not known.

Perspectives

There has been a recent explosion in the understanding of the role of drug transporters in mediating pharmacokinetic and pharmacodynamic relationships. Novel transporters are still being identified and much work remains on characterizing the expression, regulation, and functional properties of many of the transporters previously discussed. Interest in understanding the functional and clinical significance of genetic polymorphisms in drug transporters is high but the area is clearly in its infancy. The development of specific substrates and inhibitors for the individual transporters will greatly enhance the ability to evaluate the clinical significance of transporter polymorphisms. Detailed characterization of haplotype structure and the consideration of gene-gene and gene-environment interactions also will be important. Although much work remains, it is likely that for many drugs transporter polymorphism data will be considered in the individualization of drug therapy.

References

1. Dean M, Rzhetsky A, Allikmets R. The human ATP-binding cassette (ABC) transporter superfamily. Genome Res 2001;11:1156–66.

2. Ambudkar SV, Dey S, Hrycyna CA, Ramachandra M, Pastan I, Gottesman MM. Biochemical, cellular, and pharmacological aspects of the multidrug transporter. Annu Rev Pharmacol Toxicol 1999;39:361–98.

3. Borst P, Evers R, Kool M, Wijnholds J. A family of drug transporters: the multidrug resistance-associated proteins. J Natl Cancer Inst 2000;92:1295–302.

4. Konig J, Nies AT, Cui Y, Leier I, Keppler D. Conjugate export pumps of the multidrug resistance protein (MRP) family: localization, substrate specificity, and MRP2-mediated drug resistance. Biochim Biophys Acta 1999;1461:377–94.

5. Adachi M, Reid G, Schuetz JD. Therapeutic and biological importance of getting nucleotides out of cells: a case for the ABC transporters, MRP4 and 5. Adv Drug Deliv Rev 2002;54:1333–42.

6. Chen ZS, Hopper-Borge E, Belinsky MG, Shchaveleva I, Kotova E, Kruh GD. Characterization of the transport properties of human multidrug resistance protein 7 (MRP7, ABCC10). Mol Pharmacol 2003;63:351–8.

7. Bates SE, Robey R, Miyake K, Rao K, Ross DD, Litman T. The role of half-transporters in multidrug resistance. J Bioenerg Biomembr 2001;33:503–11.

8. Matheny CJ, Lamb MW, Brouwer KR, Pollack GM. Pharmacokinetic and pharmacodynamic implications of P-glycoprotein modulation. Pharmacotherapy 2001;21:778–96.

9. Burckhardt G, Wolff NA. Structure of renal organic anion and cation transporters. Am J Physiol Renal Physiol 2000;278:F853–66.

10. Dresser MJ, Leabman MK, Giacomini KM. Transporters involved in the elimination of drugs in the kidney: organic anion transporters and organic cation transporters. J Pharm Sci 2001;90:397–421.

11. Zhang L, Brett CM, Giacomini KM. Role of organic cation transporters in drug absorption and elimination. Annu Rev Pharmacol Toxicol 1998;38:431–60.

12. Sekine T, Cha SH, Endou H. The multispecific organic anion transporter (OAT) family. Pflugers Arch 2000;440:337–50.

13. Tirona RG, Kim RB. Pharmacogenomics of organic anion-transporting polypeptides (OATP). Adv Drug Deliv Rev 2002;54:1343–52.

14. Hyde RJ, Cass CE, Young JD, Baldwin SA. The ENT family of eukaryote nucleoside and nucleobase transporters: recent advances in the investigation of structure/function relationships and the identification of novel isoforms. Mol Membr Biol 2001;18:53–63.

15. Wang J, Schaner ME, Thomassen S, Su SF, Piquette-Miller M, Giacomini KM. Functional and molecular characteristics of Na^+-dependent nucleoside transporters. Pharm Res 1997;14:1524–32.

16. Cass C, Young J, Baldwin S, et al. Nucleoside transporters of mammalian cells. In: Amidon G, Sadee W, eds. Membrane Transporters as Drug Targets. New York, NY: Kluwer Academic/Plenum Publishers; 1999:313–52.

17. Ritzel MW, Ng AM, Yao SY, et al. Molecular identification and characterization of novel human and mouse concentrative Na^+-nucleoside cotransporter proteins (hCNT3 and mCNT3) broadly selective for purine and pyrimidine nucleosides. J Biol Chem 2001;276:2914–27.

18. Leabman MK, Huang CC, DeYoung J, et al. Natural variation in human membrane transporter genes reveals evolutionary and functional constraints. Proc Natl Acad Sci U S A 2003;100:5896–901.

19. Kroetz DL, Pauli-Magnus C, Hodges LM, et al. Sequence diversity and haplotype structure in the human *ABCB1* (*MDR1*, multidrug resistance transporter) gene. Pharmacogenetics 2003;13:481–94.

20. Kim RB, Leake BF, Choo EF, et al. Identification of functionally variant *MDR1* alleles among European Americans and African Americans. Clin Pharmacol Ther 2001;70:189–99.

21. Kimchi-Sarfaty C, Gribar JJ, Gottesman MM. Functional characterization of coding polymorphisms in the human *MDR1* gene using a vaccinia virus expression system. Mol Pharmacol 2002;62:1–6.

22. Conrad S, Kauffmann HM, Ito K, et al. A naturally occurring mutation in *MRP1* results in a selective decrease in organic anion transport and in increased doxorubicin resistance. Pharmacogenetics 2002;12:321–30.

23. Ito S, Ieiri I, Tanabe M, Suzuki A, Higuchi S, Otsubo K. Polymorphism of the ABC transporter genes, *MDR1*, *MRP1* and *MRP2/cMOAT*, in healthy Japanese subjects. Pharmacogenetics 2001;11:175–84.

24. Toh S, Wada M, Uchiumi T, et al. Genomic structure of the canalicular multispecific organic anion-transporter gene (*MRP2/cMOAT*) and mutations in the ATP-binding-cassette region in Dubin-Johnson syndrome. Am J Hum Genet 1999;64:739–46.

25. Tsujii H, Konig J, Rost D, Stockel B, Leuschner U, Keppler D. Exon-intron organization of the human multidrug-resistance protein 2 (*MRP2*) gene mutated in Dubin-Johnson syndrome. Gastroenterology 1999;117:653–60.

26. Keitel V, Kartenbeck J, Nies AT, Spring H, Brom M, Keppler D. Impaired protein maturation of the conjugate export pump multidrug resistance protein 2 as a consequence of a deletion mutation in Dubin-Johnson syndrome. Hepatology 2000;32:1317–28.

27. Itoda M, Saito Y, Soyama A, et al. Polymorphisms in the *ABCC2* (*cMOAT/MRP2*) gene found in 72 established cell lines derived from Japanese individuals: an association between single nucleotide polymorphisms in the 5'-untranslated region and exon 28. Drug Metab Dispos 2002;30:363–4.

28. Struk B, Cai L, Zach S, et al. Mutations of the gene encoding the transmembrane transporter protein *ABC-C6* cause pseudoxanthoma elasticum. J Mol Med 2000;78:282–6.

29. Honjo Y, Hrycyna CA, Yan QW, et al. Acquired mutations in the *MXR/BCRP/ABCP* gene alter substrate specificity in MXR/BCRP/ABCP-overexpressing cells. Cancer Res 2001;61:6635–9.

30. Kerb R, Brinkmann U, Chatskaia N, et al. Identification of genetic variations of the human organic cation transporter *hOCT1* and their functional consequences. Pharmacogenetics 2002;12:591–5.

31. Leabman MK, Huang CC, Kawamoto M, et al. Polymorphisms in a human kidney xenobiotic transporter, *OCT2*, exhibit altered function. Pharmacogenetics 2002;12:395–405.

32. Iida A, Saito S, Sekine A, et al. Catalog of 258 single-nucleotide polymorphisms (SNPs) in genes encoding three organic anion transporters, three organic anion-transporting polypeptides, and three NADH:ubiquinone oxidoreductase flavoproteins. J Hum Genet 2001;46:668–83.

33. Kullak-Ublick GA, Beuers U, Fahney C, Hagenbuch B, Meier PJ, Paumgartner G. Identification and functional characterization of the promoter region of the human organic anion transporting polypeptide gene. Hepatology 1997;26:991–7.

34. Tamai I, Nezu J, Uchino H, et al. Molecular identification and characterization of novel members of the human organic anion transporter (OATP) family. Biochem Biophys Res Commun 2000;273:251–60.

35. Nozawa T, Nakajima M, Tamai I, et al. Genetic polymorphisms of human organic anion transporters *OATP-C* (*SLC21A6*) and *OATP-B* (*SLC21A9*): allele frequencies in the Japanese population and functional analysis. J Pharmacol Exp Ther 2002;302:804–13.

36. Tirona RG, Leake BF, Merino G, Kim RB. Polymorphisms in *OATP-C*: identification of multiple allelic variants associated with altered transport activity among European- and African-Americans. J Biol Chem 2001;276:35669–75.

37. Hoffmeyer S, Burk O, von Richter O, et al. Functional polymorphisms of the human multidrug-resistance gene: multiple sequence variations and correlation of one allele with P-glycoprotein expression and activity in vivo. Proc Natl Acad Sci U S A 2000;97:3473–8.

38. Becquemont L, Verstuyft C, Kerb R, et al. Effect of grapefruit juice on digoxin pharmacokinetics in humans. Clin Pharmacol Ther 2001;70:311–6.

39. Sakacda T, Nakamura T, Horinouchi M, et al. *MDR1* genotype-related pharmacokinetics of digoxin after single oral administration in healthy Japanese subjects. Pharm Res 2001;18:1400–4.

40. Gerloff T, Schaefer M, Johne A, et al. *MDR1* genotypes do not influence the absorption of a single oral dose of 1 mg digoxin in healthy white males. Br J Clin Pharmacol 2002;54:610–6.

41. Horinouchi M, Sakaeda T, Nakamura T, et al. Significant genetic linkage of *MDR1* polymorphisms at positions 3435 and 2677: functional relevance to pharmacokinetics of digoxin. Pharm Res 2002;19:1581–5.

42. Kurata Y, Ieiri I, Kimura M, et al. Role of human *MDR1* gene polymorphism in bioavailability and interaction of digoxin, a substrate of P-glycoprotein. Clin Pharmacol Ther 2002;72:209–19.

43. Johne A, Kopke K, Gerloff T, et al. Modulation of steady-state kinetics of digoxin by haplotypes of the P-glycoprotein *MDR1* gene. Clin Pharmacol Ther 2002;72:584–94.

44. Drescher S, Schaeffeler E, Hitzl M, et al. *MDR1* gene polymorphisms and disposition of the P-glycoprotein substrate fexofenadine. Br J Clin Pharmacol 2002;53:526–34.

45. Fellay J, Marzolini C, Meaden ER, et al. Response to antiretroviral treatment in HIV-1-infected individuals with allelic variants of the multidrug resistance transporter 1: a pharmacogenetics study. Lancet 2002;359:30–6.

46. Hitzl M, Drescher S, van der Kuip H, et al. The C3435T mutation in the human *MDR1* gene is associated with altered efflux of the P-glycoprotein substrate rhodamine 123 from CD56$^+$ natural killer cells. Pharmacogenetics 2001;11:293–8.

47. Calado RT, Falcao RP, Garcia AB, Gabellini SM, Zago MA, Franco RF. Influence of functional *MDR1* gene polymorphisms on P-glycoprotein activity in CD34$^+$ hematopoietic stem cells. Haematologica 2002;87:564–8.

48. Moriya Y, Nakamura T, Horinouchi M, et al. Effects of polymorphisms of *MDR1*, *MRP1*, and *MRP2* genes on their mRNA expression levels in duodenal enterocytes of healthy Japanese subjects. Biol Pharm Bull 2002;25:1356–9.

49. Tanabe M, Ieiri I, Nagata N, et al. Expression of P-glycoprotein in human placenta: relation to genetic polymorphism of the multidrug resistance *(MDR)-1* gene. J Pharmacol Exper Ther 2001;297:1137–43.

50. Siegsmund M, Brinkmann U, Schaffeler E, et al. Association of the P-glycoprotein transporter *MDR1*(C3435T) polymorphism with the susceptibility to renal epithelial tumors. J Am Soc Nephrol 2002;13:1847–54.

51. Illmer T, Schuler US, Thiede C, et al. *MDR1* gene polymorphisms affect therapy outcome in acute myeloid leukemia patients. Cancer Res 2002;62:4955–62.

52. Roberts RL, Joyce PR, Mulder RT, Begg EJ, Kennedy MA. A common P-glycoprotein polymorphism is associated with nortriptyline-induced postural hypotension in patients treated for major depression. Pharmacogenomics J 2002;2:191–6.

53. Yamauchi A, Ieiri I, Kataoka Y, R, et al. Neurotoxicity induced by tacrolimus after liver transplantation: relation to genetic polymorphisms of the *ABCB1* (*MDR1*) gene. Transplantation 2002;74:571–2.

54. Furuno T, Landi MT, Ceroni M, et al. Expression polymorphism of the blood-brain barrier component P-glycoprotein (*MDR1*) in relation to Parkinson's disease. Pharmacogenetics 2002;12:529–34.

55. Trip MD, Smulders YM, Wegman JJ, et al. Frequent mutation in the *ABCC6* gene (R1141X) is associated with a strong increase in the prevalence of coronary artery disease. Circulation 2002;106:773–5.

56. Nezu J, Tamai I, Oku A, et al. Primary systemic carnitine deficiency is caused by mutations in a gene encoding sodium ion-dependent carnitine transporter. Nat Genet 1999;21:91–4.

333

Self-Assessment Questions

1. Which one of the following transporters is most likely to limit bioavailability of large, hydrophobic neutral or cationic drugs?

    A. MRP2.
    B. OCT1.
    C. P-glycoprotein (Pgp).
    D. ENT1.

2. Which one of the following transporters plays a crucial role in maintaining cellular homeostasis?

    A. OCT1.
    B. Mitoxantrone resistance protein.
    C. P-glycoprotein.
    D. ENT1.

3. Pravastatin is an organic anion, a poor substrate for drug metabolizing enzymes and is excreted unchanged in the bile and urine. Which one of the following phenotypes is *least* likely after administration of pravastatin to patients with Dubin-Johnson syndrome?

    A. Increased plasma levels of pravastatin.
    B. Decreased fecal excretion of pravastatin.
    C. Increased urinary excretion of pravastatin.
    D. Increased neurotoxicity.

4. Which one of the following statements is *least* consistent with known patterns of genetic variability in membrane transporters?

    A. The degree of genetic variation in the transmembrane domains is less than that in the loops.
    B. Nucleotides encoding evolutionarily conserved amino acids are less likely to be variant than nonconserved nucleotides.
    C. Genetic variation in neurotransmitter transporters is low relative to that in xenobiotic transporters.
    D. Nonsynonymous changes are more likely than synonymous changes.

5. Linkage disequilibrium describes the nonrandom association of multiple alleles of a given gene or different genes. A significant degree of linkage disequilibrium in transporter genes would be most likely under which one of the following conditions?

    A. When two alleles have a similar frequency in the population of interest.

B. When a silent mutation is associated with a clinical phenotype.
C. When alleles with different frequencies are associated with a common clinical phenotype.
D. When two genes with similar function are located in close proximity on a chromosome.

6. Opposing effects of a C3435T variant in the *MDR1* gene on the plasma levels of the Pgp substrates digoxin and fexofenadine have been reported in the recent literature. Which one of the following strategies best addresses these discrepancies?

   A. Additional studies in ethnically diverse populations.
   B. Consideration of the genotypes of uptake transporters and drug metabolizing enzymes.
   C. Selection of study populations based on haplotype instead of genotypes.
   D. Studies with increased sample sizes.

7. The usefulness of drug transporter phenotypes in predicting drug response and/or toxicity depends on the characteristics of the substrates for these transporters. Which one of the following attributes is *least* likely to influence whether transporter genotypes will predict a pharmacokinetic or pharmacodynamic response?

   A. The drug is a substrate for efflux transporters expressed in the intestinal epithelium and largely escapes first-pass intestinal and liver metabolism.
   B. The major route of elimination is renal secretion.
   C. An estimated 20 percent of a dose of a drug is secreted into the bile and the remainder is metabolized by cytochrome P450 3A4 to inactive metabolites.
   D. The drug is a Pgp substrate and has limiting neurotoxicity.

8. The multidrug resistance transporters, nucleoside transporters, and organic cation transporters all have been implicated in the resistance of tumor cells to cancer chemotherapeutic agents. In a lung cancer cell line, resistance to gemcitabine has been associated with overexpression of nucleoside transporters and MRP5. Which one of the following is the most plausible explanation for the role of these transporters in gemcitabine resistance?

   A. The nucleoside transporters increase intracellular gemcitabine levels.
   B. Gemcitabine resistance depends on intracellular levels of nucleotide metabolizing enzymes.
   C. Sensitivity of the cells to gemcitabine depends on the host cell genetics.

D. Increased gemcitabine efflux decreases intracellular levels.

9. P-glycoprotein is the best characterized transporter with respect to function and clinical significance. Which one of the following phenotypes would be most significant in a patient who is homozygous for a *MDR1* variant that results in complete loss of Pgp function?

A. Increased neurotoxicity of a Pgp substrate that acts as a peripheral opiate agonist.
B. Increased bioavailability of a CYP3A and Pgp substrate.
C. Increased urinary excretion of digoxin.
D. Decreased biliary excretion of digoxin.

10. Passive permeability of organic anions and organic cations is often limited by their hydrophilicity. In considering the determinants of hepatic levels of an organic anion which one of the following transporters is least likely to play a significant role?

A. MRP2.
B. CNT3.
C. MRP3.
D. OATP1.

Drug Target Pharmacogenetics

Julie A. Johnson, Pharm.D., BCPS, FCCP

Key Words

Drug target, pharmacological action, pharmacogenetics, pharmacogenomics, candidate gene, individualized therapy, polymorphisms.

Abstract

The study of drug metabolism pharmacogenetics has been ongoing for nearly 5 decades, whereas drug targets pharmacogenetics is relatively new. Drug target is defined as any protein involved in the pharmacological action of the drug, and not just the protein to which the drug binds. Drug target pharmacogenetics seeks to identify the contribution of genetic variability in drug targets to either variable drug efficacy or toxicity. This chapter highlights some of the similarities and differences between drug metabolism versus drug target pharmacogenetics, and then discusses representative examples from the drug target pharmacogenetics literature. Although there currently is substantial literature supporting the concept that genetic polymorphisms in drug targets contribute to variable drug response, moving drug pharmacogenetics to the clinical setting presents certain challenges, which are discussed. One of the major challenges of the clinical application of drug target pharmacogenetics is the complexity of the drug response and the numerous proteins (and thus genes) involved in drug action. Although most studies to date have focused on polymorphisms in single genes, it seems likely that a more comprehensive (genomic) approach will be needed. Genomic approaches may use either candidate gene or genome scanning approaches, and the advantages and disadvantages to each of these are discussed. There is clear evidence that genetic polymorphisms in drug targets contribute to variable drug response; the challenge is to move this field to the point that genetic information can be used to guide drug therapy.

Despite the challenges ahead, it seems likely that information on genetic polymorphisms in drug targets will be used in the future to individualize drug therapy.

Outline

Learning Objectives

1. Apply knowledge to explain or predict the role of genetic variability in drug targets on drug efficacy and toxicity.
2. Demonstrate an understanding of the complexity of most drug responses (i.e., the drug response cascades), and the influence this has on the contribution of genetic variability to drug response.
3. Evaluate the current and future potential applications of drug target pharmacogenetics to individualization of drug therapy.

Abbreviations in this Chapter

ACE	Angiotensin-converting enzyme
βAR	β-Adrenergic receptor
β₂AR	β₂-Adrenergic receptor
GNB3	G protein β3 subunit
HER-2	Human estrogen receptor-2
SNP	Single nucleotide ploymorphism

Introduction

Response to most drugs exhibits a high degree of interpatient variability, which leads to certain patients receiving prescriptions for drugs that are not efficacious or that cause serious adverse effects. Pharmacogenetics and pharmacogenomics aim to elucidate the genetic basis for the interpatient variability in drug response. Thus, the long-term goal is that drug therapy be individualized based on a patient's genetic makeup, resulting in better efficacy rates and lower toxicity rates. There are numerous recent reviews that summarize the current pharmacogenetics/pharmacogenomics literature (References 1, 2) and the potential future impact of pharmacogenetics (References 3–6). This chapter focuses on drug target pharmacogenetics literature, identifies potential limitations with current approaches in this area, and discusses how drug target pharmacogenetics is likely to be used in the future by clinicians to aid in drug therapy decision-making.

In general, information about drugs can be divided into two broad categories: pharmacokinetics (what the body does to the drug) and pharmacology or pharmacodynamics (what the drug does to the body). Study of the influence of the inherited basis for variability in pharmacokinetics, particularly hepatic drug metabolism, has been ongoing since the 1950s. However, it was not until the late 1990s that studies were published on the influence of genetic variability on pharmacology or pharmacodynamics. This latter research area has been coined "drug target pharmacogenetics." The Pharmacogenetics of Oxidative Drug Metabolism and Its Clinical Applications and Drug Transporter Pharmacogenetics chapters in this module focus on the influence of genetic variability on drug metabolism and drug transport, both of which influence the pharmacokinetis of drugs. This chapter focuses on drug targets and the effects of genetic variability on them. Drug targets are defined as the direct protein target of a drug (e.g., a receptor or enzyme); proteins involved in the pharmacological response (e.g., signal transduction proteins or down-stream proteins); or proteins associated with disease risk, pathogenesis, or toxicity risk (References 1, 7). The specific focus of drug target pharmacogenetics is to identify the inherited basis for interindividual variability in drug response and toxicity, particularly when this variability is not explained by differences in drug concentration (pharmacokinetics) that might be because of genetic variation in drug metabolizing enzymes or drug transporters.

Some confusion exists about the differences between pharmacogenetics and pharmacogenomics. There are several definitions of these two terms in the literature, and in many settings, the terms are used interchangeably. The definitions most consistent with the distinction in genetics and genomics are: pharmacogenetics describes studies that evaluate the relationship between variability in a single gene and drug response, whereas pharmacogenomics describes studies that evaluate the impact of polymorphisms in multiple genes (or eventually, across the entire genome) to try to explain drug response variability (Reference 1). Even these terms are awkward from a practical perspective. Therefore, in this chapter, the term pharmacogenetics is used throughout.

Drug Target Versus Drug Metabolism Pharmacogenetics: Comparisons and Contrasts

As previously discussed, work in the area of drug metabolism pharmacogenetics predates work in drug target pharmacogenetics by nearly four decades. There are several reasons for this large gap that are important to understanding drug target pharmacogenetics, and will influence how drug target pharmacogenetics enters clinical practice.

Functional Consequences of Genetic Polymorphisms

The primary explanation for the drug metabolism-drug target discrepancy lies in the genetic mutations in the genes of interest. There are several different kinds of mutations or polymorphisms (those occurring with a frequency greater than 1 percent), with consequences of varying severity. The most common form of polymorphism is the single nucleotide polymorphism (SNP). If located in an intronic region, it typically is not expected to have functional consequences. Exonic SNPs can have one of several consequences. Those that do not change the coded amino acid (silent or synonymous SNPs) are not expected to have functional consequences. Those that result in a different amino acid (nonsynonymous or missense SNPs) have the potential for functional consequences, the magnitude of which depends on the location of the SNP in the protein and the degree to which the characteristics of the two amino acids differ. Single nucleotide polymorphisms that occur in the promoter or regulatory regions of the gene can influence protein expression. The most severe consequence that results from an SNP is the creation of a stop codon. In this latter case, the SNP leads to a truncated, and usually abnormal or nonfunctional protein.

Other types of polymorphisms include insertion/deletion polymorphisms and variable number tandem repeats, in which a set of nucleotides repeats a variable number of times. When these occur in exonic regions, they create frameshifts, and also have extreme consequences, such as unstable or nonfunctional protein.

Phenotypes Resulting from Genetic Polymorphisms

The phenotypic consequences of different polymorphisms are highlighted in Figure 1. Polymorphisms that result in the complete, or near complete, loss of functional protein result in two very distinct phenotypes, as shown in the panel at the left of the figure. Many of the widely studied drug metabolism polymorphisms, such as thiopurine methyltransferase, cytochrome P450 2D6, or cytochrome P450 2C19, are inactivating mutations (References 1, 8). Thus, the resulting phenotypes from these polymorphisms

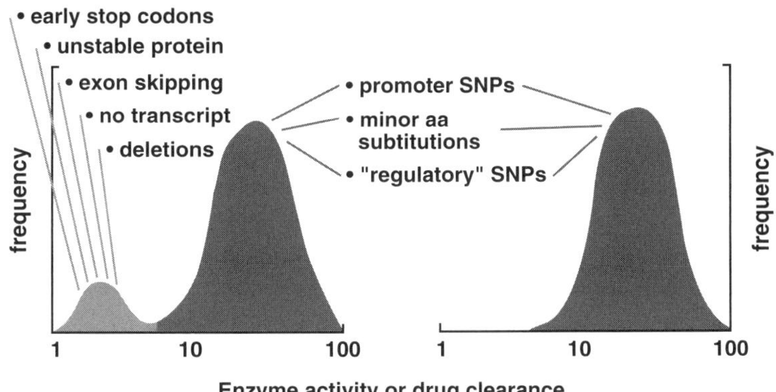

Figure 1. Influence of mutation/polymorphism type on population distribution of phenotypes. The left panel highlights the types of mutations/polymorphisms that result in absent or nonfunctional proteins. These types of polymorphisms typically result in two distinct phenotype populations. These types of polymorphisms are typical of many of the well-known drug metabolizing enzyme polymorphisms. The right panel highlights the polymorphisms that result in more subtle phenotypes, and which fail to result in two distinct populations. In contrast, these polymorphisms may help to explain the variability across the single population distribution curve. These are more representative of the types of polymorphisms observed in drug targets. SNP = single nucleotide polymorphism.
Reproduced from Evans WE, Johnson JA. Pharmacogenomics: the inherited basis for interindividual differences in drug response. Annu Rev Genomics Hum Gent 2001;2:9–39, with permission.

are quite distinct, and easily recognized through clinical or pharmacokinetic information.

In contrast, the genetic polymorphisms of drug targets typically are not inactivating, but rather are polymorphisms with more subtle effects, such as amino acid changes, or effects on protein expression. As a consequence, the resulting phenotypes are more subtle than those observed with inactivating mutations. These are more accurately reflected by the right-hand portion of Figure 1, where the polymorphisms do not result in two distinct populations of phenotypes, but help explain the variability across the single distribution curve. It is interesting to speculate that there is a teleological basis for the relative absence of inactivating mutations in drug targets (e.g., receptors or signal transduction proteins) because such mutations might be lethal, or strongly selected against.

Differences between the drug target and drug metabolism polymorphisms, and the resulting phenotypes also have influenced the approach to pharmacogenetic studies. In the case of most of the drug metabolism polymorphisms, an extreme phenotype was clinically noted, which led to the search for the molecular genetic basis for the phenotype, an approach referred to as phenotype to genotype. In contrast, the approach with drug targets commonly is identification of genetic polymorphisms, followed by study of the association between these polymorphisms and different phenotypes, an approached described as genotype to phenotype. Finally, for drugs whose metabolism occurs mainly by a single enzyme, genetic variations for a single protein can have a marked impact on the drug's pharmacokinetics. In contrast, there typically are numerous proteins involved in the pharmacological effect of the drug; thus, variability in a single protein is less likely to have profound clinical effects. This concept is discussed in greater detail in the Moving Drug Targets section because it may influence how rapidly genetic tests for drug metabolizing enzymes versus drug targets are adopted into clinical practice

Drug Target Pharmacogenetics

The typical approach to drug target pharmacogenetics research is a candidate gene approach. This approach relies on existing knowledge for selection of genes to be studied, and in the case of drug target pharmacogenetics, relies primarily on knowledge of the pharmacology of the drug, and the proteins involved in the pharmacological effects. Representative examples from the literature of drug target pharmacogenetics studies are summarized in Tables 1 and 2.

Polymorphisms of Direct Drug Targets and Association with Drug Response

Candidate genes for drug target pharmacogenetics are broken into three categories. The first category is the direct protein to which the drug binds, referred to in Table 1 as the direct drug target. The direct drug target is the logical first place to study the effects of genetic variability on drug response; thus, there are numerous examples in the literature of pharmacogenetic studies of direct drug targets. The majority of examples in this category are studies of associations between genetic variability in receptors and responses of drugs that bind to those receptors. Receptors whose genetic variability are associated with drug response include β-adrenergic receptors (βAR), dopamine receptors, serotonin receptors, estrogen receptor, and sulfonylurea receptor.

The βAR polymorphisms, particularly those of the β_2-adrenergic receptor (β_2AR), are studied extensively (Reference 9). The β_1AR polymorphisms were identified only a few years ago; thus, the pharmacogenetics literature is somewhat limited. In a study of patients with hypertension, it was recently shown that the β_1AR genetic polymorphisms at codons 389 and 49 are associated with the daytime and 24-hour antihypertensive effect of metoprolol (Reference 10). For example, patients who were *Arg389* homozygotes had a nearly 3-fold greater lowering in daytime diastolic blood pressure than those who carried a *Gly389* allele (Diastolic blood pressure: -13.3 percent vs. -4.5 percent; p<0.002). Comparisons of response by codon 49 genotype did not reveal statistical significance. However, analysis by haplotype provided additional information over the single polymorphism analysis. Haplotype is the genetic information on a single allele, thus, in this case, represents genetic information at β_1AR codon 49 and 389 as inherited from mother or father. As such, each person has two haplotypes, and this pair of haplotypes is called the diplotype. When the analysis was conducted by diplotype, blood pressure lowering was -14.5 mm Hg for patients with the *Ser49Arg389/Ser49Arg389* diplotype, compared to -0.5 mm Hg for those with the *Gly49Arg389/Ser49Gly389* diplotype. There were two other diplotypes, which had intermediate blood pressure lowering. This example is not one where it is only through haplotype analysis that an association was found; thus, these results primarily represent the additive effects of the single polymorphisms. However, even if this is the case, haplotype analysis remains a meaningful way to account for the contributions of multiple polymorphisms.

Of importance, these data are consistent with the in vitro functional studies, which showed the *Arg389* form of the β_1AR to have higher adenylyl cyclase activity than the *Gly389* form, (Reference 11) and the *Ser49* form to undergo less down-regulation than the *Gly49* form (Reference 12). Thus, this example represents a typical candidate gene approach to drug target pharmacogenetics. First, the β_1AR gene is of interest because its protein is the direct target of β-blockers. Thus, interest in pharmacogenetic

Table 1. Examples of Associations between Drug Response and Direct Drug Targets, Signal Transduction Proteins, or Downstream Proteins

Gene/gene product	Drug/drug class	Clinical effects category	Protein	Polymorphism type/location	Reference
CARDIOVASCULAR					
• β_1AR	β-Blockers	Antihypertensive response	DT	NS SNP/exonic	95
• ACE	ACE inhibitors	Renoprotective effects, blood pressure reduction, left ventricular mass reduction, endothelial function improvement, ACE inhibitor-induced cough	DT	I/D/intronic	32–3
• Glyco-protein IIIa subunit of glycoprotein IIb/IIIa receptor	Aspirin/ glycoprotein IIIa IIb/IIIa inhibitors	Antiplatelet effect	DT/ST/DP	NS SNP/exonic	96–98
• Bradykinin B2 receptor	ACE inhibitors	ACE inhibitor-induced cough	ST/DP	SNP/promoter	48
• Gs protein α	β-Blockers	Antihypertensive effect	ST/DP	S SNP/exonic	47
• G protein β3	Thiazide diuretics	Antihypertensive effect	ST/DP	SNP-splice vanant/exonic	89
• Platelet FC receptor (FCRII)	Heparin	Heparin-induced thrombocytopenia	ST/DP	NS SNP/exonic	99
• α-Adducin	Diuretics	Risk of nonfatal myocardial infarction or stroke in patients with hypertension	DT?	NS SNP/exonic	100
• Aldosterone synthase	AT_1-receptor blocker	Antihypertensive effect	ST/DP	SNP/promoter	101

Table 1. Examples of Associations between Drug Response and Direct Drug Targets, Signal Transduction Proteins, or Downstream Proteins (continued)

Gene/gene product	Drug/drug class	Clinical effects category	Protein	Polymorphism type/location	Reference
PULMONARY					
• β_2-Adrenergic receptor	β_2-Agonists	Bronchodilation, susceptibility to agonist-induced desensitization, cardiovascular effects (e.g., increased heart rate, cardiac index, and peripheral vasodilation)	DT	NS SNP/exonic	14–21
• ALOX5	Leukotriene biosynthesis inhibitors (e.g., ABT-761-zileuton-derivative)	Improvement in FEV$_1$	DT	VNTR/promoter	88
CANCER					
• *HER-2*	Trastuzumab	Responsiveness to therapy	DT	Protein expression tested	76
• BCR-ABL	Imatinib	Resistance to therapy	DT	SNP/exonic	77–80
• TNF-α2	Bleomycin	Chemotherapy-induced pulmonary fibrosis	ST/DP	MHC haplotype	81
IMMUNOLOGY					
• FCgamma RIIA	Immunosuppressive therapy (e.g., corticosteroids and other agents)	Response to therapy in idiopathic thrombocytopenia purpura	DT	NS SNP/exonic	102
• Interferon-γ	Post-transplant immunosuppression	Organ rejection	DT	VNTR/exonic	103
• IL-10 and TNF-α	Post-transplant immunosuppression	Successful weaning from immunosuppression	DT	IL-10: SNPs/promoter TNFα: SNP/promoter	104

Table 1. Examples of Associations between Drug Response and Direct Drug Targets, Signal Transduction Proteins, or Downstream Proteins (continued)

Gene/gene product	Drug/drug class	Clinical effects category	Protein	Polymorphism type/location	Reference
ENDOCRINOLOGY					
• Estrogen receptor	Conjugated estrogens	Bone mineral density , increases, increases in HDL	DT	SNP/intronic	105, 106
• Sulfonylurea receptor	Sulfonylureas	Sulfonylurea-induced insulin release, fasting triglyceride levels	DT	SNP/intronic	107, 108
PSYCHIARTY/NEUROLOGY					
• Dopamine receptors (D2, D3, D4)	Antipsychotics	Antipsychotic response (D2, D3, D4), antipsychotic-induced tardive dyskinsia (D3), antipsychotic-induced acute akathisia (D3), NMS (D2)	DT	D2: I/D/ promoter D3: NS SNP/exonic D4: VNTR/exonic	22–28, 109
• Dopamine receptor	Levodopa & dopamine	Drug induced hallucinations	DT	Above	68
• Serotonin receptors (5HT2A, 5HT2C)	Antipsychotics (e.g., clozapine and typical antipsychotics)	Antipsychotic response and long-term outcomes, antipsychotic-induced tardive dyskinesia (5HT2A), antipsychotic-induced weight gain (5HT2C)	DT	5HT2A: SNP/ promoter and S SNP/exonic 5HT2C: SNP/ promoter and NS SNP/exonic	28–31
• Serotonin transporter (5-HTT)	Antidepressants	5-HT neurotransmission, antidepressant response	DT	I/D/promoter	40, 41, 46
• G protein β3	Antidepressants	Response to antidepressant therapy	ST/DP	SNP-splice variant/exonic	110
• Inositol-p1p	Lithium	Response of manic depressive illness	ST/DP	NS SNP/exonic	111
• TNFα, TNFβ, LTβ	Clozapine	Clozapine-induced agranulocytosis	ST/DP	MHC Haplotypes/ VNTRs	112

Table 1. Examples of Associations between Drug Response and Direct Drug Targets, Signal Transduction Proteins, or Downstream Proteins (continued)

Gene/gene product	Drug/drug class	Clinical effects category	Protein	Polymorphism type/location	Reference
OTHER					
• Ryanodine receptor	Anesthetics	Malignant hyperthermia	DT	Multiple NS SNPs/exonic	113–116

ACE = angiotensin-converting enzyme; ALOX5 = 5-lopoxygenase; AT_1 = angrotensin receptor type I; $\beta_1 AR$ = β1-adrenergic receptor; BP = blood pressure; DT = direct drug target; I/D = insertion/deletion polymorphism; FEV_1 = forced expiratory volume in 1 second; HDL = high-density lipoprotein; *HER-2* = human estrogen receptor-2; IL = interleukin; MHC = major histocompatability complex proteins; NS = monsynonymous; S = synonymous; SNP = single nucleotide polymorphism; ST/DP = signal transduction or downstream protein; TNF = tumor necrosis factor; VNTR = variable number tandem repeat.

investigation was raised when common, nonsynonymous genetic polymorphisms for the $\beta_1 AR$ were identified (Reference 13). Functional effects of the receptor variants were documented through in vitro site-directed mutagenesis studies. This was followed by study of the association of the $\beta_1 AR$ polymorphisms with drug response in a patient population where interpatient variability in the drug response is recognized. This progression is highlighted in Figure 2. Further studies are required, but these data provide early evidence that it might be possible to predict antihypertensive response to β-blockers based on the genetic profile.

Numerous studies also were conducted on the associations between the β2-receptorpolymorphisms and both the bronchodilator (forced expiratory volume in 1 second) and cardiovascular responses (such as increased heart rate, cardiac output, and vasodilation) to β2-agonists (References 14–21). There are data suggesting that consideration of the β2AR haplotype is more informative than individual genetic polymorphisms. Specifically, one study found no association between single polymorphisms and bronchodilation response to albuterol, but did note a significant association when the β2AR haplotypes were compared for β2-agonist response (Reference 18).

Other receptors that are studied extensively for genetic associations with drug response include receptors that are direct targets for antipsychotic drugs, namely the dopamine and serotonin receptors (References 22–31). These studies reported associations between these polymorphisms and antipsychotic response, and antipsychotic-induced side effects (e.g., tardive dyskinesia, acute akathisia, weight gain, and neuroleptic malignant syndrome).

Enzymes are another common direct drug target. One of the most extensively studied of polymorphisms is the insertion/deletion polymorphism of the angiotensin-converting enzyme (ACE). Angiotensin-converting enzyme is responsible for conversion of angiotensin I to angiotensin II, and ACE inhibitors work by blocking this conversion. The *D/D* genotype for ACE (those who carry two copies of the ACE deletion

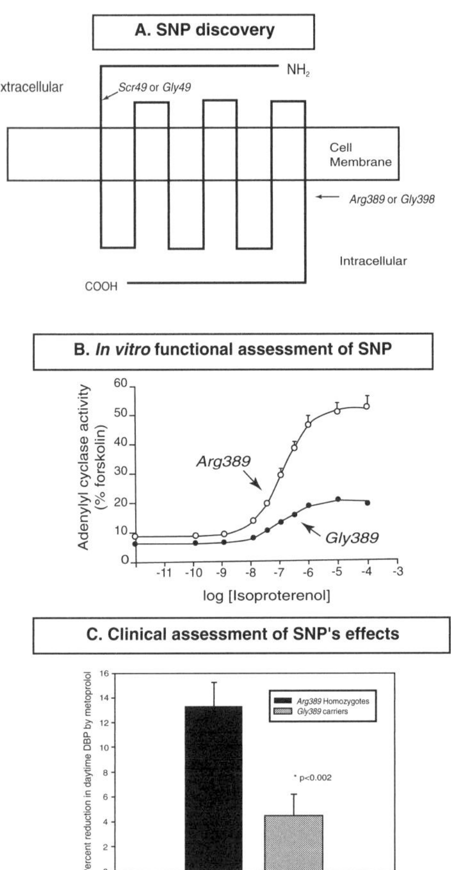

Figure 2. β_1AR codon 389 genetic polymorphism as representative example of candidate gene approach to pharmacogenetics.

A. Representation of the β_1AR, including the sites of the two common, nonsynonymous polymorphisms. The discovery of these polymorphisms signalled the beginning of pharmacogenetic work with the β_1AR.

B. In vitro assessment of the functional consequences of the β_1AR codon 389 polymorphism. These data depict the higher basal and agonist-stimulated adenylyl cyclase activity for the *Arg389* form of the β_1AR. Reprinted with permission. Mason DA, Moore JD, Green SA, Liggett SB. A gain-of-function polymorphism in a G-protein coupling domain of the human bate1-adrenergic receptor. J Biol Chem 1999;274:12670–4

C. Assessment of the influence of the β_1AR codon 389 polymorphism on the antihypertensive response to β-blockers. These data depict the greater antihypertensive response to metoprolol in patients who were β_1AR *Arg389* homozygous genotype.

SNP = single nucleotide polymorphism.

Derived from data by Johnson JA, Zineh I, Puckett BJ, McGorray SP, Yarandi HM, Pauly DF. Beta 1-adrenergic receptor polymorphisms and antihypertensive response to metoprolol. Clin Pharmacol Ther 2003;74:44–52.

allele) consistently is associated with increased ACE activity. Angiotensin-converting enzyme insertion/deletion genotypes are associated with various clinical effects of ACE inhibitors, including renoprotective effects, blood pressure lowering, left ventricular hypertrophy reduction, cough, and improvements in endothelial function (References 32–39).

Transporters, such as the serotonin transporter for selective serotonin reuptake inhibitors, represent another type of drug target. The serotonin transporter is another example of a direct drug target with numerous examples in the literature documenting an association between genetic variation and response. Specifically, these studies have documented associations between genotype and antidepressant response, prolactin response to antidepressants, and antidepressant-induced switch to mania (References 40–46). The pharmacogenetics of numerous other direct drug targets that are less well studied also are highlighted in Table 1.

Polymorphisms of Signal Transduction/Downstream Proteins and Associations with Drug Response

Table 1 also provides examples of signal transduction or downstream proteins whose genetic variability are associated with drug response variability (indicated in Table 1 by signal transduction or downstream protein). An example from this group comes from data on $G\alpha_S$ polymorphisms and β-blocker response. The βARs are Gs protein-coupled receptors and the G proteins are composed of three subunits: α, β, and γ. A recent study found that a polymorphism in the $G\alpha_S$ subunit was associated with the antihypertensive response to β-blockers. (Reference 47). Thus, these data provide evidence that the signal transduction proteins, in addition to the direct drug target, can contribute to drug response variability. A study of bradykinin B2 receptor polymorphisms and ACE inhibitor therapy provides an example of how a downstream protein influences drug response. It is recognized that ACE inhibitors block conversion of angiotensin I to angiotensin II, along with preventing the breakdown of bradykinin. Bradykinin binds to its own G protein-coupled receptor, and polymorphisms in this receptor's gene are associated with ACE inhibitor-induced cough (Reference 48). Thus, although ACE inhibitors do not directly act at the bradykinin B2 receptor, this protein contributes to the overall drug response, and thus, variability in its gene contribute to variability in the ACE inhibitor response.

Polymorphisms of Disease Pathogenesis Proteins and Associations with Drug Response

A pharmacogenetic study approach that diverges somewhat from studying the proteins known to be involved in the pharmacological effects of a drug is one that focuses on genetic polymorphisms described to be associated with disease risk. Table 2 provides examples of these types of studies. The first examples in Table 2 highlight how a drug known to cause

Table 2. Examples of Associations between Disease Risk Polymorphisms and Drug Toxicity or Efficacy

Gene/gene product	Disease association	Medication	Impact of polymorphism on drug effect/toxicity	Reference
• Prothrombin and Factor V	Deep vein thrombosis and cerebral vein thrombosis	Oral contraceptives	Increased deep vein and cerebral vein thrombosis risk with oral contraceptives	49, 50, 117
• *HERG, KvLQT1, Mink, MiRP1*	Congenital long QT syndrome	Various such as: erythromycin, terfenadine, cisapride, clarithromycin, antiarrhythmic drugs	Increased risk of drug-induced torsade de pointes	51–53, 55, 56
• MHC proteins	Hypersensitivity reactions	Abacavir	Risk of abacavir-induced hypersensitivity	57, 58
• APOE	Atherosclerosis progression; ischemic cardiovascular events	Statins	Enhanced survival prolongation with simvastatin	59–61
• APOE	Alzheimer's disease	Tacrine	Clinical improvement with tacrine	65, 66, 118
• Stromelysin-1	Atherosclerosis progression	Statins	Reduction in cardiovascular events by pravastatin (e.g., death, myocardial infarction, stroke, and angina), reduction in repeat angioplasty	63
• Parkin	Parkinson's disease	Levodopa	Clinical improvement and L-dopa-induced dyskinesias	67

ApoE = apolipoprotein E; MHC = major histocompatability complex.

a certain adverse event, in combination with a genetic polymorphism associated with the same adverse event, lead to a marked increase in risk of drug toxicity. For example, a meta-analysis of 2310 cases and 3204 controls estimated that the odds ratio for risk of developing venous thrombosis is 5.9 in patients with a Factor V Leiden gene mutation. Oral contraceptive use carries a 2.3-fold increased risk of venous thrombosis. However, the risk for venous thrombosis rises to 10.3 times in those with both the mutation and oral contraceptive use (Reference 49). These data suggest at least an additive effect of the polymorphism plus oral contraceptive use, and other studies have suggested the effect may be synergistic (Reference 50). Similar findings are shown for the prothrombin mutation, oral contraceptive use, and thrombosis risk (References 49, 50).

Similarly, gene mutations in cardiac potassium and sodium channels are associated with congenital long QT syndrome. There is mounting evidence that in some patients with these mutations, there are no overt clinical manifestations of the mutation until the patient is challenged with a drug that also causes QT prolongation (References 51–56). Intensive investigation is now under way to identify the genetic determinants of the highly unpredictable, drug-induced torsades de pointes (Reference 54). The ability to predict this adverse event (and, thus, avoid therapy in at-risk patients) is particularly appealing given that risk of QT prolongation and torsades de pointes is the basis for withdrawing many drugs from the market over the past decade.

Major histocompatability complex proteins are thought to be associated with "idiosyncratic" hypersensitivity reactions to drugs. The reverse transcriptase inhibitor abacavir is associated with a 5 percent risk of hypersensitivity; thus, there was interest in determining whether major histocompatability complex protein haplotypes are associated with hypersensitivity risk. Two recent reports found certain major histocompatability complex protein haplotypes to be highly predictive of hypersensitivity risk, such that these genetic screens might be useful in the future for identifying patients who should not receive abacavir (References 57, 58).

The three examples highlighted above use long-recognized information about genetic risk for an adverse event. The advance is coupling knowledge of the genetic risk with the drug-induced risk. Thus, these examples provide a useful paradigm for understanding the genetic basis for serious drug-induced adverse effects.

The remaining examples in Table 2 highlight how disease-associated polymorphisms also impact drug efficacy, even when the proteins of interest are not directly involved in the pharmacological actions of the drug. Many such studies with statins were conducted in large populations with specific clinical end points (beyond lipid changes). These studies focused on genetic polymorphisms in proteins not directly involved in the pharmacological mechanism of the drug, such as apolipoprotein E, cholesteryl ester transfer protein, stromelysin-1, and β-fibrinogen (References 59–64). The studies consistently show in the placebo arm that the genetic polymorphism was associated with an adverse clinical outcome (e.g., greater atherosclerosis progression, cardiovascular event, or death). In addition, the studies consistently documented that patients who carried the "higher risk" polymorphism derived the greatest benefit from statin therapy, whereas the lower risk genotype group derived less or no benefit from the statin. Similar findings are documented with apolipoprotein E polymorphisms and tacrine response in Alzheimer's disease (References 65, 66), and parkin polymorphisms and efficacy or adverse effects of levodopa therapy in Parkinson's disease (References 67, 68).

Drug Targets in Infectious Disease and Cancer

The drug targets for treating infectious diseases and cancers are different than those for most other conditions. For most diseases, the drug target is a human protein which has not undergone mutation during the patient's life. In the case of infectious diseases, the drug target is a nonhuman protein, namely a pathogen protein. Thus, understanding the genetic basis for variable drug response in infectious diseases is more complicated than for most diseases. This is because it is genetic variability of the pathogen, not the human, that is likely to contribute to variable responses. In fact, there are numerous studies of the role of pathogen genetic variability on drug resistance, particularly in human immunodeficiency virus (References 69–72), but also with other pathogens (References 73–75). However, this chapter focuses on human variations in genomic deoxyribonucleic acid; thus, these examples are not discussed. These issues, however, are discussed in detail in the Infectious Diseases chapter in Module 3 of this curriculum. Human genetic variability influences a patient's susceptibility to infection by a pathogen, and also may be related to adverse events associated with anti-infective therapy. Recent studies showing association of haplotypes of the major histocompatability complex proteins with risk of abacavir-induced hypersensitivity represent an example of this latter concept (References 57, 58).

Understanding the pharmacogenetics of the drug targets for cancer agents also requires a different approach, in many cases, than for most drugs. Although cancer cells are human cells, they are cells that have undergone, in most cases, somatic mutations during the patient's lifetime. These mutations are, therefore, not evident in the genomic deoxyribonucleic acid; thus, this is not the source for understanding the genetic basis for variable drug response. Rather, gene expression studies, measuring messenger ribonucleic acid or protein in the cancer cells, may hold the keys to understanding variable drug response in cancer.

A classic example in this area is trastuzumab, used for treating metastatic breast cancer. It was discovered in early clinical trials of this drug that the only women who responded well to trastuzumab were those who overexpressed the human estrogen receptor-2 (*HER-2*) protein (Reference

76). Thus, later premarketing studies focused on this population, and the package insert for trastuzumab indicates that testing for *HER-2* overexpression in the breast cancer cells should be done before patients receiving the drug.

The ABL-selective tyrosine kinase inhibitor imatinib, used to treat Philadelphia chromosome-positive leukemias, is another example where mutations in cancer cells are being investigated to gain understanding of resistance to the drug. Early studies in this area suggest that certain mutations may confer resistance to imitinab (References 77–80). Additional studies are needed to determine whether it is possible to predict sensitivity or resistance to imitinab *a priori*.

These examples highlight that much of the genetic basis for variable efficacy of cancer chemotherapy lies in mutations in cancer cells. However, some (or perhaps much) of the genetic contribution to toxicity risk with chemotherapeutic agents may arise from variability in genomic deoxyribonucleic acid. This is particularly true for those toxicities that are not a direct extension of the pharmacology of the drug. For example, a recent study found an association between bleomycin-induced pulmonary fibrosis and a polymorphism in the tumor necrosis factor 2a gene (Reference 81).

In many respects, hematology and oncology are ahead of most other medical disciplines in that many diseases are classified at a cellular or molecular level, and treatments are guided by these classifications. Although the challenges of pharmacogenetics are greater in cancer than in other medical disciplines, the potential benefits also are greater. Thus, the pharmacogenetics of cancer is an area where important advances were made for the drug metabolizing enzymes, and substantial further advances are likely with the drug targets.

Limitations of Current Literature

Similar to most disease-gene association literature for complex diseases, there is discordance in some literature regarding the influence of genetic polymorphisms on drug response. This is best exemplified by the literature on the ACE insertion/deletion polymorphism, for which there is a wealth of literature. Studies are consistent in showing that the *D/D* genotype is associated with higher levels of ACE activity. Based on this, it could be anticipated that the *D/D* genotype would show the greatest response to ACE inhibitors or angiotensin receptor blockers. Although this is the case in many studies, (References 34, 35, 39, 82) there also are examples from the literature where the *I/I* genotype had the greatest response, (References 32, 33, 83, 84) or where there was no association between genotype and response (Reference 85).

There are many potential explanations for these discrepancies, including differences in populations or diseases studied, differences in the response evaluated, differences in the drugs evaluated, and lack of statistical power. These problems are confounded by polymorphisms that have small effects on the phenotype and, thus, contribute a smaller percentage to the variable drug response. In addition, the contribution of multiple proteins in the signal transduction cascade complicates this issue further, as discussed in greater detail in the next section. Thus, those studying drug target pharmacogenetics face some of the same challenges as those trying to unravel the genetic basis for common complex (or polygenic) diseases (Reference 86). This is where functional studies assist in the interpretation of pharmacogenetic study results. Specifically, consistency of the findings of a pharmacogenetics study with the in vitro or in vivo functional assessments for the specific polymorphism lead to greater acceptance of those data than in those cases where there is no functional understanding of the polymorphism, or the data are inconsistent with the known functional effects.

Moving Drug Target Pharmacogenetics from Proof of Concept to Clinical Practice

Using Genotype Information to Predict Response

The previously discussed studies and the information provided in Tables 1 and 2 provide "proof of concept" that genetic variability in drug targets contributes to variable drug response. Although these studies documented that some variability in drug response is explained by genetic variability, they do not, in most cases, provide a level of predictability that is clinically useful.

Assessment of Clinical Value of Genetic Tests

Genetic testing to guide drug therapy is not necessarily superior to other types of medical testing, but it needs to provide data that are clinically useful. Thus, issues of sensitivity, specificity, positive predictive value, and negative predictive value of the test become important (Reference 87).

Sensitivity describes the ability of the test to identify true-positives. In the case of a pharmacogenetic test aimed at identifying responders to therapy or those at toxicity risk, this would represent the percent of patients who are predicted to respond or have toxicity, based on the genetic test, relative to the number who actually respond or have toxicity (i.e., the true-positives). Thus, a high sensitivity means that the test has a high true-positive rate, or in other terms, a low false-negative rate. In contrast, specificity describes the ability of the test to identify true-negatives. Thus, in the case of a pharmacogenetics tests, this would mean the percent of patients predicted at low toxicity risk, or nonresponders, relative to the actual rate of toxicity or nonresponse.

Other statistical calculations that are useful in determining the value of a test, including a pharmacogenetic test, are the positive predictive value and the negative predictive value. Positive predictive value provides insight into the predictiveness of a positive test, and negative predictive value provides insight into the predictiveness of a negative test. Positive predictive value is calculated as the ratio of true-positives to total positives. Similarly, negative predictive value is calculated as the ratio of true-negatives to total negatives.

For clinical purposes, the values for these parameters that are acceptable vary depending on the situation. For example, the values deemed acceptable for a test used to predict for risk of a serious, life-threatening toxicity might be different than if the test is used to predict response/nonresponse.

Predictability of Response Based on Genotype—Examples from the Literature

Although few studies in the literature to date reported sensitivity, specificity, positive predictive value, or negative predictive value, it is possible to calculate these data for some studies. For example, a cited pharmacogenetics study evaluated responses of 221 patients with asthma to a 5-lipoxygenase inhibitor relative to genotype for a tandem repeat in the promoter region of the 5-lipoxygenase gene (Reference 88). Five copies of the tandem repeat is considered the wild-type, whereas three, four, or six copies are considered variant or mutant alleles. The results from this study are shown in Figure 3.

Based on the data provided, it is possible to calculate the parameters of interest with the assumption, based on the study's findings, that those with a wild-type allele are predicted as responders, whereas those without a wild-type allele are nonresponders. The numbers from this study that are necessary for calculating the parameters of interest are shown in Table 3. Of the 221 study participants, 204 carried a wild-type allele, thus, are predicted to be responders; however, only 106 of them met the criteria for response, a 12-percent increase in forced expiratory volume in 1 second. All 17 of the patients who did not carry a wild-type allele failed to achieve the target response. Thus, the sensitivity of the test was 100 percent and the specificity was 15 percent. This resulted in a positive predictive value of 52 percent and a negative predictive value of 100 percent. Thus, only 52 percent of those with a positive test (predicted responder) are actual responders. If the patient was predicted as a nonresponder, this is correct, but the test would

Table 3. Example of Sensitivity Analysis using Data from Reference 88

Response predicted by genetic test	Actual response Responder	Nonresponder
Responder	106 (TP)	98 (FP)
Nonresponder	0 (FN)	17 (TN)

Numbers represent the number of patients.
FN = false-negative; FP = false-positive; TN = true-negative; TP = true-positive.

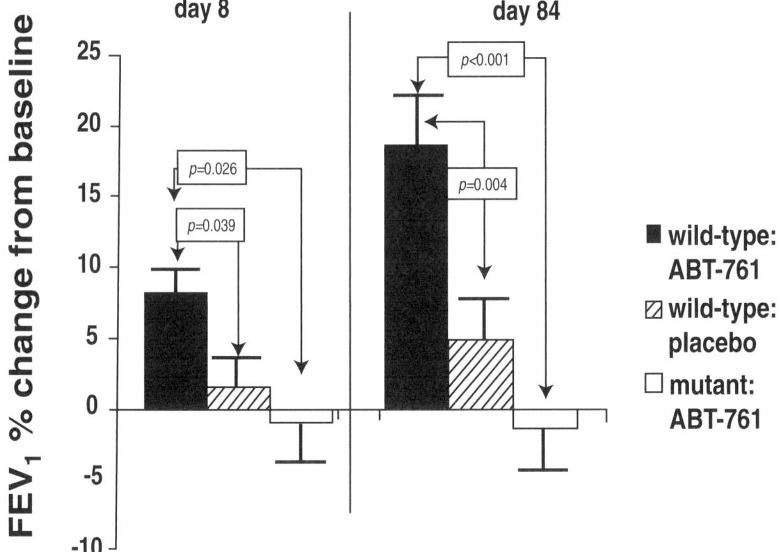

Figure 3. FEV_1 response to 5-lipoxygenase inhibitor by 5-lipoxygenase genotype.
Change in FEV_1 from baseline in 5-lipoxygenase wild-type patients given the study drug (ABT-761) (solid bars); in 5-lipoxygenase wild-type patients given placebo (hatched bars); and in 5-lipoxygenase variant patients given ABT-761 (open bars).
ALOX5 = 5-lipoxygenase; FEV_1 = forced expiratory volume in 1 second.
Reprinted with permission from Nature Publishing Group.

only detect 15 percent of all nonresponders. Thus, without testing other genetic markers, such a genetic test is probably of little value for clinical decision-making.

Such sensitivity analyses are useful in the setting where response is considered a dichotomous variable, such as response/nonresponse or toxicity/no toxicity. However, the response to drugs is a continuous variable, in which case sensitivity analysis is of little value. In this case, the most informative data comes from regression modeling, where an estimate of the relative contribution of genotype (R^2) to variable response can be tested. This was done in a few pharmacogenetic studies.

The first example of such a modeling approach comes from the study which showed a significant association between the G protein β3 subunit (*GNB3*) genotype and antihypertensive response to thiazide diuretics. In this study, the authors documented a clear association between blood pressure lowering and *GNB3* genotype (Reference 89). The authors performed multivariate regression analysis to determine relative contribution of various factors to response variability. G protein β3 subunit genotype was a significant predictor of systolic and diastolic blood pressure response, but only accounted for 3.1 percent and 4.5 percent of response variability, respectively. Thus, although contributing to the variability in response to diuretics, genotype information on this gene alone would not provide sufficient information to be predictive in the clinical setting.

Similarly, multiple regression analysis of the antihypertensive response to β-blockers relative to $β_1AR$ genotype revealed that along with baseline diastolic blood pressure, codon 389 and codon 49 genotype were significant predictors of response variability, accounting for 15 percent and 5 percent, respectively, of the observed variability in response (Reference 10). Thus, 20 percent of response variability to β-blockers might be explained by genotype at these two $β_1AR$ SNPs. And although this represents more accountability for variable response than the *GNB3* genotype—diuretic response example above—it is still insufficient predictive value to be used clinically.

Moving Drug Target Pharmacogenetics/Genomics from Proof of Concept to Clinical Practice

The previous discussion highlighted the advances in drug target pharmacogenetics in recent years. However, it also illustrates that, in most cases, the currently available information is not of sufficient predictive value for drug target pharmacogenetics to enter clinical practice. Thus, an important question is what is necessary for the predictive value of genotype information to be useful in guiding drug therapy.

All of the studies highlighted are consistent in that the studies investigated the influence of variability in a single gene on drug response. And in most cases, the studies focused on a single polymorphism in a single gene. A more sophisticated approach is needed to move drug target pharmacogenetics into clinical practice. For example, most genes are highly polymorphic, with a recent resequencing study of 313 genes revealing an average of 12.5 polymorphisms per gene (Reference 90). Thus, an approach that considers haplotype is more informative than one that focuses on single SNPs, as was evident from the β-blocker pharmacogenetic data (Reference 10) and that of the $β_2$-agonist pharmacogenetic analysis by haplotype (Reference 18).

To fully understand the genetic contribution to variable drug response, it is important to consider the complexity of the drug response. G protein-coupled receptors are the target for greater than 50 percent of the currently marketed drugs in the United States (Reference 91). Figure 4 highlights the complexity of the signal transduction cascade for G protein-coupled receptor that couple to $Gα_s$ or $Gα_i$. The β-adrenergic receptors are examples of drugs that couple to $Gα_s$. When the pharmacogenetics literature relative to $β_2$-agonists is considered, there is some discrepancy in the findings (Reference 92). However, these papers focused on variability in the $β_2AR$ gene only, yet it is clear that the $β_2AR$'s signal transduction

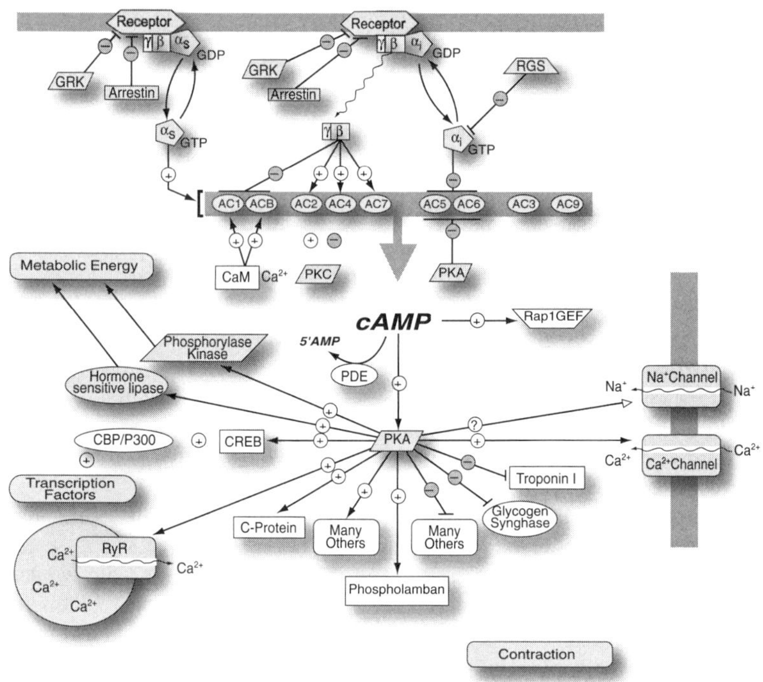

Figure 4. Representative signal transduction cascade for G protein-coupled receptors. Cartoon highlights signal transduction cascade for G protein-coupled receptors that couple to $G\alpha_i$ and $G\alpha_s$. Schematic highlights the numerous proteins, downstream from the receptor, that are involved in elciting a response to agonists.

5'AMP = 5' adenosine monophosphate; AC = adenylyl cyclase; Ca^{2+} = calcium; CaM = calmodulin; cAMP = cyclic adenosine monophosphate; GRK = G protein receptor kinases; Na^+ = sodium; PDE = phosphodiesterase; PKA = protein kinase A.

From *www.afcs.org/cm2/camp.html.*

cascade has numerous genes that contribute to variability in the β_2-agonist response. For example, there are the three protein subunits of the G protein (α, β, γ), to which the β_2AR couples. G protein receptor kinases and arrestins influence receptor regulation. Adenylyl cyclase activity influences the amount of cyclic adenosine monophosphate, phosphodiesterase metabolizes cyclic adenosine monophosphate, thus, reducing the generated second messenger. Protein kinase A is activated by cyclic adenosine monophosphate and results in activation of down stream proteins to produce the pharmacological response. Variability in the genes for any of these proteins could contribute to the variable response to β_2-agonists.

Most drugs have actions that are tied to signal transduction cascades that are similarly or more complex than that of the β_2AR. Thus, polygenic approaches that take into account the numerous proteins involved in the pharmacological response might provide information that has higher predictive value, and it is likely such an approach is needed to move pharmacogenetics into the clinical arena.

The complexity of the pharmacological effects of a drug represent another area where drug target pharmacogenetics diverges from that of drug metabolism. In the case of drug metabolism, a single protein (i.e., enzyme) plays a critical role in the metabolism of the drug, such that variability in that single protein's gene has profound effects on the drug's pharmacokinetics. Although it is possible that genetic variability for a single drug target protein has a profound effect on the drug action, this is less likely than with drug metabolizing enzymes, given the large number of proteins involved in the drug's pharmacological effects. Therefore, it seems likely that genetic tests of drug metabolizing enzyme polymorphisms will become commonplace in clinical practice before such tests for drug targets.

Genomic Approaches to Describing Drug Response Variability

Candidate Gene Approach

The previously discussed approach, where the selected genes of interest are based on knowledge of the pharmacology and pharmacokinetics of a drug, is considered a candidate gene approach. Although most studies in the literature used a single gene candidate approach, there are limited examples where a polygenic (pharmacogenomics) candidate gene approach was taken elucidate drug response variability. One such example of this approach is a study that investigated the association between response of patients with schizophrenia to clozapine and variability in 10 genes known to be involved in the pharmacology of the drug (Reference 28). These included genes for α-adrenergic receptors, dopamine receptors, serotonin receptors, histamine receptors, and the serotonin transporter. The investigators found that of the 19 polymorphisms studied, six showed the strongest association with response. The combination of these six polymorphisms provided a positive predictive value of 0.76, a negative predictive value of 0.82, with a sensitivity of 96 percent for identifying patients with schizophrenia showing improvement with clozapine and a specificity of 38 percent for identifying patients with minimal response to clozapine. Additional studies are needed to validate this model in a larger patient population, and to expand the repertoire of genes and polymorphisms investigated. These data suggest that such an approach could be useful in predicting response to clozapine.

There are insufficient examples in the literature on which to judge the superiority of a pharmacogenomic (polygenic) approach as compared to a pharmacogenetic (single gene) approach. Time will tell whether the pharmacogenomic approach is superior, but it is a logical approach, which seems to prove more powerful in the quest to move drug target pharmacogenetics into the clinical setting.

Genome Scanning Approach

An alternative approach to drug target pharmacogenetics is the genome scanning approach. The advantage of such an approach is that it does not rely on knowledge of the drug's pharmacological actions, as does the candidate gene approach. Thus, it is a particularly useful approach for drugs that are in the drug development stage, where the precise mechanisms of benefit are not well understood. Such an approach is useful for drugs whose effects seem to extend beyond their pharmacology, such as the ACE inhibitors or statins. The disadvantage of the genome scanning approach is that it requires evaluation of substantially more polymorphisms. Specifically, use of such an approach requires creation of a map of polymorphisms across the human genome (SNP map), and then this SNP map is evaluated for associations with drug response or toxicity (References 3, 93). Given that there are at least 3–4 million SNPs in the human genome, the SNP map would not include all SNPs but would be based on selected SNPs. Thus, representative SNPs, somewhat evenly spaced across the genome, are selected for testing (i.e., some have suggested 200,000–300,000 SNPs). Although the technology for genotyping has improved in recent years and the costs have fallen (to $1–2 per SNP), such an approach remains technically and financially difficult. It is presumed with such an approach that those SNPs showing an association with response or toxicity are not necessarily causative or functional polymorphisms, but in linkage disequilibrium with the functional SNP(s). However, the risk of this approach is that the functional polymorphisms are not in the SNP map or are in weak linkage disequilibrium with SNPs in the map, resulting in an inability to detect genetic associations that are present. The promise of this approach is that SNPs associated with drug response or toxicity are localized to a certain chromosomal region, and a better understanding of the precise mechanisms of benefit (or toxicity) for a drug are gained. This is an approach in the proof of concept stage, and for which pharmaceutical companies are likely to afford. Nonetheless, as further technological advances are made, this approach holds increasing appeal.

Clinical Potential for Drug Target Pharmacogenetics

It seems clear that pharmacogenetics has the potential to allow clinicians to develop individualized drug regimens for patients, based on their genetic information. Figure 5 depicts a schematic for the potential clinical utility of pharmacogenetics. Currently, there are two common approaches to drug therapy. The first approach is trial and error, an approach used for such

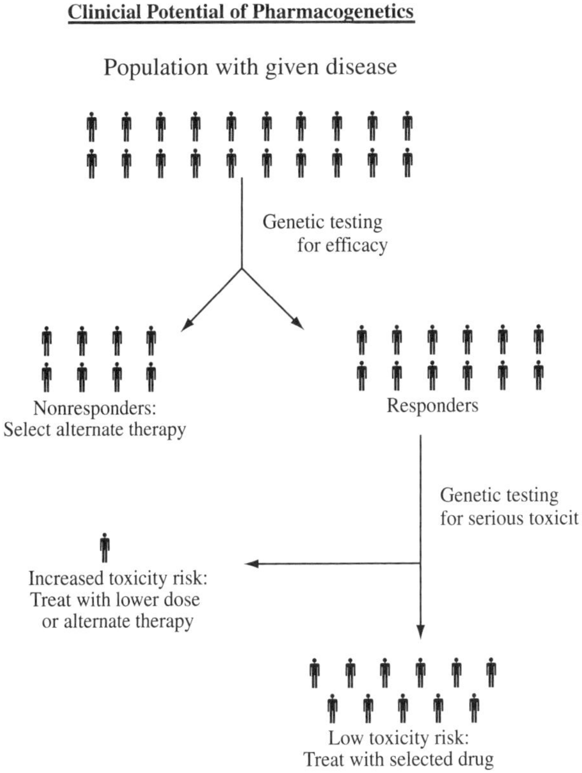

Figure 5. Clinical potential for pharmacogenomics.
A representative population with a given disease is highlighted. Current treatment with the hypothetical drug is by trial and error and results in a response rate of 60 percent. Pharmacogenomic testing for efficacy will allow identification of responders and nonresponders. Nonresponders would be prescribed an alternative therapy. Responders could undergo subsequent testing for genetic/genomic risk for serious toxicity. Those identified as being at high risk of toxicity would be given a lower dose, or alternative therapy. The remaining patients would be ideal candidates for the therapy–at low risk of toxicity with high likelihood for a beneficial response.

treatments as hypertension, diabetes, depression, schizophrenia, asthma, seizure disorders, and infectious diseases, among others. The other approach is one in which all patients with a given disease receive essentially the same drug therapy. Common disease states and clinical situations managed by this approach include most cancers, post-transplant patients, heart failure, acute myocardial infarction, among others. Both approaches have the potential of improvement by addition of pharmacogenetics to help guide drug therapy.

For diseases managed by the trial and error approach, the potential benefit of pharmacogenetics is that effective therapy for the patient is more easily identified, resulting in earlier appropriate management of the patient's disease. This is particularly important for silent diseases, such as hypertension or diabetes, where failure to find effective therapy leads to some patients losing faith or interest in the drug therapy management of their disease. The benefits of pharmacogenetics are easier to document in this category, given that response is easy to measure in a relatively short time frame. Thus, it seems that drug target pharmacogenetics is likely to first enter clinical practice for diseases managed by a trial and error approach.

The benefits of pharmacogenetics are more difficult to document for diseases managed by standard regimens, in part because in many cases the response is more difficult or takes longer to measure (e.g., prolonged survival or response to chemotherapy). The benefits of pharmacogenetics in this group of diseases are more individualized therapy, avoiding drugs (and their toxicity) that are of little benefit to the patient, and perhaps allowing for additional therapy that is beneficial. And either approach (trial and error or standard protocol) has the potential to benefit from recognition of patients at toxicity risk from a particular drug.

Pharmacogenetics also potentially allows practitioners to move away from the practice of using race/ethnicity in determining drug therapy. For example, for treating hypertension, racial differences in responses to various antihypertensives are cited as the basis for choosing initial therapy in a given patient. There is recent debate about the role of race on response to heart failure therapies. Although race has been a reasonable surrogate in the pregenomics era, it has clear flaws in the genomics era (Reference 94). When taking this approach, a clinician is using one set of variant alleles (i.e., those controlling skin pigmentation or hair texture) to predict another set of variant alleles (i.e., those associated with a drug response). Recent pharmacogenetic studies of β-blockers and diuretics highlight that much of the clinically observed difference in drug response by race is because of racial differences in the frequencies of the polymorphisms associated with drug response (References 9, 10, 89). In both cases, race and genotype are significant predictors of response in univariate regression analysis. However, in multivariate analysis, race is no longer a significant response predictor, suggesting that it is genotype, not race that is the major determinant of the clinically observed differences in response by race or ethnicity.

In summary, pharmacogenetics will enter into the practice of pharmacy and medicine in an important way in the next decade. If it meets its potential, pharmacogenetics will lead to safer and more effective use of drugs to treat disease.

References

1. Evans WE, Johnson JA. Pharmacogenomics: the inherited basis for interindividual differences in drug response. Annu Rev Genomics Hum Genet 2001;2:9–39.

2. Evans WE, McLeod HL. Pharmacogenomics–drug disposition, drug tables, and side effects. N Engl J Med 2003;348:538–49.

3. Roses AD. Pharmacogenetics and the practice of medicine. Nature 2000;405:857–65.

4. Shi MM, Bleavins MR, de la Iglesia FA. Pharmacogenetic application in drug development and clinical trials. Drug Metab Dispos 2001;29:591–5.

5. Spear BB, Heath-Chiozzi M, Huff J. Clinical application of pharmacogenetics. Trends Mol Med 2001;7:201–4.

6. Johnson JA, Evans WE. Molecular diagnostics as a predictive tool: genetics of drug efficacy and toxicity. Trends Mol Med 2002;8:300–5.

7. Johnson JA. Drug target pharmacogenomics: an overview. Am J Pharmacogenomics 2001;1:271–81.

8. Weinshilboum R. Inheritance and drug response. N Engl J Med 2003;348:529–39.

9. Johnson JA, Terra SG. Beta-adrenergic receptor polymorphisms: cardiovascular disease associations and pharmacogenetics. Pharm Res 2002;19:1779–87.

10. Johnson JA, Zineh I, Puckett BJ, McGorray SP, Yarandi HN, Pauly DF. Beta 1-adrenergic receptor polymorphisms and antihypertensive response to metoprolol. Clin Pharmacol Ther 2003;74:44–52.

11. Mason DA, Moore JD, Green SA, Liggett SB. A gain-of-function polymorphism in a G-protein coupling domain of the human beta1-adrenergic receptor. J Biol Chem 1999;274:12670–4.

12. Rathz DA, Brown KM, Kramer LA, Liggett SB. Amino acid 49 polymorphisms of the human beta 1-adrenergic receptor affect agonist-promoted trafficking. J Cardiovasc Pharmacol 2002;39:155–60.

13. Maqbool A, Hall AS, Ball SG, Balmforth AJ. Common polymorphisms of beta1-adrenoceptor: identification and rapid screening assay [letter]. Lancet 1999;353:897.

14. Israel E, Drazen JM, Liggett SB, et al. The effect of polymorphisms of the beta(2)-adrenergic receptor on the response to regular use of albuterol in asthma. Am J Respir Crit Care Med 2000;162:75–80.

15. Lima JJ, Thomason DB, Mohamed MHN, Eberle LV, Self TH, Johnson JA. Impact of genetic polymorphisms of the beta2-adrenergic receptor on albuterol bronchodilator pharmacodynamics. Clin Pharmacol Ther 1999;65:519–25.

16. Martinez FD, Graves PE, Baldini M, Solomon S, Erickson R. Association between genetic polymorphisms of the beta2-adrenoceptor and response to albuterol in children with and without a history of wheezing. J Clin Invest 1997;100:3184–8.

17. Tan S, Hall IP, Dewar J, Dow E, Lipworth B. Association between beta 2-adrenoceptor polymorphism and susceptibility to bronchodilator desensitisation in moderately severe stable asthmatics [see comments]. Lancet 1997;350:995–9.

18. Drysdale CM, McGraw DW, Stack CB, et al. Complex promoter and coding region beta 2-adrenergic receptor haplotypes alter receptor expression and predict in vivo responsiveness. Proc Natl Acad Sci U S A 2000;97:10483–8.

19. Gratze G, Fortin J, Labugger R, et al. Beta-2 Adrenergic receptor variants affect resting blood pressure and agonist-induced vasodilation in young adult Caucasians. Hypertension 1999;33:1425–30.

20. Hoit BD, Suresh DP, Craft L, Walsh RA, Liggett SB. Beta2-adrenergic receptor polymorphisms at amino acid 16 differentially influence agonist-stimulated blood pressure and peripheral blood flow in normal individuals. Am Heart J 2000;139:537–42.

21. Cockcroft JR, Gazis AG, Cross DJ, et al. Beta(2)-adrenoceptor polymorphism determines vascular reactivity in humans. Hypertension 2000;36:371–5.

22. Suzuki A, Kondo T, Mihara K, et al. The -141C Ins/Del polymorphism in the dopamine D2 receptor gene promoter region is associated with anxiolytic and antidepressive effects during treatment with dopamine antagonists in schizophrenic patients. Pharmacogenetics 2001;11:545–50.

23. Suzuki A, Mihara K, Kondo T, et al. The relationship between dopamine D2 receptor polymorphism at the Taq1 A locus and therapeutic response to nemonapride, a selective dopamine antagonist, in schizophrenic patients. Pharmacogenetics 2000;10:335–41.

24. Eichhammer P, Albus M, Borrmann-Hassenbach M, et al. Association of dopamine D3-receptor gene variants with neuroleptic induced akathisia in schizophrenic patients: a generalization of Steen's study on DRD3 and tardive dyskinesia. Am J Med Genet 2000;96:187–91.

25. Lerer B, Segman RH, Fangerau H, et al. Pharmacogenetics of tardive dyskinesia: combined analysis of 780 patients supports association with dopamine D3 receptor gene Ser9Gly polymorphism. Neuropsychopharmacology 2002;27:105–19.

26. Basile VS, Masellis M, Badri F, et al. Association of the MscI polymorphism of the dopamine D3 receptor gene with tardive dyskinesia in schizophrenia. Neuropsychopharmacology 1999;21:17–27.

27. Hwu HG, Hong CJ, Lee YL, Lee PC, Lee SF. Dopamine D4 receptor gene polymorphisms and neuroleptic response in schizophrenia. Biol Psychiatry 1998;44:483–7.

28. Arranz MJ, Munro J, Birkett J, et al. Pharmacogenetic prediction of clozapine response [letter]. Lancet 2000;355:1615–6.

29. Joober R, Benkelfat C, Brisebois K. T102C polymorphism in the 5HT2A gene and schizophrenia: relation to phenotype and drug response variability [see comments]. J Psychiatry Neurosci 1999;24:141–6.

30. Tan EC, Chong SA, Mahendran R, Dong F, Tan CH. Susceptibility to neuroleptic-induced tardive dyskinesia and the T102C polymorphism in the serotonin type 2A receptor. Biol Psychiatry 2001;50:144–7.

31. Reynolds GP, Zhang ZJ, Zhang XB. Association of antipsychotic drug-induced weight gain with a 5-HT2C receptor gene polymorphism. Lancet 2002;359:2086–7.

32. Kohno M, Yokokawa K, Minami M, et al. Association between angiotensin-converting enzyme gene polymorphisms and regression of left ventricular hypertrophy in patients treated with angiotensin-converting enzyme inhibitors. Am J Med 1999;106:544–9.

33. Penno G, Chaturvedi N, Talmud PJ, et al. Effect of angiotensin-converting enzyme (ACE) gene polymorphism on progression of renal disease and the influence of ACE inhibition in IDDM patients: findings from the EUCLID Randomized Controlled Trial. EURODIAB Controlled Trial of Lisinopril in IDDM. Diabetes 1998;47:1507–11.

34. Perna A, Ruggenenti P, Testa A, et al. ACE genotype and ACE inhibitors induced renoprotection in chronic proteinuric nephropathies1. Kidney Int 2000;57:274–81.

35. Ha SK, Yong Lee S, Su Park H, et al. Angiotensin-converting enzyme D/D genotype is more susceptible than ACE II and ID genotypes to the antiproteinuric effect of ACE inhibitors in patients with proteinuric non-insulin-dependent diabetes mellitus. Nephrol Dial Transplant 2000 Oct;15:1617–23.

36. Takahashi T, Yamaguchi E, Furuya K, Kawakami Y. The ACE gene polymorphism and cough threshold for capsaicin after cilazapril usage. Respir Med 2001;95:130–5.

37. Stavroulakis GA, Makris TK, Krespi PG, et al. Predicting response to chronic antihypertensive treatment with fosinopril: the role of angiotensin-converting enzyme gene polymorphism. Cardiovasc Drugs Ther 2000;14:427–32.

38. Hernandez D, Lacalzada J, Salido E, et al. Regression of left ventricular hypertrophy by lisinopril after renal transplantation: role of ACE gene polymorphism. Kidney Int 2000;58:889–97.

39. Prasad A, Narayanan S, Husain S, et al. Insertion-deletion polymorphism of the ACE gene modulates reversibility of endothelial dysfunction with ACE inhibition. Circulation 2000;102:35–41.

40. Whale R, Quested DJ, Laver D, Harrison PJ, Cowen PJ. Serotonin transporter (5-HTT) promoter genotype may influence the prolactin response to clomipramine. Psychopharmacology (Berl) 2000;150:120–2.

41. Smeraldi E, Zanardi R, Benedetti F, Di Bella D, Perez J, Catalano M. Polymorphism within the promoter of the serotonin transporter gene and antidepressant efficacy of fluvoxamine. Mol Psychiatry 1998;3:508–11.

42. Serretti A, Zanardi R, Rossini D, Cusin C, Lilli R, Smeraldi E. Influence of tryptophan hydroxylase and serotonin transporter genes on fluvoxamine antidepressant activity. Mol Psychiatry 2001;6:586–92.

43. Rausch JL, Johnson ME, Fei YJ, et al. Initial conditions of serotonin transporter kinetics and genotype: influence on SSRI treatment trial outcome. Biol Psychiatry 2002;51:723–32.

44. Pollock BG, Ferrell RE, Mulsant BH, et al. Allelic variation in the serotonin transporter promoter affects onset of paroxetine treatment response in late-life depression. Neuropsychopharmacology 2000;23:587–90.

45. Mundo E, Walker M, Cate T, Macciardi F, Kennedy JL. The role of serotonin transporter protein gene in antidepressant-induced mania in bipolar disorder: preliminary findings. Arch Gen Psychiatry 2001;58:539–44.

46. Kim DK, Lim SW, Lee S, et al. Serotonin transporter gene polymorphism and antidepressant response. Neuroreport 2000;11:215–9.

47. Jia H, Hingorani AD, Sharma P, et al. Association of the G(s)alpha gene with essential hypertension and response to beta-blockade. Hypertension 1999;34:8–14.

48. Mukae S, Aoki S, Itoh S, Iwata T, Ueda H, Katagiri T. Bradykinin B(2) receptor gene polymorphism is associated with angiotensin-converting enzyme inhibitor-related cough. Hypertension 2000;36:127–31.

49. Emmerich J, Rosendaal FR, Cattaneo M, et al. Combined effect of factor V Leiden and prothrombin 20210A on the risk of venous thromboembolism—pooled analysis of 8 case-control studies including 2310 cases and 3204 controls. Study Group for Pooled-Analysis in Venous Thromboembolism. Thromb Haemost 2001;86:809–16.

50. Martinelli I, Sacchi E, Landi G, Taioli E, Duca F, Mannucci PM. High risk of cerebral-vein thrombosis in carriers of a prothrombin-gene mutation and in users of oral contraceptives. N Engl J Med 1998;338:1793–7.

51. Napolitano C, Schwartz PJ, Brown AM, et al. Evidence for a cardiac ion channel mutation underlying drug-induced QT prolongation and life-threatening arrhythmias. J Cardiovasc Electrophysiol 2000;11:691–6.

52. Drici MD, Barhanin J. Cardiac K+ channels and drug-acquired long QT syndrome. Therapie 2000;55:185–93.

53. Abbott GW, Sesti F, Splawski I, et al. MiRP1 forms IKr potassium channels with HERG and is associated with cardiac arrhythmia. Cell 1999;97:175–87.

54. Roden DM. Pharmacogenetics and drug-induced arrhythmias. Cardiovasc Res 2001;50:224–31.

55. Escande D. Pharmacogenetics of cardiac K(+) channels. Eur J Pharmacol 2000;410:281–7.

56. Splawski I, Timothy KW, Tateyama M, et al. Variant of SCN5A sodium channel implicated in risk of cardiac arrhythmia. Science 2002;297:1333–6.

57. Hetherington S, Hughes AR, Mosteller M, et al. Genetic variations in HLA-B region and hypersensitivity reactions to abacavir. Lancet 2002;359:1121–2.

58. Mallal S, Nolan D, Witt C, et al. Association between presence of HLA-B*5701, HLA-DR7, and HLA-DQ3 and hypersensitivity to human

immunodeficiency virus-1 reverse-transcriptase inhibitor abacavir. Lancet 2002;359:727–32.

59. Gerdes LU, Gerdes C, Kervinen K, et al. The apolipoprotein epsilon4 allele determines prognosis and the effect on prognosis of simvastatin in survivors of myocardial infarction: a substudy of the Scandinavian simvastatin survival study. Circulation 2000;101:1366–71.

60. Nemeth A, Szakmary K, Kramer J, et al. Apolipoprotein E and complement C3 polymorphism and their role in the response to gemfibrozil and low fat low cholesterol therapy. Eur J Clin Chem Clin Biochem 1995;33:799–804.

61. Ordovas JM, Lopez-Miranda J, Perez-Jimenez F, et al. Effect of apolipoprotein E and A-IV phenotypes on the low density lipoprotein response to HMG CoA reductase inhibitor therapy. Atherosclerosis 1995;113:157–66.

62. Kuivenhoven JA, Jukema JW, Zwinderman AH, et al. The role of a common variant of the cholesteryl ester transfer protein gene in the progression of coronary atherosclerosis. The Regression Growth Evaluation Statin Study Group [see comments]. N Engl J Med 1998;338:86–93.

63. de Maat MP, Jukema JW, Ye S, et al. Effect of the stromelysin-1 promoter on efficacy of pravastatin in coronary atherosclerosis and restenosis. Am J Cardiol 1999;83:852–6.

64. de Maat MP, Kastelein JJ, Jukema JW, et al. -455G/A polymorphism of the beta-fibrinogen gene is associated with the progression of coronary atherosclerosis in symptomatic men: proposed role for an acute-phase reaction pattern of fibrinogen. REGRESS group. Arterioscler Thromb Vasc Biol 1998;18:265–71.

65. Farlow MR, Lahiri DK, Poirier J, Davignon J, Schneider L, Hui SL. Treatment outcome of tacrine therapy depends on apolipoprotein genotype and gender of the subjects with Alzheimer's disease. Neurology 1998;50:669–77.

66. Poirier J, Delisle MC, Quirion R, et al. Apolipoprotein E4 allele as a predictor of cholinergic deficits and treatment outcome in Alzheimer disease. Proc Natl Acad Sci U S A 1995;92:12260–4.

67. Lucking CB, Durr A, Bonifati V, et al. Association between early-onset Parkinson's disease and mutations in the parkin gene. French Parkinson's Disease Genetics Study Group. N Engl J Med 2000;342:1560–7.

68. Makoff AJ, Graham JM, Arranz MJ, et al. Association study of dopamine receptor gene polymorphisms with drug-induced hallucinations in patients with idiopathic Parkinson's disease. Pharmacogenetics 2000;10:43–8.

69. Van Vaerenbergh K, Harrer T, Schmit JC, et al. Initiation of HAART in drug-naive human immunodeficiency virus type 1 patients prevents viral breakthrough for a median period of 35.5 months in 60 percent of the patients. AIDS Res Hum Retroviruses 2002;18:419–26.

70. Grossman Z, Vardinon N, Chemtob D, et al. Genotypic variation of human immunodeficiency virus-1 reverse transcriptase and protease: comparative analysis of clade C and clade B. AIDS 2001;15:1453–60.

71. Demeter L, Haubrich R. International perspectives on antiretroviral resistance. Phenotypic and genotypic resistance assays: methodology, reliability, and interpretations. J Acquir Immune Defic Syndr 2001;26 Suppl 1:S3–9.

72. Weinstein MC, Goldie SJ, Losina E, et al. Use of genotypic resistance testing to guide hiv therapy: clinical impact and cost-effectiveness. Ann Intern Med 2001;134:440–50.

73. Wolle K, Leodolter A, Malfertheiner P, Konig W. Antibiotic susceptibility of *Helicobacter pylori* in Germany: stable primary resistance from 1995 to 2000. J Med Microbiol 2002;51:705–9.

74. Owen RJ, Slater ER, Gibson J, Lorenz E, Tompkins DS. Effect of clarithromycin and omeprazole therapy on the diversity and stability of genotypes of *Helicobacter pylori* from duodenal ulcer patients. Microb Drug Resist 1999;5:141–6.

75. Kruuner A, Pehme L, Ghebremichael S, Koivula T, Hoffner SE, Mikelsaar M. Use of molecular techniques to distinguish between treatment failure and exogenous reinfection with Mycobacterium tuberculosis. Clin Infect Dis 2002;35:146–55.

76. Shak S. Overview of the trastuzumab (Herceptin) anti-HER2 monoclonal antibody clinical program in HER2-overexpressing metastatic breast cancer. Herceptin Multinational Investigator Study Group. Semin Oncol 1999;26:71–7.

77. Hofmann WK, de Vos S, Elashoff D, et al. Relation between resistance of Philadelphia-chromosome-positive acute lymphoblastic leukaemia to the tyrosine kinase inhibitor STI571 and gene-expression profiles: a gene-expression study. Lancet 2002;359:481–6.

78. von Bubnoff N, Schneller F, Peschel C, Duyster J. BCR-ABL gene mutations in relation to clinical resistance of Philadelphia-chromosome-positive leukacmia to STI571: a prospective study. Lancet 2002;359:487–91.

79. Hofmann WK, Jones LC, Lemp NA, et al. Ph(+) acute lymphoblastic leukemia resistant to the tyrosine kinase inhibitor STI571 has a unique BCR-ABL gene mutation. Blood 2002;99:1860–2.

80. Roche-Lestienne C, Soenen-Cornu V, Grardel-Duflos N, et al. Several types of mutations of the Abl gene can be found in chronic myeloid leukemia patients resistant to STI571, and they can pre-exist to the onset of treatment. Blood 2002;100:1014–8.

81. Libura J, Bettens F, Radkowski A, Tiercy JM, Piguet PF. Risk of chemotherapy-induced pulmonary fibrosis is associated with polymorphic tumour necrosis factor-a2 gene. Eur Respir J 2002;19:912–8.

82. Sasaki M, Oki T, Iuchi A, et al. Relationship between the angiotensin converting enzyme gene polymorphism and the effects of enalapril on left ventricular hypertrophy and impaired diastolic filling in essential hypertension: M-mode and pulsed Doppler echocardiographic studies. J Hypertens 1996;14:1403–8.

83. Okamura A, Ohishi M, Rakugi H, et al. Pharmacogenetic analysis of the effect of angiotensin-converting enzyme inhibitor on restenosis after percutaneous transluminal coronary angioplasty. Angiology 1999;50:811–22.

84. Ohmichi N, Iwai N, Uchida Y, Shichiri G, Nakamura Y, Kinoshita M. Relationship between the response to the angiotensin converting enzyme inhibitor imidapril and the angiotensin converting enzyme genotype. Am J Hypertens 1997;10:951–5.

85. Cannella G, Paoletti E, Barocci S, et al. Angiotensin-converting enzyme gene polymorphism and reversibility of uremic left ventricular hypertrophy following long-term antihypertensive therapy. Kidney Int 1998;54:618–26.

86. Ioannidis JP, Trikalinos TA, Ntzani EE, Contopoulos-Ioannidis DG. Genetic associations in large versus small studies: an empirical assessment. Lancet 2003;361:567–71.

87. Dawson B, Trapp RG. Methods of evidence-based medicine. In: Dawson B, Trapp RG, eds. Basic and clinical biostatistics. New York, NY: McGraw-Hill, 2001:262–81.

88. Drazen JM, Yandava CN, Dube L, et al. Pharmacogenetic association between 5-lipoxygenase promoter genotype and the response to anti-asthma treatment. Nat Genet 1999;22:168–70.

89. Turner ST, Schwartz GL, Chapman AB, Boerwinkle E. C825T polymorphism of the G protein beta(3)-subunit and antihypertensive response to a thiazide diuretic. Hypertension 2001;37:739–43.

90. Stephens JC, Schneider JA, Tanguay DA, et al. Haplotype variation and linkage disequilibrium in 313 human genes. Science 2001;293:489–93.

91. Marinissen MJ, Gutkind JS. G-protein-coupled receptors and signaling networks: emerging paradigms. Trends Pharmacol Sci 2001;22:368–76.

92. Johnson JA, Terra SG. Beta-adrenergic receptor polymorphisms: Cardiovascular disease associations and pharmacogenetics. Pharm Res 2002;19:1779–87.

93. McCarthy JJ, Hilfiker R. The use of single-nucleotide polymorphism maps in pharmacogenomics. Nat Biotechnol 2000;18:505–8.

94. Schwartz RS. Racial profiling in medical research. N Engl J Med 2001;344:1392–3.

95. Szczeklik A, Sanak M, Undas A. Platelet glycoprotein IIIa pl(a) polymorphism and effects of aspirin on thrombin generation. Circulation 2001;103:E33–4.

96. Michelson AD, Furman MI, Goldschmidt-Clermont P, et al. Platelet GP IIIa Pl(A) polymorphisms display different sensitivities to agonists. Circulation 2000;101:1013–8.

97. Cooke GE, Bray PF, Hamlington JD, Pham DM, Goldschmidt-Clermont PJ. PlA2 polymorphism and efficacy of aspirin. Lancet 1998;351:1253.

98. Brandt JT, Isenhart CE, Osborne JM, Ahmed A, Anderson CL. On the role of platelet Fc gamma RIIa phenotype in heparin-induced thrombocytopenia. Thromb Haemost 1995;74:1564–72.

99. Psaty BM, Smith NL, Heckbert SR, et al. Diuretic therapy, the alpha-adducin gene variant, and the risk of myocardial infarction or stroke in persons with treated hypertension. JAMA 2002;287:1680–9.

100. Kurland L, Melhus H, Karlsson J, et al. Aldosterone synthase (cytochrome P450 11B2) -344 C/T polymorphism is related to antihypertensive response: result from the Swedish Irbesartan Left Ventricular Hypertrophy Investigation versus Atenolol (SILVHIA) trial. Am J Hypertens 2002;15:389–93.

101. Fujimoto TT, Inoue M, Shimomura T, Fujimura K. Involvement of Fc gamma receptor polymorphism in the therapeutic response of idiopathic thrombocytopenic purpura. Br J Haematol 2001;115:125–30.

102. Asderakis A, Sankaran D, Dyer P, et al. Association of polymorphisms in the human interferon-gamma and interleukin-10 gene with acute and chronic kidney transplant outcome: the cytokine effect on transplantation. Transplantation 2001;71:674–7.

103. Mazariegos GV, Reyes J, Webber SA, et al. Cytokine gene polymorphisms in children successfully withdrawn from immunosuppression after liver transplantation. Transplantation 2002;73:1342–5.

104. Herrington DM, Howard TD, Hawkins GA, et al. Estrogen-receptor polymorphisms and effects of estrogen replacement on high-density lipoprotein cholesterol in women with coronary disease. N Engl J Med 2002;346:967–74.

105. Ongphiphadhanakul B, Chanprasertyothin S, Payatikul P, et al. Oestrogen-receptor-alpha gene polymorphism affects response in bone mineral density to oestrogen in post-menopausal women. Clin Endocrinol (Oxf) 2000;52:581–5.

106. Meirhaeghe A, Helbecque N, Cottel D, et al. Impact of sulfonylurea receptor 1 genetic variability on non-insulin- dependent diabetes mellitus prevalence and treatment: a population study. Am J Med Genet 2001;101:4–8.

107. Hansen T, Echwald SM, Hansen L, et al. Decreased tolbutamide-stimulated insulin secretion in healthy subjects with sequence variants in the high-affinity sulfonylurea receptor gene. Diabetes 1998;47:598–605.

108. Suzuki A, Kondo T, Otani K, et al. Association of the TaqI A polymorphism of the dopaminc D2 receptor gene with predisposition to neuroleptic malignant syndrome. Am J Psychiatry 2001;158:1714–6.

109. Zill P, Baghai TC, Zwanzger P, et al. Evidence for an association between a G-protein beta3-gene variant with depression and response to antidepressant treatment [In Process Citation]. Neuroreport 2000;11:1893–7.

110. Steen VM, Lovlie R, Osher Y, Belmaker RH, Berle JO, Gulbrandsen AK. The polymorphic inositol polyphosphate 1-phosphatase gene as a candidate for pharmacogenetic prediction of lithium-responsive manic-depressive illness. Pharmacogenetics 1998;8:259–68.

111. Turbay D, Lieberman J, Alper CA, et al. Tumor necrosis factor constellation polymorphism and clozapine-induced agranulocytosis in two different ethnic groups. Blood 1997;89:4167–74.

112. Girard T, Urwyler A, Censier K, Mueller CR, Zorzato F, Treves S. Genotype-phenotype comparison of the Swiss malignant hyperthermia population. Hum Mutat 2001;18:357–8.

113. Sambuughin N, McWilliams S, de Bantel A, Sivakumar K, Nelson TE. Single-amino-acid deletion in the RYR1 gene, associated with malignant hyperthermia susceptibility and unusual contraction phenotype. Am J Hum Genet 2001;69:204–8.

114. Sambuughin N, Sei Y, Gallagher KL, et al. North American malignant hyperthermia population: screening of the ryanodine receptor gene and identification of novel mutations. Anesthesiology 2001;95:594–9.

115. McCarthy TV, Quane KA, Lynch PJ. Ryanodine receptor mutations in malignant hyperthermia and central core disease. Hum Mutat 2000;15:410–7.

116. Martinelli I, Taioli E, Bucciarelli P, Akhavan S, Mannucci PM. Interaction between the G20210A mutation of the prothrombin gene and oral contraceptive use in deep vein thrombosis. Arterioscler Thromb Vasc Biol 1999;19:700–3.

117. Farlow MR, Lahiri DK, Poirier J, Davignon J, Hui S. Apolipoprotein E genotype and gender influence response to tacrine therapy. Ann N Y Acad Sci 1996;802:101–10.

Self-Assessment Questions

1. Atenolol is a β_1-selective blocker that is eliminated primarily by the kidneys. It is well recognized that when used to treat hypertension, 30–50 percent of patients have inadequate blood pressure lowering with atenolol. Which one of the following has the greatest potential for contributing to this variability in response?

   A. A nonsynonymous single nucleotide polymophism (SNP) in the cytochrome P450 2D6 enzyme gene.
   B. A synonymous SNP in the β_1-adrenergic receptor (B_1AR) gene.
   C. A nonsynonymous SNP in the β_1AR gene.
   D. An intronic insertion/deletion polymorphism in the angiotensin-converting enzyme (ACE) gene.

2. A receptor that is the target of drug X recently was resequenced in a large population to describe its variability. The following polymorphisms were discovered: polymorphism A–a nonsynonymous SNP; polymorphism B–a synonymous SNP; polymorphism C–a 4 base pair tandem repeat in exon 2 (with 2, 3, or 4 repeats); polymorphism D–an 152 base pair insertion/deletion polymorphism located 87 base pair into intron 6. Which one of the following is most likely to influence a response to the drug X?

   A. Polymorphism A.
   B. Polymorphism B.
   C. Polymorphism C.
   D. Polymorphism D.

Questions 3–5 pertain to the following case.

Drug B is used to treat human immunodeficiency virus/acquired immune deficiency syndrome and is associated with a rare (0.5 percent), but serious side effect. Although there are alternative therapies to drug B, it is considered to have superior efficacy to the alternatives in the treatment of human immunodeficiency virus/acquired immune deficiency syndrome. Thus, there is a desire to uncover a possible genetic basis for this adverse effect.

3. A study designed to assess this would compare polymorphism allele frequencies between which one of the following?

   A. Patients with the side effect and patients exposed to drug without the side effect.
   B. Patients with the side effect and the general population.

   C. Patients with the side effect and a general population of human immunodeficiency virus/acquired immune deficiency syndrome patients.
   D. Patients with human immunodeficiency virus/acquired immune deficiency syndrome and random individuals from the general population.

4. Based on the case, which polymorphism is *most likely* associated with the side effect?

   A. A nonsynonymous polymorphism with an allele frequency of 0.20.
   B. A combination of polymorphisms (haplotype) that occurs in less than 1 percent of the population.
   C. A synonymous polymorphism with an allele frequency of 0.005.
   D. A polymorphism in the 3' untranslated region with an allele frequency of 0.10.

5. A study was performed to identify the genetic risk factor(s) for the adverse effect of drug B. The authors identified a combination of polymorphisms that showed statistically significant association with the adverse effect. The authors reported that the positive predictive value was 87 percent and the negative predictive value was 21 percent. Which one of the following is the best interpretation?

   A. Patients with the polymorphism combination should not receive drug B.
   B. Patients without the polymorphism combination can receive drug B with minimal to no risk of the toxicity in question.
   C. This information is of no value in the clinical use of drug B.
   D. The likelihood of the patients with the combination of polymorphisms *not* experiencing the adverse effect is 21 percent.

6. Some genetic polymorphisms in drug metabolizing enzymes result in profound changes in the pharmacokinetics of a drug, whereas in most cases, the effect of genetic polymorphisms in most drug targets are more subtle. All except which one of the following may be explanations for this finding?

   A. Some of the drug metabolism polymorphisms result in absent or nonfunctional protein.
   B. Functional polymorphisms in drug targets most commonly involve changes in a single amino acid or a SNP in the promoter region that influences protein expression.
   C. Most genes for drug targets lack genetic polymorphisms, whereas the genes for drug metabolizing enzymes have numerous polymorphisms.

D. Numerous proteins typically are involved in the pharmacological response, whereas a single protein may be primarily involved in the elimination of a drug.

7. It has been noted clinically that about 40 percent of patients who receive drug Q have little or no response to it. Studies were undertaken to determine whether there was a genetic association between the drug targets and poor response. Which one of the following best describes this approach?

   A. Phenotype to genotype approach.
   B. Genotype to phenotype approach.
   C. Clinical observation to clinical trial to molecular diagnostics.
   D. Genome scanning approach.

8. Studies have suggested that ACE inhibitor-induced cough is associated with a genetic polymorphism in the bradykinin B2 receptor. Which one of the following best describes this genetic association?

   A. It likely represents a type 1 statistical error since there is no pharmacological basis for this protein being involved in the ACE inhibitor-induced cough.
   B. Genetic association with the direct drug target.
   C. Genetic association with a drug transporter.
   D. Genetic association with a protein that is not a direct drug target but is involved in the pharmacological response cascade.

9. Routine use of pharmacogenetic information in clinical decision-making has the potential to do which one of the following?

   A. Eliminate the need for intensive follow-up of patients after initiation of drug therapy.
   B. Replace other approaches that currently are used in choosing a patient's drug therapy, and represent the sole factor used in drug therapy selection.
   C. Be highly accurate in predicting drug efficacy and/or toxicity.
   D. Reduce health care expenditures.

10. Incorporation of pharmacogenomics into the drug development process is likely to result in which one of the following?

    A. Larger Phase II trials.
    B. Larger Phase III trials.
    C. Increased numbers of blockbuster drugs.
    D. Fewer restrictions on product labeling.

Pharmacogenomics in Drug Discovery and Drug Development

John M. Valgus, Pharm.D., BCOP

Key Words

Pharmacogenomics, drug development, drug discovery, microarray analysis, toxicogenomics.

Abstract

Pharmacogenomics has the potential to revolutionize the drug discovery and development process. The ideal way to use pharmacogenomics in drug discovery and development has yet to be determined. However, rapid progress is being made in this field and the number of genomic-driven medicines on the market is on the rise. Clinicians are now seeing the first generation of genomic-based drugs with novel mechanisms of action, improved efficacy, and reduced toxicities. Therefore, it is imperative for pharmacists and health care professionals to be aware of this arising technology. By measuring gene expression profiles in various disease states, microarray technology is aiding researchers in identifying new potential drug targets and screening new compounds for potential toxicities. Pharmacogenomic analysis currently is being implemented broadly throughout the preclinical and clinical development phases of drug development. Pharmacogenomic analysis in clinical trials can identify patients who receive therapeutic benefit or those who are at increased risk of toxicity. Pharmacogenomic analysis incorporated into postmarketing surveillance is a powerful tool that may aid in identifying patients who experience rare but serious adverse reactions that were not evident in clinical trials. Before pharmacogenomics is incorporated into mainstream medicine, health care professionals and regulators also will need to identify and develop policies regarding the ethical, legal, and pharmacoeconomic issues that will accompany this science.

Outline

Learning Objectives

1. Describe the risks and values that genomic information brings to the drug discovery and development process.
2. Understand how pharmacogenomics and genomic technology will lead to an increased number of drug targets.
3. Identify how pharmacogenomics could be implemented and used in each phase of preclinical and clinical trials.
4. Identify key regulatory issues that pharmacogenomics raise in the drug development process.

Abbreviations in this Chapter

ADR   Adverse drug reaction
BCR-ABL   Translation products of a fusion messenger ribonucleic acid derived from the breakpoint cluster region (bcr) gene and a cellular abl (c-abl) gene translocated to chromosome 22
CML   Chronic myeloid leukemia
DNA   Deoxyribonucleic acid
FDA   Food and Drug Administration

HIV	Human immunodeficiency virus
HLA-B	Human lymphocyte antigen B
IND	Investigational new drug
NDA	New drug application
PhRMA	Pharmaceutical Research and Manufacturers of America
PWG	Pharmacogenetics Working Group
RNA	Ribonucleic acid
SACGT	Secretary's Advisory Committee on Genetic Testing
SNP	Single nucleotide polymorphism
UGT1	Uridine diphosphate glucuronosyltransferase 1

Introduction

Rooted in chemistry and guided by pharmacology, biochemistry, and medical sciences, drug discovery and development has arguably had more impact on the progress of medical sciences than any other discipline. Looking back over the past 2 centuries of drug discovery and development, there are several monumental scientific breakthroughs that have left lasting impressions on this field. Select examples include the isolation of morphine from opium extract by F.W. Serturner in 1815; Paul Ehrlich's theory of chemoreceptors in 1872, which led to the birth of modern chemotherapy; and the discovery of penicillin by Alexander Flemming in 1929, which opened the door to a new era in infection treatment. Many experts feel that recent advances in genomic technology will be the next breakthrough to bring a paradigm shift in the way novel therapeutic agents are discovered and developed.

In the past 2 decades, the influence of molecular biology on drug discovery and development has been profound. The number of recombinant proteins and monoclonal antibody-based drugs being developed is rapidly growing and has opened a new era of targeted drug therapy. Much like the days of Ehrlich and Flemming, this day and age is an era where the drug discovery and development process is being revolutionized. The explosion of data and technological advances in the field of genomics is giving researchers new insights into disease mechanisms and better ideas for novel drug targets. In this "postgenomic" era, the pharmaceutical and biotechnology industry is scrambling to figure out how best to use this technology to aid in the discovery and development of novel therapeutic agents, which will offer maximal efficacy profiles while minimizing adverse drug reactions (ADRs). With advancements in discovering the roles of proteins and pathways relevant to cellular pathophysiology and disease, the industry has identified hundreds of novel drug targets which are now entering preclinical and clinical trials. For agents already on the market or in clinical trials, pharmacogenomics has helped identify those populations that are most likely to respond or who may be more susceptible to ADRs.

Now, pharmacogenomics is being implemented across all phases of drug discovery and development—from target discovery to postmarketing surveillance. This chapter provides an overview of how and where pharmacogenomics is aiding the drug development and discovery process, and what regulatory and social issues this new technology raises.

Pharmacogenomics in Drug Discovery
New Target Discovery

The entire biopharmaceutical industry currently is based on less than 500 drug targets (Reference 1). With an estimated 5000–10,000 of our genes being possible therapeutic targets, it is obvious that the surface of potential targets has barely been scratched. By giving new insights into disease mechanisms, genomic technology promises to produce several hundred to thousands more. Although this potential seems massive, the percentage of these targets that will be therapeutically useful and pharmacologically manipulatable is debated and remains to be determined (Reference 2). To mine these new targets, the biopharmaceutical industry has taken a multidisciplinary genomic approach, which includes rapid deoxyribonucleic acid (DNA) sequencing, molecular profiling, proteomics, and predictive toxicogenomics to name a few. When these new technologies are combined with the latest advances in combinatorial chemistry and automated high-throughput screening, the result will be a large influx of hypothetical targets to be validated in in vitro, cell-based assays and in silico experiments.

It is estimated that it takes about 15 years to bring a new compound through the discovery and development process. By targeting smaller, more specific populations with enhanced efficacy and reduced toxicity profiles, pharmacogenomics promises to reduce this amount of time by several years. On average, the cost to bring a new compound to market is estimated to range from $100 million up to $800 million. By reducing the number of failed compounds, decreasing time of development, and building smaller, higher powered clinical trials, pharmacogenomics will reduce the attrition costs by millions of dollars. These are the promises of pharmacogenomics which have lured pharmaceutical and biotechnology companies alike to invest billions into this new science. However, many experts have warned the biopharmaceutical industry that this time and cost savings will only come after up-front, large scale investments that may, in actuality, first drive research and development costs upward and increase the cost of each new chemical entity or drug chosen for development (Reference 3).

The main driver for this increase in research and development costs may be the lack of supporting data behind new targets. Traditionally, before a target was identified for development, there would be a plethora of in vitro and animal model studies supporting its efficacy. Traditional studies also often were supported by clinical trials of compounds which were similar in mechanism of action to existing marketed agents with proven efficacy.

Currently, the number of supporting literature references for a given target is less than 10 compared to more than a hundred references per target being developed a decade ago (Reference 3). In general, what this means for the drug development industry is higher risk targets; and the higher the risk of failure of a given target, the higher the potential attrition costs will be. Although genomics may be bringing a higher element of failure in a certain capacity, there also are several genomic technologies aimed at reducing much of the risk that was associated with drug discovery in the past. Toxicogenomics, which is the marriage of functional genomics and toxicology, is one of the most exciting new technologies with this promise.

Toxicogenomics

The drug discovery process begins with identifying disease targets and designing novel chemical compounds with potency toward these targets. Once a chemical compound has been identified, it then enters the development phase where a therapeutic index will be evaluated. The therapeutic index is the ratio of the dose needed to produce a beneficial effect versus the relative safety of this dose. The higher the therapeutic index, the safer a drug will be at a given dose. Traditionally, there has been a wide gap between the chemical discovery phase and evaluating the compound for possible toxicity. The development phase often can follow by several months to years after the chemical entity has been chosen. The safety of the chemical compound or drug candidate begins with in vitro and animal model testing and later is tested in humans in Phase I trials. Often, it is here where many drug candidates fail because of an unacceptable therapeutic index. At this point, the compound is terminated from development and back-up compounds must be chosen. As can easily be seen, this can be an inefficient process and the later in the development phase that this occurs, the more costly this failed candidate becomes. In an ideal environment, researchers would be able to evaluate both efficacy and toxicity simultaneously early in the discovery process. Toxicogenomics is giving researchers new insights on how to make this model environment a reality.

The ultimate purpose of toxicogenomics is to predict toxicity early in the discovery phase before a compound is even tested in humans. In turn, this will improve the prioritization of lead compounds and subsequently reduce total drug development time and research and development costs. Gene expression technologies currently are being tested in this area with the promise of giving new insights into the mechanisms behind both efficacy and toxicity. Deoxyribonucleic acid microarrays in particular, allow researchers to quantify gene expression through examining levels of messenger ribonucleic acid (RNA) in certain tissues. These gene expression profiling techniques now allow for genome-wide analysis of gene expression at the RNA and protein level and are being incorporated widely throughout the drug discovery and development process. Preliminary research has indicated that if expression was measured before and after exposure to specific drugs, gene expression profiles or fingerprints could be developed. By using these DNA fingerprints, the drugs' effects to certain biological pathways could be traced, depending on which genes were over- or underexpressed after exposure. The pharmaceutical industry is using this same technology to explore the toxic effects of chemical compounds on specific biological systems. The utility of these techniques has been validated by testing compounds with already known toxicity mechanisms such as acetaminophen, carbamazepine, carbon tetrachloride, and etoposide. The results of gene expression trials have shown that expression profiles do correlate with already known toxicity mechanisms as well as provide insight in new possible details regarding toxicity pathways. Researchers also have been able to cluster known hepatotoxins based on their mechanism of toxicity and the results of gene expression experiments (Reference 4). With a growing database of such gene expression data, compounds early in development may be compared to these known hepatotoxins early in the screening process. If similar expression profiles are seen, this may be a red flag that the new agent also may have the same properties in humans as the known hepatotoxins. However, it is most likely that this technology will have to be coupled with histopathologic and chemical experiments to delineate true mechanisms of toxicity and to determine if these experiments will correlate with clinical outcomes.

Gene expression experiments hold much more promise than just predictive toxicogenomics and will undoubtedly also feed much information into drug discovery's search for novel compounds. By comparing the expression profiles of patients with or without specific disease states, researchers may be able to hypothesize genetic roots of disease. Researchers also can examine diseased and healthy tissue in the same patient to determine what molecularly makes the tissue different. Much work is being published on expression profiles predicting response to therapy and survival in patients with breast cancer and certain types of non-Hodgkin's lymphoma (References 5,6). Whether these and other examples will eventually be used clinically remains to be determined.

There is little doubt that expression profiling will contribute significantly to the drug discovery and development process; however, at the present, this technology is still in its infancy. Before gene expression profiling leads researchers to delineating mechanisms of action and prediction of toxicity in humans, there will need to be a better understanding of the complexities that accompany gene expression (Reference 7). Such complexities include time and dose relationships to expression profiles, the need for better statistical analysis tools to interpret the resulting massive amounts of data derived from expression profiles, and better techniques for mining which expression changes are clinically most significant in humans.

In addition to helping to create safer compounds earlier in the development phase, pharmacogenomics will bring a flurry of new compounds to the benchtop with completely novel mechanisms of action. Clinicians are already seeing the first phase of these new genetic-based drugs being introduced into clinical practice. An example can be seen with the agent imatinib mesylate (Gleevec), which was developed by Novartis pharmaceuticals and is used to treat Philadelphia chromosome-positive chronic myeloid leukemia (CML). Chronic myeloid leukemia is characterized by a reciprocal translocation between chromosome 9 and 22 which, when discovered, provided the first evidence of a specific genetic mutation associated with a human cancer (Reference 8). The consequence of this mutation is the formation of the BCR-ABL (translation products of a fusion messenger RNA derived from the breakpoint cluster region [bcr] gene and a cellular abl [c-abl] gene translocated to chromosome 22) gene, which encodes a protein with increased tyrosine kinase activity and has been linked as the oncogenic event responsible for the pathogenesis of CML. Imatinib mesylate is a selective tyrosine kinase inhibitor which inhibits proliferation and induces apoptosis in cell lines with this genetic abnormality. Imatinib mesylate has not only proven to be a tremendous scientific breakthrough in the laboratory, but has proven to be just as remarkable in the clinic. Imatinib mesylate is a truly targeted therapy with tremendous efficacy proven in clinical trials to be superior to any other agent used to treat CML (References 9, 10). In addition, because of its specificity toward leukemic cells, the side effect profile also is benign, with patients usually only experiencing mild side effects, if any at all. The success of imatinib mesylate has set the stage in drug discovery for similar agents and other proposed targeted novel therapies for cancer therapy. Discovering and understanding the key molecular differences in various diseases may allow for the discovery of similar breakthrough compounds with tremendous potential for positive impacts for patient care.

Pharmacogenomics in Drug Development

Although genomics is revolutionizing the way novel drug compounds are discovered, the more immediate impact of pharmacogenomics will probably come from those compounds already in the development stage. Once the research efforts shift to clinical trials, the goal is to identify genetic markers for drug safety and efficacy, although certain information may still feed back into the pipeline to provide information on novel targets and next generation compounds. Mainly because of the cost of implementing pharmacogenomics into clinical trials, controversy remains over where in the drug development process that pharmacogenomics best fits. There are opportunities for pharmacogenomics to impact all phases of clinical trials. By defining the desired outcome, frequency of variant alleles of interest, and frequency of desired phenotype, the most appropriate and cost-efficient use of pharmacogenomic analysis can be used. Table 1 describes potential advantages to implementing pharmacogenomics across various phases of drug development.

In Phase I clinical trials, the goal is to test a new drug or treatment in a small group of patients for the first time to evaluate safety, determine the safe dosage range, and identify ADRs. Implementing pharmacogenomics early in Phase I studies has several advantages. A Phase I trial is the first opportunity to evaluate safety in humans. If any results of preclinical pharmacogenomic information raised concerns for possible populations that may be of increased risk of toxicity, they can be evaluated here before the compound moves to larger, more costly clinical trials. Also, if a patient demonstrates toxicity at an unexpectedly low-dose or if the toxicity was not expected, then the patient may be screened to evaluate if he or she may have been genetically susceptible to this adverse event. In theory, this could prevent the premature termination of a compound, which may have been otherwise continued in development. For example, a patient who takes drug X develops a specific side effect. From previous pharmacogenetic data, patients with a specific polymorphism are more likely to develop this side

Table 1. Pharmacogenomics in Various Phases of Drug Development

Phase I	• Correlation between genotype, phenotype, and pharmacokinetic and pharmacodynamics of drug candidate
	• First opportunity in humans to evaluate those who may be more genetically susceptible to adverse events
	• For unexpected adverse events, can explore genetic explanations before moving drug target further in development
Phase II	• First opportunity to evaluate if pharmacogenomics can influence efficacy in humans
	• First opportunity to evaluate influence of pharmacogenomics in target population
	• Can give valuable information on strategies for further development in Phase II trials
Phase III	• Large scale evaluation of influence of pharmacogenomics on specific efficacy parameters
	• Large scale evaluation of influence of pharmacogenomics on those who may be more susceptible to adverse events
	• Gain valuable information about possible genetic drivers of disease and how this may influence response
	• Information on those who do and do not benefit can feed back into the pipeline to develop novel targets and strategies
Phase IV	• Evaluation of relatively rare adverse events that may not have been seen in clinical trials
	• Overall market impact of pharmacogenomics

effect when exposed to drugs either related or unrelated to drug X. This patient is then screened for the polymorphism that has put patients at risk for this particular ADR. Based on this evaluation, the drug may only exhibit this effect in this specific subpopulation. Normally, without this pharmacogenomic information, the compound would probably be stopped here in development and eliminated. However, after pharmacogenomic analysis, the developers can make a decision if development should continue with screening for patients with this susceptibility gene or if development should be halted.

The main advantage of implementing pharmacogenomic testing in early Phase I studies is to determine if any ADRs associated with this phase can be explained genetically. Phase I also is an excellent opportunity to test or generate information that can be validated in Phase II trials. One example is to evaluate the effect of polymorphic cytochrome P450 enzymes on the pharmacokinetics of a new compound metabolized through this pathway. If in Phase I trials, there is a significant effect, then in Phase II trials, investigators can screen for patients with these drug metabolism polymorphisms and adjust the doses accordingly and evaluate outcomes with this strategy. The regular use of pharmacokinetic samples in Phase I trials in addition to the broad dosing ranges usually seen make this an ideal situation to evaluate pharmacogenetic/kinetic interactions. Of course, the main drawback of using pharmacogenomic analysis in Phase I is the small amount of patients in each study. If the polymorphisms that are selected for analysis only occur in a small percentage of the population, then there is a low likelihood that a patient with the polymorphism would even be enrolled. One way to overcome this limitation is to combine the analysis to include all Phase I trials that the compound will go through. Another option is to specifically screen for patients with a specific polymorphism of interest and test the hypothesis in this population separately from an unscreened population. Depending on the allele frequency of the variant, this could be both time- and resource-consuming to screen a general population for a less frequently occurring variant. Regardless if results demonstrated the polymorphism to have significance, this information would have most likely to be confirmed in larger Phase II or III trials which would be much better suited to test the robustness of the pharmacogenomic test.

In Phase II trials, the goal is to evaluate the study drug or treatment in a larger, more defined group of patients to evaluate efficacy and further evaluate safety. A Phase II trial is the first time clinicians can truly evaluate efficacy in humans and determine if pharmacogenomics can be used to better predict response. The advantages of Phase II trials are a larger, more defined population, while still being much smaller and less costly than Phase III trials. In the current system, if a drug progresses to Phase III trials, even if Phase II trials showed a low percentage of responders, the Phase III trial is powered to show significant results by predicting the low percentage of responders. This method results in a much larger trial than if there were a higher percentage of responders. Large, less selective clinical trials also expose the majority of patients to the risk of ADRs in face of the fact that most will not respond to the drug. If the results of pharmacogenomic analysis of Phase I and II trials demonstrated strong correlation with clinical outcomes, then follow-up phase III trials could incorporate pharmacogenomics to better tailor the study population. Patients could then be stratified by their "response profiles". This stratification could reduce interpatient variability in response, limit unnecessary exposure to ineffective or dangerous therapies, increase the chance of statistically significant results of the clinical trial, and decrease the cost of development by reducing the size of the Phase III pivotal trials. Pharmacogenomics also would help identify patients who do not respond to conventional therapy and would expedite the process of finding novel therapies to reach the unmet medical needs of these patients.

Whether these potential benefits of using pharmacogenomics in Phase I and II trials will truly yield clinical benefit remains to be determined. Many experts suggest that targeting smaller populations goes against the current philosophy of drug development, which is dominated by the drive to produce the next "blockbuster" agent that will be used in the majority of patients with a common, chronic disease, such as asthma, diabetes, and hypertension. What pharmacogenomics does to this philosophy is to drive the market toward developing several "minibusters". These agents would not be used to treat everyone with a common disease, just specific subpopulations within this larger group. Pharmacogenomics will likely provide clues as to why not all patients respond in the same manner to a blockbuster agent. By using pharmacogenomics, patients will be more selectively chosen based on likelihood of response or susceptibility to side effects. In the subsequent Phase III trials, the target population will be based on the results of the earlier Phase I and II trials, which will ultimately mean smaller, less expensive Phase III trials. Also, Phase I and II data can be fed back into the pipeline so that a compound can be developed to specifically target the subpopulations in which the current compound was ineffective.

To date, pharmacogenomics most commonly has been implemented in Phase III trials and beyond. It is common across many large pharmaceutical company-sponsored Phase III trials to institute genetic sample collections for all participants in the trial. Phase III studies have the advantage of having a homogeneous, well-defined patient population, specific therapeutic outcomes being measured, and a large number of patients to be evaluated. This information could be beneficial to the developers by identifying potential "super-responders" or identifying a subpopulation that may be at a higher risk of an ADR. Identifying subpopulations of responders may be especially beneficial if the results in the overall population were inferior to competitor compounds in regard to efficacy or toxicity. In this case, the likelihood of approval would be slim. If it is shown that there are subpopulations with superior efficacy to competitor compounds, then approval may be granted at least for this specific subpopulation.

The main drawback of implementing pharmacogenomic analysis in Phase III studies is the cost associated with collecting, storing, and genotyping this large number of samples. Also, because this information is generated so late in development, there is concern that any relevant information may actually complicate the approval process. It would be detrimental if the results of the overall trial were equal or superior to the competitor compounds but pharmacogenomic data demonstrated different responses in subpopulations. In this scenario, without the pharmacogenomic data, the compound would probably be approved for the overall population if the Phase III results were equal to or better than the competitor. Adding the pharmacogenomic data could possibly hold this process up by complicating the issues. Pharmacogenomics also could dissect the market of the compound demonstrating subpopulations that would either not respond as well or be at increased risk of an adverse drug reaction. Pharmacogenomics may potentially raise conflicts of interest between those with more of a commercial focus and those who are truly most interested in what is most beneficial for the patient. These potential risks are discussed in more detail in the Regulatory Concerns and Ethical Concerns sections.

A clear example of how pharmacogenomics could be used in Phase III trials was briefly described with an experimental agent, Tranilast, which was being developed by GlaxoSmithKline to treat restenosis after percutaneous transluminal coronary revascularization (Reference 11). During the Phase III pivotal trial, about 10 percent of patients experienced hyperbilirubinemia. Although no patients progressed to hepatic failure, a 10-percent incidence of hyperbilirubinemia most likely would have raised regulator concerns over the safety of this drug. Pharmacogenomic analysis discovered that patients with a specific polymorphism within the uridine diphosphate glucuronosyltransferase 1 (*UGT1*) gene were particularly susceptible to Tranilast-induced hyperbilirubinemia. Polymorphisms within this region were previously linked with Gilbert's syndrome, a spontaneously occurring benign form of hyperbilirubinemia. Because the pharmacogenomic analysis determined that Tranilast could induce Gilbert's syndrome in patients already susceptible and not result in more severe hepatic dysfunction, drug development termination or black box label warning for the potentially serious hepatic ADR could have been prevented. Unfortunately, it will never be known how this scenario would have resulted because Tranilast did not prove efficacy in preventing restenosis of coronary vessels and was subsequently terminated in development.

With more pharmacogenomic data being generated in Phase I and II trials, the future methodology of Phase III trials may, in the not too distant future, routinely use pharmacogenomics in the inclusion and exclusion criteria. In the meantime, many investigators are analyzing pharmacogenetic data from Phase III trials retrospectively. Such analysis can be conducted by reanalyzing data once a clinical trial is complete and restratifying patients based on results of genetic samples taken during the study. Retrospective analysis also could be done by going back to patients who were enrolled in a previously completed trial, genotyping them with a specific pharmacogenetic hypothesis in mind, then going back to reanalyze the data. There is controversy about whether this type of study should be labeled prospective, retrospective, or both. There also is controversy about whether this type of trial is suitable for regulatory purposes. To date, there have been no submissions including this type of information so there is no information about whether this type of information would be acceptable for regulatory purposes.

In a recent article summarizing the major discussion points of a pharmacogenomic workshop cosponsored by the Food and Drug Administration (FDA), the Pharmacogenetics Working Group (PWG), the Pharmaceutical Research and Manufacturers of America (PhRMA), and the PhRMA Preclinical Safety Committee, the authors stated that if such studies met several specific conditions then this trial may be acceptable for regulatory purposes (Reference 12). Some of the specific conditions included adequate power in the genetically defined subsets, adequately validated genotyping test, clear biologic relation between response and the gene, a prospective hypothesis for assessing the response-genotype relationship, and follow-up by an independent prospective trial.

Postmarketing Surveillance

There have been an alarming number of approved drugs pulled from the market because of rare but serious idiosyncratic ADRs. The drugs that cause more frequent serious ADRs will usually fail somewhere along one of the clinical trial phases. However, the agents that cause serious ADRs occurring less frequently (less than one in 1000) may not cause these ADRs seen in the clinical trials, which may be limited to a few thousand patients. When the drug is approved and is used for the first time by tens of thousands to hundreds of thousands of people, then the rare adverse event may surface, resulting in a market withdrawal or black box warning, depending on the risk-to-benefit ratio of the drug. A few recent examples of safety-based drug withdrawals include cerivastatin (Baycol), alosetron (Lotronex), cisapride (Propulsid), troglitazone (Rezulin), and terfenadine (Seldane). By using pharmacogenomic surveillance of these agents, patients who experience rare, serious ADRs could be genotyped and compared to controls who did not experience ADRs. If the results of the analysis were highly predictive, could this information then be used to screen out patients who may be genetically predisposed to the ADR and allow patients who may receive benefit to have continued access to the effective drugs? Unfortunately for the majority of these cases, it may never be known if pharmacogenomics had a role in these ADRs.

By reflecting on these previous drug withdrawals because of life-threatening ADRs, the potential value of Phase IV and postmarketing pharmacogenetic surveillance studies can clearly be seen. An example of pharmacogenetics making an impact in postmarketing surveillance can be seen with the drug abacavir, a reverse transcriptase inhibitor used to treat human immunodeficiency virus (HIV). Abacavir is associated with a hypersensitivity reaction characterized by multisystem involvement and occurs in about 4 percent of the population (Reference 13). Symptoms usually manifest within 6 weeks from the initiation of treatment and consist of fever, rash, gastrointestinal symptoms, and respiratory symptoms. The reaction worsens with continued therapy and symptoms usually improve within 24 hours of drug discontinuation. Rechallenging patients who previously demonstrated abacavir hypersensitivity results in recurrence of symptoms within hours.

Two independent research groups have published results on candidate gene analysis aimed at determining if there is a genetic predisposition to abacavir hypersensitivity reactions (References 14, 15). One retrospective, case-control study was conducted to identify multiple markers in the vicinity of the human lymphocyte antigen B (HLA-B) associated with hypersensitivity which included 85 cases of hypersensitivity and 115 controls (Reference 15). Many polymorphisms within the HLA-B region occurred more frequently in cases than controls. In particular 39 (46 percent) cases had the HLA-B5701 polymorphism compared to only four (4 percent) of controls. In a separate trial, a cohort study, which included the first 200 patients participating in the Western Australian HIV Cohort Study, was conducted (Reference 14). In the cohort of 200 patients, 18 confirmed cases of abacavir hypersensitivity were identified. This study found that the HLA-B5701 polymorphism was present in 14 (78 percent) of the cases of abacavir hypersensitivity and in four (2 percent) of the patients who tolerated abacavir.

These studies both demonstrated the possibility that genetic factors can be used to identify patients at increased risk of serious ADRs. The utility of these data is still being debated by clinicians and regulators because of the low sensitivity of these markers in predicting abacavir hypersensitivity in the more heterogenous population of the retrospective, case-controlled study It is hoped that a follow-up study using whole genome single nucleotide polymorphism (SNP) mapping will provide a more sensitive tool to identify patients at increased risk of abacavir hypersensitivity by evaluating thousands of markers across the genome. These data show the promise of using postmarketing survcillance to track possible ADRs with drugs on the market. If all of the cases of a particular ADR could be collected and pharmacogenetic markers for ADRs were identified, then it would be possible to screen out patients who are genetically predisposed to the adverse event and keep the drug available for those who benefit from it.

In summary, pharmacogenomics has the potential to impact drug development at all phases. Instituting pharmacogenomics early in Phase I and II trials has the advantages of giving clues early to subpopulations that may have a varied response to a drug while still early in development. This information could help better tailor Phase III trials and identify patients who may have been genetically predisposed to certain ADRs. The major disadvantage would be the small number of patients evaluable in these earlier trials. The pharmacogenomic results of Phase III trials have the potential to truly tailor therapy to the patient by being able to predict those most likely to respond and those who are at most risk of ADRs. By using pharmacogenomics prospectively, the size of Phase III clinical trials could possibly be reduced. If the results of Phase III pharmacogenomic analysis show benefit, then labeling and identifying the targeted patient population will be impacted significantly. Postmarketing pharmacogenomic surveillance holds the highest hope for being able to predict and explain the biology behind serious idiosyncratic ADRs. This will help clinicians to identify patients who are at increased risk of certain ADRs. Postmarketing surveillance also may help prevent useful drugs from being pulled from the market because of rare ADRs at the expense of losing a potentially useful drug for a large population who responded well to that same agent.

Regulatory Concerns

As genomics rapidly moves to the forefront of discovering new therapies, regulatory agencies have begun preparing for what challenges this new science will bring. In June 1998, in response to the recommendations of Human Genome Project task forces, the Secretary's Advisory Committee on Genetic Testing (SACGT) was chartered by the Department of Health and Human Services. The duty of the SACGT was to advise the government about all aspects of the development and use of genetic tests, including the complex medical, ethical, legal, and social issues raised by genetic testing, which also has the potential to apply to pharmacogenetic testing.

The FDA also has begun developing steps to handle the potential influx of pharmacogenomic information that may accompany many investigational new drugs (INDs) and new drug applications (NDAs) in the near future (References 12, 16). The FDA currently is accepting pharmacogenomic information submitted by the industry to use in regulatory decision-making; however, to date, the FDA has had limited experience with submissions with pharmacogenomic data. The FDA has released interim results of a survey identifying the extent to which pharmacogenomics has been used in submitted data (Reference 16). The results demonstrate that the scope of research was limited mostly to evaluate pharmacokinetic interindividual variability and did not result in any specific dosing recommendations for a genetic subgroup of the populations studied.

Because the FDA has seen such limited pharmacogenetic data, the question of how the FDA will address issues raised by pharmacogenomics is still uncertain and is of major concern to those involved in drug discovery and development. Potential issues include: Is it acceptable to stratify patients *a priori* by genotype? How would stratifying by genotype affect the product label? Would a diagnostic test have to be submitted with the drug? What are the specificity/sensitivity requirements of a pharmacogenomic test? and What data need to be collected from patients who were excluded from the trial based on a specific genotype? These issues are only a few of the issues the FDA and the pharmaceutical industry will have to address before pharmacogenomics becomes a routine part of the drug development process. In preparation for this potential influx of pharmacogenomic data, the FDA has initiated several steps to ensure that the agency will be ready to handle these data. Educational programs for staff, regular meetings with representatives within the pharmaceutical industry, organization of internal working groups, and collaborating with other regulatory agencies are some examples of how the FDA is moving forward to prepare for pharmacogenomic data submissions.

Ethical Concerns

Incorporating pharmacogenomics into the drug development process also has several ethical ramifications (Reference 17). Whenever patients are preselected or excluded from a clinical trial based on their genetic make-up, issues must be addressed as to the fate of the population that was excluded. This genetic screening may lead to medically ignored populations and, to some extent, genetic discrimination. Not only will there not be many data to support the efficacy of specific drugs in these populations, but there also will be a lack of safety data in case clinicians would like to use the drug off-label in patients with an unmet medical need.

If the field of pharmacogenomics matures into its expected role in to mainstream medicine, then it will only be a matter of time until the field of pharmacogenomics meets the field of pharmacoeconomics. Public health experts will have to provide guidance as to how all citizens will be able to benefit from these potentially costly therapies which require genetic testing before the prescription is written. As is the case with already approved costly agents on the market, drug manufacturers will play a substantial role in providing access to patients who may not be able to afford the specific therapy but who would benefit from it. In a system where the underprivileged already do not receive appropriate health care, it is possible that genomic medicine may widen the gap even further among those social classes that may vary in access the health care.

If it is found through pharmacogenomic research that patients have an untreatable subclassification of a common disease, such as diabetes, what will the psychological impact be on the patient? How would this information affect the friends and family of the patient? What if a private insurer were to learn of this? These are all unresolved issues that are being brought up as the science of pharmacogenomics develops. As advances are made in developing this science, progress also must be made in developing public policy and ethical guidelines to deal with the issues that accompany the science.

Conclusions

In summary, the field of pharmacogenomics will have a significant impact on the discovery and development of new drugs. Many researchers feel that pharmacogenomics will revolutionize this process. Pharmacogenomics has the potential to aid researchers early in the pipeline to choose safer compounds for development and also to identify thousands of novel drug targets.   Once a compound is in development, pharmacogenomics will help identify patients who are more or less likely to respond to or have ADRs with a given agent. Across all phases of drug development, pharmacogenomics has potential advantages and disadvantages, and the single best manner to use this technology has yet to be determined. Along with the science, come several regulatory and ethical issues, which drug developers will have to address for the benefits of pharmacogenomics to be integrated into the health care system. Although there are only a handful of examples of genetically derived compounds on the market currently, the science is progressing rapidly with billions of dollars being spent by drug developers to figure out how this technology can best be used. Only time will tell how this revolution will end.

References

1.   Drews J. Drug discovery: a historical perspective. Science 2000;287:1960–4.

2.   Hopkins AL, Groom CR. The druggable genome. Nat Rev Drug Discov 2002;1:727–30.

3.   Fruits of genomics: drug pipelines face indigestion until the new biology ripens. Lehman Brothers/McKinsey & Co. Research, 2001.

4.   Waring JF, Jolly RA, Ciurlionis R, et al. Clustering of hepatotoxins based on mechanism of toxicity using gene expression profiles. Toxicol Appl Pharmacol 2001;175:28–42.

5.   van de Vijver MJ, He YD, van't Veer LJ, et al. A gene-expression signature as a predictor of survival in breast cancer. New Engl J Med 2002;347(24):1999–2009.

6.   Shipp MA, Ross KN, Tamayo P, et al. Diffuse large B-cell lymphoma outcome prediction by gene expression profiling and supervised machine learning. Nat Med 2002;8(1):68–74.

7.   Fielden MR, Zacharewski TR. Challenges and limitations of gene expression profiling in mechanistic and predictive toxicology. Toxicol Sci 2001;60:6–10.

8. Nowell PC, Hungerford DA. A minute chromosome in human granulocytic leukemia. Science 1960;132:1497.

9. O'Brien SG, Guilhot F, Larson RA, et al. Imatinib compared with interferon and low-dose cytarabine for newly diagnosed chronic-phase chronic myeloid leukemia. N Engl J Med 2003;348:994–1004.

10. Kantarjian H, Sawyers C, Hochhaus A, et al. Hematologic and cytogenetic responses to imatinib mesylate in chronic myelogenous leukemia. N Engl J Med 2002;346:645–52.

11. Roses AD. Genome-based pharmacogenetics and the pharmaceutical industry. Nat Rev Drug Discov 2002;1:541–9.

12. Lesko LJ, Salerno RA, Spear BB, et al. Pharmacogenetics and pharmacogenomics in drug development and regulatory decision-making: report of the first FDA-PWG-PhRMA-DruSafe Workshop. J Clin Pharmacol 2003;43:342–58.

13. Hewitt RG. Abacavir hypersensitivity reaction. Clin Infect Dis 2002;34:1137–42.

14. Mallal S, Nolan D, Witt C, et al. Association between presence of HLA-B*5701, HLA-DR7, and HLA-DQ3 and hypersensitivity to HIV-1 reverse-transcriptase inhibitor abacavir. Lancet 2002;359:727–32.

15. Hetherington S, Hughes AR, Mosteller M, et al. Genetic variations in HLA-B region and hypersensitivity reactions to abacavir. Lancet 2002;359:1121–2.

16. Lesko LJ, Woodcock J. Pharmacogenomic-guided drug development: regulatory perspective. Pharmacogenomics J 2002;2:20–4.

17. Issa AM. Ethical perspectives on pharmacogenomic profiling in the drug development process. Nat Rev Drug Discov 2002;1(4):300–8.

Self-Assessment Questions

1. The entire biopharmaceutical industry currently is based on less than 500 drug targets. Pharmacogenomics will most likely cause which one of the following to happen?

    A. There will be no impact to drug target numbers.
    B. Number of drug targets will decrease.
    C. Number of new drug targets will increase significantly.
    D. Significantly increase the number of potential new drug targets.

2. Which one of the following drug-disease state combinations is the best example of how pharmacogenomics can lead to rational drug design resulting in superior clinical outcomes?

    A. Imatinib and chronic myelogenous leukemia (CML).
    B. 6-Mercaptopurine and acute lymphocytic leukemia.
    C. Tranilast and restenosis.
    D. Abacavir and human immunodeficiency virus (HIV).

3. Which one of the following steps are examples of how the Food and Drug Administration (FDA) is preparing to deal with the future influx of pharmacogenomic data?

    A. Meeting with industry pharmacogenomic working groups to listen to concerns and identify issues that need resolution.
    B. Surveillance of investigational new drugs (INDs) and new drug applications (NDAs) to find new examples of usage of pharmacogenomic information.
    C. Development of educational programs for current FDA staff.
    D. By meeting with industry pharmacogenomic groups, surveying INDs and NDAs, *and* developing educational programs.

4. Which one of the following is the primary concern with incorporating pharmacogenomics into Phase I clinical trials?

    A. Patients will not accept pharmacogenomics at this stage of research.
    B. Small number of patients enrolled in Phase I trials makes analysis difficult.
    C. Pharmacogenomic information will only be useful in Phase III trials where efficacy is the primary objective.
    D. Pharmacogenomic information will only be useful in Phase II trials and beyond, where safety and efficacy are being evaluated in specific disease states.

5. Full-scale incorporation of pharmacogenomics into drug discovery and development would most likely lead to a market dominated by which one of the following types of drug?

   A. Several agents within a therapeutic category, each having high efficacy and low toxicity in small genetic subgroups of patients.
   B. A large number of blockbuster agents that are highly efficacious and have low toxicity for a high percentage of populations with common diseases such as diabetes and hypertension.
   C. Several agents that will be genetically engineered to meet the specific genome of each individual patient.
   D. Gene therapy that will alter or replace defective disease susceptibility genes.

6. Pharmacogenomics has the potential to add value to which one of the following phases of drug development?

   A. Only preclinical target discovery and evaluation.
   B. Only Phase I–III clinical trials.
   C. Only postmarketing surveillance.
   D. All phases of drug development.

7. Implementing pharmacogenomics into which one of the following phases of drug development has the best chance of explaining serious adverse drug reactions (ADRs), which occur in a very small percentage (less than one in 1000) of the population?

   A. Phase I.
   B. Phase II.
   C. Phase III.
   D. Postmarketing surveillance.

8. An ethical dilemma that may arise as a result of incorporating pharmacogenomics into clinical trials includes which one of the following?

   A. May create medically ignored, genetic subpopulations.
   B. Lack of safety data in populations that have been genetically screened out of studies but who may still receive the drug off-label.
   C. Genetic discrimination.
   D. Creation of genetic subpopulations, lack of safety data, *and* genetic discrimination.

9. The ultimate purpose of toxicogenomics is which one of the following?

   A. Predict patients who are most likely to respond to a given therapy.
   B. Predict potential ADRs early on in the drug discovery phase before a compound is tested in humans.

C. Identify novel drug targets based on gene expression patterns, which can be used in the drug discovery process.

D. Compare diseased versus normal tissue to elucidate genetic drivers of disease.

10. Which one of the following statements is incorrect regarding gene expression profiles?

A. The results of gene expression trials have shown that expression profiles correlate with already known toxicity mechanisms.

B. Gene microarrays quantify gene expression through examining levels of messenger ribonucleic acid in certain tissues.

C. A major barrier that exists with using gene expression profiles is that only a limited number of genes can be examined with this technique.

D. The pharmaceutical industry currently is using gene expression to explore the toxic effects of chemical compounds on specific biological systems.

Societal and Ethical Issues in Pharmacogenomics

Pilar Ossorio, Ph.D., J.D.

Key Words

Ethnicity, equality, eugenics, fairness, genetic variation, health disparities, justice, law, miscegenation, pharmacogenetics, pharmacogenomics, race, and regulation.

Abstract

Modern genetic findings do not support the antiquated notion of human races as separate subspecies or genetically distinct categories. Even though human races cannot be defined genetically, the concept of race may provide an important tool in treatment or research. In United States society, race is such an important stratifying practice that it plays a role in determining many features of people's lives, features that affect health. Not all of these features are known or can be measured as separate variables. Scientists and physicians must determine when and how to use race, so that they obtain the most informative data and the best treatment outcomes. But using race is always dangerous because assumptions about the nature of race can undermine researchers' and physicians' abilities to conduct valid science or draw justified conclusions. The possibility that pharmacogenetics could result in racially stratified medicine, in which people of different races have different access to drugs, raises concerns about injustice. This chapter discusses some theories of justice and how each would contend with racially differentiated pharmacology research and treatment. It proposes that researchers and physicians apply a rebuttable presumption that any observed racial differences in treatment outcomes are not due to racial differences in allele frequencies.

Outline

Learning Objectives

1. Understand that although modern anthropology and genetics show that there are no genetically distinguishable human racial groups, that does not mean that races do not exist. Races exist as social constructs—race is "real" even though it is not genetic.
2. Understand that race is relevant in biomedical research because the social interactions that create race can have profound affects on human health.
3. Understand the several different conceptions of justice that support the twin propositions that researchers should pay attention to race, and that researchers should be careful about attributing observed differences in biomedical outcomes to genetic differences among races.
4. Understand the several different conceptions of justice, as well as the human subjects research regulations, that generate ethical imperatives for researchers to conduct and report their research in a manner that minimizes harms to subjects.

Abbreviations in this Chapter

A-HeFT	African-American Heart Failure Trial
ApoE	Apolipoprotein E
CDC	Centers for Disease Control and Prevention
CHF	Congestive heart failure
CYP	Cytochrome P450
DNA	Deoxyribonucleic acid
FDA	Food and Drug Administration
HBC	Hereditary breast cancer
IND	Investigational new drug
NDA	New drug application
NIH	National Institutes of Health
OMB	Office of Management and Budget
SES	Socioeconomic status

Societal and Ethical Issues in

Pharmacogenomics

Current Controversies over Race in Science

Since the early 1990s, the scientific literature has blossomed with articles about the use of race in biomedical research and clinical practice (References 1–7). Some argue that popular racial terms and concepts, such as "white", "Caucasian", "black", and "Asian", should be abandoned because they are unscientific and do not reflect current understandings of human genetics. One commentator referred to research in which race variables are used as "black box epidemiology," and stated that such research has "seldom given fundamental new understanding of disease" (Reference 2). Other commentators argue that race should be used because it is an important proxy for ancestry, genetic susceptibility, or epidemiological exposures, and because the use of racial categorization in research could diminish costs or improve the sensitivity and/or specificity of an experiment (References 6–8). Although some molecular biologists argue that data from the genome project undermine the entire notion of race, (Reference 9), others claim to have developed "the only race-determining set of (ancestry informative genetic markers)" (Reference 10).

There is a great deal of confusion and unclarity regarding the role of race in pharmacokinetics, pharmacodynamics, and drug safety. One study concluded that groups created by clustering people according to genotype were better predictors of drug metabolism than were clusters based on subjects' geographic origins, racial, or ethnic labels (Reference 11). Investigators reached this conclusion after studying 39 different microsatellite markers in 354 individuals from eight populations. However, other researchers dispute this conclusion (Reference 7).

Some commentators claim that most observed clinical differences among racial groups reflect racially distributed patterns of allelic variation, and that race should always be a consideration in pharmacogenetic research (Reference 12). For instance, the authors of a 1999 article in Science (Reference 8) stated that:

> "All pharmacogenetic polymorphisms studied to date differ in frequency among ethnic and racial groups. In fact, the slow acetylator phenotype was originally suspected to be genetically determined because of the difference in frequency of isoniazid-induced neuropathies observed in Japan versus those observed in the United States. The marked racial and ethnic diversity in the frequency of functional polymorphisms in drug- and xenobiotic-metabolizing enzymes dictates that race be considered in studies aimed at discovering whether specific genotypes or phenotypes are associated with disease risk or drug toxicity."

On the other hand, the authors of an often cited review article reached no definitive conclusions regarding the relationship between race and the expression or activity of any drug-metabolizing or transporting enzyme (Reference 13). The article contains a substantial discussion of cytochrome P450 (CYP) 2C9, a gene encoding a CYP responsible for the metabolism of numerous clinically relevant substrates. This cytochrome's substrates include anticoagulants, such as warfarin; oral hypoglycemics, such as tolbutamide; and the anticonvulsant phenytoin. Investigators determined that the relationship between ethnicity and CYP2C9 expression and activity is unclear, even though some allelic variants differ in frequency among different racial or ethnic groups. The data are contradictory, with some studies yielding clinical or in vivo results opposite of those predicted from the observed racial and ethnic pattern of allele frequency variation.

These examples are indicative of the state of the field of pharmacogenomics with respect to elucidating relationships among pharmacology, race or ethnicity, and allelic variation. Strong claims often are made about the relevance of race and ethnicity, even when data supporting these claims are lacking or contradictory.

Researchers now face legal requirements—statutes, regulations, and guidelines—for the inclusion of racial and ethnic minorities in human subjects research (Reference 14). National Institutes of Health (NIH)-funded research that involves humans must include racial and ethnic minorities and their subpopulations, unless there are valid reasons to exclude some group(s). For NIH-defined Phase III clinical trials, minorities must be included in a manner that allows for valid analyses of differences among subpopulations (note that the phrase "valid analyses" does not mean statistically valid) (Reference 15). Cost is not an acceptable reason for failing to meet this requirement. The NIH guidelines state that racial data should be collected in a manner that allows researchers to use the racial and ethnic categories developed by the Office of Management and Budget (OMB) in 1997; data must be capable of being collapsed into these categories.

The Food and Drug Administration (FDA) regulations require sponsors of investigational new drug (IND) applications and new drug applications (NDAs) to report data analyzed by racial subgroups (Reference 16). Recent FDA draft guidelines, which were published for comment in January 2003, take the same approach as the NIH guidelines in suggesting that race and ethnicity should be reported according to the OMB categories. Likewise, the Centers for Disease Control and Prevention (CDC) has a policy, stating that women and racial and ethnic minorities must be included in studies unless there is a clear and compelling reason to exclude any group, and that the OMB race and ethnicity categories should be used as "basic minimum guidance" (Reference 17). These guidelines reflect the government's interests in standardizing data so that meta-analyses, cross-agency comparisons, and longitudinal studies can be performed.

Laws and regulations regarding collecting and reporting data using OMB race and ethnicity categories may contribute to confusion among researchers and clinicians. They focus scientists on the search for racial differences, elevating racial differences to the status of the more interesting and important scientific story while simultaneously de-emphasizing racial similarities and implying that they are the less important outcome. Furthermore, the requirement for inclusion can easily be understood as reflecting an *a priori* assumption that people of different races or ethnicities are likely to differ from each other in ways that are medically consequential.

Legal requirements for minority inclusion in research were instituted in response to studies showing that racial and ethnic minorities were largely absent from federally funded clinical studies, and that there are significant racially patterned differences in morbidity and mortality in the United States. Minorities typically are worse-off (Reference 18). Minority inclusion requirements were a response to the fear that minorities were being deprived of the direct benefits of participating in some protocols and the long-term benefits of having their problems studied. Nonetheless, inclusion for the wrong reasons, inclusion that mindlessly reinforces or reproduces antiquated racial stereotypes, can be more harmful than beneficial (Reference 19).

The remainder of this chapter addresses the nature of race and discusses justice issues associated with racially patterned practices of prescribing drugs or conducting research. However, before addressing race some discussion about nomenclature is in order.

Biomedical scientists have not been careful to distinguish among the terms "race," "ethnicity," "population," and various designations of nationality (e.g., Chinese and Japanese). This practice both reflects and produces analytic confusion. It produces analytic confusion because using the same term (such as ethnicity) in reference to different types of human collectives—groups that are constituted through different social and/or biological mechanisms—may result in comparisons among incomparable groups. It also may result in the unjustified generalization of results (e.g., generalization of results obtained by studying a small, localized, closely related population to claims about an entire race).

The biomedical literature is replete with debate about whether scientists and clinicians should use the terms "race" or "ethnicity." Commentators note that the meaning of "ethnicity" or "ethnic group" should or could incorporate culture, language, socioeconomic status (SES), and other environmental information, along with some notion of shared origins (References 13, 20, 21). However, in the genomics and genetics literature, the label "ethnicity" is rarely accompanied by any description of the culture, environment, or social status of study subjects. Ethnicity is frequently substituted for race, but with no alteration of the conceptual framework for allocating people to one group or another. This substitution is apparent in articles that use the term "ethnicity" but label data with terms, such as "black" or "Asian," thus reverting to racial categories and tropes. Alternatively, articles use the term "ethnicity" but then present data using categories of race and nationality, such as "Asian-Chinese" and "Asian-Korean".

In this chapter, the term "population" usually is avoided, because it has both nontechnical and technical meanings, and the two are easily confused. Evolutionary and population biologists use the term "population" for geographically localized, relatively small, interbreeding groups within a much larger, common gene pool (species) (Reference 22). In the nontechnical sense, the term "population" can refer to any identifiable group of organisms, no matter what common characteristics signal their collective identity. Those studying pharmacogenetics or pharmacogenomics rarely study human populations in the technical sense.

This chapter primarily is concerned with claims about race (as defined in the next section) and genetics. However, examples occasionally are drawn from articles that use the terms "ethnicity" and "population". The examples chosen are illustrative of particular modes of reasoning and methods of categorizing human groups, regardless of label. The term "human group" is used to denote any type of human collective, when no judgment is being made as to how that group was or is constituted.

A Brief History of Race

"When we talk about the concept of race, most people believe that they know it when they see it but arrive at nothing short of confusion when pressed to define it."
—Evelyn Brooks Higginbotham (Reference 23)

The 18th century French naturalist George-Louis Leclerc, the Comte de Buffon, is credited with introducing the term "race" into the scientific discussion of human groups (Reference 24). He introduced the term in an article published in 1749. Nine years later, the Swedish naturalist Carolus Linneaus described four human races—*Americanus rubescus* (red), *Europaeus albus* (white), *Asiaticus luridus* (yellow), and *Afer niger* (black)—in a revised version of his momentous work on organismal classification (Reference 24). Linneaus and Leclerc used skin color, physiognomy, and geography as criteria for classification.

As 18th and 19th century scientists encountered and studied a greater variety of human populations and groups, these scientists continued to categorize and explain human variation using the notion of race. In attempting to define and distinguish race, scientists focused particularly on skull shape and size. They believed that skull form was highly resistant to environmental influences and, thus, would be more constant among members of any particular racial group. Scientists believed that every race had an "ideal type," and that their theories should explain how and why individual members of any race failed to conform to the ideal type (Reference 22).

Attempts to apprehend race scientifically have gone through many different iterations and used several different methodological approaches, including craniometry, blood typing, and now, measurements of allele frequencies in different human groups. During the 19th century, anthropologists and other scientists attempted to introduce analytical rigor into the measurement of human diversity. They devised scales of skin color, measures of hair texture, and complex methodologies for determining the size and shape of bodily features.

The researchers' aim was to identify features, or ranges of them, that captured "common sense" notions of race and that could be used to define racial ideal types. However, the more carefully scientists measured and the more people and populations they studied, the less clear cut racial boundaries and racial characteristics became. They could not identify distinct morphological boundaries among human populations. Researchers found few members of any race who conformed to the ideal type, howsoever defined. When they measured combinations of features, such as height, nose shape, hair texture, skin/hair color, and eye shape to define human races, anthropologists discovered that human features vary independently of each other. Dark skin does not always coincide with a particular height range, nose shape, or head shape.

Throughout the 19th and 20th centuries, the number of races identified by various anthropologists grew from the four categories set forth by Linneaus to 13, 30, and even more. Anthropologists were discovering what geneticists would later rediscover—there is biological and genetic variation among human individuals and human populations, but this variation does not fit neatly into a few discrete, separable categories of people. The observation that different surface traits vary independently of each other was an early observation of a phenomenon that modern geneticists refer to as nonconcordance. Nonconcordance is observed because traits encoded by unlinked genes are inherited independently of each other. By the early and mid 20th century, many anthropologists were coming to the conclusion that the prevailing conception of race was deeply flawed, and that perhaps there were no human races if race meant discrete, natural categories of people.

The history of the science of race provides an excellent example of the manner in which ideologies from the broader society shape the scientific process, and how the scientific process helps shape broader social ideologies. From its inception, the notion of race developed by Linneaus and subsequent researchers incorporated negative value judgments about non-European people, and a hierarchy of superiority and inferiority with Europeans as the preeminent race. Linneaus described people from Europe as active, smart, inventive, and governed by the rule of law; people from Asia as severe, haughty, melancholy, and governed by belief; people from the Americas as ill-tempered, obstinate, happy, liberty-loving, and governed by custom; and people of Africa as crafty, slow, foolish, and in need of governance by others (Reference 24). Surface physical traits used to designate race were thought to indicate or correlate with innate psychological traits, such as character, behaviors, and aptitudes. Each member of a group was thought to have the physical and psychological traits assigned to her or his race.

This categorical, essentialist, hierarchical understanding of race had political implications; it was used to justify colonialism, and later, the enslavement of blacks. Furthermore, this notion of race was tied to eugenics and beliefs about miscegenation. Many scholars and policy-makers in 19th- and early 20th-century United States and Europe abhorred "race mixing" because interracial procreation would supposedly taint the white race with inferior qualities, both physical and psychological. Such views culminated in the mass murder of Jewish people and other groups deemed biologically inferior by the Nazis during the Third Reich.

In 19th- and early 20th-century United States, scientific and "folk" understanding of races as discrete categories of people with essential physical and psychological differences provided the underpinning for antimiscegenation laws, laws that prohibited interracial marriage. It was not until 1967 that the United States Supreme Court declared antimiscegenation laws unconstitutional in the case of Loving v. Virginia (Reference 25). At the time, 16 states still had antimiscegenation laws on the books, and Virginia's highest court had previously concluded that Virginia's statute embodied the state's "legitimate purposes" of preserving "the racial integrity of its citizens" and preventing "the corruption of blood" that might produce "a mongrel breed of citizens" and obliterate "racial pride" (Reference 25). In an opinion authored by then Chief Justice Earl Warren, the United States Supreme Court held that antimiscegenation statutes violate both the equal protection clause and the due process clause of the 14th Amendment, and that they serve no state purpose independent of invidious racial discrimination.

The eugenics movements of the United States, the United Kingdom, and Europe have been superbly described and analyzed elsewhere (References 26–28). For purposes of this chapter, it is enough to note that eugenics movements around the world were supported by early human geneticists, and although some may have viewed the political movements and policies that grew out of the science with lukewarm enthusiasm or ambivalence, few spoke out against eugenics until the 1920s or later. Eugenics views were widely held by well-educated members of society and by opinion leaders of both conservative and liberal bent.

In the United States eugenics movement, the underpinning for a variety of criminal and disreputable social behavior was believed to be a genetic tendency to feeblemindedness. People behaved badly, in violation of Anglo-Protestant middle class norms, because they were too stupid to know better. The notion of race fit in here in several ways. First, it was people of Anglo-Saxon and Nordic ancestry who considered themselves a superior but beleaguered and endangered race. Second, not only were people of recent Asian, African, or Native American ancestry considered as different races from the Anglo and Nordic whites, but so were Jewish, Irish, and Polish immigrants. Collectively, these nonwhite races were viewed as being more prone to live in slums and engage in criminal behavior. They also were perceived as voracious breeders, who would take command of the social and material resources if not restrained. In the United States, restraints, or negative eugenics, took the form of restrictive immigration laws, eugenic sterilization laws, and antimiscegenation laws.

Eugenics movements gained steam in concert with the increasing social strains brought about by industrialization at the end of the 19th century and the beginning of the 20th century. The movements began to experience strong opposition in the 1920s, and lost almost all social support after World War II. Explicit scientific discussion of race and human biological or genetic variation was largely absent in the period between World War II and the 1980s. Some theorize that scientists, geneticists in particular, avoided studying or discussing race precisely because the notion was infested with beliefs about the innate superiority of some racial groups and the innate inferiority of others. The Holocaust of the 1940s and the United States Civil Rights movement of the 1960s created a social backlash against the notion that some human groups were innately superior or inferior.

But population genetic studies of humans were quietly taking place, even if geneticists were not discussing race. By the early 1990s, data suggested that most human genetic variation, about 75 percent of all deoxyribonucleic acid (DNA) variants, could be found in any small, localized group of people (Reference 24). Data also suggested that when human population groups differ in allele frequencies at a particular genetic locus, each population tends to be quite similar to nearby populations, and dissimilar to geographically distant populations. Allele frequency difference increases with geographic distance. The variation is gradual; distinct discontinuities are rarely observed. This pattern is referred to as clinal variation (Reference 20).

Research of the past 10 years has shown that any two individual human beings are 99.9 percent genetically alike, no matter what continent, nation, city, or village they come from, and no matter what their racial and ethnic designations. Any two (unrelated) people will differ from each other about once in every 1000 nucleotides. The human species is exceptionally genetically homogeneous compared to other mammals and even to *Drosophila*. "The chimpanzees living on a single hillside in Africa have twice as much variety in their DNA as do the 6 billion people scattered across the globe" (Reference 29). With respect to race, no genetic marker is found in all people of one race and no people of other races.

The most common explanation for humanity's unusual genetic homogeneity—the explanation accepted by the majority of population biologists, geneticists, and anthropologists—is that modern humans are a young species that originated from one small group of ancestors, probably not more than 20,000 people living in eastern Africa. Humans began with a relatively restricted gene pool and expanded rapidly to our current world population without much genetic differentiation (References 24, 30, 31). Fewer than 10,000 generations separate every human alive today from that small group of ancestors. In evolutionary time spans, this is a short time for mutations to occur and accumulate (References 24, 30). The commonly identified human races do not represent distinct evolutionary lineages, they are not discrete populations, and there never were "pure" human races (Reference 31).

This is not to say that all human groups are genetically indistinguishable. In comparing the genetic similarities and differences of groups, scientists look for loci that demonstrate interindividual variation, and then determine whether the frequency of alleles at any of those loci differ between two groups of interest. Groups can be characterized by the frequencies of alleles at variable loci. When comparing widely separated groups on the same continent, such as two isolated small towns in different parts of Europe, studies find that about 10 percent of loci will show allele frequency differences between the two groups. When comparing two isolated groups from different continents, such as a small, isolated town in rural east Africa and a small, isolated town on a reservation in the United States, studies find that about 15 percent of loci will show allele frequency differences between the two groups. On occasion, a genetic variant is found at a discernible (typically low) frequency in one group, but is not found in other groups studied.

When scientists compare a group of people whose known ancestors are from one continent to a group whose ancestors are from another continent, they find that about 5 percent of loci show allele frequency differences between the two groups, differences that typically are not found between two groups from the same continent (References 24, 32). Using some genetic markers drawn from this 5 percent, computer programs can infer a person's ancestry, or create clusters of people, all of whose ancestors likely originated on the same continent. Traditional notions have tied race to continent of origin, and, therefore, some people may view this 5 percent of DNA as the genetic location of race. However, contemporary genetic findings are not consistent with folk notions of race or the antiquated scientific one.

One difference is that, although folk notions construct races as categorically distinct, the genetic differences between continental groups are statistical. Genetic markers that show between-continent variation do not identify two substantially separate or clearly distinctive genetic categories of people. It is not the case that all people with origins on one continent will have allele A at locus X, while all people with origins on a different continent will have allele B at locus X. And if people are grouped using standard racial taxonomies, it is not the case that all people of one race will have allele A at locus X, while all people of another race will have allele B at locus X.

Furthermore, there is no reason to believe that those 5 percent of loci that can be used to cluster people according to continents of origin are particularly important for defining human identity or elucidating medically significant information. The same data that can distinguish groups by continent of origin also can be used to create subcontinental clusters

(Reference 32). Most loci cannot be used to cluster people at all because there is little or no between-group variation at these loci. There is no reason to believe that continent-level clusters are more significant than subcontinental clusters, or that loci which can produce clusters are more relevant for defining human identity or understanding human history than loci which cannot be used to cluster people.

Researchers and physicians should avoid assumptions about the medical relevance of loci that are used to create clusters. Most such loci are microsatellite markers, hypervariable regions in noncoding DNA. There is no *a priori* reason to think that these noncoding markers will be linked to genes of relevance for drug metabolism, drug transport, drug receptors, or particular diseases.

Perhaps the most important issue to consider is the vast amount of within-group genetic variation. Groups comprised of millions of people, such as the four or five commonly recognized races, contain about 95 percent of all human genetic variation. Thus, people who share a racial identity (either by self-report or by attribution) may be quite different genetically. Although researchers can make statistical distinctions among human groups, researchers and physicians are not justified in assuming that most people within any racial group are relevantly alike with respect to medically important alleles.

Black people apparently possess the highest degree of within-group genetic variation. At any particular locus, black people are likely to possess alleles not found at high frequency in other human groups (References 24, 33, 34). Although genetic and other biomedical studies often categorize some participants as "black," this is a particularly incoherent category from a genetic standpoint.

Races are composed of numerous populations, and populations' genetic structures are constantly changing through gene flow, genetic drift, genetic bottlenecks, and merger with other populations (Reference 22). Because many different genetically important phenomena have occurred within each race, scientists ought to use extreme care when inferring from data on a few samples or a single study of people from any race. Such generalizations may not be valid, and even if valid, may be misleading to the extent that they obscure important genetic substructure within a race. Furthermore, average allele frequency numbers for an entire race may not provide the most illuminating information from which to generate further research hypotheses or make treatment decisions because they may obscure a population within the race that has a high frequency of disease-causing or pharmacologically relevant alleles.

Some have argued that the usefulness of race as a research and clinical category is shown by the fact that the group of people of Ashkenazi Jewish descent possesses a higher than average frequency of alleles that predispose carriers to several serious medical conditions, including hereditary breast cancer (HBC) (Reference 7). Although information about people of

Ashkenazi Jewish descent is certainly information about a population of white people, it would be inappropriate to generalize from studies on HBC allele frequencies in this population to claims about the frequency of such alleles in white or Caucasian people. It would not necessarily be helpful either to sample several different Caucasian populations and then generate an average number for the frequency of HBC alleles in Caucasians. Such race aggregate numbers would not help clinicians to provide optimal health care for people of Ashkenazi Jewish descent or for other Caucasians, an average frequency for a racial group of tens or hundreds of millions would not likely reveal anything interesting about human population history or migration patterns.

If race cannot be found in our genes, then what is it? Contemporary race scholars do not view race as being definable through genetics or genetic categories. Rather, race is a set of meanings and distinctions that people impose on the continuous spectrum of human genetic and social variation. Through social interactions and institutions, people and cultures create and maintain racial demarcations; they create categories and allot people to them. Race is a social process or relationship through which some groups are subordinated to others, a set of practices and beliefs through which people are stratified in a social hierarchy. Decades of careful research have illuminated the ways in which people create, recreate, and decreate racial categories and have shown how the same person can be black in one country and white in another, how the Irish and the Italians became "white" in the United States although they were not always considered so (Reference 35). This contemporary understanding is often referred to as the view that race is a social construct.

Many argue that if race is a social construct then racial categories should not be used in research or clinical practice. Some commentators argue that using race confuses genetic categories with social ones, and reifies antiquated and incorrect beliefs about race (References 1, 3, 9). This claim often is framed in the following manner: modern genetics has shown that race is not real, and if race is not real then it should not be used as a variable in research or medicine. Stated this way, the claim confuses things genetic with things real. Many real things cannot be defined or identified through genetics. Social constructs can be real and relevant in at least some area of biomedical research or clinical practice. For instance, "family" is a social construct that may be useful in biomedical research or clinical practice even though the precise meaning of the term is geographically and historically contingent.

Even if race is "only" a social construct, it still has great relevance for health states, and, therefore, in some instances biomedical scientists may legitimately study or take account of it. In the United States, race has significant consequences over a wide range of institutions and social practices. People interact on the basis of their beliefs about race and in doing so create residential segregation, racially differentiated access to health insurance, employment segregation, racially differentiated exposures to toxins and dangers (e.g., gunshot wounds, racially differentiated treatment in and by health care institutions) etc (References 18, 36). The lifetime, accumulated pattern of exposures and experiences that result from living in the United States at a particular historical juncture as a person of a particular race may have physiological consequences. Such cumulative effects, or interactions among several race-related variables, might be difficult to detect as separable, easily decomposed causes of treatment outcomes and health states. The cumulative social circumstances can feed back and create racialized bodies.

Data indicate that racial and ethnic minorities are disproportionately burdened by health problems. In a recent report, the Institute of Medicine noted that, "despite steady improvement in the overall health of the United States population, racial and ethnic minorities, with few exceptions, experience higher rates of morbidity and mortality than nonminorities" (Reference 18). African Americans have the highest rates of mortality from cancer, cerebrovascular disease, heart disease, and human immunodeficiency virus/acquired immune deficiency syndrome. American Indians and Hispanics suffer from disproportionately high rates of diabetes and diabetes-related complications, and some Asian-American subpopulations experience disproportionately high rates of stomach, liver, and cervical cancer (Reference 18).

The causes of particular health disparities, and the means for their elimination, vary tremendously. In 1998, President Bill Clinton set a national goal of eliminating racial and ethnic health disparities in six areas by 2010 (References 37, 38). The president's five-step plan ended a practice in which agencies and health care providers set lower goals for minority health (Reference 38). Society will not know whether health disparities exist, or whether they are diminishing in response to particular interventions, if race cannot be used as a variable in research. Yet, using race can have its drawbacks—erroneous causal attributions or treatment schemes based on simplistic assumptions about race could produce more harm than benefit.

With respect to eliminating health disparities, one currently controversial question is whether drugs, vaccines, or other interventions should be developed for and targeted to particular racial or ethnic groups. For instance, claims that blacks suffer from heart failure at twice the rate of whites (Reference 39) and that blacks do not respond as well as whites to some heart failure drugs (References 40, 41) have led to the first clinical trial of a drug intended to treat congestive heart failure (CHF) only in African Americans. The African-American Heart Failure Trial (A-HeFT) aims to enroll between 600 and 800 African Americans to study the efficacy of the drug BiDil, a combination of the vasodilators hydralazine and isosorbide dinitrate (Reference 39).

Perhaps BiDil will prove efficacious for treating CHF in black patients and the FDA will approve its labeled indications; however, this outcome might not prove an unmitigated benefit. Enthusiasm of researchers and the public for a race-based drug could divert resources from the development of drugs that provide unambiguous benefits for many or most patients, regardless of race. It could wrongly reinforce genetic determinist notions of both race and drug response. If A-HeFT had segmented the study population according to genotype or pathophysiology rather than race, perhaps it would have better identified which patients could benefit from BiDil, regardless of race. If BiDil proves efficacious in blacks, the reasons could be many, but A-HeFT will not help elucidate them.

In a racially stratified society such as the United States, causes of racial disparities in health or racial differences in pharmacodynamics are difficult to ascertain because of the many confounders that covary with race. Too often, researchers observe a correlation between race and a drug response or side effect and immediately assume that the cause of the observed racial difference is genetic. This assumption seems to follow from the widely held but incorrect notion that people of the same race are closely related and likely to have the same alleles at relevant loci.

One challenge for researchers is to devise better measures of environmental factors that may have causal connections to health outcomes. Socioeconomic status variables, for instance, often are poorly conceived, and the data relating to them are wrongly interpreted (References 5, 42). Researchers have not yet devised sophisticated methods for measuring racism, or the degree to which it is directed toward particular individuals. They do not possess good methods for measuring cumulative and interactive effects of various exposures. Race variables almost certainly capture aspects of SES and environmental exposures that scientists do not or cannot currently measure through more direct assessments.

For these reasons, a binary approach to the issue of race in science may not prove particularly enlightening. Rather than debating whether race should be used as a variable in research, the scientific community ought to engage in discussion concerning when and how race may be used as a variable. In any particular case, researchers should consider whether analyzing the data by race is the most informative approach, and what alternative analytic frameworks might be applied. Even when the use of race is consistent with a well-developed scientific consensus, studies must be designed to use this variable with much greater sophistication.

Race and Justice in Pharmacogenomics

"Justice is the first virtue of social institutions ..." (Reference 43). So begins John Rawls' influential book, A Theory of Justice. Justice is not simply a virtue of people, but of the systems of explicit rules, implicit rules (habits and internalized norms), material structures, and material circumstances that societies create. Social cooperation and the institutions through which it is mediated create and allocate benefits and burdens or harms, rights and duties, privileges, and disadvantages. Social justice theories evaluate the creation and distribution of benefits, burdens, and harms, and ask whether the distributions are based on legitimate criteria and allocated through fair processes. These theories are concerned not simply with the aggregate good, but with questions about who benefits or obtains privilege, and who is harmed or disadvantaged. Often, justice is concerned with the processes and systems that produce inequality, and whether those inequalities are justifiable.

According to some theories, health is a subject of justice because reasonable health is instrumental in creating and maintaining opportunities for individuals to achieve a variety of life plans and social goods (Reference 44, 45). According to other theories, health is a subject of justice because it is one of the valuable capabilities that a society should protect and facilitate among its members (Reference 46). Health care and biomedical research are subjects of justice to the extent that they are important for achieving health, and because society has limited resources for providing health care or conducting research. Because resources are limited, everybody cannot have as much health care or conduct as much research as they would like. Members of society, collectively, must make difficult decisions about which interventions or research projects will be undertaken.

The ethics regulations for federally funded research (the Common Rule, codified at 45 Code of Federal Regulations 46) embody a conception of justice that focuses on protecting vulnerable individuals or groups, and ensuring that the burdens and benefits of research are fairly distributed. One group in society should not carry a disproportionate share of the research burdens if a different group is likely to reap most of the benefits. Subjects should not be exposed to unnecessary risk, regardless of the benefits to be achieved by the research.

The regulations' focus on preventing additional burdens on, or exploitation of, vulnerable individuals and social groups is consistent with the idea that the operation of social institutions is not just if those at the bottom of the social hierarchy are made less well-off for the benefit of those who are at the pinnacle of the social hierarchy or who are better-off. On some views, institutions are only permitted to increase inequality if doing so actually works to the benefit of those who are least well-off (a stringent requirement). Conducting research in which the least well-off are exposed to more risk than potential benefit and allocating the resulting health care benefits to those who are better-off arguably exacerbates inequalities of many sorts. If health is a prerequisite for obtaining many other social goods, then exacerbating health inequalities may increase inequality in other spheres of activity, such as employment.

The Common Rule was promulgated in response to reports of abusive and unethical research projects, the most notorious of which was the United States Public Health Service study of untreated syphilis

(Reference 47). This study was conducted in Tuskegee, Alabama, and the research subjects were poor, poorly educated African Americans. The study ran for 40 years and was stopped in 1972, after accounts of it were published in the national press. Given this history, it is not surprising that the regulations reflect more concern with protecting potential subjects from harms and burdens than with ensuring that potential subjects and the greater society receive the benefits of research.

For many years after the research ethics regulations were adopted, racial and ethnic minorities were largely absent from biomedical research. Publicity about the syphilis study probably made researchers leery of recruiting minority subjects, and also exacerbated distrust of biomedical researchers among minorities who were potential subjects. The protective focus of the regulations also may have discouraged researchers from making extensive efforts to recruit minority subjects out of fear that ethics review committees (termed institutional review boards) would look on such efforts with heightened suspicion. However, throughout the past several years, the public and regulatory conception of justice in research has altered; the pendulum has swung from a focus on protection to a focus on equality of access and to fair distribution of both direct and long-term research benefits. Legal requirements for inclusion of women and minorities in research stem from this new focus on equal access.

Justice theories that emphasize equality must always address the central question, equality of what? Some conceptions of justice require nothing more than formal equality before the law—for instance, the removal of laws, regulations, or institutional policies that make invidious racial distinctions—so that people of similar talents and characteristics will have similar chances to achieve their life plans. Other conceptions require that our social institutions create a more robust equality of opportunity. Among those, some hold that equality of opportunity is satisfied when no formal or informal barriers of discrimination are present. Other theories require not only elimination of barriers, but some efforts to eliminate the effects of bad luck in the social lottery. For instance, the latter type of theory requires that society offset or compensate for the fact that some people, through no fault of their own, will receive much poorer schooling than others. Theories of health care justice tend to focus on "equality of respect and concern for each person or patient," or on the ways in which health care might be necessary for ensuring equality of opportunity.

Racial inequalities raise ethical flags because race, alone, typically is not viewed as a characteristic on which judgments of merit or desert should be based. Race is not a characteristic on which distributive patterns should depend. Patterns of racial inequality raise an inference that social institutions are unjustifiably treating people with relevantly similar characteristics, such as talents or health care needs, differently from each other. For instance, if three applicants for a laboratory technician job had the same degree, from the same quality of school, and each had the same prior job experience, but one was Asian and two were Caucasian, an observer might suspect that the irrelevant characteristic of race was being used in hiring decisions if only the Caucasians received job interviews. Such a use of race would be unjustified because race, alone, is not a characteristic that should determine the distribution of employment opportunities.

Both in ethics and law, scholars look with particular suspicion on unequal treatment of different racial groups, and many also look with suspicion on racially unequal outcomes of social processes, in part, because of this country's history of invidious racial discrimination. A disproportionate number of the least well-off people in society are members of racial and ethnic minority groups, which also raises concerns about practices and processes that increase their burdens or disadvantages. Thus, reports that people with the same health insurance and the same medical condition but different races do not receive the same services (Reference 18) invite heightened moral scrutiny.

Biomedical studies that focus on racial differences confront the dilemma of difference (Reference 48). On the one hand, if scientists do not use race as a variable, they will not identify or develop responses to differences in health or treatment outcomes. For society to show equal respect and concern for the health of all of its members, it must have evidence as to whether some groups are experiencing disproportionate burdens of particular diseases, disproportionate total or cumulative burdens of disease, lack of access to health care, or discriminatory treatment by health professionals. On the other, if scientists do use race as a variable, they run the risk of reinforcing antiquated beliefs and stereotypes about race.

One of these stereotypes is that some races are constitutionally inferior, prone to disease and dissolution. Another mistaken belief, discussed at length previously, is that races are fundamentally, biologically different. Too often, any observation of racial differences in health states or treatment outcomes is assumed to reflect genetic or other fundamental biological divisions among people, despite lack of data supporting this assumption. Deeply embedded notions about the nature of race make assumptions of fundamental racial differences credible and unexceptional. Acknowledging the "dilemma of difference" may help the scientific community to develop and implement practices that will tilt the balance of benefits and harms in the net positive direction, if and when researchers do use race as a variable in research.

Although there are many conceptions of justice, there are some biomedical concerns about which proponents of divergent ethical traditions would likely come to similar conclusions, even if for different reasons. Identifying conclusions and fair processes that would be ethically acceptable to individuals who use a broad range of ethical theories and who hold a variety of values, is desirable in a pluralistic society such as ours. Identifying such domains of agreement is sometimes referred to as reaching "overlapping consensus." This section examines some justice issues at the intersection of A) notions of race, B) research or medical treatment, and C) pharmacology, about which people with diverse viewpoints might reach overlapping consensus.

When evaluating the justice of pharmacogenomics and pharmacogenetics research or treatments that incorporate pharmacogenetic information, analysts must determine which social institutions are relevant, what processes these institutions use, and what outcomes they produce. The relevant social institutions are, at least, those that fund, regulate, and conduct biomedical research; those that market and pay for pharmaceutical products; and those through which health care is delivered. Do these institutions produce unjustifiable, racially patterned inequalities in access to drugs? Do they produce unjustifiable medical burdens for those who are least well-off in society? Do they disproportionately and unfairly fail to ameliorate health burdens for those who are least well-off? Do these institutions fail to exhibit equal concern for the problems of all individuals, including racial and ethnic minorities? These are the types of questions that a justice analysis should address.

Pharmacogenetics and Access to Health Care

Pharmacogenetics and pharmacogenomics may help researchers and clinicians better understand pharmacodynamics, variability in drug metabolism, or genetic diversity of disease pathogenesis. The advent of these sciences has raised people's expectations that individualized assessments of drug responsiveness or adverse drug reactions will soon become a routine step in prescribing drugs. The medical community could likely prevent some harm by making such individual genetic determinations. However, given the current economic realities, few commentators believe that genetic tests soon will become available for every pharmacologically relevant allele. Furthermore, if pharmacogenetic tests are to be paid for by health insurance, Medicare, or other public programs, it is unlikely that payers will reimburse the costs of all possible tests, for all people. How will physicians decide which drugs or which pharmacogenetic tests to offer patients? How will payers determine which drugs or tests to reimburse? How will drug companies and governmental agencies determine their research and development agendas with respect to drugs and pharmacogenetic tests?

The belief that race and ethnicity will play a role in determining access to drugs and pharmacogenetic tests is fostered by scientists' and physicians' claims about the strong correlation between race or ethnicity and frequency differences in known pharmacogenetic polymorphisms. Commentators have theorized that pharmacogenomics and genetics will result in substantial segmentation of markets for pharmaceuticals; will one aspect of that segmentation be racial? As previously discussed, there currently is one drug, BiDil, undergoing clinical trials to determine efficacy in black people. If the FDA approves this drug's labeled indications, the label will describe its demonstrated efficacy only in black people (although physicians could still engage in off-label prescribing to people of other races). The specter of racially segregated drugs raises fears that different groups will be given different shares of the available health care resources, that medicine will become separate and unequal. However, if equal attention is given to the health problems of all racial groups, and attention to race produces medical interventions that are more effective, then it would be difficult to find injustice.

Pharmacogenetics could affect access to drugs in several ways. One obvious possibility is that, in the absence of a genetic test approved for clinical use, data about the concentration of responder or nonresponder alleles in one racial group could cause physicians to engage in racially differentiated prescribing patterns. Such data could cause payers to engage in racially differentiated reimbursement practices. Would such practices be unjust? The answer to this question is contingent on many factual predicates, suggesting the necessity for case-by-case assessments of justice.

A crucial factual predicate concerns the robustness of the correlation between particular alleles and a drug response phenotype. A careful examination of existing data reveals observations of racial or ethnic differences in drug responsiveness, and observations that some pharmacogenetic polymorphisms vary among different racial or ethnic groups, but rarely unearths data unambiguously linking alleles to racially differentiated phenotypes. On the contrary, the in vivo pharmacology frequently contradicts predictions based simply on genotypes.

For instance, groups of Caucasians studied to date possess higher frequencies than Asians of two CYP alleles associated with slow metabolism of warfarin (CYP2C9*2 and CYP2C9*3). A researcher reviewing these data might hypothesize that, on average, Caucasians would require lower doses of warfarin than Asians to achieve anticoagulant effects; yet surprisingly, white patients typically require higher warfarin doses than Asians (Reference 13). With respect to another CYP, one review article notes that "ethnic comparisons with different CYP3A4 substrates have yielded inconsistent results that are difficult to interpret and may reflect an interplay of genetic and environmental factors" (Reference 13). The article also notes that interindividual variation in the in vivo levels of CYP3A4 expression may be 20-fold or greater. In the face of such significant interindividual variation, population-aggregate results may provide little clinically useful information, regardless of whether the means differ among racial or ethnic groups.

These data suggest that race may be irrelevant in many prescribing decisions, and, if race is relevant, it may be a marker of unknown environmental influences, rather than a useful surrogate for genotype. The unknown environmental influences could include (but are in no way limited to) diet, exposures to toxins, comorbidities, levels of stress, or some combination of these. At the least, researchers and physicians should not assume that information about the frequency of a pharmacogenetic allele in a racial or ethnic group can be used to make unambiguous predications about phenotype, or that information about phenotype can be used to predict racial differences in allele frequencies.

To complicate matters further, correlations of race with drug-response phenotypes may be temporally and geographically unstable, precisely because many of the causal factors in the distribution of drug responses are environmental. In an interesting study, investigators showed that environmental differences between Sweden and Ethiopia influence the activity of CYP2D6 enzymes (Reference 20). The authors examined debrisoquine metabolic ratio values for black Ethiopians living in Ethiopia, blacks from Ethiopia but now living in Sweden, and whites living in Sweden. From each of these groups, the investigators compared enzyme activity among individuals with the same CYP2D6 genotype. For almost all genotypes, enzyme activity was lowest for black Ethiopians living in Ethiopia, significantly higher for black Ethiopians living in Sweden, and highest for whites living in Sweden.

Looking beyond pharmacogenetics, there are other examples of racial differences with respect to a particular genotype-phenotype correlation. For instance, whites in the United States exhibit a dose-dependent relationship between particular variants of apolipoprotein E (ApoE) and increased risk of developing Alzheimer's disease—whites who are homozygous for the ApoE4 allele have the greatest risk. On the other hand, neither blacks nor Hispanics exhibit this relationship (Reference 49). Perhaps some environmental exposure that is more common among black and Hispanic people swamps the effects of ApoE4; or perhaps some exposure that is more common in whites enhances the significance of ApoE4 alleles.

The above examples should serve to warn researchers and physicians that there often is not a robust correlation between genotype and phenotype. People with the same genotype are not necessarily alike in all of the characteristics relevant for prescribing decisions. People of the same genotype and the same race may still respond differently to a particular drug. The above results should call into question the ease with which commentators draw broad generalizations about the relationships among genotype, race, and phenotype from one or a few studies. Regardless of whether racial or ethnic groups possess different frequencies of pharmacogenetic alleles, the lack of a robust correlation between genotype and drug-response phenotype should cause scholars and other interested members of the society to doubt the justice of any system that routinely allocated access to drugs based on race.

In determining whether racially differentiated prescribing was just, scholars also would want to determine what was at stake for patients. Are the alleles concentrated in a particular racial group ones that predict poor response or nonresponse to the drug? Limiting access to a drug based on the likely presence of nonresponder alleles would appear more justified than denying access based on poor responder alleles.

What kinds of side effects do this drug typically induce? Are the alleles correlated with adverse reactions rather than nonresponse, and if so, how severe are these reactions? Is this a situation in which the physician could prescribe a standard dose and then adjust it until she observed the desired therapeutic response and acceptable toxicity? Is there an alternative drug that could be similarly effective? If there were alternative effective drugs to which she had access, then prescribing those based on crude racial or ethnic group statistics of drug-response genotype might not violate the requirements of justice. A system that shows equal concern for all patients, or promotes equality of opportunity, does not necessarily owe each and every drug to each and every patient.

Analysts also should pay attention to the reported frequencies of pharmacogenetic alleles, and not simply to observations of racial or ethnic differences in these frequencies. In many cases, there may be a statistically significant difference in allele frequency, but the majority of people from any racial or ethnic group will possess the same allele or exhibit the same phenotype. For instance, if a "poor-metabolizer" allele for drug D is found in 9 percent of Asians studied, 14 percent of Caucasians, and 21 percent of African Americans and Native Americans, then the majority of people of all races will be extensive metabolizers (assuming that there is a robust correlation between genotype and phenotype and that all non-poor metabolizer genotypes correlate with the extensive metabolizer phenotype). If a physician relied on these data to prescribe the relevant drug to Caucasians and Asians but not to African Americans and Native Americans, then many people who are relevantly alike would be treated differently. Among African Americans and Native Americans, many people who could benefit from the drug would be denied access unnecessarily.

Given all of the above information, an ethically favorable approach might be to start deliberation about prescribing with the <u>rebuttable presumption</u> that the drug believed to be most efficacious should be prescribed for all patients with a similar disease phenotype, regardless of race. This presumption is, of course, intended to operate in the context of reasonable medical judgment concerning appropriate therapy; for instance, physicians, patients, and payers should still take into account comorbidities, documented drug allergies, and possible interactions with other drugs already prescribed. The point is that clinicians and other relevant decision-makers should start with the presumption that race is <u>not</u> a relevant characteristic in determining who is alike or different with respect to prescribing. If two or more similarly effective drugs are available to treat a particular condition, and data show some racial differences in drug-response phenotype or the distribution of pharmacogenetic alleles, then the presumption could be eliminated so long as no group of people would systematically be denied treatment.

The presumption could be rebutted. It might be rebutted when a reasonable quantity and quality of data show that A) there is a robust correlation between genotype and phenotype, <u>and</u> B) a particular racial or ethnic group possesses a high concentration of alleles that would predict a serious, adverse drug response. Under these circumstances, the patient's risk from taking the drug might outweigh her risk from not taking it. A physician demonstrates equal concern for all patients by attempting to optimize the benefit-harm ratio in each case. Optimizing does not necessarily entail treating each patient exactly alike. At the least, if such data exist, the physician should explain this to the patient, so that if the drug is offered she can make a well-informed choice about her treatment options.

The presumption also might be rebutted by data showing that within the physician's cachement area people of different racial or ethnic groups respond differently to a particular drug, regardless of whether genotype information is available. Data generated by studying Japanese people in Japan are far less likely to apply to a patient population of Japanese people in Atlanta, Georgia, than are data from studying Japanese people in Atlanta. Use of such locally generated data need not incorporate monolithic, categorical notions of a particular group, such as Asians or Japanese. One who acts on the basis of such data ought not assume that all people who can be labeled with the same race or nationality are the same for all time and in all places. Rather, such data may reflect current, local conditions that create racial patterning in a drug response.

The presumption focuses on decisions to offer or prescribe a drug, rather than on dosage decisions. Using available information about race, ethnicity, and drug responsiveness to determine starting doses of a drug is more easily justified than using such information to withhold a drug altogether. Such an approach might permit a good balance between ethical concerns about fair access to treatment and the ethical requirement of minimizing harm.

The approach discussed above promotes an institutional environment in which health care providers act out of equal concern and respect for all patients, regardless of race. It increases the likelihood that medicine functions to diminish inequalities of opportunity in society, rather than the reverse. The presumption is justified by the state of existing data, in which there are few cases of a robust correlation among genotype, race, and drug-response phenotype. The presumption could be woven into the fabric of health care institutions through explicit policies, such as quality management procedures and practice guidelines.

The presumption also is justified by the history of science and medicine. This history is replete with examples in which racial biases undermined scientific and medical judgment. People who were not perceived as white frequently were found to be morally and physically inferior to whites, and constitutionally incapable of achieving the same social status. Past scientific claims about race now seem absurd; from our current vantage point, research design and methodologies appear deeply flawed and the conclusions unjustified. However, those studies were taken seriously and considered quite credible in their time. Many flawed studies on race and health outcomes were conducted by virtuous people with good intentions.

Despite technical advances, today's researchers, health care providers, and scholars ought not assume that they are better at recognizing or resisting bias than their predecessors. When race and genetics are involved, United States society operates with such strong and deeply buried assumptions that, regardless of researchers' personal beliefs or ideologies, and even with the noblest of intentions, their judgment may be compromised. Deeply imbedded assumptions may operate to make certain claims about race and health seem reasonable and credible, even in the absence of strong empirical support. Such assumptions may increase the salience of information that supports them while decreasing the salience of contradictory information. All people use heuristics, mental shortcuts, to process the vast quantities of information they confront. These shortcuts may incorporate racial biases or prevent well-meaning people from noticing their own or their institution's biases.

The presumption recommended here reverses "common sense" understandings about the importance of race in health. By forcing biomedical researchers and physicians to justify the use of race rather than assume its relevance, the presumption may help the medical community to identify unsubstantiated assumptions, and to focus on the many other relevant aspects of a person's life and health before making treatment decisions.

The Nuffield Council on Bioethics, an advisory committee in the United Kingdom, recently released a report (Reference 50) in which it recommends that race never be used as a proxy for genotype or as a substitute for actual pharmacogenetic testing, even when relevant genetic variants are known to be more or less prevalent in particular racial or ethnic groups. The council further recommends that some federal agency should monitor access to treatment to determine whether inequalities emerge along racial or ethnic lines. The council recommendation is more stringent than the previously discussed presumption.

Thus far, this section has addressed the situation in which data are available about pharmacogenetic variations, but clinical genetic tests are unavailable. However, it should be clear that even if clinical genetic tests are available, physicians should not assume that the correlation between genotype and drug-response phenotype is robust. Genetic information is only one kind of information necessary for making good clinical decisions; it is not necessarily dispositive. Mistaken beliefs about genotype-phenotype correlations and race-phenotype correlations may result in treatment decisions that routinely, systematically, and unnecessarily deny an effective drug to patients of one race but not to patients of a different race.

It is the physician's duty to educate herself regarding the complexities involved in interpreting these tests. Acting ethically does not require anybody to do the impossible or to know the unknowable, and in every treatment decision there are unknowns. However, professionals are morally culpable for not educating themselves and for not using good professional judgment.

Pharmacogenetics in Research and Development

Pharmacogenomics and pharmacogenetics can play several roles in pharmaceutical research and development. These sciences may improve candidate drug selection; help researchers to develop new biomarkers for drug toxicity in animals and humans; aid researchers, particularly in stage II and stage III clinical trials, in determining who will likely respond to a drug and who will likely experience adverse side effects; and help rationalize drug dosing. These sciences may facilitate a paradigm shift in drug development, from current empirical approaches to mechanism-based, hypothesis-driven research. By comparison to current drug development, the hope and promise of pharmacogenetics and pharmacogenomics is that they will result in faster, lower cost, more effective, less toxic drugs that are appropriate for a smaller group of people. Whether this promise becomes reality remains to be seen, and as the Nuffield Council on Bioethics report states, "At this stage, it is not possible to predict the impact of pharmacogenetics on the cost of medicines" (Reference 50).

The United States FDA currently does not require submission of pharmacogenetic or pharmacogenomic data for clinical trials. The agency is developing policies for using and submitting these data. In April 2003, the director of the FDA's Center for Drug Evaluation and Research stated that any pharmacogenetic data actually used by sponsors in protocol decision-making in a human trial should be submitted (Reference 51). Also, a sponsor may submit pharmacogenetic or pharmacogenomic data to bolster a claim or scientific position. The agency will request voluntary submission of pharmacogenetic and pharmacogenomic information, not to be used for regulatory decision-making, but to aid regulators in developing a knowledge base. The FDA plans to create an Interdisciplinary Pharmacogenomics Review Group that would review pharmacogenetic and pharmacogenomic information and engage in ongoing policy development. Other regulatory authorities, such as the European Medicines Evaluation Agency, also are developing policies for using pharmacogenetic and pharmacogenomic data. However, recall that the FDA does require that safety and efficacy data be analyzed for demographic subgroups (previously discussed), regardless of whether pharmacogenetics is involved.

Any type of genetics research raises numerous ethical questions, which have been addressed at great length and with admirable thoughtfulness in other articles and reports. With respect to pharmacogenetics research in particular, concerns about informed consent, subject privacy and confidentiality, reporting clinically relevant results to subjects, and the use of stored tissue samples have been discussed (References 50, 52, 61). Here, this chapter focuses on justice issues raised by pharmacogenetics research, particularly in the context of the differential distributions of pharmacogenetic and pharmacogenomic variants in different racial groups. Clearly, access to drugs will depend on the data generated regarding the suitability of any particular drug for any particular individual or group of people, and on the development of drugs suitable for as many people as possible. One general ethical concern about pharmacogenetic and pharmacogenomic research is that it will stratify patients with respect to their suitability for entire classes of existing drugs. Research could do this by determining that some groups of people are likely to be nonresponders or poor responders to a particular class of drugs, or that some groups are likely to suffer a high proportion of particularly adverse side effects.

Another means by which genetic research could stratify patient populations is by distinguishing among similar pathological processes. The same or similar symptoms may be caused by different pathological processes and biochemical pathways. Genetic research might reveal that some patients who share symptoms do so as a result of different causal mechanisms, and may, therefore, not respond to the same drugs.

In some cases, the drugs at issue will be those already labeled and on the market. In other cases, genetic research will occur parallel to drug development. In the latter, genetics could be used to determine who is included in clinical trials, with predicted responders or those with no predicted adverse side effects being included in Phase II and Phase III trials. This genetic stratifying process would then determine for whom drugs are developed and approved. If the stratifying process mapped onto race, ethnicity, then it could result in people of a particular race or ethnicity being largely excluded from the population for whom drugs were being developed.

Wholesale racial and ethnic exclusion from a protocol is unlikely to occur if the inclusion or exclusion criteria involve actual pharmacogenetic tests because, as previously discussed, when genetic differences occur among racial and ethnic groups, they are differences in the frequency of relevant alleles. Rarely does a pharmacogenetic variant appear in only one human group and no others. The problem of wholesale exclusion would be much greater if researchers simply used race as a proxy for genotype. This approach has been viewed as ethically problematic for the practice of medicine (previously discussed) and should be similarly viewed in the research context.

Race as a proxy for genotype should never count as a justification acceptable to regulatory authorities. When research is subject to regulatory requirements of inclusion (publicly funded research), and researchers must justify categorical exclusions of any racial or ethnic group, only actual genotype should be an acceptable justification. Using the actual genotype might result in the exclusion of more individuals from one race or ethnicity, but it would not deny research participation to individuals who would be acceptable participants but for race. Using actual genotype will help avoid the possibility that individuals who could benefit from research participation, or from the generalized knowledge developed, do not benefit because of categorical exclusion. It also will help avoid the possibility that some racial or ethnic groups have their health problems differentially and unjustly undervalued by public agencies or researchers. Also, where NIH is involved, researchers cannot argue that including people of different races will make the research more expensive, because the law explicitly rules out cost as a justification for excluding minorities or women from research.

There is a more insidious pathway through which pharmacogenetics and pharmacogenomics research could result in racial disparities with respect to drug development. To the extent that the genetic likelihood of reacting to a class of drugs varies in a manner that could be mapped on to race, ethnicity, or other socially relevant categories, then the genetics also stratifies groups based on which would present the most and least attractive markets. After all, a market is not determined by need or by how many people have a medical condition, but by ability to pay. Race and socioeconomic class covary in society, with non-whites possessing, on the average, lower incomes and less wealth. Furthermore, whites in the United States have greater access to health insurance and health care. A firm deciding among several research programs might make the economic decision to focus its resources on a program to develop a drug or class of drugs for those most likely to be insured or to have the economic resources to purchase the drug.

Thus, with respect to access to drugs there are two ways in which a racial or ethnic group might be affected by pharmacogenetic or pharmacogenomic tests. The first is if the group appeared to contain a large proportion of nonresponders or poor responders, or a high proportion of those predicted to experience adverse side effects. The second is if the group is likely to contain a high proportion of all responders, but is economically disadvantaged. In either case, this segmentation of patient populations, when combined with crude cost-benefit analysis done by public or private research sponsors, might avert research on potentially useful new drugs. Of course, in some instances, stratification also may lead to the development and labeling of drugs that would not otherwise have been developed, because it may be possible to show safety and efficacy in a subgroup even when no statistically valid effects are observed in the total patient pool.

Pharmacogenetic stratification is not necessarily bad or suspect. It becomes suspect if it works consistently to the disadvantage of one or more social groups. It becomes suspect if it results in researchers and the medical profession classifying some groups as "innately difficult to treat."

How should biomedical research institutions respond to the fact that genetic differences influence people's drug responsiveness? Genomes are immutable, and result from the working of a "natural lottery." Nobody has chosen her own genome; however, people in society collectively can choose how institutions respond to any individual's genetic endowment. Does justice require that medical institutions minimize the effects of genetic inequality on people's opportunities to compete for the goods of society? Does a showing of equal concern and respect for all people require medical institutions to conduct research and drug development in a manner that minimizes differential access to drugs or a manner that minimizes health disparities? Even if society arrives at overlapping consensus on the general proposition that justice requires attempts to respond equally to the health needs of all social groups and to mitigate health disparities, that consensus may not extend to agreement as to the specific responses required. Members of society may not agree on which kinds of research programs to undertake and which social institutions are responsible for bearing the financial burden of achieving a more just society.

Some theories of equal opportunity dictate that social institutions aim to create a "level playing field" from which members of society could compete for goods and positions (Reference 44). Creating a level playing field involves removing formal legal barriers, removing informal or *de facto* discriminatory barriers, and further, removing impediments caused by accidents of birth. Typically, the accidents of birth theories have focused on poverty and lack of education. (Level playing field versions of equal opportunity are quite demanding, and may require redistribution of wealth or governmental intrusion in institutional practices; for this reason they are not attractive to some equality theorists.) Is access to health care, and the research that makes it possible, another feature of social institutions that must be leveled to produce genuine equality of opportunity? The answer to this question might depend on a person's justification for the level playing field approach.

Some theorists argue for a level playing field because they believe that current inequalities are caused by past and continuing unjust social structures. Thus, the current distribution of social assets represents the cumulative effect of ongoing, illegitimate discrimination. Can the same be said for health care and biomedical research?

Some level playing field theorists would hold that justice does not require the remedy of many health-related inequalities, particularly those arising from genetics (Reference 44). That people are born with different genetic endowments is not attributable to past discrimination by unjust social institutions; rather, it is a natural fact about the world and is not a subject of justice.

Other theorists would note that health disparities among minorities and whites do not stem primarily from differential distributions of genetic variants, but from social factors that are properly the subject of justice. They would note the well-documented history of racial and ethnic discrimination in biomedical research and medical care. They also might note the history of discrimination that has led to racial stratification in access to the social determinants of health, such as high-quality housing without lead-based paint and fulfilling, stable employment. Furthermore, attributing health inequalities solely or primarily to genes would be to use an overly simplistic model of the genotype-phenotype relationship. Phenotypes such as health outcomes typically arise through the complex interplay between genes and the environment. Although society cannot change people's genes, it can attempt to ensure that people with a broad variety of genotypes can thrive. Thus, noting that the composition of a particular person's genome, or any group's distribution of alleles, are natural facts about the world, does not necessarily indicate that the responses to these facts are irrelevant to producing a justice society.

Those concerned about racial inequalities produced by past and continuing invidious discrimination have a sordid research history at which to point. Although the best-known instance of racial abuse in research may be the previously discussed United States Public Health Service syphilis experiment at Tuskegee, historians of medicine have documented many others. For instance, at early medical school clinics and infirmaries free blacks, black slaves, and other poor members of society were considered suitable research subjects for experiments done without their knowledge and consent (Reference 53). Black slaves were used in early research on gynecological surgery, research that was done without anesthetic because physicians of the time believed that slaves did not experience pain the same way that white people do (Reference 54). The governor of the Zuni Indian Tribe states that researchers performed kidney biopsies, against medical advice, on Zuni research subjects (Reference 55). Many of the secret radiation experiments conducted during the cold war apparently involved people who were poor and minority (Reference 56). Most of this research was conducted to address the needs and further the goals of people who were well-off and white, not because the society or researchers had a particular concern for the lives and health of minority people.

After the disclosure of racial abuses in research and the introduction of federal regulations governing research ethics, the United States entered several decades during which minorities were largely excluded from research. This widespread exclusion may have led to less research on problems of particular concern to minority communities. Documentation of differential incidence and prevalence of disease largely took place in the 1990s, subsequent to federal legislation mandating inclusion.

The well-documented current health disparities, and the differential treatment of minorities in health care institutions, (Reference 18) may partially reflect the previous century's and decades' legacy of discriminatory research and lack of concern for minority health. For some level playing field theorists, ameliorating this past and continuing illegitimate discrimination would require that contemporary social institutions do what they can to remove impediments to equal opportunity caused by inadequate health care and inadequate research. At a minimum, for research to help produce a more level playing field, research programs would have to focus on the health care needs of all groups, and produce treatments (some of which would be drugs) that were responsive to the needs of all. This is not to say that any one treatment should be efficacious for everybody (an impossibility in many cases), but rather that enough treatments should be developed that people with different constitutions would have a similar probability of having their opportunity-limiting health problems addressed.

A second, different justification for the level playing field concept of equal opportunity is the moral intuition that people should not have lesser opportunity because of factors beyond their control. A person's claim on a share of social goods should not depend on the "natural lottery" (Reference 44). This view requires that society do what is possible to equalize the initial distribution of assets, regardless of whether the initial inequality was created by social institutions or by nature. Under this view, it would not matter whether patterns of racial and ethnic health and health care inequality reflected past discrimination or genetic endowments, society should respond as a matter of justice. A criticism of this second view is that it would seem to require an endless investment in biomedical research and interventions in the attempt to equalize opportunity (Reference 44). Under this conception, society would have to respond to all genetic and biological inequalities that limit a person's competitiveness for goods and positions, even if these inequalities could not be characterized as diseases or poor health states.

One philosopher has argued for a theory of health care justice in which equal opportunity requires that health care institutions direct their resources toward bringing as many individuals as possible into a range of health described as "normal species functioning." (Reference 45). Under this view, a health care system should aim to place as many as possible in the position of a normal or average competitor for goods and positions. Of course, one problem with the concept of normal species functioning is that, among humans, normal has often been defined with respect to a narrow range of individuals, a range that does not include women and minorities. Presuming that the concept of normal species functioning did take account of the variety of human forms and biologies, it still seems the case that a disproportionate number of minority individuals suffer from a compromised ability to compete due to untreated disease. A reasonable person could argue that justice requires that extra resources be directed toward developing treatments for minorities.

Some scholars who have studied the works of the great justice philosopher John Rawls argue that his theory would not address "natural" inequalities through the principle of equality of opportunity, but through another principle of justice, the difference principle. The difference principle requires social and economic inequalities to be arranged so that they are "reasonably expected to be to everyone's advantage," insofar as this arrangement is consistent with the greatest liberty for all (Reference 43). The social order should not secure more attractive life prospects for those who are naturally or socially better-off unless doing so is to the advantage of those less fortunate. According to Rawlsian theory, a just society is one in which social institutions operate according to principles that all rational people would agree to if none of them knew their place in society when they made the agreement. These principles would be necessary to create a society in which those who were least well-off had rational reasons for cooperating with those who were better-off.

People concerned about justice could reasonably argue that an approach to determining research priorities, or inclusion and exclusion criteria, that consistently disadvantaged minority members of society would not fulfill the difference principle. Whether measured by SES or health status, minorities typically are less well-off than whites in the United States. There is little reason to think that improving the health of whites by comparison to minorities would operate to increase the overall position of minorities in society. A pharmaceutical research program that aimed to produce drugs for the social and racial stratum with the greatest resources, and, therefore, chose to study or produce drugs that operated effectively in conjunction with alleles commonly found in whites, could become a research program that increased the advantages of the best-off without improving the lot of the least well-off.

Even if many views of equal opportunity require that society focus more resources on the health of minority individuals than it currently does, there are still many conceptual problems in determining what a just health care system, including biomedical and pharmaceutical research, would look like. Ontological and epistemological problems (problems concerning what exists and how people know what exists) arise from the fact that there is no consensus on what constitutes a good measure of health states or health quality. However, even with such problems, under most theories of justice, moral suspicion will arise if biomedical research and drug development priorities result in a pattern whereby more drugs are developed for majority racial or ethnic groups, or more pharmacogenetic tests are developed to prevent adverse side effects in majority racial or ethnic groups.

No justice theory is likely to produce a fully determined set of criteria for determining research priorities, and more than one set of priorities could meet the requirements of any justice theory. Should a just system aim for an equal number of drugs per disease for people of every racial and ethnic group? Such an approach may inadequately account for the fact that different groups are disproportionately affected by different diseases. Should the program aim to equalize the opportunity-limiting impact of disease burdens in different racial and ethnic groups? Such a system could result in a large proportion of the limited pool of research dollars being spent on a small number of people. Is it ethically acceptable to develop different amounts and kinds of drugs for different racial and ethnic groups but to compensate for any resulting health inequalities or inequalities in opportunity through some other means?

When developing a pharmacogenetic test for clinical use, how do researchers and program directors decide exactly which alleles to include?

For some drugs or some diseases, there may be thousands of alleles, not all of which can be screened for (for financial or technical reasons), and not all of which are at equal frequency in all racial or ethnic groups. So how do policy-makers and firms decide which alleles to include in a multiplex genetic test that will be administered to all of the people in a state or country? Do firms create different tests for different geographic regions? Should a state mandate tests tailored to the genetic make up of people within its jurisdiction or surveillance area?

To the extent that the previously discussed questions require the weighing and balancing of values and priorities, such questions may not be soluble by more refined application of ethical theory. Such problems may be more appropriately dealt with by creating institutional mechanisms through which many different segments of society can come together and engage in priority-setting. To be legitimate, such mechanisms should be widely accessible and the processes should be transparent. Decision-makers should expect to justify their decisions, particularly to participants who feel that the decision did not go their way. Justification should include a description of what information decision-makers took into account, what reasoning strategies were followed, and what means of weighing and valuing competing interests were used.

Several different genetics research projects currently are or recently have attempted to engage relevant publics in discussions and decision-making processes. The relevant publics are, at least, people from groups about whom scientific claims may be made. These typically are people who could participate in the research, but inevitably, not all of them will. Members of these groups may be affected by the research claims, even though they are not actual subjects and will not have the opportunity to provide individual informed consent.

Activities to involve broader publics in research design and priority-setting go under a variety of labels, including community consultation, community engagement, participatory research, and community dialogue. They also involve numerous methods, including exchanges of information and questions at town hall meetings, ethnographic study of members of the relevant groups, focus groups, interviews, and surveys. Consultation activities are designed to inform relevant social groups about the research, and to elicit from them some mixture of values, preferences, concerns, attitudes, and beliefs. These activities may not yet fulfill all of the criteria necessary for creating just decision-making procedures in research, but they are a start.

Policy-makers and ethics committees are beginning to recommend that some form of community consultation be undertaken when genetic research will likely make claims about members of identifiable or "named" social groups. An NIH guidance document titled, Points To Consider When Planning a Genetic Study that Involves Members of Named Populations, encourages investigators to consider whether and how the relevant group should be consulted (Reference 58). The National Bioethics Advisory Commission recommended that community consultation should take place when research on stored tissues (quite often some form of genetics research) could prove risky to "groups" (Reference 59).

Pharmacogenetics or pharmacogenomics may, on occasion, segment drug markets to the extent that there is no incentive for private firms to develop beneficial drugs. This situation would occur when the predicted market would be so small that the firm could not recoup its research and development investments during the patent term (the time when firms can charge higher-than-competitive prices). One law professor argues that despite their small markets, some drugs will provide overall benefit commensurate with the costs of their development (Reference 60). This is because drugs do not lose their efficacy when the patent expires, so they are still beneficial to society even if they are not making money for the initial developer.

Governments may need to provide additional incentives to encourage drug development. If, for some class of drugs, pharmacogenetic market segmentation coincides with racial or ethnic divisions in society, governmental intervention may be essential to ensure that beneficial drugs become available to people of all races and ethnicities. One suggested approach is to expand the Orphan Drug Act to subsidize manufacturers of some drugs that would otherwise appear unattractive because of pharmacogenetic-driven market segmentation (Reference 60).

Other direct and indirect incentives that could improve the likelihood that no group is systematically disadvantaged by pharmacogenetics include tax incentives for firms that carry out research on and development of drugs with small markets, and patent extensions.

Finally, there exists another domain of concern regarding justice and pharmacogenetic or pharmacogenomic research. Researchers with incomplete pharmacogenetic information, with unsophisticated understandings of race and ethnicity, or with an inadequate understanding of the social and political implications of their statements, may conduct research or report results in a manner that unnecessarily reinforces negative stereotypes and incorrect beliefs about race. Research that produces inaccurate data will ultimately be corrected through the scientific process. Incorrect interpretations of data will ultimately be corrected. On the other hand, public policy recommendations based on such inaccuracies can irrevocably devastate people's lives. For instance, scholars estimate that as many as 50,000 people in the United States were subjected to eugenic sterilization under laws designed to prevent the United States gene pool from being corrupted by the poor hereditary material of "feebleminded" people (Reference 27). Inaccurate scientific understandings behind the eugenic notion of a "feeblemindedness genes" have been corrected, but individuals who were sterilized cannot recover their fertility.

Avoiding such outcomes is required by the basic research ethics requirement that scientists refrain from creating unnecessary harms, although the people harmed by inadequately justified and wrongheaded public policy will include many beyond those who are or were research subjects. Principles of justice that reach beyond research ethics also would counsel that scientific institutions, including those involved in research, refrain from creating additional burdens on and barriers to those who are already disadvantaged, and refrain from unjustifiably diminishing the opportunities of particular human groups.

One tremendously insightful and amusing book on the meanings of human genetic similarity and difference states that scientists have some moral responsibility to learn from the past mistakes of their predecessors (Reference 24). The author particularly addresses scientists who engage in genetics research, and their responsibilities to study and learn from the mistakes of early 20th century geneticists who articulated and supported the eugenics agenda in the United States and abroad. "In science, you do not have the right to make the same mistakes over and over—you only have the right to make new and creative mistakes" (Reference 24). Such education also might include a study of the history of the concepts of race and ethnicity, and some current social science on race, ethnicity, and identity formation.

In addition to a general education on the history of eugenics, and education on the nature of race, researchers will run less risk of creating injustice if they devise strategies to detect and avoid some common mistakes found in the contemporary scientific literature pertaining to race, ethnicity, and genetic variation. Chief among these is the tendency to attribute interracial or interethnic health differences to genetics, even in the absence of data. The gathering of data describing differences between races or ethnic groups is viewed as an end in itself, with few studies designed to actually identify an etiology, perhaps because the genetic etiology is presumed. Observations of difference are not necessarily incorrect; however, they often do nothing more than restate a social reality as a putative biologic one (Reference 5).

The logical constructs necessary for proving that racial differences in complex health states are caused by innate biological differences are quite complex. The counterfactual framework that justifies certain causal claims in randomized, controlled trials cannot necessarily be applied to retrospective, observational studies (Reference 5). If an investigator takes a group of similar individuals, randomly divides them in half, and exposes half to an experimental treatment and half to a control, the investigator is justified in concluding that the collective outcome observed in the treatment arm was caused by the treatment only if the individuals in the treatment arm are truly interchangeable with the individuals in the control arm.

But suppose the investigator is doing a retrospective or observational study on the degree to which Asians are more susceptible to developing depression than are other racial groups. Controls for confounding variables can only be done through statistical adjustments. But such adjustments "become suspect when used to identify the independent effects of attributes that define the essential character of an individual, such as gender or race" (Reference 5). The counterfactual framework would reduce to the question, "What would the risk of depression have been for this individual if she were not Asian?" Is such a question coherent?

As a general matter, attempting to infer the genetic effects of race from observational, epidemiological studies may be impossible in many cases because of the vast number of social factors that correlate with race. These social influences are confounders that overwhelm extant statistical techniques. Many of these influences may not be observable or easily measurable. Exposures that produce developmental effects also may be difficult to measure as variables distinct from race. Thus, studies that control for one or two socioeconomic variables and then observe a residual influence of race do not justify claims about the likely genetic influences of race (Reference 42).

As previously discussed, a corollary logical problem arises when scientists observe racial or ethnic differences in the pharmacogenetic alleles at some locus, and then assume that these differences must lead to racial differences in in vivo pharmacology. And a problem arises when researchers assume, without further experimentation, that allelic differences explain any observed racial differences in in vivo pharmacology. As previously discussed, such assumptions are unjustified and should be avoided. Connecting genotype to phenotype requires data. Pharmacogenetic alleles may have less than full penetrance or may not always be expressed. Dietary factors may undermine simple allele-phenotype correlations by up-regulating or down-regulating enzymes, or otherwise altering drug response.

Another significant problem in the literature is the failure to adequately specify the groups or populations being studied. Labels such as Asian, Chinese, Hispanic, Caucasian, Spanish, and African American are not sufficiently informative. Within the constraints of respect for agreements pertaining to the confidentiality of individuals and study populations, researchers should describe what is known about the culture and migration patterns of study subjects drawn from geographically localized groups. Researchers should be explicit about subjects who are of the same race or nationality but from more than one cultural group. They should make clear when the study involves members of more than one nationality but from the same race. And when using race or ethnicity, they should describe how those identities were determined. Researchers should characterize study samples with respect to the proportions of immigrants and United States-born individuals. A more complete description of study subjects will allow all scientists to better judge when and to what degree generalizations can be drawn, and which studies are comparable.

One commentator suggests that researchers could minimize injustices associated with research on racial differences if they adopted a rebuttable presumption that any observed differences are not due to innate biological differences (Reference 19). Adopting such a presumption might lead to more studies in which an observed racial difference was followed up by studies of the same group of people in different environments. For instance, studies could compare a relevant outcome, such as drug response, in people who emigrated from a particular canton in Sweden to Northern Wisconsin, rural Colorado, a city in Japan, and a city in Jamaica, to determine whether each group showed similar pharmacokinetic or pharmacodynamics profiles. Although identifying specific environmental influences will be difficult, such studies would show that environmental influences exist and play a role in creating observed racial differences in pharmacology.

Conclusions

Pharmacogenetics and pharmacogenomics hold the promise of improving health care delivery and rationalizing drug development. Use of these technologies may allow physicians to maximize the effectiveness of the drugs they prescribe while minimizing adverse side effects. In research, these technologies may allow investigators to minimize harm to human subjects while demonstrating safety and effectiveness more quickly or for more drugs. However, the development and use of these technologies also holds perils. This chapter focused on the perils associated with racial disparities in access to drugs, and the perils of undertaking and reporting scientific research in a manner that unjustifiably reinforces incorrect beliefs about race and promotes racial prejudices.

In their clinical and research activities, scientists and physicians should apply a rebuttable presumption that innate, genetic differences among races are <u>not</u> the cause or explanation for any observed racial differences. Applying this presumption may help clinicians and researchers overcome the deep and unconscious assumptions that they absorb simply by living in a racially stratified society. Commentators should not conclude that injustice has occurred simply because an action or policy produces different consequences for people of different races; however, given this country's history of invidious racial discrimination, and given the current inequalities in health and health care, racial disparities should raise ethical flags. Racial distinctions in access to medicines or inclusion in research should generate ethical scrutiny.

References

1. Schwartz RS. Racial profiling in medical research. N Engl J Med 2001;344(18):1392–3.

2. Bhopal R. Is research into ethnicity and health racist, unsound, or important science? BMJ 1997;314:1751–68.

3. Witzig R. The medicalization of race: scientific legitimization of a flawed social construct. Ann Intern Med 1996;125:675–9.

4. Cooper RS, Kaufman JS, Ward R. Race and Genomics. N Engl J Med 2003;348(12):1166–70.

5. Cooper RS, Kaufman JS. Race and hypertension: science and nescience. Hypertension 1998;32:813–16.

6. Burchard EG, Ziv E, Coyle N, et al. The importance of race and ethnic background in biomedical research and clinical practice. N Engl Med 2003;348(12):1170–75.

7. Risch N, Burchard E, Ziv E, Tang H. Categorization of humans in biomedical research: genes, race and disease. Genome Biol 2002;3(7):1–12.

8. Evans WE, Relling MV. Pharmacogenomics: translating functional genomics into rational therapeutics. Science 1999;286:487–91.

9. Haga SB, Venter JC. Genetics. FDA races in the wrong direction. Science 2003;301(5632):466–7.

10. Gaskin Z. Determining race proportions from crime scene DNA. DNAPrint Genetics. Available at *http://www.dnaprint.com/dnawitness.htm*. Accessed June 9, 2003.

11. Wilson JF. Population genetic structure of variable drug response. Nat Genet 2001;29:265–9.

12. Wood AJ. Racial differences in the response to drugs-pointers to genetic differences. N Engl J Med 2001;344(18):1393–5.

13. Xie HG, Kim RB, Wood AJ, Stein CM. Molecular basis of ethnic differences in drug disposition and response. Ann Rev Pharmacol Toxicol 2001;41:815–50.

14. National Institutes of Health Revitalization Act. 1994. Public Law 103–43, 1993 S 1. 103rd Congress. Approved June 10, 1993.

15. Guidelines on the inclusion of women and minorities as subjects in clinical research. Fed Regist 1994;59:14508.

16. Clayton EW, Steinberg KK, Khoury MJ, et al. Consensus statement: informed consent for genetic research on stored tissue samples. JAMA 1995;274(22):1786–92.

17. United States Centers for Disease Control and Prevention; United States Agency for Toxic Substances and Disease Registry. Available at *http://www.atsdr.cdc.gov*.

18. Policy on the inclusion of women and racial and ethnic minorities in externally awarded research. Fed Regist 1995;60:47947–51.

19. Smedley BD, Stith AY, Nelson AR, eds. Unequal treatment: confronting racial and ethnic disparities in health care. Washington, D.C.: Institute of Medicine; 2002.

20. King PA. Race, justice, and research. In: Sugarman J, Kahn JP, Mastroianni AC, eds. Beyond consent: seeking justice in research. New York, NY: Oxford University Press; 1998:88–110.

21. Macbeth H. What is an ethnic group? A biological perspective. In: Parsons E, Clark A, eds. Culture, kinship, and genes: toward cross-cultural genetics. New York, NY: St. Martin's Press; 1997:54–66.

22. Loue S. Gender, ethnicity, and health research. New York, NY: Klewer Academic/Plenum Publishers; 1999.

23. Molnar S. Human variation: races, types and ethnic groups, 4th Ed. Upper Saddle River, NJ: Prentic Hall, Inc.; 1998.

24. Higginbotham EB. African-American women's history and the metalanguage of race. Signs 1992;17:253–68.

25. Marks J. What it means to be 98 percent chimpanzee. Berkeley, CA: University of California Press; 2002.

26. Loving v. Virginia. Supreme Court Reporter 1967;87:1817.

27. Kevles DJ. In the name of eugenics: genetics and the use of human heredity. Cambridge, MA: Harvard University Press; 1985.

28. Mazumdar PMH. Eugenics, human genetics, and human failings: the eugenics society, its sources and its critics in Britain. New York, NY: Routledge; 1992.

29. Ordover N. American eugenics: race, queer anatomy, and the science of nationalism. Minneapolis, MN: University of Minnesota Press; 2003.

30. Olson S. The genetic archeology of race. Atlantic Monthly April 2001.

31. Olson S. Mapping human history: discovering the past through our genes. New York, NY: Houghton Mifflin Company; 2002.

32. Templeton AR. Human races: a genetic and evolutionary perspective. Amer Anthrop 1999;100:632–50.

33. Rosenberg NA, Pritchard JK, Weber JL, et al. Genetic structure of human populations. Science 2002;298:2381–5.

34. Relethford JH. Genetics of modern human origins and diversity. Ann Rev Anthropol 1998;27:1–23.

35. Reich DE, Cargill M, Bolk S, et al. Linkage disequilibrium in the human genome. Nature 2001;411:199–204.

36. Lopez IH. White by law. New York, NY: New York University Press; 1996.

37. Statement of the American Sociological Association on the importance of collecting data and doing social scientific research on race: American Sociological Association; 2002. Available at *http://www.asanet.org/governance/racestmt.html*. Accessed June 1, 2003.

38. Root M. The problem of race in medicine. Philo Soc Sci 2001;31(1):20–39.

39. Sheet WHF. President Clinton announces new racial and ethnic health disparities initiative; 1998. Available at

http://raceandhealth.hhs.gov/sidebars/sbinitPres.htm. Accessed September 20, 2003.

40. Kahn J. Getting the numbers right: statistical mischief and racial profiling in heart failure research. Perspect Biol Med 2003;46(4):473–83.

41. Exner DV, Dries DL, Domanski MJ, Cohn JN. Lesser response to angiotensin-converting enzyme inhibitor therapy in black as compared with white patients with left ventricular disfunction. N Engl J Med 2001;344:1351–7.

42. Dries DL, Strong M, Cooper R, Drazner M. Efficacy of angiotensin-converting enzyme inhibition in reducing progression from asymptomatic left ventricular dysfunction to symptomatic heart failure in black and white patients. J Am Coll Cardiol 2002;40(4):311–17.

43. Kaufman JS, Cooper RS, McGee DL. Socioeconomic status and health in blacks and whites: the problem of residual confounding and the resiliency of race. Epidemiology 1997;8(6):621–8.

44. Rawls J. A theory of justice. Cambridge, MA: Harvard University Press; 1971.

45. Buchanan A, Brock DW, Daniels N, Wikler D. From chance to choice: genetics and justice. Cambridge, MA: Cambridge University Press; 2000.

46. Daniels N. Just health care. New York, NY: Cambridge University Press; 1985.

47. Sen A. Inequality reexamined. Cambridge, MA: Harvard University Press; 1992.

48. Brandt AM. Racism and research: the case of the Tuskegee syphilis study. Hastings Center Report 1978:21–9.

49. Aklillu E, Herrlin K, Gustafsson LL, Bertilsson L, Ingelman-Sundberg M. Evidence for environmental influence on CYP2D6-catalysed debrisoquine hydroxylation as demonstrated by phenotyping and genotyping of Ethiopians living in Ethiopia or in Sweden. Pharmacogenetics 2002;12(5):375–83.

50. Tang MX, Stern Y, Marder K, et al. The APOE-E4 allele and the risk of Alzheimer disease among African Americans, whites and Hispanics. JAMA 1998;279(10):751–5.

51. Pharmacogenetics: ethical issues. London, England: Nuffield Council on Bioethics; September 2003. Available at *http://www.nuffieldbioethics.org/ publications/pp_0000000018.asp*. Accessed January 22, 2004.

52. Woodcock J. Drug development and regulation in the age of pharmacogenomics; 2003. Food and Drug Administration Web site. Available at *http://www.fda.gov/ohrms/dockets/ac/03/briefing/3964B1_02_Woodcock.pdf*. Accessed September 22, 2003.

53. Buchanan A, Califano A, Kahn JP, McPherson E, Robertson J, Baruch B. Pharmacogenetics: ethical issues and policy options. Kennedy Inst Ethics J 2002;12(1):1–15.

54. Savitt T. The use of blacks for medical experimentation and demonstration in the Old South. J South His August 1982;48:331–48.

55. Richardson DA. Ethics in gynecologic surgical innovation. Am J Obstet Gynecol January 1994;170:1–6.

56. Bowekaty MB. Perspectives on research in American Indian communities. Jurimetrics 2002;42:145–8.

57. Cincinnati Radiation Litigation. District Court for the Southern District of Ohio. F Supp 1995;874:796.

58. NIH. Points To Consider When Planning a Genetic Study That Involves Members of Named Populations. National Institutes of Health Web site. April 01, 2002. Available at *http://www.nih.gov/sigs/ bioethics/named_populations.html*. Accessed September 01, 2003.

59. National Bioethics Advisory Commission. Research Involving Human Biological Materials: Ethical Issues and Policy Guidance. Volume I: Report and Recommendations of the National Bioethics Advisory Commission. Rockville, MD: National Bioethics Advisory Commission; August 1999.

60. Rai AK. Pharmacogenetic interventions, orphan drugs, and distributive justice: the role of cost-benefit analysis. Soc Philoso Policy 2002;19(2):246–70.

61. Allen, WL. Ethical, legal, and social issues in pharmacogenomics. In: Allen, WL, Johnson JA, Knoell DL, et al, eds. Pharmacogenomics: Applications to Patient Care. Kansas City: American College of Clinical Pharmacy, 2004:227–52.

Self-Assessment Questions

1. Which one of the following does federal law require?

    A. Scientists whose research is funded by any federal agency must include racial and ethnic minorities in their human subjects research.
    B. Scientists whose research is funded by the National Institutes of Health (NIH) must include racial and ethnic minorities in their human subjects research, unless doing so is not cost-effective.
    C. Scientists who conduct NIH-sponsored Phase III clinical trials must include sufficient numbers of racial and ethnic minorities so that valid analyses of the intervention's effect on different subgroups can be performed.
    D. Scientists whose research is sponsored by the NIH or Centers for Disease Control and Prevention (CDC) should include racial and ethnic minorities in all of their human subjects research, if data from prior studies indicate the existence of differences in intervention effect among racial or ethnic groups.

2. Agencies recommend that data on the race and ethnicity of research subjects should do which one of the following?

    A. Reflect the researcher's assessment of each subject's ancestry.
    B. Be collected using as many different categories as possible.
    C. Include the birthplace of each grandparent, if known.
    D. Be reported using the Office of Management and Budget (OMB) race and ethnicity categories.

3. Which one of the following was the purpose of antimiscegenation laws in the United States?

    A. To preserve the so-called purity of the white race.
    B. To prevent the birth of feebleminded people.
    C. To prevent non-white people from immigrating to the United States.
    D. To prevent non-white people from naturalizing as United States citizens.

4. Which one of the following statements is the most common explanation for the unusually low genetic diversity of the human species?

    A. Several distinct populations of modern humans arose at different geographic locations around the world, but these separate populations later merged to form one, large indistinguishable human species.
    B. All modern humans arose from a small population in eastern Africa that rapidly expanded and generated the current world population.

C. Those humans who had more Neanderthal genes became extinct.
D. The progenitor population for modern humans arose in Asia, and then expanded around the world; some went back to repopulate Africa.

5. Clinal genetic variation describes which one of the following?

A. In comparisons of one population to another, dramatic discontinuities in allele frequencies between populations that are geographically proximate.
B. A high degree of within-group genetic variation in a single population.
C. In comparisons of one population to another, a high degree of between-group genetic variation.
D. In comparisons of one population to another, gradual variation in allele frequencies that increases with geographic distance.

6. About 75 percent of all human genetic variation is found within any human population. Which one of the following statements is true of the remaining 15 percent?

A. All of it is scientifically useful in distinguishing among people from different continents.
B. About 10 percent is useful in distinguishing among people from different continents.
C. About 5 percent is useful in distinguishing among people from different continents.
D. None of it can be used to distinguish among people from different continents.

7. Generally speaking, which one of the following statements is true of social justice theories?

A. They are concerned with whether a social system creates the greatest possible aggregate good for society.
B. They are theories about how to produce equality of outcomes.
C. They are Aristotelian theories.
D. They are concerned with the generation of benefits, burdens, or harms, and with the fairness of their distribution.

8. Which one of the following justice concerns is raised by the possibility that pharmacogenetics could be used to discover, develop, and market race-targeted drugs?

A. That a health care system will be developed in which people of some races will have less access than people of other races to medically beneficial pharmaceuticals.

B. That drug markets will become so segmented that drug development in the private sector will no longer be economically viable.
C. That people of different races will receive different drugs for the same conditions.
D. That too many drugs will be developed that are only effective for a small group of people.

9. The level playing field conception of equal opportunity could require that social institutions remove barriers to competition that result from people's "unequal genetic endowments." Which one of the following statements supports this claim?

A. Under a level playing field theory, past discrimination does not justify present remedial actions.
B. People's genomes are the result of a "natural lottery" so they should not dictate people's life chances.
C. An individual's claim on a share of social goods should depend only on his or her character and on whether he or she has adequately developed the appropriate virtues, such as industriousness. Genes are irrelevant in determining a person's fair share.
D. With the expenditure of enough resources, anybody could be brought within a range of health states that would make him or her a normal competitor for the scarce positions and goods of society.

10. "The dilemma of difference" refers to which one of the following problems?

A. The problem of finding drugs that can be efficacious in a multiracial, multiethnic patient population.
B. The problem that, by its nature, the type of research that may be necessary to help eradicate health in equalities runs a high risk of exacerbating those inequalities instead.
C. The problem that scientists do not have adequate statistical tools or research methods to distinguish among the many possible causes of racial differences in drug response.
D. The problem that scientists do not know, *a priori*, when pharmacogenetic stratification of patients or research subjects is wrong. Such stratification is only ethically suspect when it works consistently or systematically to the disadvantage of one or more racial groups.

Oncology and Hematology

Jill M. Kolesar, Pharm.D., FCCP, BCPS

Key Words

Pharmacogenomics, oncology, carcinogenesis, genetic testing, thiopurine methyltransferase (TPMT) deficiency, dihydropyrimidine dehydrogenase (DPD) deficiency, multidrug resistance polymorphisms, and cytochrome P450 polymorphisms.

Abstract

Cancer represents a complicated genetic picture. Genetic mutations in genes, such as *p53*, both cause cancer and influence response to treatment. Analysis of cancer-causing genes may be performed to assess risk of cancer, institute preventive strategies, or to diagnose and classify disease, and assist in determining prognosis. Genetic mutations also become targets for cancer therapies and are driving current drug development. For example, imitinab was developed to target the Philadelphia chromosome, the characteristic mutation of chronic myelogenous leukemia. Polymorphisms in drug metabolizing enzymes, such as the cytochrome P450 enzymes, influence an individual's response to both chemotherapy and supportive care agents, and polymorphisms in drug efflux pumps, such as P-glycoprotein, can influence drug concentrations and response. Given the multitude of genes that affect a single drug and the number of different genes potentially important in the carcinogenesis process, it appears likely that combinations of genes will need to be considered to determine the best management of a patient.

Outline

Learning Objectives

1. Describe the role of pharmacogenetics in carcinogenesis.
2. Understand the role of genetic mutations in the diagnosis and prognosis of cancer and hematological disorders.
3. Describe the clinical use of pharmacogenomics and pharmacogenetics in oncology pharmacotherapy.
4. Appreciate the use of pharmacogenomics in developing new antineoplastic agents.

Abbreviations in this Chapter

5-FdUMP	5-Fluoro-2-deoxyuridine monophosphate
5-FU	5-Fluorouracil
5-HT$_3$	Serotonin type 3
6-MP	6-Mercaptopurine
AAPC	Attenuated adenomatous polyposis coli
ALL	Acute lymphoblastic leukemia
AML	Acute myelogenous leukemia
APC	Adenomatous polyposis coli
ASCO	American Society of Clinical Oncology
bcr	Breakpoint cluster region
BER	Base excision repair
CLL	Chronic lymphocytic leukemia
CMF	Cyclophosphamide, methotrexate, and 5-FU
CML	Chronic myelogenous leukemia
CR	Complete remission
CYP	Cytochrome P450
DHFU	5$_1$b Dihydrofluorouracil
DNA	Deoxyribonucleic acid
DPD	Dihydropyrimidine dehydrogenase

ERCC	Excision repair cross complementing
FAB	French, American, and British (classification)
FAP	Familial adenomatous polyposis
GST	Glutathione S transferase
HNPCC	Hereditary nonpolyposis colon cancer
IFN	Interferon
MDR	Multidrug resistance
MDS	Myelodysplasia
MHFR	Methylenetetrahydrofolate reductase
MMC	Mitomycin-c
MMR	Mismatch repair
mRNA	Messenger ribonucleic acid
MSI	Microsatellite instability
MTD	Maximum tolerated dose
NER	Nucleotide excision repair
Pgp	P-glycoprotein
Ph	Philadelphia (chromosome)
PM	Poor metabolizer (genotype)
RAR-α	Retinoic acid receptor-alpha
TI	Topoisomerase I
TPMT	Thiopurine methyltransferase
TS	Thymidylate synthase
UGT	UDP-Glucuronosyltransferase

Introduction

Cancer is a group of disorders characterized by uncontrolled cellular growth and caused by the combination of inherited genetic and acquired environmental exposures. Taking all cancers together, the American Cancer Society estimated that in 2003 there would be more than 1,330,000 new cases and 556,500 deaths due to cancer in the United States. This estimate corresponds to 25 percent of all deaths and a death rate of 1500 people/day.

Despite the "war on cancer" declared by Richard Nixon's signing of the National Cancer Act on December 12, 1971, cancer continues to claim the lives of Americans in record numbers, second only to heart disease, and, unless there is a significant medical breakthrough, cancer is expected to overtake heart disease as the leading killer in the next 10–15 years. Since 1971, more than 12.5 million Americans have died of cancer, and more than $45 billion has been spent by the National Cancer Institute alone for studying cancer. This number does not include health care and treatment-related costs, which were estimated by the National Institutes of Health for 2002 to be $60.9 billion for direct medical costs of patients with cancer.

The tide may be turning in the war on cancer; in fact, testicular cancer, acute lymphomas, and childhood leukemias, once almost uniformly and rapidly fatal, are routinely cured today. These advances are in a large part related to the use of aggressive combination chemotherapy and stem cell transplants, with advanced supportive care. In addition, in breast cancer, the second leading cause of cancer death in women, mortality declined by 1.4 percent/year between 1989 and 1995 and by 3.2 percent/year thereafter. The largest reductions were noted in younger women and are attributed to earlier detection through screening programs and better therapies.

Prevention and genomics are likely the next major frontiers in cancer. Lifestyle factors, including smoking, which is directly linked to lung cancer (male smokers are at 20 times the risk for developing lung cancer), and obesity, as recently reported in the New England Journal of Medicine, are responsible for increased death rates for most cancers. If Americans could maintain an ideal weight (body mass index less than 25) and stop smoking, it is estimated that more than 250,000 deaths could be prevented annually.

Cancer is a genetic disorder, and our genes hold the answers to our overall risk for cancer as well as our likelihood of benefiting from a given therapy. Individuals not only have inherited cancer susceptibility, but also the mutations they acquire in somatic cells drive the development of cancer. Finally, both their inherited genetic makeup and the acquired mutations may influence how they respond to a given intervention. Genomic information is being used to guide anticancer drug development, individualize drug therapy, and assess cancer risk.

Carcinogenesis

Overview

It is well accepted that most cancers are acquired genetic diseases, and many years of research have identified the multistage process of carcinogenesis as the mechanism of acquiring a cancer. The first and irreversible step is initiation, or the interaction of a carcinogen with a target tissue. Although the results of an initiation event typically are unobservable in pathological specimens, initiated cells are thought to be the precursor cells for future neoplasms. The next step is that of promotion, which is a reversible process that facilitates the expression of the initiated cells. Cells in this stage are still premalignant and conversion to a malignant stage (progression) is the longest stage of carcinogenesis. The final step, or development of metastatic potential, occurs quite rapidly in the development of a tumor.

Genetic Susceptibility to Cancer

Although many individuals are exposed to carcinogens, few actually develop a cancer. Predicting who will develop a cancer and why are important applications of pharmacogenomics information. Differences in carcinogen metabolism, as well as cell susceptibility, may make significant contributions in the carcinogenesis process.

Xenobiotic Drug Metabolizing Enzymes

Xenobiotic drug metabolizing enzymes, including the cytochrome P450s (*CYPs*), are essential not only in metabolizing clinically useful drugs, but in detoxifying environmental and chemical carcinogens. Therefore, a long-standing, yet largely still unproven, hypothesis for carcinogenesis is that polymorphisms in these metabolizing enzymes lead to altered metabolism, either increased activation or decreased inactivation of environmental carcinogens, prolonged exposure to genotoxic compounds, and hence cancer. Numerous case-control and epidemiological studies have been reported.

What is well known is that *CYP* enzymes are involved in the activations of numerous carcinogens. The role of CYP1A1 in benzo pyrene metabolism; CYP1A2 in toluene and the heterocyclic amines found in broiled meat; CYP1B1 in nitropyrenes; CYP2E1 in benzene, butadiene, chloroform, and vinyl chloride; and CYP3A4 in aflatoxin metabolism are well established.

There is substantial evidence from animal models that susceptibility to cancer induced by chemical carcinogens is greatly influenced by variations in CYPP450 enzymes. Although not as conclusive as the animal studies, population epidemiological evidence supports the association of CYP1A1 inducibility, potentially related to the *2B genotype, with susceptibility to tobacco-induced cancers in Japanese populations, but not in Caucasian or other populations, including lung and head and neck cancers, and the CYP1A2 *2F genotype with an increased risk of colon cancer and bladder cancer. The significance of these polymorphisms is still unclear, as most are rare, with allelic frequencies of less than 10 percent.

The family of glutathione S transferases (GST) are enzymes, including alpha, (A), mu (M), pi (P), and theta (T) that catalyze reduced glutathione-dependent reactions with compounds containing an electrophilic center, including occupational and environmental carcinogens such as solvents, pesticides, and polycyclic aromatic hydrocarbons. One polymorphism has been identified in each of GSTM1 and GSTT1 that results in a loss of functional gene product. Two polymorphisms in *GSTP1* have been discovered (I105V and A114V) for which effects on function have not been fully evaluated, although those with the 105 valine allele appear to have some degree of decreased enzyme activity, which varies with the substrate. The GSTM1 polymorphisms occur in about 50 percent of Caucasians and are associated with an increased risk of lung cancers, as is the *GSTP1* I105V.

A recent large case-control genotyping study evaluated multiple genotypes and identified 1A1*2C and the GSTM1*2/*2 genotype, both involved in the metabolism of polycyclic aromatic hydrocarbons, such as benzpyrene, as predictors of high risk for lung cancer. See Table 1.

Deoxyribonucleic Acid Repair Enzymes

After a carcinogen causes a lesion in deoxyribonucleic acid (DNA), DNA repair enzymes are on hand to repair it. Therefore, a more recently generated hypothesis is that polymorphisms in DNA repair pathways also may contribute to carcinogenesis.

The DNA repair enzymes have been evaluated extensively in the past 10 years, with four different pathways of DNA repair identified. Each of the four pathways involves multiple molecules and repair specific types of damaged DNA. Base excision repair (BER) repairs small lesions such as oxidized or reduced bases, fragmented or nonbulky adducts, or those produced by methylating agents. Other involved molecules include apurinic endonuclease and apyrimidinic endonuclease, polynucleotide kinase, DNA polymerase-β, and XRCC1. Nucleotide excision repair (NER) acts on larger lesions, such as large chemical adducts or cross-links. Nucleotide excision repair involves lesion recognition, formation of the TFIIH complex, unwinding, incision, and removal of 25–30 nucleotides. Mismatch repair (MMR) recognizes mismatched bases (e.g., A paired with C) and uses MLH1, MSH2, PMS2, and MSH6 in damage recognition, followed by excision, polymerization, and ligation. Double-strand breaks, like those caused by ionizing radiation, are repaired by two pathways: the first involves Rad52 and Rad51, XRCC2 and XRCC3, and BRCA1 and BRCA2; the second involves DNA-PK, XRCC4, and LIG4.

Of these enzymes involved in DNA repair, OGG1, XRCC, and BRCA2 exhibit polymorphisms in up to 50 percent of reference population controls and have been evaluated in epidemiological studies in the United States, Asia, and Europe to test the hypothesis that defects in DNA repair lead to the inability to repair damaged DNA and carcinogenesis.

Table 1. Human Drug Metabolizing Enzymes Potentially Important in Cariogenesis

Allele	Variant	Population	Cancer Risk	Strength of Association
1A1	M1, M2	Caucasians	Lung	Controversial
1A1/GST	GST/M1	Japanese smokers	Lung	Strong consistent association in multiple studies
NQO1	*2	Benzene exposed	Aplastic anemia, leukemia	Strong association in one large population study
NQO1	*2	Prior chemotherapy	MDS, AML	Consistent effect in multiple studies

AML = acute myeloid leukemia; GST = glutathione transferase; MDS = myelodysplasia.

OGG1, responsible for excising oxidized guanine from DNA, has 10 common polymorphisms with an allele frequency ranging from 0.15–0.50 in reference population controls. OGG1 polymorphisms have been evaluated for lung and prostate cancer risk, and consistently show increased risk for lung and prostate cancer with the variant genotypes in both Caucasian and Asian populations. XRCC is responsible for stimulating endonuclease activity after the damaged base is removed. A characteristic polymorphism is present, R194W, in 0.06-0.35 of control populations. When evaluated in breast cancer, lung cancer, and bladder cancer risk, the presence of the W allele is associated with a decreased risk of cancer with odds ratios ranging from 0.6 to 07. Of interest, BRCA2 gene product is important in DNA double-strand repair. A polymorphism at N372H present in 0.22–0.27 of controls is associated with an increased risk of breast cancer in one small American study and one large population-based study evaluating more than 2000 Australian women.

Overall, there is no polymorphism that is commonly accepted to predispose an individual to cancer or to cause cancer, and there is no clinically used screening test. Therefore, the current in vitro and epidemiological data appear to support another long held notion that carcinogenesis is multifactorial and suggesting that haplotypes, most likely in combination with environmental exposures, will have better predictive power. It appears likely that assessing a "chemoprevention haplotype" will be necessary to develop a tailored cancer prevention plan.

Treatment-related or Secondary Malignancies

Treatment-related, or secondary malignancies are a complication of malignancies successfully treated with chemo- or radiotherapy. Treatment-related malignancies occur in about 1 percent of individuals within 1 year of completion of initial chemotherapy. Long-term survivors of breast cancer, testicular cancer, pediatric leukemias, and lymphomas are at the greatest risk; however, this risk is most likely because these cancers are the potentially curable malignancies; should other cancers be cured with chemotherapy, patients with those cancers also would be at risk for treatment-related malignancies. The most common secondary malignancies are acute myelogenous leukemia (AML) and myelodysplasia (MDS). Unfortunately, treatment-related AML and MDS respond very poorly to standard therapies, and there is no commonly accepted or efficacious therapy for them. In one retrospective evaluation of treatment-related malignancy after treatment for lymphoma, the 5-year survival rate was only 4 percent, regardless of whether they had AML or MDS and regardless of whether patients received a stem cell transplantation or supportive care.

Although this complication is rare, outcomes are so dismal that efforts focus on identifying risk for treatment-related malignancies. A variety of clinical risk factors associated with the development of secondary AML/MDS have been found, including the cumulative dose of alkylating agents or topoisomerase II inhibitors, and previous radiation exposure. Older age, number and type of prior courses of chemoradiotherapy, exposure to radiotherapy before transplantation, and use of total-body irradiation in the conditioning regimen also are related to the development of secondary AML/MDS after high-dose chemotherapy and stem cell transplantation.

In addition to clinical risk factors, the genetic predisposition to secondary malignancies is being evaluated. To date, the most evidence supports polymorphisms in enzymes that regulate the intracellular redox potential, with the general hypothesis that null polymorphisms in these enzymes result in prolonged intracellular half-lives of free radicals and subsequently more DNA damage. NADP(H)Quinone:oxidoreductase (NQO1) is a two-electron reductase with a characteristic null polymorphism, the *2 allele, that has been associated with both benzene toxicity and the development of leukemia. In a case-control study conducted in Shanghai, China, patients homozygous for the *2 allele had a 7.6-fold (95% confidence interval = 1.8–31.2) increased risk of benzene poisoning, and increased risk for leukemia after benzene exposure compared to patients who carried one or two wild-type NQO1 alleles. In a series of infant leukemias with mixed lineage leukemia rearrangements versus unselected cord blood controls, mixed lineage leukemia-rearranged leukemias were more likely to have genotypes with low NQO1 function (heterozygous CT or homozygous TT at nucleotide 609) than controls (odds ratio = 2.5; p=0.015). In addition, Caucasian patients who are nonsmall cell lung cancer homozygous for the *2 allele have much poorer survival than those who are wild-types or heterozygotes. In addition, in a retrospective study, 44 patients with treatment-related AML/MDS (breast cancer primary) were analyzed for GSTM1 and GST1 null polymorphisms. Only 8.8 percent of the control group compared with 55 percent of the patients with AML/MDS had the null polymorphisms in both GSTM1 and GST1 (p=0.0003).

Although the genetic assessment of predisposition to treatment-related malignancies is in its infancy, should genotypes that predict outcome be identified, a subset of patients who should not be treated with topoisomerase II inhibitors and alkylating agents may be identified.

Genetic Mutations in the Diagnosis of Disease

The era of genetic diagnosis of solid tumors began in 1969 when Li and Fraumeni published a retrospective analysis of children who were diagnosed with rhabdomyosarcoma. The investigators found from extended family histories that four children's histories were significant for other cancers, particularly sarcomas, breast cancers, and leukemia at young ages.

Subsequent studies have demonstrated that Li-Fraumeni cancer syndrome is a highly penetrant cancer syndrome, with segregation analysis revealing cancer risks of 50 percent by 40 years of age and up to 90 percent by 60 years of age. An additional study calculated age-specific cancer risks and found a 42 percent risk between 0 and 16 years of age, a 38 percent risk between 17 and 45 years of age, and a 63 percent risk after 45 years of age. The overall lifetime risk for cancer development was calculated to be 85 percent, corresponding to an estimated relative risk of 100 times the reference population.

Germline mutations in the *p53* gene are found in more than 50 percent of families with Li-Fraumeni cancer syndrome, with clinical testing for germline mutations in *p53* available in since 1993. Fortunately, the Li-Fraumeni cancer syndrome is rare, with less than 300 families worldwide affected. However, the lessons learned from patients with Li-Fraumeni have been important in discovering and evaluating additional and more common hereditary cancer.

American Society of Clinical Oncology Guidelines

The American Society of Clinical Oncology (ASCO) Policy Statement for Genetic Testing of Cancer Susceptibility was approved on February 20,1996, and updated on March 1, 2003. Available online at *www.asco.org* it is a policy written for clinical genetic testing related to cancer predisposition, and in its revised version begins to address pharmacogenetics. The revised version states that the genetic basis of cancer is the foundation of diagnosis and monitoring and has given rise to new therapies for treating both solid tumors and hematological malignancies.

Genetic testing should be preceded by adequate genetic education and counseling. The actual education may be carried out by a genetic counselor, physician, or other health care providers who have adequate knowledge and training to provide such education. Adequate education and counseling should include the benefits of genetic testing, which typically is earlier identification of the carrier state and implementation of surveillance or risk reduction strategies that would decrease a patient's risk of cancer, or in the event the test were negative in a patient with a strong family history, the benefit of decreased psychological stress and the absence of risk makes increased intervention and surveillance unnecessary. The risks of genetic testing, including psychological stress, the false-positive and false-negative rates of a given test, and the risk of insurance or employer discrimination also must be conveyed to the patient. The genetic counseling process should culminate in the patient being fully informed before consenting or not consenting to genetic testing. Table 2 summarizes the elements of informed consent for genetic testing.

Criteria for a Genetic Test

First, ASCO recommends that genetic testing be performed only when the following criteria are met:
1) The individual has personal or family history features suggestive of a hereditary cancer condition.
2) The test can be adequately interpreted.

Table 2. Elements of Informed Consent for Genetic Testing

1. Information of the specific test being performed
2. Implications of a positive and negative result
3. Possibility the test will not be informative
4. Options for risk assessment without genetic testing
5. Risk of passing a mutation to children
6. Technical accuracy of the test
7. Fees involved in testing and counseling
8. Psychological implications of the test results
9. Risks of insurer or employer discrimination
10. Confidentiality issues
11. Options and limitations of medical surveillance strategies
12. Importance of sharing genetic test results with at-risk relatives so that they may benefit from the information

3) The results will affect the management of the patient or his or her family.

Furthermore, ASCO recommends that genetic testing only be performed in the setting of pre- and post-test counseling, which should include discussion of possible risks and benefits of early cancer detection and prevention modalities.

The earlier version of the ASCO guidelines categorized genetic tests by their clinical usefulness and listed several tests for syndromes, including hereditary nonpolyposis colon cancer (HNPCC), and familial adenomatous polyposis (FAP) as category 1 tests, or tests that should be considered part of routine clinical management. The revised ASCO recommendations do not categorize specific tests, but rely on the clinical judgment of the practitioner in ordering and interpreting a genetic test.

Autosomal Dominant Cancer Syndromes

The most common autosomal dominant cancer syndromes include FAP, HNPCC, BRCA1, and BRCA2. The rarer autosomal recessive disorders include ataxia-telangiectasia, Fanconi's anemia, and Bloom's syndrome.

Hereditary Colon Cancer. Familial adenomatous polyposis is an autosomal dominant syndrome caused by mutations in the adenomatous polyposis coli (APC) gene, in which affected individuals develop more than 100 adenomas. The incidence is about one in 10,000 and accounts for about 1 percent of colon cancers. The average age of first adenoma appearance is 16 years, with a risk of colon cancer approaching 100 percent and an average age of onset of 39 years. A variant of FAP called attenuated APC (AAPC) is associated with a variable number of adenomas, usually 20–100, a tendency toward right-sided colonic adenomas, an age of onset of colorectal cancer that is about 10 years later than for FAP, and mutations near the 5' or 3' end of the APC gene.

Genetic testing for the APC gene should be considered routinely in a person with an FAP phenotype (more than 100 adenomas) if there are unaffected first-degree relatives younger than 40 years of age. The first person to be tested should be the individual with the FAP phenotype, to identify the specific disease producing mutation. After this test is complete, all first-degree relatives younger than 40 should be tested, although testing of children can be delayed until 10 years of age. First-degree relatives older than 40 years of age are assumed not to carry the APC mutation and have the reference population risk of colon cancer. Family members who test negative for the APC mutation also have the reference population risk for colon cancer. Family members who test positive are followed by sigmoidoscopy until polyps develop, and a prophylactic colectomy is then performed. Individuals who develop polyps may be started on celecoxib, a specific cyclooxygenase-2 inhibitor that decreases the number of polyps in patients with APC; however, it is important to note that sulindac is not more effective than placebo in preventing polyp formation in individuals with FAP and should not be started routinely, although it may be effective in preventing recurrence in retained rectal segments after colectomy.

In an analysis of prospectively collected data from the Hereditary Gastrointestinal Cancer Registry, Hong Kong, individuals who presented with clinical symptoms and an FAP phenotype were tested for mutation in the APC gene. Eligible family members were subsequently screened for APC mutations. Familial adenomatous polyposis was diagnosed earlier (mean age of 29 years) by screening compared to symptoms (mean age of 40 years). Of the patients who presented with symptoms and were found to have FAP, 47 of 77 already had colon cancer, and 39 of these 47 patients died shortly after diagnosis. In the 31 patients diagnosed with FAP by genetic screening, only three had colon cancer, all of whom were still alive. This highlights the importance of APC mutation screening in families predisposed to FAP because those who present with symptoms are likely to already have cancer. Early identification of susceptible family members can lead to diagnosis before malignancy, increased surveillance and early intervention, and is expected to improve survival. However, it is important to note that testing is only for at-risk families and not the general population because FAP is a relatively rare disorder and the mutations occur over a wide area of the APC gene, making it difficult to detect without knowing the founder mutation.

Hereditary Nonpolyposis Colon Cancer. Current literature suggests that HNPCC accounts for between 0.86 percent and 2.0 percent of colon cancer cases. The Finnish Cancer Registry evaluated cumulative incidence of HNPCC-related cancers in HNPCC gene carriers up to 70 years of age in the registry. Although colorectal cancer was the most common, occurring in 82 percent of individuals; a variety of other common cancer syndromes were identified, including endometrium, 60 percent; stomach, 13 percent; ovary,

12 percent; bladder, urethra, and ureter, 4.0 percent; brain, 3.7 percent; kidney, 3.3 percent; and biliary tract and gallbladder, 2.0 percent.

Hereditary nonpolyposis colon cancer typically is clinically defined by these criteria and individuals who fit the modified Amsterdam criteria should be tested for mutations in the DNA mismatch repair genes. Germline MMR mutations are found in 45–64 percent of families meeting the modified Amsterdam criteria. In an analysis of 59 United States families with HNPCC for MSH2, MLH1, and MSH6 mutations, in 45 (92 percent) of the 49 Amsterdam criteria-positive families and in seven (70 percent) of the 10 Amsterdam criteria-negative families, a mutation was detected in one of the three analyzed MMR genes. Forty-nine mutations were in MSH2 or MLH1, and only three were in MSH6.

Colon tumors that fit the Bethesda criteria should be tested for microsatellite instability (MSI), which is found in more than 95 percent of colorectal cancers from HNPCC patients, but in only about 15 percent of colorectal cancers from those with sporadic colorectal cancer. If MSI is identified, genetic testing for MMR should proceed. If a mutation in MMR is identified, the first-degree relatives of the affected individual should then be tested.

Individuals in families with a history of HNPCC, regardless of mutation status, should undergo screening colonoscopy every 3 years, based on the efficacy of screening identified in a controlled trial conducted over 15 years. Colonic screening at 3-year intervals was performed for 133 patients from families with a history of HNPCC; 119 patients in the control group also from families with a history of HNPCC had no screening. Colorectal cancer developed in eight screened patients (6 percent) compared with 19 patients in the control group (16 percent; p=0.014); thus, the rate of colorectal cancer was reduced by 62 percent in the screened group. All cancers in the screened group were identified in a local stage, causing no deaths, compared with nine deaths caused by colorectal cancer in the control group. The overall death rates were 10 versus 26 patients in the study and control groups (p=0.003).

In addition to the genes associated with FAP and HNPCC, many genes now have been identified that seem to play a role in this more common but less penetrant category of inherited colon cancers, including the I1307K APC mutation in Jewish people of Ashkenazi descent, the HRAS1-VNTR polymorphism in the general population, the methylenetetrahydrofolate reductase val/val polymorphism (protective), and the TGFβR-1(6A) polymorphism. These and other genes may soon be included in a routine screening panel for colon cancer susceptibility testing and the targets of yet to be developed new therapies.

Hereditary Medullary Carcinoma. Hereditary medullary thyroid carcinoma occurs as part of three familial syndromes: multiple endocrine neoplasia type IIA, multiple endocrine neoplasia type IIB, and isolated familial medullary thyroid carcinoma. Multiple endocrine neoplasia type IIA is most common, representing two-thirds of the hereditary cases.

Diagnosis and management of hereditary thyroid carcinoma rely on genetic testing for the *RET* proto-oncogene. Genetic testing should begin by no later than 6 years of age in families with multiple endocrine neoplasia type IIA and shortly after birth in multiple endocrine neoplasia type IIB (because of the earlier onset and greater virulence of the latter).

The current standard of care is to recommend surgical treatment for medullary thyroid carcinoma family members diagnosed with *RET* mutations. Affected individuals should undergo prophylactic total thyroidectomy and central compartment lymph node dissection, as young as 2 years of age for those with multiple endocrine neoplasia IIA and by 1 year of age in those with the IIB form.

Breast Cancer and Ovarian Cancer. Annually, more than 200,000 cases of breast cancer and about 25,000 cases of ovarian cancer are diagnosed in the United States. Hereditary predisposition, inherited in an autosomal dominant manner, is thought to account for between 5 percent and 10 percent of all cases of breast cancer. Although many yet unrecognized genes may substantially contribute to inherited breast cancer, currently best studied is the BRCA1 gene, with mutations of BRCA1 thought to account for about 45 percent of families with a family history of breast cancer and at least 80 percent of families with an increased incidence of both early-onset breast cancer and ovarian cancer. Although the penetrance of BRCA1 and BRCA2 has not been precisely determined, these genes are considered highly penetrant genes, and individuals who carry a mutation in BRCA1 or BRCA2 are at as much as 92-percent lifetime risk of developing breast and/or ovarian cancer.

The precise physiological function of BRCA1 and BRCA2 is under investigation; however, current evidence suggests that both are important in double-strand break repair and maintaining integrity of the genome. Both genes are essential to cellular development, with deletions in either leading to embryonic lethality in mice. In addition, emerging evidence suggests that BRCA1 mutations may lead to radiation and chemotherapy insensitivity.

Genetic testing of BRCA1 and BRCA2 is routinely recommended for women from high-risk breast and ovarian cancer families. Although there are several founder mutations that are well characterized, new mutations may be identified in almost any region of the BRCA1 or BRCA2 gene. Therefore, it is recommended that in the incident case of breast cancer, the entire BRCA1 and BRCA2 gene sequences be analyzed. Should a mutation be identified, first-degree relatives may be tested subsequently in the region identified to contain the family-associated mutation. Family members who test negative may be considered at normal or population risk, whereas those who test positive are at high risk for breast and ovarian cancer and should be offered risk reduction strategies.

The currently accepted risk reduction strategies are prophylactic oophorectomy and bilateral mastectomy; several studies support their use. In one evaluation of breast cancer risk reduction, 176 women with a strong family history of breast cancer who underwent prophylactic bilateral mastectomy were subsequently analyzed for mutations in the BRCA1 or BRCA2 genes. Of the 176 women tested, 26 had an alteration in BRCA1 or BRCA2, and none developed breast cancer after a median of 13.4 years of follow-up (range = 5.8-28.5 years). The predicted risk for BRCA1 or BRCA2 mutation carriers at 13 years is 13–34 percent, which translates into a risk reduction, after bilateral prophylactic mastectomy, of 89.5–100 percent (95% confidence interval = 41.4–100). In an evaluation of ovarian cancer risk reduction, 551 women with disease-associated germline BRCA1 or BRCA2 mutations were identified from registries. The incidence of ovarian cancer in 259 women who had undergone bilateral prophylactic oophorectomy and in 292 matched controls who had not undergone the procedure was analyzed, with a median follow-up from prophylactic surgery of 8 years. Of the women undergoing prophylactic oophorectomy, six (2.3 percent) women were diagnosed with stage I ovarian cancer at the time of the procedure, and two (0.8 percent) women were diagnosed with papillary serous peritoneal carcinoma after 3.8 and 8.6 years after bilateral prophylactic oophorectomy. Among the controls, those with BRCA1 or BRCA2 mutations who did not have a prophylactic oophorectomy, 58 women (19.9 percent) were diagnosed with ovarian cancer, after a mean follow-up of 8.8 years, demonstrating that prophylactic oophorectomy significantly reduced the risk of coelomic epithelial cancer (hazard ratio = 0.04; 95% confidence interval = 0.01–0.16).

Based on available data on the incidence and prognosis of cancer in BRCA1- and BRCA2-positive women, and the efficacy of prophylactic mastectomy and oophorectomy in preventing breast and ovarian cancer in this population, a decision analysis comparing prophylactic mastectomy and prophylactic oophorectomy with no prophylactic surgery among women with BRCA1 or BRCA2 gene mutations was performed. A 30-year-old woman with BRCA1 or BRCA2 mutations was expected to gain from 2.9 to 5.3 years of life expectancy from prophylactic mastectomy and from 0.3 to 1.7 years of life expectancy from prophylactic oophorectomy. Overall, women from families that carry the BRCA1 or BRCA2 mutation are likely to undergo genetic testing and request prophylactic surgical procedures. In one consecutive and prospective assessment of 220 women from 112 high-risk families, 192 (87 percent) underwent genetic testing, and among eligible women (BRCA1- or BRCA2-positive, surgical candidate, younger than 60 years of age), 35 of 101 (35 percent) requested bilateral or contralateral mastectomy, and 47 of 95 (49 percent) requested oophorectomy.

BRCA1 and BRCA1 mutations also have been evaluated in sporadic cases of breast cancer, with essentially no mutations identified, and rare mutations identified in cases of sporadic ovarian cancer. BRCA1 messenger ribonucleic acid (mRNA) is reduced and the BRCA1 promotor region is hypermethylated in breast cancer cells, compared to normal breast epithelium, suggesting the importance of BRCA1 in sporadic cancers. However, there is no currently available or routinely recommended genetic screening test for sporadic breast cancers.

Molecular Characterization of Hematological Malignancies
Chronic Myelogenous Leukemia

Chronic myelogenous leukemia (CML) is a relatively rare disorder; the American Cancer Society estimated 4400 new cases and 2000 deaths for 2003. Chronic myelogenous leukemia is unique in that it is cytogenetically characterized by the Philadelphia (Ph) chromosome. The Ph chromosome was the first consistent genetic abnormality noted in a human cancer, arising from a reciprocal translocation, t(9;22)(q34;q11), and molecularly by the fusion of the proto-oncogene *ABL*, located on the long arm of chromosome 9, with the *BCR* gene of chromosome 22, known as the breakpoint cluster region (bcr). See Table 3. The diagnosis of CML is made routinely by a pathological and cytogenetic evaluation of the bone marrow and finding the Ph chromosome is diagnostic of the disorder. In fact, patients with CML-like features, but without the Ph chromosome, should be evaluated further diagnostically.

Also unique to CML is the development of a therapy, designed to a specific genetic abnormality, the 9;22 translocation. Imatinib (STI571, Gleevec) is an oral inhibitor of tyrosine kinases, such as the fusion protein of *BCR-ABL*, and has demonstrated substantial activity in treating CML.

Table 3. Frequent Chromosomal Abnormalities in Leukemias

Chromosomal Reaarangement	Leukemia	Clinical Implications
t(8;21)(q22;q22)	AML-M2 (20%)	Improved prognosis
t(12;21)(p13;q22)	Childhood ALL (20%)	Improved prognosis
t(15;17)(q22;q12)	AML-M3 (95%)	Excellent prognosis Induction with tretinoin
t(9;22)(q34;q11) The Philadelphia chromosome	CML (more than 95%) Adult ALL (25%)	Excellent prognosis for those with CML and an indication for imitinab Poor prognostic factor for ALL
t(1;19)(p23;p13)	Childhood ALL (2–5%)	Intermediate prognosis
t(6;9)(p23;q24)	AML preceeded by MDS	Unfavorable prognosis
Inv(16)(p13;22) or t(16;16)(p13q22)	AML-M4 with eosinophilia	Favorable prognosis

ALL = acute lymphoblastic leukemia; AML = acute myeloid leukemia; CML = chronic myelogenous leukemia; MDS = myelodysplasia.

Imatinib currently is recommended as first-line therapy for CML in the chronic phase, as it has demonstrated higher initial response rates and longer time to progression than interferon (IFN) and cytarabine. In patients resistant to or who did not benefit from IFN, imatinib still demonstrates significant response rates.

Chronic Lymphocytic Leukemia

In contrast to the single genetic event defining CML, in chronic lymphocytic leukemia (CLL), genetic abnormalities are common, but heterogenous. Chronic lymphocytic leukemia may be of either B-cell or T-cell origin with the B-cell type more common. In B-cell CLL, trisomy of chromosome 12 is one of the most common cytogenetic abnormalities and is associated with atypical morphology of lymphocytes, progressing disease, and poor survival rates. A deletion of chromosome 13 (13q14) occurs in 51 percent of the patients with CLL and in up to 70 percent of patients with mantle-cell lymphoma. Chromosome 14 abnormalities—usually the translocation t(11;14)(q13;q32)—correlate with a high leukocytes count, adverse response to cytostatic therapy, and increased risk of prolymphocytic proliferation. Mutations of *p53* also are reported for CLL and are associated with rapid progression, aggressive course, poor prognosis, and low survival. In T-cell CLL, characteristic deletions are 11q22-q23 and a.14q23.1, as well as the inversion, inv(14)(11q32), and some rarer aberrations. Despite the multitude of genetic events in CLL, none is considered essential in the diagnosis of this disease.

Myelodysplasias

The MDSs are a heterogeneous group of clonal hematopoietic stem cell disorders, and typically are a precursor to AML, with about a 1 percent/year risk of conversion. The diagnosis of MDS is based on a morphological examination of bone marrow aspirate and marrow chromosome analysis. In general, the genetic abnormalities are independent prognostic indicators, and patients with MDS may have single or multiple chromosome changes. The deletion of 20q carries a poor prognosis in myeloid disorders, with a high rate of transformation of MDS to AML. Another nonrandom abnormality, t(5;12)(q31-33;p12-13), fuses the TEL (12p) and PDGFR*b* (5q). The 5q– syndrome is a distinct hematological disorder that affects primarily elderly women with refractory macrocytic anemia and normal or elevated platelet counts. Patients with 5q– as the sole abnormality have long survival times.

Currently, cytogenetics is a routine feature of diagnosis of MDS, and is under evaluation as a prognostic indicator. In the future, it seems likely that therapeutic decisions will be based on cytogenetic evaluation of MDS.

Acute Myeloid Leukemia

Acute myeloid leukemia is a heterogeneous disease; about 10,600 new cases and 7400 deaths were estimated for 2003 by the American Cancer Society. Cellular morphology was the basis for the first widely accepted classification system that was developed by the joint efforts of French, American, and British (FAB)—known as the FAB classification—hematologists in 1976.

The World Health Organization recently proposed a revision is this classification, based on the following three major determinants: cytogenetics, the presence of dysplastic features, and the preceding history. For cases that cannot be categorized by these criteria, the FAB classification is used.

In two recent studies, various factors relating to AML prognosis were evaluated. In a cohort of 300 patients, the presence of blast cells did not affect 5-year mortality. Categories of AML with recurrent cytogenetic abnormalities of t(15;17), t(8;21), inv(16)/t(16;16), and 11q23 showed significant differences in 5-year survival, suggesting that recurring cytogenetic abnormalities and multilineage dysplasia are the most significant features of current AML classification. In a subsequent multivariate analysis of 614 patients with de novo AML, only cytogenetics, age, and high lactate dehydrogenase had prognostic significance and dysplastic features did not predict prognosis when cytogenetics was considered.

Identification of the t(15;17) or M3 variant of AML has played an important role in changing the natural history of this disease. Before 1980, patients with M3 AML routinely died of early complications related to coagulopathies, with less than 20 percent of patients enjoying long-term survival. In the late 1970s, the RAR-PML fusion protein generated by the t(15;17) was identified. Further work identified its function in cell differentiation and the discovery that tretinoin-induced differentiation of affected cells without causing the related coagulopathies. Currently, patients with the M3 variant are treated with a course of tretinoin, followed by daunorubicin and cytarabine, with 80 percent of patients becoming long-term survivors.

Therefore, cytogenetic variations in AML are important in diagnosis, prognosis, and selection of therapy.

Acute Lymphoblastic Leukemia

Acute lymphoblastic leukemia is a relatively rare disorder with 3800 new cases and 1400 deaths annually as estimated by the American Cancer Society. Acute lymphoblastic leukemia occurs primarily in children, but sometimes in adults and is categorized as L1, L2, and L3 subtypes. Cytogenetics plays an important role in predicting prognosis; however, there are multiple genetic lesions. The t(12;21)(p13;q22) is the most common, found in 25 percent of patients with childhood ALL. The t(12;21) translocation results in a fusion protein call TEL-AML1 that may be important in leukemogenesis and results in a good prognosis.

The t(8;14)(q24;q32) translocation is detected in 75–85 percent of cases of Burkitt's lymphoma and less frequently in L3 ALL, indicating a possible commonality of ALL-L3 and Burkitt's lymphoma. Patients with this translocation have an increased incidence of central nervous system involvement and a poor prognosis. The Ph chromosome, t(9;22), is found in 6 percent of childhood ALL, 17 percent of adult cases of ALL, up to 44 percent of ALL occurring in adults older than 50 years of age, and is associated with a very poor prognosis. Imatinib is being evaluated as a therapy to achieve an initial complete remission (CR) before transplantation in patients with Ph chromosome plus ALL, as being in a CR before transplantation is an important predictor of success. Preliminary evidence suggests that this may be an effective strategy. Although the full impact of this drug on this chromosomal abnormality has not been elucidated, it is expected to change the course of disease.

Use of Pharmacogenetics and Pharmacogenomics in Oncology

6-Mercaptopurine

Thiopurine methyltransferase (TPMT) is the enzyme responsible for the catabolism of 6-mercaptopurine (6-M), an agent routinely used to treat pediatric leukemias. Thiopurine methyltransferase deficiency is inherited as an autosomal recessive trait, with 89–94 percent of Caucasians having high activity, 6–11 percent with intermediate activity, and 0.3 percent with very low or no activity. This deficiency is largely explained by three polymorphisms in the TPMT gene (*2, *3A, and *3C), which also have a profound influence on 6-MP tolerance and dose intensity in children with ALL. Although these polymorphisms are rare, they are certainly important with case reports of toxic deaths attributed to 6-MP dating back several decades. In a recent clinical trial, children who were homozygous for one of the variant alleles required 6-MP dose reductions of 91 percent, whereas heterozygotes required a dose reduction of about 50 percent. Children with dose reductions had equivalent overall survival compared with children receiving full doses of 6-MP, suggesting that TPMT polymorphisms are important for drug metabolism and toxicity, but play no role in the pathogenesis of ALL. See Tables 3 and 4.

Thiopurine methyltransferase screening is recommended for children starting therapy with 6-MP with empiric dose reductions for those with genotypes associated with a deficiency.

5-Fluorouracil and Capecitabine

5-Fluorouracil (5-FU) is a uracil analog that is widely used to treat solid tumors, such as colorectal and breast cancer. 5-Fluorouracil itself is a prodrug that requires activation to 5-fluoro-2-deoxyuridine monophosphate (5-FdUMP). 5-Fluoro-2-deoxyuridine monophosphate inhibits tumor cell replication by inhibiting thymidylate synthase (TS), an enzyme that is required for de novo pyrimidine synthesis. Capecitabine is a recently available oral prodrug of 5-FU that also is widely used to treat solid tumors.

Dihydropyrimidine Dehydrogenase

Dihydropyrimidine dehydrogenase (DPD) is the first and rate-limiting enzyme in the three-step catabolic pathway for the endogenous pyrimidine bases uracil and thymine and is the enzyme primarily responsible for converting 85 percent of an intravenous dose of 5-FU to its inactive form 5_1b dihydrofluorouracil (DHFU). Dihydropyrimidine dehydrogenase is widely expressed in both normal and tumor tissue, including the liver, gastrointestinal mucosa, and peripheral blood mononuclear cells.

Familial DPD deficiency is an inborn error of metabolism inherited in an autosomal recessive manner with widely variable penetrance. Affected children present with a variety of neurological syndromes. Dihydropyrimidine dehydrogenase deficiency is reported in about 3–5 percent of Caucasians and results from one of more than 20 reported polymorphisms in the DPD gene, although the *2A appears to be one of the most significant. Patients with low DPD activity cannot effectively inactivate 5-FU, leading to excessive amounts of 5-FdUMP, causing gastrointestinal, hematopoietic, and neurological toxicities that are potentially fatal.

Table 4. Clinically Important Polymorphism in Predicting Toxicity in Patients with Cancer

Gene	Variant	Phenotype	Drug	Clinical Use
TPMT	*2, *3A, *3C	Increased toxicity	6-MP, pediatric ALL	Routine screening Homozygous variants receive emperic dose reduction of 90%
DPD	*2A	Increased toxicity	5-FU	Not clinically useful, low sensitivity
UGT1A1	*28	Increased toxicity	Irinotecan	Under investigation
MTHFR	C677T	Severe myelo-suppression	CMF regimen	Under investigation

5-FU = 5-fluorouracil; 6-MP = 6-mercaptopurine; ALL = acute lymphoblastic leukemia; CMF = cyclophosphamide, methotrexate, and 5-FU; DPD = dihydropyrimidine dehydrogenase; MTHFR = methyl tetra hydrofolate reductase; TPMT = Thiopurine methyltransferase.

More than 350 cases of DPD deficiency in patients receiving 5-FU and seven toxic deaths have been documented. However, other investigators have shown that only 33–66 percent of individuals with severe myelotoxicity related to 5-FU administration actually have a known polymorphism, underscoring the complexity of this phenotype. Therefore, routine clinical screening for DPD polymorphisms currently is not recommended.

Thymidylate Synthase

Thymidylate synthase is the intracellular target of 5-FU and several studies have demonstrated that TS induction is associated with resistance to 5-FU and that decreases in tumor TS are associated with improved sensitivity to 5-FU. The endogenous level of TS expression is controlled by polymorphic variation in the enhancer region of the TS gene (Table 5). Two, three, four, and nine copies of 28-base pair tandem repeated sequences (TSER*2, TSER*3, TSER*4, and TSER*9) have been identified. Compared to the TSER*2 allele, in vitro assays demonstrate that TS expression of the TSER*3 is 2.6 times that of the TSER*2 allele. In an analysis of genomic DNA from patients with colon cancer, 29 percent of patients were homozygous for TSER*3, 16 percent were homozygous for the TSER*2, and 55 percent were heterozygous. In 24 patients who received 5-FU, 40 percent of responders were homozygous for the TSER*2, compared to 20 percent of nonresponders, and those with the TSER*2 polymorphism had improved median survival of 16 months compared to the TSER*3 those who had a 12-month median survival.

Table 5. Clinically Important Pharmacogenetics in Predicting Efficacy in Patients with Cancer

Gene	Variant	Phenotype	Drug	Clinical Use
TS	*2, *3 tandem repeat	*3 with increased expression, *2 with improved survival	5-FU	Under investigation
2D6	UM EM PM	UM with increased emesis, PM with no emesis	Ondansetron Tropisetron	Under investigation
2D6	UM EM PM	Non responder	Codiene	Under investigation
TI	Induction	Improved response	Irinotecan	Under investigation

5-FU = 5-fluorouracil; EM = extensive metabolizer; PM = poor metabolizer; TI = topoisomerase I; TS = thymidylate synthase; UM = ultra-extensive metabolizer.

When the TS polymorphic status of 24 patients with advanced colon carcinoma was evaluated and their response to capecitabine treatment was determined, finding that three of four patients (75 percent) with the TSER*2 variant responded to capecitabine, compared with two of eight patients (25 percent) and one of 12 patients (8 percent) with the TSER*2 heterozygotes and TSER *3 variants, respectively (p=0.026; Fisher exact test).

Irinotecan
UDP-Glucuronosyltransferase
Irinotecan's active metabolite, SN-38, is glucuronidated by the 1A1 isoform of UDP-glucuronosyltransferase (UGT). The *28 variant is best studied and occurs in 3–10 percent of the population. Several groups have shown both prospectively and retrospectively that the *28 variant is a risk factor for both severe neutropenia and diarrhea in patient's receiving irinotecan, most likely due to a decreased capacity to glucuronidate SN-38, associated with a longer half-life and area under the curve of SN-38. However, like DPD, not all individuals with severe toxicity have the genotype, indicating that other factors in addition to this genotype are important in determining irinotecan toxicity. Ongoing clinical trials are investigating many aspects of irinotecan disposition, including CYP3A, MDR1, MRP-1, MRP-2, BCRP, and carboxyesterases. Currently, routine clinical assessment of UGT polymorphisms is not yet recommended.

Topoisomerase I
Numerous in vitro evaluations suggest that increased topoisomerase I (TI) predicts a better response to irinotecan and that mitomycin-c (MMC) can induce TI expression. A recent Phase I trial tested the hypothesis that MMC could induce TI in vivo and that TI induction would predict response to therapy. Forty patients were enrolled in this Phase I trial, where MMC was given as a 6 mg/m^2 dose on the day before irinotecan with escalating doses every 21 days. The maximum tolerated dose (MTD) of irinotecan was 125 mg/m^2 and responders had an 8-fold induction in TI gene expression in peripheral blood lymphocytes compared to nonresponders.

This regimen currently is under evaluation in Phase II trials for breast and esophageal cancer.

Platinum Agents
Deoxyribonucleic Acid Repair Polymorphisms
Platinum agents, including cisplatin, carboplatin, and oxaliplatin, cause cytotoxicity by induction of DNA intrastrand, interstrand, and protein cross-links as well as intrastrand bidentate N7 adducts with the bases guanine and adenine. Excision repair cross complementing (ERCC), in addition to being important in DNA repair and carcinogenesis, may be important in tumor resistance to cisplatin. Because ERCC prevents

mutations and injuries to DNA through a pathway of nucleotide excision and repair, ERCC makes the same repairs after administration of a platinum agent, and decrease its efficacy. In fact, in vitro investigations have demonstrated that high tumor levels of DNA repair enzymes lead to cisplatin resistance, and relatively low levels of DNA repair enzymes have been associated with cisplatin sensitivity.

Polymorphisms are present in many of the DNA repair enzymes. The ERCC1 contains a common polymorphism at codon 118 that results in a single nucleotide change, C to T, but does not result in an amino acid change. Although this is a silent mutation, a preliminary evaluation in 32 patients with metastatic colon cancer treated with 5-FU and oxaliplatin showed that those with the polymorphism had higher ribonucleic acid concentrations. This polymorphism may be helpful in predicting response to oxaliplatin. In a recent evaluation, patients with ERCC1 expression levels greater than 7.4×10^3 (44 of 50 patients) had a median survival of 292 days, compared with 150 days for patients with ERCC1 expression levels of less than 7.4×10^3 (6 of 50 patients) (p= 0.0098).

Many polymorphisms with unknown functional significance have been identified in the XPD gene. Probably best studied is a single nucleotide polymorphism in codon 751 (A to C) that causes an amino acid change of Lys to Gln. In an evaluation of 69 patients with metastatic colorectal carcinoma, patients with the Lys/Lys genotype had a higher response rate to chemotherapy and better overall survival when they were treated with the combination of 5-FU and oxaliplatin compared with patients who had the Lys/Gln and Gln/Gln genotypes.

GSTP1-1 Polymorphism

Glutathione transferases consist of a super family of Phase II metabolic enzymes that catalyze the conjugation of reduced glutathione, a reaction necessary for preventing damage from carcinogens. One of the members of the glutathione transferase family is GSTP-1, and increased levels of GSTP1-1 in tumors have been associated with chemotherapy resistance. A characteristic polymorphism at nucleotide 313, results in a protein sequence change from isoleucine to leucine and is associated with a reduced GSTP-1 activity. Clinical evaluations of this polymorphism have shown that the polymorphisms influence response to platinum-based chemotherapy in patients with head and neck cancer as well as those with advanced colorectal tumors receiving 5-FU and oxaliplatin.

Purines and Pyrimidine Analogs

A common polymorphism, occurring as a homozygous variant in up to 10 percent of Caucasians, occurs as a C677T in the methylenetetrahydrofolate reductase (MHFR) gene. The normal function of MHFR is to regulate the intracellular folate pool used in DNA and protein synthesis. Individuals homozygous for the MHFR polymorphism have only 35 percent of normal enzyme capacity and accumulate 5,10-methylenetetrahydrofolate, in purine and pyrimidine synthesis.

Severe toxicity, primarily myelosuppression, was reported in patients with breast cancer with this polymorphism receiving cyclophosphamide, methotrexate, and 5-FU (CMF). The toxicity may be explained by an excess of 5,10-methylenetetrahydrofolate that increases the ability of 5-FU to inhibit TS and therefore increased myelosuppression. The relationship between this polymorphism and TS-based therapy appears convincing, as a recently reported Phase I trial with the TS inhibitor, raletrexid, found that individuals without the polymorphism had no toxicities associated with raletrexid.

Cytochrome P450 Polymorphisms and Drug Response
Cytochrome P450 2D6

Although serotonin type 3 (5-HT$_3$) receptor antagonists represent a major advance in the treatment of chemotherapy-induced nausea and vomiting, there is still a substantial minority of individuals who do not respond to antiemetic therapy, up to 30 percent. Many characteristics associated with poor response to antiemetics have been identified, including female sex, young age, and no prior history of alcohol consumption. Variations in 2D6 metabolism may be responsible for some patients who do not respond to antiemetics when receiving the 2D6 substrates tropisetron and ondansetron. In 270 patients evaluated, 7.8 percent were categorized as poor metabolizers (PMs), 32.6 percent had one active allele, and 58.1 percent had two actives alleles and were extensive metabolizers and 1.5 percent were ultraextensive metabolizers. Individuals who were ultraextensive metabolizers experienced significantly more episodes of vomiting and those who were poor metabolizers had no episodes of vomiting. These results suggest that the ultraextensive metabolizers may require other approaches to emesis control or higher doses of ondansetron and tropisetron. However, before these results may be applied routinely, further studies should evaluate them prospectively.

In addition to 5-HT$_3$ receptor antagonists, CYP2D6 polymorphisms are important in activation of the prodrug codeine to its active form morphine. Individuals with a PM genotype—up to 6–10 percent of Caucasian populations—have been identified as nonresponsive to codeine.

Drug Efflux Pumps
P-glycoprotein

P-glycoprotein (Pgp) is a large transmembrane protein encoded by the MDR-1 gene that confers multidrug resistance (MDR) against antineoplastic agents. Recently, many polymorphisms in the MDR-1 gene were identified, and the T/T genotype at position 3435 in exon 26 was found to correlate with decreased intestinal Pgp expression and increased bioavailability of digoxin after oral administration. The T/T genotype appears common, with an allele frequency of 88 percent in African-American populations and more than 50 percent in Caucasian-American populations. A recent analysis of the T/T genotype in 68 patients with locally advanced breast cancer treated by preoperative chemotherapy consisting of anthracyclines alone or in combination with taxanes revealed an overall clinical response rate (clinical complete response and clinical partial response) of 68 percent but only seven patients (10.3 percent) achieved pathological complete response. Heterozygous (C/T genotype) occurred in 57 percent of the patients and 22 percent had the T/T genotype. Those with the T/T genotype were more likely to respond to preoperative chemotherapy (p=0.029).

Drug Development

Acute Myelogenous Leukemia-M3 and the Development of Tretinoin

One of the earliest successes in the use of genetic information to treat disease was the use of tretinoin for treating the M3 variant of AML. The M3 variant of AML, before about the 1990s, had a very poor prognosis. Early mortality associated with coagulopathies, disseminated intravascular coagulation, and bleeding occurred in many patients and long-term survivors numbered less than 20 percent of all those with the disease. In 1977, a consistent chromosomal translocation involving the long arms of chromosomes 15 and 17 was identified. Identification of the specific molecular lesion that produced the t(15;17) translocation occurred in 1990 and was shown to involve the retinoic acid receptor-alpha (RAR-α) gene. Currently, all patients with this subtype are treated with an induction course of tretinoin, followed by conventional therapy with daunorubicin and cytarabine. Treatment with tretinoin has changed the course of this disease to the AML variant with the best prognosis, and more than 80 percent of patients are long-term survivors.

Chronic Myelogenous Leukemia and the Development of Imatinib

The availability of the small molecular imatinib, STI-571, for first-line therapy of CML in March 2003 capped one of the most rapid drug developments in oncology and hematology history. The story began with the identification of the Ph chromosome in 1960 and the characterization of the function of the fusion protein *BCR-ABL* as a tyrosine kinase during the 1990s. Imatinib was developed as an inhibitor of tyrosine kinase, entering clinical trials in 2000, and available in May 2001 as a treatment for patients with CML who did not benefit from IFN. In clinical trials, imatinib demonstrated hematological response rates of 88 percent and cytogenetic

Table 6. Commercially Available Monoclonal Antibodies

Name	Target Antigen	Indication	Mechanism
Alemtuzumab	CD52	B-cell CLL	ADCC, CDC
Gemtuzumab	CD33	AML	Complex internalization and cell death
Ibritumomab	CD20	NHL	Local radiation therapy
Rituximab	CD20	NHL	ADCC, CDC
Trastuzumab	HER-2-neu	Breast	ADCC, CDC

ADCC = antigen-dependent cellular cytotoxicity; AML = acute myeloid leukemia; CD = cell determinant; CDC = cell determined cytotoxicity; CLL = chronic lymphocytic leukemia; CMF = cyclophosphamide, methotrexate, and 5-fluorouracil; NHL = nonhodgkin's lymphoma.

response rates of 49 percent in patients with chronic phase CML who did not benefit from IFN.

Monoclonal Antibodies

There currently are five monoclonal antibodies available for treating cancers (see Table 6). A detailed discussion is outside the scope of this chapter; however, it is important to note that the development of monoclonal antibodies is another successful use of understanding genetic changes unique to tumor cells and designing a drug that targets the cancer cell specifically. The ability to target therapy has important advantages in that it decreases toxicity and may improve efficacy.

Conclusion

Pharmacogenomics, while still in its infancy, is central to both the current and future practice of oncology and hematology. Genetic changes are essential in the development of cancers and serve as diagnostic criteria and risk assessment tools, aid in monitoring and dosing anticancer drugs and supportive care agents, and serve as targets for new drug discovery.

References

1. American Society of Clinical Oncology. American Society of Clinical Oncology policy statement update: genetic testing for cancer susceptibility. Adopted on February 20, 1996. J Clin Oncol 1996;14:1730–6.

2. Arber DA, Stein AS, Carter NH, Ikle D, Forman SJ, Slovak ML. Prognostic impact of acute myeloid leukemia classification. Importance of detection of recurring cytogenetic abnormalities and multilineage dysplasia on survival. Am J Clin Pathol 2003;119:672–80.

3. Bartsch H, Nair U, Risch A, et al. Genetic polymorphism of *CYP* genes, alone or in combination, as a risk modifier of tobacco-related cancers. Cancer Epidemiol Biomarkers Prev 2000;9:3–28.

4. Goode EL, Ulrich CM, Potter JD. Polymorphisms in DNA repair genes and associations with cancer risk. Cancer Epidemiol Biomarkers Prev 2002 Dec;11(12):1513–30.

5. Ingelman-Sundberg M, Oscarson M, Daly AK, Garte S, Nebert DW. Human cytochrome P-450 (*CYP*) genes: a Web page for the nomenclature of alleles. Cancer Epidemiol Biomarkers Prev 2001;10:1307–8.

6. Lander ES, Linton LM, Birren B, et al; International Human Genome Sequencing Consortium. Initial sequencing and analysis of the human genome. Nature 2001;409:860–921.

7. Jarvinen HJ, Aarnio M, Mustonen H, et al. Controlled 15-year trial on screening for colorectal cancer in families with hereditary nonpolyposis colorectal cancer. Gastroenterology 2000;118:829–34.

8. Kaiser R, Sezer O, Papies A, et al. Patient tailored antiemetic treatment with 5-hydroxytryptamine type 3 receptor antagonists according to cytochrome P450 genotypes. J Clin Oncol 2002;20:2805–11.

9. McLeod HL, Krynetski EY, Relling MV, Evans WE. Genetic polymorphism of thiopurine methyltransferase and its clinical relevance for childhood acute lymphoblastic leukemia. Leukemia 2000;14:567–72.

10. Meijers-Heijboer H, Brekelmans CT, Menke-Pluymers M, et al. Use of genetic testing and prophylactic mastectomy and oophorectomy in women with breast or ovarian cancer from families with a BRCA1 or BRCA2 mutation. J Clin Oncol 2003;21:1675–81.

11. Nebert DW, Roe AL, Vandale SE, Bingham E, Oakley GG. NAD(P)H:quinone oxidoreductase (NQO1) polymorphism, exposure to benzene, and predisposition to disease: a HuGE review. Genet Med 2002;4:62–70.

12. Langebrake C, Reinhardt D, Ritter J. Minimising the long-term adverse effects of childhood leukaemia therapy. Drug Saf 2002;25:1057–77.

13. Lazzeroni LC, Karlovich CA. Genotype to phenotype: associations, errors and complexity. Trends Genet 2002;18:283–4.

14. Sawyers CL. Rational therapeutic intervention in cancer: kinases as drug targets. Curr Opinion Genet Dev 2002;12:111–5.

15. Scheuer L, Kauff N, Robson M, et al. Outcome of preventive surgery and screening for breast and ovarian cancer in BRCA mutation carriers. J Clin Oncol 2002;20:1260–8.

16. Weinstein IB. Cancer. Addiction to oncogenes-the Achilles heal of cancer. Science 2002;297:63–4.

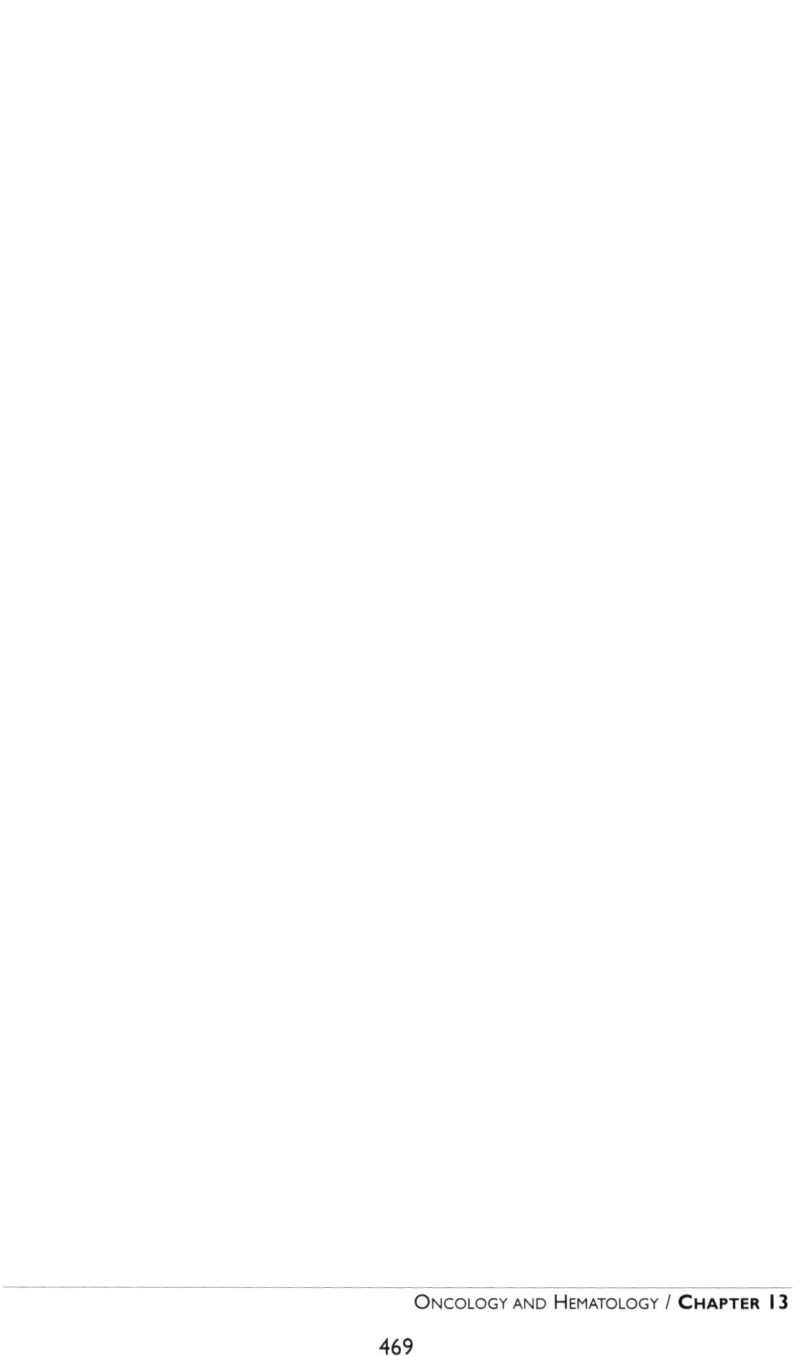

Self-Assessment Questions

1. A.M. is a 62-year-old Chinese woman with a work history consistent with benzene exposure. Which one of the following alleles is most important to genotype to assess her risk for leukemia?

    A. Cytochrome P450 (*CYP*) 1A1.
    B. NQO1.
    C. Cytochrome P450 2D6.
    D. Multidrug resistance (MDR).

2. C.C. is a 47-year-old woman who develops the familial adenomatous polyposis (FAP) variant of colon cancer and tests positive for the attenuated adenomatous polyposis coli (APC) gene. Which one of the following family members is most important to test for the APC gene?

    A. 49-year-old spouse.
    B. 86-year-old grandmother.
    C. 65-year-old mother.
    D. 19-year-old daughter.

3. B.B. is a 79-year-old woman with newly diagnosed chronic myelogenous leukemia (CML) who tests positive for the Philadelphia (Ph) chromosome. Based on her test results, the best course of action is which one of the following?

    A. Stem cell transplantation.
    B. Imatinib.
    C. Hydroxyurea.
    D. Interferon (IFN).

4. A.V. is a 6-year-old child with acute lymphocytic leukemia (ALL). She tests positive as a heterozygote for the thiopurine methyltransferase (TPMT) gene. Which one of the following is the best clinical course of action?

    A. Do not administer dose.
    B. 91 percent dose reduction.
    C. 50 percent dose reduction.
    D. Administer full dose.

5. V.V. is a 67-year-old woman with stage III breast cancer starting her second cycle of cyclophosphamide, doxorubicin, 5-fluorouracil (5-FU). With her first cycle, she had intractable nausea and vomiting despite the recommended dose of ondansetron and dexamethasone as antiemetic

prophylaxis. Which one of the following is the most plausible explanation for her failure to respond to standard antiemetic therapy?

A. Noncompliance with antiemetic regimen.
B. Cytochrome P450 2D6 ultraextensive metabolizer.
C. Cytochrome P450 2D6 poor metabolizer.
D. Cytochrome P450 2D6 average metabolizer.

6. D.D. is a 48-year-old man with metastatic colon cancer. He is enrolled in a research study to evaluate polymorphisms in the thymidylate synthase (TS) gene. He is determined to carry the TSER*2 allele. Which one of the following is the most clinically significant outcome you can expect in *2 carriers compared to the *3 carriers?

A. Higher TS expression.
B. Improved response rates when treated with 5-FU.
C. Improved survival when treated with 5-FU.
D. Decreased susceptibility to colon cancer.

7. F.F. is a 57-year-old woman with metastatic breast cancer about to receive single agent taxotere, a known substrate for the MDR or P-glycoprotein (Pgp). As part of a research study, F.F. is tested and determined to have TT exon 26 variant of the MDR gene. Compared to an individual with the wild-type gene, which one of the following describes F.F.'s expected plasma maximum concentration levels of taxotere?

A. Increased.
B. Decreased.
C. Same.
D. Greatly reduced when rifampin is administered.

8. Which one of the following is an appropriate candidate for TPMT testing as part of routine clinical management?

A. Neonatal screening.
B. Children with ALL who will receive 6-mercaptopurine (6-MP).
C. Adults with rheumatoid arthritis receiving azathioprine.
D. Children with ALL being evaluated for a bone marrow transplantation.

9. Which one of the following individuals is the best candidate for BRCA1 testing as part of routine clinical management?

A. A 25-year-old woman with no family history of cancer.
B. A 36-year-old woman whose sister has breast cancer but who tested negative for BRCA1.
C. A 36-year-old woman with a sister and mother with breast cancer who have not been tested for BRCA1.

D. A 36-year-old woman with a sister and mother with breast cancer who have tested positive for BRCA1.

10. Which one of the following best describes the advantages of monoclonal antibodies over standard cytotoxic chemotherapy?
    A. Increased efficacy and decreased toxicity.
    B. Decreased efficacy and decreased toxicity.
    C. Increased efficacy and increased toxicity.
    D. No advantage of standard cytotoxic chemotherapy.

Infectious Diseases

P. David Rogers, Pharm.D., Ph.D.

Key Words

Anti-infective resistance, drug discovery, functional genomics, genetic polymorphism, genomics, innate immune response, microarray analysis, pharmacogenomics, proteomics, reverse vaccinology, vaccine, virulence.

Abstract

The application of pharmacogenomics to clinical practice in the area of infectious diseases is in its infancy. Scientists and clinicians are only beginning to make use of the recent information derived from the sequencing of both human and pathogen genomes. The field of genomics has enhanced the understanding of genetic predisposition to infection; expanded the knowledge of microbial physiology, virulence, and anti-infective resistance; and shed new light on the interaction that occurs between the pathogen and the host at a molecular and cellular level. Genomics has radically altered the anti-infective drug discovery process as well as vaccine development, and has made possible the evolution of the field of pharmacogenomics. This chapter addresses how genomics impacts the triad of the host-pathogen-drug interaction.

Outline

Learning Objectives

1. Describe host genetic factors that contribute to susceptibility to infectious diseases.
2. Analyze the role of genomics in understanding the virulence of pathogenic organisms.
3. Recognize the contributions and utility of genomics to the understanding of the host-pathogen relationship.
4. Evaluate the application of genomics to the anti-infective drug discovery and development process.
5. Discuss the potential clinical utility of pharmacogenomics in the management of infectious diseases.
6. Describe the role of genomics in vaccine development.

Abbreviations in this Chapter

CYP	Cytochrome P450
DNA	Deoxyribonucleic acid
HBV	Hepatitis B virus
HCV	Hepatitis C virus
HIV	Human immunodeficiency virus
HLA	Human leukocyte antigen
INH	Isoniazid
mRNA	Messenger ribonucleic acid
PAGE	Polyacrylamide gel electrophoresis
PCR	Polymerase chain reaction
RT	Reverse transcriptase
SDS	Sodium dodecyl sulfate
SNP	Single nucleotide polymorphism
TNF	Tumor necrosis factor
TNFA	Gene encoding TNF-α

Introduction

In most disease processes, pharmacogenomics makes use of information relating to the human genome. In contrast, its application to the management of infectious diseases must take into account the genomes of both the host and the infecting pathogen(s). The amount of genomic sequence information that has become available to the scientific community has grown exponentially in recent years. At the time this chapter was written, more than 100 genomes had been completely sequenced (Reference 1). In addition to the human genome, these included the genomes of pathogenic bacteria, fungi, and viruses, as well as model organisms (e.g., mice and yeast) used in the study of infectious diseases and anti-infective therapies.

Pharmacogenomics has had a significant impact in specialties such as oncology and cardiology; however, its application to the study of infectious diseases is still in its infancy. The field of genomics has made great contributions to the understanding of the host immune response, the physiology and virulence of pathogenic organisms, and the interaction between host and pathogen. It has expanded the repertoire of potential anti-infective and vaccine targets for drug development, changed the way clinicians consider drug disposition, and revealed opportunities for the improvement of the safety and efficacy of anti-infective pharmacotherapy. This chapter addresses how genomics impacts the triad of the host-pathogen-drug interaction.

Genetic Predisposition to Infection in the Host

Interindividual Variation and Genetic Association with Susceptibility to Infectious Diseases

It has long been recognized that individual responses to similar infectious processes vary greatly. This is particularly true for severe infection such as nosocomial pneumonia and sepsis (References 2–4). Although this variability can be attributed to many factors, genetics clearly makes a significant contribution. A single defect in a gene that is essential to fighting infection, although uncommon, could have devastating consequences. Such defects in the genes encoding interferon-gamma, the interleukin-12 p40 subunit, and the interleukin-12 receptor β1 chain have been associated with severe mycobacterial and *Salmonella* infections (Reference 2). Of broader clinical significance are polygenic traits inclusive of genetic variants with more subtle effects on specific mediators of immune response (References 2, 3). This is demonstrated by genetic polymorphisms observed in genes involved in the innate immune response in association with severe sepsis in humans (Table 1).

One of the genes most studied in the context of predisposition to sepsis is that encoding the pro-inflammatory cytokine tumor necrosis factor (TNF)-α. Tumor necrosis factor-α is one of the first mediators produced in response to a wide range of infectious stimuli, and it is a critical factor in both inflammation and the innate immune response. Although TNF-α is necessary for resolving a variety of infections, due to many pathogens, it also has been implicated in the progression to severe sepsis and multiple organ failure. Substantial interindividual variability in TNF-α production has been documented in healthy subjects in response to various stimuli, and it has been estimated that as much as 60 percent of this variability is genetic in nature (References 3, 4).

Polymorphisms in the gene encoding TNF-α *(TNFA)* have been associated with increased production of this cytokine and linked to severe infection. One such polymorphism occurs as a single nucleotide polymorphism (SNP) at position -308 and is the result of a substitution of adenine for guanine. This promoter has been associated with a 6- to 9-fold increase in *TNFA* expression in vitro and with elevated TNF-α plasma

Table 1. Association of Genetic Polymorphisms with Human Infectious Diseases

	Gene	Polymorphisms	Infectious Disease
Pathogen detection	*Mannose binding lectin*	Codons 52, 54, 57	Meningococcal bacteremia Respiratory infections
	Toll-like receptor 4	D299G	Gram-negative septic shock
	Fc gamma IIA receptor	H131R	Meningococcal bacteremia Pneumococcal bacteremia
	CD14	C160T	Septic shock
Inflammation	*TNFA*	TNF2	Meningococcal bacteremia Cerebral malaria Septic shock
	TNFB	TNFB2	Severe sepsis
	IL-1B	IL-1B (511)	Meningococal dosease
	IL-1Ra	IL-1 RN2	Severe sepsis
Coagulation	*PAI-1*	4G/4G	Meningococcemia Severe sepsis

CD4 = cluster of differentiation 4; IL = interleukin; PAI-1 = plasminogen activator inhibitor type 1; *TNFA* = gene encoding tumor necrosis factor-α; *TNFB* = gene encoding tumor necrosis factor-β. Reprinted with permission from Lippincott, Williams & Wilkins. Cariou A. Critical Care Medicine 2002;30(5):S341–S3.

levels in vivo. Another promoter SNP in the *TNFA* gene is at position -376 and is also the result of a substitution of adenine for guanine. Both of these SNPs have been implicated as independent risk factors for cerebral malaria, and both impact predisposition to and resolution of septic shock (References 3, 4).

As more SNPs are identified in host immune response genes, and as stronger associations or cause-and-effect relationships are found between specific SNPs and specific infectious diseases, this information will become more clinically useful. When practitioners know the infectious diseases for which a patient is at risk, they can take more aggressive preventive steps to minimize that risk.

Pathogen Genomics

Microbial Physiology

Functional genomics can be applied quite effectively to the study of common biosynthetic and metabolic functions of a microorganism. Such functions may be essential to microbial viability, and hence serve as potential targets for anti-infective drug development. By understanding the transcriptional regulation of each of the genes encoding proteins that make up the pathways critical to these functions, drug development efforts can be tightly focused on areas with the highest likelihood of success (Reference 5).

This approach has been used to study the effects of isoniazid (INH) on the biosynthesis of cell envelope mycolic acids in *Mycobacterium tuburculosis*. Investigators characterized the gene expression profiles of cultures of *M. tuburculosis* treated with INH and found 14 genes to be differentially expressed. These included *AcpM* and *KasA*, both components of the fatty acid synthase II complex. Other changes in gene expression were consistent with the known mechanism of action of INH. These data demonstrate that functional genomic analysis can yield useful information regarding the mechanism of action of an anti-infective agent. It also can characterize the pathogen response rapidly at the transcriptional level and provide insight to inhibit essential biosynthetic pathways (Reference 5).

The utility of functional genomics in the identification of genes required for microbial growth has been demonstrated in *Candida albicans*. Investigators created a *C. albicans* antisense complementary deoxyribonucleic acid (DNA) library, under the control of an inducible promoter, to screen more than 2000 transformants for a reduced-growth phenotype. They then determined the sequence of the inserts of each plasmid recovered from transformants of interest, thereby revealing the identity of the gene that was disrupted. This strategy identified 86 genes required for *C. albicans* growth (Reference 6). The identification of pathogen-specific sets of genes required for growth will have significant implications for anti-infective drug development.

Virulence

Virulence may be defined as a pathogen's ability to cause disease. Microbial factors that contribute to this process may be considered virulence factors. Although this includes attributes that allow colonization and habitation within the host, it may be more narrowly defined as microbial attributes that mediate damage to the host. The application of genomics to the study of microbial virulence will undoubtedly enhance the understanding of these processes and contribute to the identification of novel drug targets for anti-infective drug development (Reference 5).

Several genomic-based techniques have proved useful in the study of microbial virulence. Gene expression profiling using DNA microarrays allows measurement of messenger ribonucleic acid (mRNA) for thousands of genes under multiple conditions. Using this approach, it is possible to study changes in gene expression in a specific pathogen between 30°C and 37°C, aiding in the identification of potential virulence factors. Likewise, proteomics techniques such as two-dimensional polyacrylamide gel electrophoresis, combined with peptide mass fingerprinting using matrix-assisted laser desorption/ionization time-of-flight mass spectrometry, allow similar examinations at the protein level. This approach makes use of the isoelectric point and molecular weight of proteins. The protein fractions from the above hypothetical experiment could be isolated and separated by isoelectric focusing and then resolved by molecular weight by sodium dodecyl sulfate-polyacrylamide gel electrophoresis (SDS-PAGE). Protein spots would then be stained, and spots of interest could be isolated and identified. These approaches also are useful in identifying genes and gene products that are differentially expressed between in vitro and in vivo conditions. In vivo expression technology and differential fluorescence induction allow the identification of genes that are uniquely expressed in vivo. Techniques that allow the identification of pathogen genes expressed specifically in the host during infections are particularly useful because such genes may be critical to the virulence of an organism. Other techniques such as signature-tagged mutagenesis facilitate the identification of genes that are required for in vivo growth. This approach is used for assessing disruption of a given pathogen gene, allowing the identification of genes necessary for growth or virulence. Many bacterial virulence factors have been identified and studied using these methods (Reference 5).

Virulence factors may indeed prove to be viable anti-infective targets; however, drugs with activity against such targets are expected to affect in vivo pathogenicity and, therefore, would not necessarily be cidal or static. These attributes may limit their utility for treating an active infection. Furthermore, virulence factors are often specific to a particular pathogen, resulting in a narrow spectrum of action for virulence-factor inhibitors.

Anti-infective Resistance

Anti-infective resistance is one of the most significant problems facing the field of infectious diseases today. Because most molecular mechanisms of resistance have a genetic basis, the application of genomics to this problem is ideal. As the ability to rapidly and efficiently sequence entire microbial genomes develops, functional and comparative genomics can be expected to greatly contribute to the identification of resistance genes.

Molecular mechanisms of anti-infective resistance may be because of a variety of genetic changes. This is exemplified by known mechanisms used by the pathogenic fungus *C. albicans* to develop resistance to the azole antifungal agents. Azole resistance may occur as a result of a point mutation in the *ERG11* gene that encodes its target ergosterol biosynthesis enzyme, lanosterol demethylase. A common theme in this process, however, is differential expression of key resistance genes. Overexpression of *ERG11* has been associated with the azole resistance phenotype. This presumably results in increased production of lanosterol demethylase, which exceeds the capacity of the azole antifungal agent. Two classes of efflux pumps have been implicated in this process as well: two adenosine 5'triphosphate-binding cassette transporters (encoded by *CDR1* and *CDR2*) and a major facilitator (encoded by *MDR1* [*BMR1*]). Overexpression of these genes is commonly found in association with azole resistance.

These mechanisms were elucidated over a period of years, and changes in gene expression were examined on a gene-by-gene basis. Recently, the azole resistance phenotype was examined using DNA microarray analysis (Reference 7). This has allowed virtually every gene in the *C. albicans* genome to be examined with regard to its expression level in the stepwise acquisition of azole antifungal resistance. In this study many novel resistance genes were implicated (Figure 1). Furthermore, groups of coordinately regulated genes were identified, lending insight into the overall transcriptional regulation of this process. These newly identified resistance genes may serve as targets for the development of pharmacological strategies to overcome azole resistance and improve the therapeutic index of these antifungal agents. Similar genomic approaches will allow a greater understanding of the molecular and cellular mechanisms of anti-infective resistance in other pathogens, ultimately leading to new strategies for combating this problem. Furthermore, measurement of steady-state mRNA levels for azole resistance genes by quantitative, high-throughput techniques such as real-time reverse transcriptase-polymerase chain reaction (RT-PCR) may prove useful for detecting resistance in the clinical microbiology laboratory.

Host-Pathogen Interactions

Genomic-based techniques have advanced the understanding of how a host responds to colonization and infection by a specific pathogen. Similarly, it has broadened understanding of how the pathogen responds to

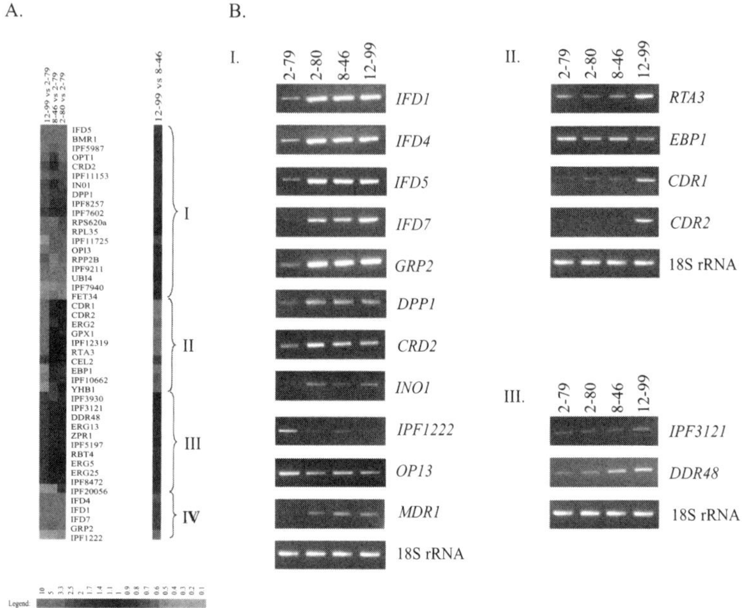

Figure 1. (A) Cluster images showing genes differentially expressed in the series of isolates. Red represents genes that are up-regulated and green represent genes that are down-regulated. Genes shown in both cluster images appear in the same order. Genes are grouped as being coodinatedly differentially expressed with (I) *CaMDR1*, (II) CDR genes, (III) neither *CaMDR1* nor CDR genes, or (IV) both *CaMDR1* and CDR genes. (B) Confirmation of differential expressions by RT-PCR of select genes found to be differentially expressed by cDNA microarray analysis. RT-PCR of *C. albicans* 18S rRNA was performed as a control. Please visit *http://aac.asm.org/cgi/content/full/47/4/1220#F1* to view the figure in full color.

cDNA = complementary deoxyribonucleic acid; CDR = Candida drug resistance; RT-PCR = reverse transcriptase-polymerase chain reaction; rRNA = ribosomal ribonucleic acid.

Reprinted with permission from the American Society for Microbiology. Antimicrob Agents Chemother. ©2003;47(11):1220–7.

contact with the host. Such interactions orchestrate the host immune response required for optimal eradication of an offending pathogen. These interactions influence the way the pathogen reacts to the host, such as activation of specific virulence factors or mechanisms for evasion of the host immune response. They also mediate the deleterious responses, such as inflammation, associated with the pathology of infection.

Innate Immune Response

Host immunity to infectious diseases is a complex genetic trait in which phenotypic expression is influenced by many environmental factors, the most important of which is the infecting pathogen. One of the most

Table 2. Host-Pathogen Interactions that have been Studied by DNA Microarray Analysis

Pathogen	Cell type	Reference
Listeria monocytogenes	THP-1 (monocytic cells)	8
Salmonella	Human macrophages	9
	Intestinal epithelial cells	10
Chlamydia pneumoniae	Endothelial cells	11
Pseudomonas aeruginosa	A549 (pulmonary epithelial cells)	12
Bordetella pertussis	BEAS-2B (bronchial epithelial cells)	13
Legionella pneumophila	Murine alveolar macrophages	14
Streptococcus pneumoniae	THP-1 (monocytic cells)	15
Candida albicans	THP-1 (monocytic cells)	16
	Dendritic cells	17

DNA = deoxyribonuclic acid.

significant contributions DNA microarray technology has made to the study of infectious diseases is the analysis of the host innate immune response. For example, cells involved in the innate immune response can discriminate among different pathogens by recognizing pathogen-associated molecular patterns through Toll-like cell surface receptors. The recognition results in a pathogen-specific response. Researchers are searching for ways to take advantage of the innate immune system's ability to discriminate among pathogens. These studies have sought to characterize the gene expression profiles of cells of the innate immune response on exposure to various pathogens (Table 2). One of the best examples of these studies involved using DNA microarrays for gene expression profiling of human peripheral blood mononuclear cells in response to strains of *Bordetella pertussis, Escherichia coli, Staphylococcus aureus, B. pertussis* lipopolysaccharide, or phobol 12-myristate 13-acetate plus ionomycin (Reference 18). In addition to providing unique insight into molecular programs involved in antigen presentation, these studies revealed a subset of genes that were stereotypically expressed in response to all pathogens and stimuli. Conversely, there were subsets of genes that were specific to each particular pathogen. This not only provides a wealth of new information about the innate immune response to different pathogens but also lays the ground work for the use of gene expression profiling for the early detection and identification of offending organisms in infected patients. Such information also may prove useful in the monitoring of patients' response to anti-infective therapy and in the discovery of pathogenic organisms yet to be identified.

Pathogen Response to Host Contact

Just as the host responds to contact with a pathogen, similar changes occur within the pathogen when it encounters the many new environments within the host. One such environment is inside a macrophage (Reference 19). On encountering a pathogen, the macrophage engulfs the microorganism via endocytosis, forming a phagosome. This compartment, along with the contained microorganism, eventually joins with lysosomes, resulting in a phagolysosome. Within this organelle is a hostile environment that includes antimicrobial substances and an acidic pH. The mechanisms by which pathogens, such as *M. tuberculosis* and *C. albicans*, survive this process and go on to cause disease is under intense investigation. Functional genomic and proteomic studies have pointed to the glycoxylate cycle as the part of the solution to this puzzle. Investigators used two-dimensional polyacrylamide gel electrophoresis to examine changes in protein expression between *Mycobacterium avium* existing inside macrophages compared with cells grown in vitro. The findings of this study implicated a key enzyme of the glycoxylate cycle in this process. Other studies examined changes in the gene expression profile of the model yeast, *Saccharomyces cerevisiae*, once engulfed by macrophages. Once again, the glycoxylate cycle was implicated, as many of its constituent genes were up-regulated while the yeast was in the macrophage. The same was true with homologous *C. albicans* genes under similar conditions. Furthermore, deletion of key genes in the glyoxylate cycle led to attenuated virulence of *C. albicans* in a murine model of infection. These studies provide significant insight into pathogen response to the host.

Genomics in Drug Discovery and Development

Novel Targets

Infections due to methicillin-resistant *Staphylococcus aureus*, vancomycin-resistant enterococci, and multiple-drug-resistant *M. tuburculosis* have become common in clinical practice. The relative lack of anti-infective drug discoveries is attributed to the obsolescence of traditional whole cell-based screening strategies. This has led to an interest in molecular target-driven discovery strategies that rely heavily on the use of genomics. With this approach, large libraries of compounds can be screened for activity against a specific gene or gene product in a high-throughput fashion (References 20–23).

The selection of optimal, "pharmaceutically relevant" targets is critical to this process. Four attributes are usually considered when defining a possible target (Reference 22). First, it must be an essential component for growth, replication, and viability of the organism in the host. Second, it must be selective for the pathogen; it should not have a host ortholog. This ensures specificity for the pathogen with minimum potential for toxicity to the host. Third, it should be common across a wide range of pathogens, allowing for the development of a broad-spectrum agent. Finally, it must lend itself to high-throughput screening for efficient identification of inhibitors.

Many target areas have led to the identification of novel lead compounds using genomic approaches. One such area is bacterial fatty acid biosynthesis. Unlike mammalian cells, bacteria make use of an extensive pathway of enzymes for the synthesis of fatty acids. Genomic approaches have identified enzymes in this pathway for pathogenic bacteria, which has led to the discovery of novel compounds that inhibit this pathway and that lack activity against the mammalian fatty acid synthase enzyme. Although the parent compounds often lack good activity against their target, medicinal chemistry approaches have led to compounds with far greater potency (Reference 20). Researchers predict that many compounds will eventually be developed into clinically useful anti-infectives though this approach.

Targeted Patient Populations

Genomics holds great promise for defining specific subsets of patient populations that would derive maximum benefit from a specific therapy. Researchers are interested in the application of genomics to elucidate target populations for reevaluation of the anti-TNF-α therapies. Sepsis is a complex disease state involving disregulation of both pro- and anti-inflammatory response pathways, leading to tissue damage and end organ failure. As noted earlier, TNF-α is one of the most critical mediators associated with sepsis and is thought to play a significant role in the pathophysiology of sepsis and septic shock. Several studies have demonstrated an association between elevated plasma TNF-α levels and poor outcome (Reference 3).

Early studies in animals suggested that anti-TNF-α therapies, such as anti-TNF-α antibodies, produced favorable responses in sepsis cases. Much effort was therefore expended toward developing both anti-TNF-α and TNF-α receptor antibodies for the treatment of sepsis and septic shock. These agents, however, failed to improve mortality in all Phase III clinical trials. Others have underscored the possibility that incorrect population selection contributed to the poor results of these trials. Subgroup analyses of several studies suggests that patients with more severe sepsis or with elevated TNF-α levels may have derived benefit from this therapeutic approach. Using SNPs that correlate with these phenotypes, it may be possible to study this therapeutic strategy in better-defined patient populations. Genomics has opened the door for investigators to revisit this and other clinical trial disappointments in specific patient populations definable by genotype (Reference 3).

Pharmacogenomics in Infectious Diseases
Drug Metabolism

Many significant drug-drug interactions are associated with anti-infective agents. Although some involve drug absorption or distribution, most involve drug metabolism. Among the major cytochrome P450 (CYP) isoforms involved in oxidative metabolism, 1A2, 2C9, 2C19, and 2D6 all have variant alleles associated with poor metabolism. The fluoroquinolones, in particular ciprofloxacin and norfloxacin, inhibit CYP1A2. Fluconazole is a potent inhibitor of both CYP2C9 and CYP2C19, and INH is an inhibitor of CYP1A2, CYP2C9, and CYP2C19. Rifampacin is a nonspecific inducer of CYP-mediated metabolism, including that mediated by CYP2C9 and CYP2C19 (Reference 24).

The potential severity of drug-drug interactions is perhaps best illustrated by the interaction between fluconazole and warfarin. Fluconazole reduces the CYP-dependent metabolic clearance of the warfarin enantiomers, in particular, isoenzyme 2C9-catalyzed 6- and 7-hydroxylation of (S)-warfarin (Reference 25). There have been case reports of drug interactions involving the azole antifungal agents, and it is clear that genetics play a significant role in their occurrence. Although genetics will not completely prevent poor clinical judgment responsible for therapeutic misadventures, screening patients for their CYP2C9 or CYP2C19 genotype could identify those at increased risk for predictable interactions *a priori*.

Drug Targets

Genomics is beginning to make a clinical impact on the management of viral infections through the use of genotyping. Mutations that confer resistance to antiviral agents have been identified and are clinically useful for at least four human viruses: hepatitis B virus (HBV), hepatitis C virus (HCV), cytomegalovirus, and human immunodeficiency virus type 1 (HIV-1). Viruses are substantially more difficult than bacterial and fungal pathogens to grow in culture. Genomic-screening approaches can be used to derive drug susceptibility information without the need for cultures and are therefore particularly appealing for viral pathogens. (Reference 26).

The development of resistance is a common occurrence in patients who have taken prolonged courses of antiviral therapy for HBV. In addition to interferon-α-2b, nucleoside analogues such as lamivudine, famciclovir, and ganciclovir can be used to treat HBV infection based on their potent inhibition of HBV polymerase. Many mutations within the RT region of this polymerase have been associated with resistance to these agents (Reference 26) (Figure 2). As the mutations' utility in the management of HBV infection expands, genotyping for these mutations will likely contribute to the selection of optimal therapeutic regimens.

Combination therapy with interferon-α-2b and ribavirin has demonstrated efficacy in the management of patients infected with HCV. However, this response differs among viral types. Infection due to HCV types 2 and 3 exhibits a similar favorable response, whereas HCV type 1 is often refractory to this regimen. Therefore, determining the HCV genotype may eventually play a role in the therapeutic decision-making process for managing HCV infections.

Common Mutations Conferring Drug Resistance in HIV-1

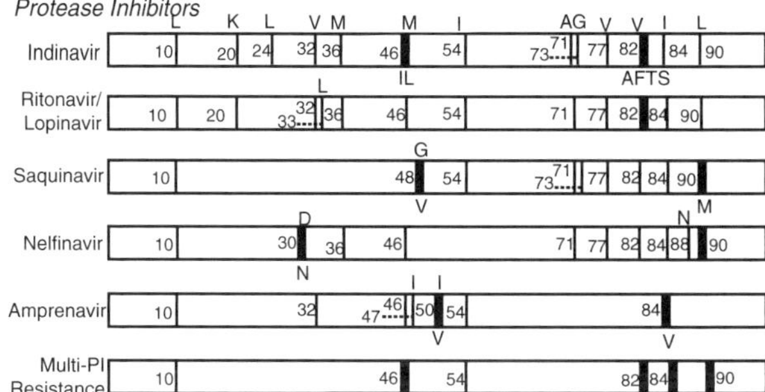

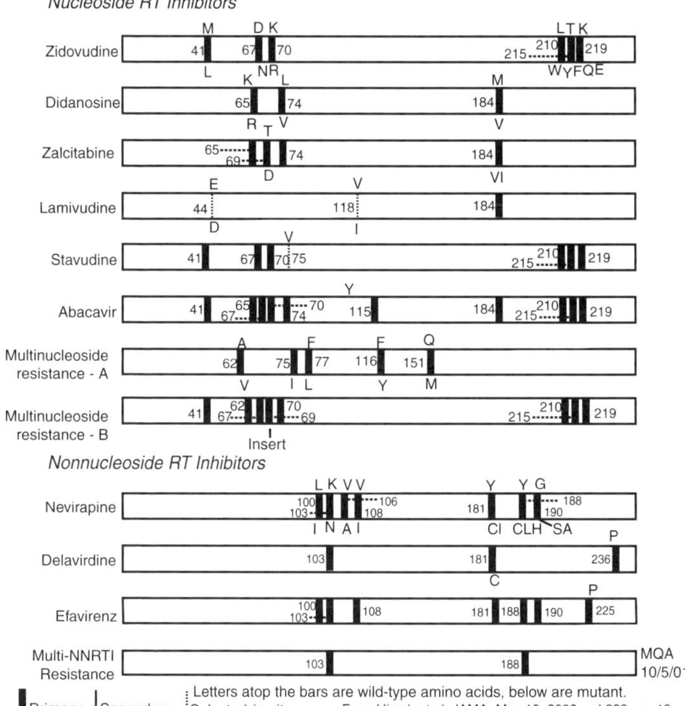

Figure 2. Common mutations conferring drug resistance in HIV-1.

HIV-1 = human immunodeficiency virus type 1; PI = protease inhibitor; RT = reverse transcriptase.

Reprinted with permission from the Journal of Clinical Virology, Vol. 22, Arens M., Clinically relevant sequence-based genotyping of HBV, HCV, CMV, and HIV, pages 11–29, 2001, with permission from Elsevier.

The HBV Polymerase and Mutations Associated With Resistance to Nucleoside Analoges

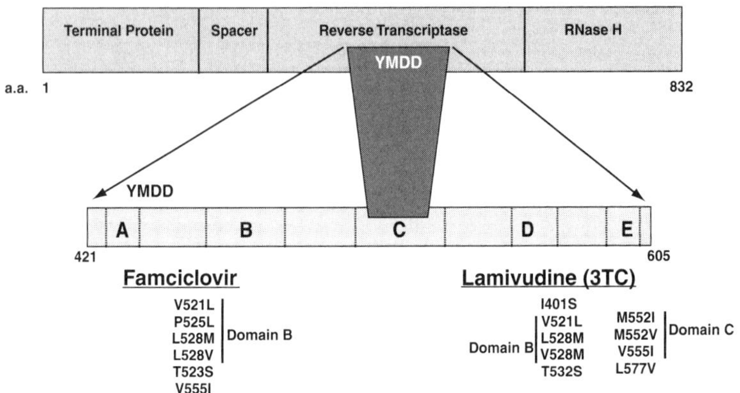

Figure 3. The HBV polymerase and mutations associated with resistance to nucleoside analoges.
HBV = hepatitis B virus; YMDD = tyrosine (Y), methionine (M), aspartate (D), aspartate (D). Reprinted with permission from the Journal of Clinical Virology, Vol. 22, Arens M., Clinically relevant sequence-based genotyping of HBV, HCV, CMV, and HIV, pages 11–29, 2001, with permission from Elsevier.

One of the current highlights of genomics in infectious diseases centers on genotyping of HIV-1. The development of resistance to antiretroviral agents has substantially hindered the pharmacological management of HIV infection and acquired immune deficiency syndrome. Therefore, genotyping for the detection of drug resistance mutations has become the standard of care for the management of breakthrough infection. Because of the absence of proofreading activity of the HIV RT, the virus exhibits a high mutation rate. Under the selective pressure of antiretroviral therapy, the stepwise acquisition of resistance mutations emerges in the viral population, culminating in high-level resistance. Mutations can directly impair the interaction between the drug and its target enzyme. These are considered primary mutations. Mutations that enhance the resistance phenotype in the presence of antiretroviral agents are considered secondary mutations (Figure 3). Compared with phenotypic assays for detecting drug resistance in HIV, genotypic assays are less costly, provide quicker results, and may allow the detection of resistance mutations before the actual resistance phenotype is exhibited. The interpretation of genotypic assays requires significant expertise. Together with the patient's viral load, cluster of differentiation 4 count, and treatment history, the determination of HIV-1 genotype promises to have significant clinical utility in guiding selection of continued anti-retroviral therapy (References 26, 27).

Vaccines and Genomics

Vaccine Response

To provide immunity, vaccination must elicit an appropriate immune response. However, vaccine response varies among individuals and appears to be partly because of genetics. Indeed, human leukocyte antigen (HLA) class I and II alleles have been associated with such variability in the response to the measles vaccine; HLA-B7, HLA-B51, HLA-DRB1*13, and HLA-DQA1*01* have been associated with a response to the vaccine, whereas homozygosity at HLA-B, HLA-DR, and HLA-DQA1 has been associated with a lack of response (Reference 28).

Reverse Vaccinology

Genomics has had a significant impact on vaccine development as well. Identification of candidate vaccine components traditionally has relied on biochemical, serological, and microbiological approaches. These strategies are time-consuming and focus efforts on antigens that can be purified in large quantities. With the availability of sequence information for entire microbial genomes, the most promising vaccine candidates can be selected using bioinformatics computational approaches for further testing. This approach, referred to as reverse vaccinology, is useful in focusing efforts on protein vaccine candidates, but it lacks utility in screening for polysaccharide or glycolipid candidates. This approach has been applied to several pathogens, including *Neisseria meningitides*, *Plasmodium falciparum*, *M. tuberculosis*, *Streptococcus pneumoniae*, and HCV (Reference 29).

One of the best examples of the application of reverse vaccinology is work directed toward vaccine target discovery in *N. meningitides*. Bioinformatics analysis of the meningococcus genome initially revealed 600 novel genes that putatively encoded cell surface or secreted proteins. Of these, 350 were successfully expressed and used to immunize mice for screening of potential vaccine candidates. This is impressive compared with the handful of such proteins identified up to this point using traditional strategies. The identification of such novel proteins provides a framework for the development of an effective vaccine against this pathogen. Reverse vaccinology has the potential to lead to the development of novel vaccines against problem pathogens.

Conclusion

In the postgenomic era, advances are expected in the basic sciences of molecular biology, genetics, bioinformatics, microbiology, immunology, biochemistry, and pharmacology that will provide the framework for great change in the approach to infectious diseases. Genomics-based technology will refine the ways in which infectious processes are diagnosed and offending pathogens are identified. New weapons against anti-infective resistance will be available, and novel anti-infective agents, immunomodulators, and vaccines will be developed. Furthermore, the design of therapeutic regimens will become more and more patient-specific, leading to improved efficacy and safety of anti-infective therapy. It will be critical for the pharmacist to maintain a working knowledge of this information and use these tools for optimal patient outcomes.

References

1. Butte A. The use and analysis of microarray data. Nat Rev Drug Discov 2002;1:951–60.

2. Kwiatkowski D. Genetic dissection of the molecular pathogenesis of severe infection. Intensive Care Med 2000;26(suppl 1):S89–97.

3. Cariou A, Chiche JD, Charpentier J, Dhainaut JF, Mira JP. The era of genomics: impact on sepsis clinical trial design. Crit Care Med 2002;30(suppl 5):S341–8.

4. Stuber F. Effects of genomic polymorphisms on the course of sepsis: is there a concept for gene therapy? J Am Soc Nephrol 2001;12(suppl 17):S60–4.

5. Alksne LE. Virulence as a target for antimicrobial chemotherapy. Expert Opin Investig Drugs 2002;11:1149–59.

6. De Backer MD, Nelissen B, Logghe M, et al. An antisense-based functional genomics approach for identification of genes critical for growth of *Candida albicans*. Nat Biotechnol 2001;19:235–41.

7. Rogers PD, Barker KS. Genome-wide expression profile analysis reveals coordinately regulated genes associated with stepwise acquisition of azole resistance in *Candida albicans* clinical isolates. Antimicrob Agents Chemother 2003;47:1220–27.

8. Baldwin DN, Vanchinathan V, Brown PO, Theriot JA. A gene-expression program reflecting the innate immune response of cultured intestinal epithelial cells to infection by *Listeria monocytogenes*. Genome Biol 2003;4:R2.

9. Detweiler CS, Cunanan DB, Falkow S. Host microarray analysis reveals a role for the *Salmonella* response regulator phoP in human macrophage cell death. Proc Natl Acad Sci U S A 2001;98:5850–5.

10. Eckmann L, Smith JR, Housley MP, Dwinell MB, Kagnoff MF. Analysis by high density cDNA arrays of altered gene expression in human intestinal epithelial cells in response to infection with the invasive enteric bacteria *Salmonella*. J Biol Chem 2000;275:14084–94.

11. Coombes BK, Mahony JB. cDNA array analysis of altered gene expression in human endothelial cells in response to *Chlamydia pneumoniae* infection. Infect Immun 2001;69:1420–7.

12. Ichikawa JK, Norris A, Bangera MG, et al. Interaction of *Pseudomonas aeruginosa* with epithelial cells: identification of differentially regulated genes by expression microarray analysis of human cDNAs. Proc Natl Acad Sci U S A 2000;97:9659–64.

13. Belcher CE, Drenkow J, Kehoe B, et al. The transcriptional responses of respiratory epithelial cells to *Bordetella pertussis* reveal host defensive and pathogen counter-defensive strategies. Proc Natl Acad Sci U S A 2000;97:13847–52.

14. Nakachi N, Matsunaga K, Klein TW, Friedman H, Yamamoto Y. Differential effects of virulent versus avirulent Legionella pneumophila on chemokine gene expression in murine alveolar macrophages determined by cDNA expression array technique. Infect Immun 2000;68:6069–72.

15. Rogers PD, Thornton J, Barker KS, et al. Pneumolysin-dependent and -independent gene expression identified by cDNA microarray analysis of THP-1 human mononuclear cells stimulated by *Streptococcus pneumoniae*. Infect Immun 2003;71:2087–94.

16. Barker KS, Filler SG, Rogers PD. Microarray analysis of differential gene expression in a human monocytic cell line in response to hyphae- and non-hyphae-producing *Candida albicans*. Infect Immun 2003 Program and Abstracts of the 42nd Interscience Conference on Antimicrobial Agents and Chemotherapy. M-207. 2002.) Manuscript is in revision.

17. Huang Q, Liu D, Majewski P, et al. The plasticity of dendritic cell responses to pathogens and their components. Science 2001;294:870–5.

18. Boldrick JC, Alizadeh AA, Diehn M, et al. Stereotyped and specific gene expression programs in human innate immune responses to bacteria. Proc Natl Acad Sci U S A 2002;99:972–7.

19. Lorenz MC, Fink GR. Life and death in a macrophage: role of the glyoxylate cycle in virulence. Eukaryot Cell 2002;1:657–62.

20. Schoolnik GK. Functional and comparative genomics of pathogenic bacteria. Curr Opin Microbiol 2002;5:20–6.

21. McDevitt D, Rosenberg M. Exploiting genomics to discover new antibiotics. Trends Microbiol 2001;9:611–7.

22. Ji Y. The role of genomics in the discovery of novel targets for antibiotic therapy. Pharmacogenomics 2002;3:315–23.

23. Buysse JM. The role of genomics in antibacterial target discovery. Curr Med Chem 2001;8:1713–26.

24. Black DJ, Kunze KL, Wienkers LC, et al. Warfarin-fluconazole. II. A metabolically based drug interaction: in vivo studies. Drug Metab Dispos 1996;24:422–8.

25. Venkatakrishnan K, von Moltke LL, Greenblatt DJ. Effects of the antifungal agents on oxidative drug metabolism: clinical relevance. Clin Pharmacokinet 2000;38:111–80.

26. Arens M. Clinically relevant sequence-based genotyping of HBV, HCV, CMV, and HIV. J Clin Virol 2001;22:11–29.

27. Hirsch MS, Brun-Vezinet F, D'Aquila RT, et al. Anti-retroviral drug resistance testing in adult HIV-1 infection: recommendations of an International AIDS Society-USA Panel. JAMA 2000;283:2417–26.

28. Hayney MS. Pharmacogenomics and infectious diseases: impact on drug response and applications to disease management. Am J Health-Syst Pharm 2002;59:1626–31.

29. Rappuoli R. Reverse vaccinology. Curr Opin Microbiol 2000;3:445–50.

Self-Assessment Questions

1. To identify proteins uniquely expressed by a pathogen under specific conditions, which one of the following approaches is the best?

   A. Differential display of reverse transcriptase polymerase chain reaction (RT-PCR) products.
   B. Serial analysis of gene expression.
   C. Microarray analysis.
   D. Two-dimensional gel electrophoresis and matrix-assisted laser desorption ionization-time of flight mass spectrometry fingerprinting.

2. Host immunity to infectious diseases can be described as a complex genetic trait in which phenotypic expression is influenced by environmental factors. Which one of the following represents the most important of these environmental factors?

   A The infecting pathogen.
   B. The geographic location in which the patient lives.
   C. Occupational factors.
   D. The lifestyle of the patient.

3. With regard to anti-infective drug development, which one of the following is most likely to be affected by application of genomic approaches to this process?

   A. Identification and validation of drug targets.
   B. Identification of novel lead compounds.
   C. Structure-activity relationship programs.
   D. Preclinical safety and efficacy trials.

4. A study was undertaken to measure the frequency of the tumor necrosis factor (TNF) 2 allele among patients with septic shock and among those who did not survive this inflammatory process. Serum TNF-α concentrations were also measured in these patients. There was a significantly greater frequency of the TNF 2 allele in patients with septic shock compared with the control group. Among patients with septic shock, the polymorphism was significantly more frequent in those who died. There was no significant difference between these groups with regard to TNF-α concentrations. Patients with the TNF 2 allele were shown to have a 3.7-fold risk of death. Which one of the following is the most reasonable conclusion?

   A. The TNF 2 allele is responsible for elevated TNF-α production in patients with sepsis.

B. The TNF 2 allele is responsible for the increased risk of death observed in these patients.

C. The TNF 2 allele is strongly associated with susceptibility to septic shock.

D. Increased production of TNF-α does not play a role in the pathogenesis of septic shock.

5. Lack of knowledge about which one of the following factors pertaining to a chosen antigen is the least likely to be an inherent limitation of reverse vaccinology?

A. Abundance of the antigen.
B. Immunogenicity of the antigen.
C. In vivo expression of the antigen.
D. Protein sequence of the antigen.

6. Which one of the following is not an advantage of genotypic assays compared with phenotypic assays for human immunodeficiency virus drug-resistance testing?

A. Lower cost.
B. Quicker results.
C. Requirement of expert interpretation.
D. Detection of mutations that precede phenotypic resistance.

7. A key area of research where genomic approaches are being applied is the development of agents that inhibit microbial virulence. Although such targets represent an untapped area for drug development, agents with activity against these targets may have limited clinical utility. Which one of the following factors is not consistent with these limitations?

A. Inhibitors of virulence will not eradicate infection by direct destruction of the invading pathogen.
B. Animal models for efficacy will be more critical in the assessment of these agents than will in vitro susceptibility testing.
C. Inhibitors of virulence will likely have broad-spectrum anti-infective activity.
D. Inhibitors of virulence will likely have the greatest utility as prophylactic agents.

8. The host-pathogen interaction exhibits significant complexity. Although there are common themes in the innate immune response to pathogenic organisms, recent work has drawn attention to the pathogen-specific responses elicited by pathogen recognition though a multitude of cell surface receptors. Application of genomics-based

technologies allows the use of this information for which one of the following?

A. Potential early indentification of the infecting pathogen based on the host gene expression profile in response to infection.
B. Detection of immunity to a given pathogen through altered expression of specific antibodies.
C. Decisions about duration of therapy based on the expression of subsets of genes encoding acute phase response proteins.
D. Therapeutic decisions based on the altered expression of ribosomal ribonucleic acid in the infected patient.

9. A common theme in azole antifungal resistance among pathogenic fungi is overexpression of the genes encoding efflux pumps of the adenosine 5' triphosphate-binding cassette transporter and major facilitator families. Which one of the following is a tool that may prove useful in identifying isolates that are overexpressing these resistance genes?

A. High-throughput deoxyribonucleic acid sequencing.
B. Real-time RT-PCR.
C. Restriction fragment length polymorphism analysis.
D. Pulsed-field gel electrophoresis.

10. Which one of the following will not be profoundly affected by the application of genomics to infectious diseases?

A. Decreased adverse drug effects through tailored drug therapy.
B. Improved outcomes through targeted patient populations.
C. Enhanced anti-infectives through identification of novel drug targets.
D. Eradication of most if not all infectious diseases.

Cardiovascular Diseases

Larisa H. Cavallari, Pharm.D., BCPS

Key Words

Pharmacogenomics, cardiovascular, drug, polymorphisms, gene.

Abstract

Currently, drug therapy decisions for patients with cardiovascular disease are largely guided by data from large-scale clinical trials and recommendations by expert consensus panels. Although a drug may have produced a positive outcome in the clinical trial population as a whole, there is no guarantee that it will provide the same beneficial effects without causing serious adverse reactions in an individual patient. Pharmacogenomics will allow clinicians to tailor cardiovascular drug therapy for an individual patient, so as to maximize the likelihood of positive outcomes while minimizing the potential for toxicity for each patient. Evidence of genetic associations with responses to different classes of cardiovascular agents is discussed in this chapter to provide a comprehensive overview of the burgeoning research in the area of cardiovascular pharmacogenomics. The applicability of these data to improve the management of cardiovascular disease and the potential for a genetic basis for other drug responses also are discussed.

Outline

Learning Objectives

1. Apply clinical data to predict the effects of drug metabolizing, drug transporter, and drug target gene polymorphisms on cardiovascular drug responses.
2. Assess the potential impact of variations in genes influencing cardiovascular disease progression on responses to cardiovascular drugs.
3. Surmise from the available literature how genetic variability might influence responses to cardiovascular drugs, including drugs that have not been specifically studied.
4. Evaluate the ultimate effects of a combination of polymorphisms in drug metabolizing, drug transporter, drug target, and/or disease progression genes on cardiovascular drug response.

5. Recognize the potential improvement in cardiovascular disease management that may arise from the application of pharmacogenomics.

Abbreviations in this Chapter

4S	Simvastatin Scandinavian Survival Trial
5A	5 adenines
ACE	Angiotensin-converting enzyme
ALLHAT	Antihypertensive and Lipid-Lowering to Prevent Heart Attack Trial
ARB	Angiotensin receptor blocker
AT_1	Angiotensin II type 1
AUC	Area under the curve
CARE	Cholesterol and Recurrent Events
CETP	Cholesteryl ester transfer protein
C_{max}	Maximum plasma concentration
CYP	Cytochrome P450
DNA	Deoxyribonucleic acid
$GN\beta_3$	G protein β_3-subunit
GP	Glycoprotein
G_s-protein	Stimulatory G protein
HDL	High-density lipoprotein
HIT	Heparin-induced thrombocytopenia
I/D	Insertion/deletion
IC_{50}	Concentration required for 50% inhibition
INR	International normalized ratio
MDR1	Multidrug resistance 1
NAPA	N-acetylprocainamide
NAT-2	N-acetyltransferase-2
RAS	Renin-angiotensin system
REGRESS	Regression Growth Evaluation Statin Study
SNP	Single nucleotide polymorphism
VA-HIT	Veterans Affairs HDL Cholesterol Intervention Trial

Introduction

Limitation to the Current Pharmacological Approach to Cardiovascular Disease Management

There are data from large randomized, controlled trials on which to base drug therapy decisions for the majority of cardiovascular diseases. However, even if a drug was shown to improve disease outcomes in a clinical trial population as a whole, there is no guarantee that it will produce the same beneficial effects without causing harm in an individual patient. This is particularly true for minorities who traditionally are underrepresented in cardiology clinical trial populations. It is difficult to predict a patient's response to a given cardiovascular drug because, as with other diseases, there is substantial interpatient variability in drug response. This interpatient variability limits the current pharmacological approach to cardiovascular disease management.

Sites of Polymorphisms that Influence the Interpatient Variability in Cardiovascular Drug Response

Polymorphisms in genes for drug-metabolizing enzymes, drug transporters, and drug target proteins likely contribute to the interpatient variability in cardiovascular drug effects. Polymorphisms for drug-metabolizing enzyme genes were the first recognized genetic variants influencing cardiovascular drug response. Indeed, genetic variation in the *N*-acetyltransferase-2 (NAT-2) gene and its association with adverse effects to hydralazine and procainamide were discovered more than 20 years ago. Much of the recent pharmacogenomic research in the area of cardiology has focused on genes for drug target proteins. For example, there are numerous published reports linking genetic polymorphisms for the renin-angiotensin system (RAS) enzymes and receptors to responses to angiotensin-converting enzyme (ACE) inhibitors and angiotensin receptor blockers (ARBs). There also has been substantial research in recent years into the effects of genes for drug transporters, such as P-glycoprotein, on drug disposition. Other studies have examined whether genes that affect cardiovascular disease severity or clinical outcomes, but do not necessarily affect drug disposition or target site sensitivity, influence clinical outcomes with drug therapy. For example, genetic determinants of coronary heart disease progression have been linked to the ability of statins to prevent recurrent coronary events.

Influence of Environmental-genetic Interactions on Cardiovascular Drug Response

Although single gene defects underlie a minority of cardiovascular diseases (e.g., hypertrophic cardiomyopathy, congenital long-QT syndrome, and some secondary forms of hypertension), it is clear that genetics contributes to the risk for most cardiovascular diseases, and these risks typically are polygenic in nature. For example, numerous genes for the RAS, the adrenergic nervous system, and renal sodium transport have been associated with the risk for essential hypertension. In addition, multiple environmental factors, including sodium intake, obesity, and physical inactivity, are known to increase blood pressure and likely interact with genetic factors to influence the overall risk for essential hypertension. Given the complexity of cardiovascular disease origin, genes linked to cardiovascular disease susceptibility are not discussed in this chapter.

Rather, the chapter focuses on genetic polymorphisms linked to responses to drugs used to manage cardiovascular diseases.

Pharmacogenomics of Drugs for Treating Hypertension and Heart Failure

Antihypertensive agents, such as diuretics, ACE inhibitors, and β-blockers, commonly are used in managing heart failure. Thus, the pharmacogenomics of drugs for treating hypertension and heart failure are discussed together in this section. Table 1 provides a summary of pharmacogenomic data to date for antihypertensive and heart failure drugs.

Table 1. Genes Linked to Effects of Drug for Treating Hypertension and Heart Failure

Drug/ Drug Class	Clinical Effect	Genes
Hydrochlorothiazide	Blood pressure reduction	G protein β_3-subunit
		α-adducin
		ACE
	Clinical outcome reduction	α-adducin
Amiloride	Blood pressure reduction	Epithelial sodium channel
ACE inhibitors	Blood pressure reduction	ACE
		Angiotensinogen
	Regression of LVH	ACE
	Improvement in LVEF	Aldosterone synthase
	Cough	ACE
		Bradykinin B_2-receptor
ARBs	Blood pressure reduction	ACE
		Aldosterone synthase
	Regression of LVH	Angiotensinogen
β-Blockers	Blood pressure reduction	β_1-adrenergic receptor
		G_s-protein α-subunit
	Transplant-free survival in heart failure	ACE

ACE = angiotensin-converting enzyme; ARB = angiotensin receptor blocker; LVEF = left ventricular ejection fraction; LVH = left ventricular hypertrophy.

Diuretics

Thiazide diuretics currently are recommended first line to manage uncomplicated hypertension. There is evidence that genes involved in renal sodium reabsorption influence antihypertensive responses to diuretic agents (Reference 1). Such genes include those for the inhibitory type guanosine triphosphate-binding protein (G protein), epithelial sodium channel, and α-adducin, which are discussed in detail below.

The G protein is heterotrimeric, of which β_3 is one component. A common synonymous single nucleotide polymorphism (SNP, *C825T*) occurs in exon 10 of the G protein β_3-subunit (*GNβ_3*) gene, located on chromosome 12p13. The *C825T* polymorphism generates a splice variant lacking 41 amino acids, which are encoded in exon 9 of the *GNβ_3* gene. The *825T* allele has been associated with enhanced sodium-hydrogen exchange and reduced plasma renin activity. The reported frequency of the *825T* allele is greater among African Americans, suggesting that this allele may contribute to the low-renin, salt-sensitive form of hypertension typically seen in this racial group.

The association between the *GNβ_3 C825T* polymorphism and response to diuretic therapy was evaluated in a study that included almost 400 patients with hypertension (Reference 2). During 4-month treatment period with hydrochlorothiazide, significantly greater blood pressure reductions were observed in patients with the *TT* genotype compared to *C* allele homozygotes. Specifically, mean systolic blood pressure decreased 16.3 mm Hg in patients with the *TT* genotype and 10.2 mm Hg with the *CC* genotype, whereas mean diastolic blood pressure reductions were 10.5 mm Hg and 5.9 mm Hg in *TT* and *CC* homozygotes, respectively. Systolic and diastolic blood pressure reductions with the heterozygous (*CT*) genotype were intermediate of the two homozygous genotypes; 13.6 mm Hg for systolic and 7.8 mm Hg for diastolic blood pressure. The association between *C825T* genotype and hydrochlorothiazide response remained significant after the adjustment for demographic factors and plasma neurohormone concentrations known to influence diuretic response. However, linear regression analysis revealed that the overall contribution of the *C825T* polymorphism to interindividual variation in thiazide response was only 5 percent. Age and plasma renin activity provided similar contributions to diuretic response, suggesting that the effects of the *C825T* genotype are additive to those of demographic and neurohormonal factors in predicting antihypertensive response to diuretic therapy.

The epithelial sodium channel plays a critical role in sodium reabsorption in the distal renal tubule. Mutations in the β- and γ-subunits of the epithelial sodium channel gene result in overactivity of the sodium channel and underlie the rare and severe salt-sensitive form of hypertension known as Liddle's syndrome. Treatment with amiloride blocks the overactive sodium channel and is used to manage blood pressure in patients with Liddle's syndrome. In addition to rare mutations in the epithelial sodium channel gene, a more common polymorphism has been described. Specifically, about 5 percent of people of African descent carry a nonsynonymous SNP in exon 12 (*T594M*) of the epithelial sodium channel β-subunit gene. The association between the *T594M* polymorphism and response to amiloride recently was examined in 14 individuals with hypertension of African origin who carried the variant *594M* allele (Reference 3). On study entry, patients were receiving an average of two antihypertensive drugs and had a mean blood pressure of 140/89 mm Hg. Withdrawal of previous drugs and institution of therapy with amiloride 20 mg/day controlled blood pressure to a similar extent as previous dual-drug therapy. These data suggest that the presence of the *T594M* polymorphism may predict a good blood pressure response to amiloride in black patients with hypertension.

To date, the most exciting genetic association with diuretic response involves a nonsynonymous SNP at codon 460 (*Gly460Trp*) of the α-adducin gene, located on chromosome 4p16. α-Adducin is a cytoskeletal protein that plays an important role in membrane ion transport. The *Gly460Trp* polymorphism has been associated with renal tubular sodium reabsorption, blood pressure responses to saline infusion, and plasma renin activity. The association between the *Gly460Trp* genotype and antihypertensive responses to 2-month treatment with hydrochlorothiazide was examined in two Italian populations with 143 total patients (Reference 4). In each population, mean blood pressure reductions were significantly greater among those who carried at least one *Trp* allele compared to *Gly/Gly* homozygotes. Specifically, mean blood pressure reductions in the two populations ranged from 12.6 to 15.9 mm Hg in *Trp* allele carriers and 6.4 to 9.3 mm Hg in *Gly/Gly* homozygotes.

In a subsequent population-based, case-control study, investigators examined the interaction between the *Gly460Trp* genotype and clinical outcomes (i.e., nonfatal myocardial infarction and nonfatal stroke) with diuretic therapy (Reference 5). The cases in this study consisted of 323 survivors of myocardial infarction or stroke who were enrolled in a large health maintenance organization and were receiving drug therapy for hypertension. The controls consisted of a random sample of 715 enrollees receiving antihypertensive drug therapy and matched to myocardial infarction cases by age and sex. Among 653 patients with the *Gly/Gly* genotype, there was no association between diuretic use and the combined end point of nonfatal myocardial infarction and stroke (odds ratio = 1.09, 95% confidence interval = 0.78–1.52). These data suggested that diuretic therapy provided similar protection against myocardial infarction or stroke as other antihypertensive agents in *Gly/Gly* homozygotes. In contrast, among the 385 individuals who carried at least one *Trp* allele, diuretic therapy was more effective at preventing myocardial infarction or stroke than other antihypertensive drugs. The odds ratio of the primary end point with diuretic therapy versus other antihypertensive treatment in those with the *Trp* allele was 0.49 (95% confidence interval = 0.32–0.77).

In the recently completed Antihypertensive and Lipid-Lowering to Prevent Heart Attack Trial (ALLHAT), treatment with diuretic therapy was associated with significant reductions in hypertension-related morbidity and mortality (Reference 6). It would be interesting to know whether ALLHAT patients who carried an α-adducin *460Trp* allele derived greater benefits from diuretic therapy compared to noncarriers. If the association between the α-adducin *Gly460Trp* genotype and reductions in clinical outcomes with diuretic therapy can be confirmed in a prospective, randomized, clinical trial, α-adducin genotype may be recognized as an important predictor not only of antihypertensive response to diuretic therapy, but more importantly, also of the effects of diuretic therapy on hypertension-related target organ damage.

Whether the *Gly460Trp* genotype interacts with the *GNβ3* and epithelial sodium channel genes in determining diuretic response remains to be determined. However, recent evidence suggests that response to hydrochlorothiazide may be influenced by the combination of the α-adducin *Gly460Trp* polymorphism and an insertion/deletion (*I/D*) polymorphism in intron 16 of the ACE gene (Reference 7). Specifically, among 87 previously untreated patients with hypertension, 2-month therapy with hydrochlorothiazide produced the greatest blood pressure reduction in carriers of at least one α-adducin *460Trp* allele and one ACE *I* allele. The odds ratio for response to hydrochlorothiazide, defined as having a mean reduction in blood pressure greater than 15 mm Hg, was 15.75 (95% confidence interval = 2.06–57.63) in ACE *I* plus α-adducin *460Trp* allele carriers compared to homozygotes for the ACE *D* plus *460Gly* genotypes.

Renin-angiotensin System Antagonists

There is evidence of interpatient variability in antihypertensive responses to ACE inhibitors, with ACE inhibitor monotherapy failing to produce adequate blood pressure control in about 50 percent of patients. African Americans, as a group, appear to derive lesser blood pressure-lowering effects from ACE inhibitor monotherapy than Caucasians. There also is evidence from retrospective analysis of heart failure studies to suggest that African Americans, compared to Caucasians, may respond less well to ACE inhibitors in heart failure, in terms of reductions in morbidity and mortality. Genetic polymorphisms commonly occur for receptors, enzymes, and intracellular signaling proteins in the RAS and may contribute to the observed interpatient variability in RAS antagonist responses.

Probably the best known and most extensively studied of the RAS polymorphisms is the ACE *I/D* polymorphism (discussed in the Diuretics section), which results in the presence or absence of a 287 basepair product in intron 16 of the ACE gene. Common polymorphisms also occur in the angiotensinogen (*T174M, M235T*), angiotensin II type 1 (AT$_1$) receptor

(*A1166C*), and aldosterone synthase (*C-344T*) genes. These polymorphisms have been linked to RAS hormone plasma concentrations and receptor sensitivity and responses to RAS antagonists (Reference 8). The frequencies of RAS gene polymorphisms differ significantly by race, as shown in Table 2, suggesting that they may contribute to the interracial variability in ACE inhibitor response.

Many studies have examined the influence of the ACE *I/D* polymorphism on antihypertensive and cardiac responses to ACE inhibitors and ARBs. However, these studies have yielded inconsistent and even conflicting results. For example, some studies have shown greater blood pressure reductions during ACE inhibitor and ARB therapy among ACE *II* homozygotes compared to *D* allele carriers. In contrast, other studies have shown either greater antihypertensive affects with ACE inhibitors in *DD* homozygotes or no association between the ACE *I/D* genotype and blood pressure responses to RAS antagonists.

Results from studies that evaluated the association between the ACE *I/D* genotype and regression of cardiac mass during ACE inhibitor therapy also are conflicting. Specifically, one study reported greater regression of cardiac wall thickness in *II* homozygotes compared to *DD* homozygotes after ACE inhibitor therapy for 2 years. This difference occurred despite similar blood pressure reductions between genotype groups. In contrast, another study conducted in a similar patient population showed a significantly greater reduction in mean left ventricular mass index after 12-month treatment with enalapril in those with the *DD* genotype compared to *II* homozygotes. Again, blood pressure reductions were similar between genotype groups.

Polymorphisms in the angiotensinogen and aldosterone synthase genes also have been linked to antihypertensive responses to RAS antagonists, with greater blood pressure reductions reported with the angiotensinogen *235T* allele and aldosterone synthase *-344TT* genotype. The link between RAS genes and regression of cardiac mass during 3-month treatment with irbesartan was studied in 41 patients with hypertension (Reference 9). The angiotensinogen *T174M*, ACE *I/D*, AT_1 receptor *A1166C*, and the

Table 2. Frequencies of Common Renin-angiotensin System Polymorphisms

Polymorphism	Chromosome	Caucasians	Africans	Asians
ACE *I/D*	17q22-q24	0.44	0.40	0.61
Angiotensinogen *M235T*	1q42-q43	0.42	0.77	0.78
Angiotensinogen *T174M*	1q42-q43	0.15	0.06	0.07
AT_1 receptor *A1166C*	3q21-q25	0.29	0.05	0.09
Aldosterone synthase *C-344T*	8q22	0.45	0.18	0.31

The frequency of the underlined allele is shown.
ACE = angiotensin-converting enzyme; AT_1 = angiotensin II type 1.

aldosterone synthase *C-344T* polymorphisms were included in the analysis. After adjustments for blood pressure changes, the angiotensinogen and AT_1 receptor polymorphisms were associated with regression in left ventricular mass index. The greatest regression occurred with the angiotensinogen *174TM* genotype and *235T* allele and the AT_1 receptor *1166AC* genotype. After stepwise multiple regression analysis, only the angiotensinogen *174TM* genotype remained an independent predictor of drug response.

The relationship between the ACE *I/D*, angiotensinogen *M235T*, and aldosterone synthase *C-344T* polymorphisms and improvements in cardiac function during heart failure treatment with an ACE inhibitor was examined in 107 African patients (Reference 10). At baseline, patients had idiopathic dilated cardiomyopathy, New York Heart Association functional class II or III heart failure, and a mean left ventricular ejection fraction of 25 percent. After a mean treatment duration of 17.4 months, individuals with the *-344C* allele of the aldosterone synthase gene had the greatest improvements in left ventricular ejection fraction. Forty-two percent of those with the *-344C* allele compared to 18 percent of those without a *-344C* allele had an ejection fraction greater than 40 percent at this time point. No other genotypes were associated with cardiac improvement in this study.

Both the ACE *I/D* polymorphism and a common SNP (*C-58T*) in the promoter region of the bradykinin B_2-receptor have been correlated with the ACE inhibitor-induced cough. Although separate studies have reported a higher incidence of cough with the ACE *II* and bradykinin B_2-receptor *-58TT* genotypes, an international multicenter trial found no significant association between either genotype and cough in a larger population of patients treated with ACE inhibitors (Reference 8). In positive gene-ACE inhibitor-induced cough studies, it is important to note that many participants with the "at-risk" genotypes remained cough free with ACE inhibitor therapy.

β-Blockers

β-Blockers commonly are used in hypertension and recommended in combination with ACE inhibitors to manage heart failure. A significant percentage of patients with hypertension do not achieve blood pressure goals with β-blocker monotherapy. When receiving treatment for heart failure, some patients experience significant blood pressure and heart rate reductions and heart failure exacerbation when low-dose β-blocker therapy is initiated, whereas others tolerate β-blocker initiation with little to no adverse effects. Genetic polymorphisms commonly occur for β-adrenergic receptors and intracellular signaling proteins and may account for some of the observed interpatient variability in β-blocker response (Reference 11).

The gene encoding the $β_1$-receptor is located on chromosome 10q24. Two common nonsynonymous SNPs occur in the $β_1$-receptor gene at codons 49 (*Ser* or *Gly*) and 389 (*Arg* or *Gly*). Site-directed mutagenesis studies have revealed enhanced receptor down-regulation with the codon 49 *Gly* allele and greater basal- and isoproterenol-mediated increases in adenylyl cyclase activity with the codon 389 *Arg* allele. Consistent with the in vitro data with the codon 389 polymorphism, two human studies found significantly higher diastolic blood pressures and heart rates in patients with the *Arg389* allele. Greater basal- and agonist-mediated effects with the *Arg389* allele in in vitro and in vivo studies suggest that patients who carry this allele may derive greater benefits from β-receptor blockade. This hypothesis was tested using data and blood samples collected during previous studies in which patients with hypertension were treated with either atenolol 50 mg/day or bisoprolol 5 mg/day. Given that β_1-receptor genotype and response to drug therapy were determined from banked blood samples and previously recorded data, this pharmacogenomic study was retrospective in design. No differences in blood pressure or heart rate reduction with β-blocker therapy were found among study patients with the *Arg/Arg*, *Arg/Gly*, or *Gly/Gly* genotypes at codon 389. However, findings from this study are limited given the retrospective study design and the fact that drug doses were not necessarily titrated to a clinical response.

More recent prospectively designed studies showed significant associations between β_1-receptor genotype at codons 49 and 389 and responses to β-blocker therapy. These studies prospectively examined subject response to β-blockade and compared response among patients with various β_1-receptor genotypes. One group of investigators reported greater reductions in resting systolic blood pressure and mean arterial pressure among *Arg389* versus *Gly389* homozygotes after a single dose of atenolol (Reference 12). Another group observed similar findings during chronic β-blocker therapy (Reference 13). Specifically, this study enrolled 40 untreated patients with hypertension who were started on metoprolol with doses titrated weekly to a maximum dose of 200 mg 2 times/day or to a diastolic blood pressure less than 90 mm Hg. A multivariate regression analysis revealed that baseline blood pressure and codons 49 and 389 genotypes were significant predictors of blood pressure response to metoprolol therapy. Specifically, the homozygous Arg389 and Ser49 genotypes were associated with the greatest blood pressure response to metoprolol. These data are consistent with the in vitro data and suggest that it may be possible to predict blood pressure response to β-blocker therapy in the future based on β_1-adrenergic receptor genotype. The codon 49 and 389 polymorphisms are in linkage disequilibrium such that the *Gly49/Gly389* haplotype rarely if ever occurs. Thus, in future studies, the β_1-receptor gene haplotype may prove to be a stronger predictor of drug response than either individual genotype.

After β-receptor stimulation, the heterotrimeric stimulatory G protein (G_S-protein) couples the receptor to intracellular signaling mechanisms to elicit a cellular response. There is a common polymorphism in the

G_S-protein α-subunit that results in the presence or absence of a restriction site for the *Fok*I enzyme, designated as *Fok*I+ if the site is present and *Fok*I- if the site is absent. A retrospective review of data from 66 patients with hypertension treated with β-blocker monotherapy for 4 weeks showed a higher frequency of the *Fok*I+ allele in those with a good blood pressure response to β-blocker therapy versus those with a poor response (good blood pressure response was defined as mean arterial pressure reductions greater than 15 mm Hg and poor blood pressure response was defined as mean arterial pressure reductions less than 11 mm Hg) (Reference 14). Prospectively designed studies are necessary to confirm these findings. In addition, the interaction between this polymorphism and β_1-receptor polymorphisms in influencing drug response should be examined. However, the separate data with the β_1-receptor and G_S-protein α-subunit gene polymorphisms imply that in many cases response to drug therapy at the receptor site is probably influenced by multiple polymorphisms for multiple proteins at the drug target level.

Although not directly involved in eliciting cellular responses to β-blockers, there is preliminary evidence to suggest that the ACE *I/D* polymorphism may be a determinant of clinical responses to β-blockers in heart failure. In a retrospective, cohort study that included 328 patients with heart failure, the association between the ACE *I/D* genotype and transplant-free survival with and without β-blocker therapy was examined (Reference 15). Among the 208 patients who were not receiving a β-blocker, transplant-free survival at 2 years was 78 percent with the ACE *II* genotype, 65 percent with the *ID* genotype, and 60 percent with the *DD* genotype (p=0.044). The association between the ACE genotype and survival was evident despite the widespread use of vasodilator therapy with ACE inhibitors or ARBs among patients. Treatment with a β-blocker appeared to negate the poorer prognosis associated with the *D* allele. Specifically, among the 120 patients with heart failure receiving a β-blocker, the 2-year transplant-free survival was 70 percent for the *II* genotype, 71 percent for the *ID* genotype, and 77 percent for the *DD* genotype (p=0.73). A plausible explanation for the association between the ACE gene and β-blocker effects in heart failure is centered on the fact that angiotensin II promotes norepinephrine release (and norepinephrine increases renin release). Thus, increased ACE activity and angiotensin II concentrations associated with the *D* allele of the ACE gene may lead to increased activation of the sympathetic nervous system. If this is the case, then patients with the ACE *D* allele may derive greater benefits from attenuation of sympathetic nervous system activity with β-blocker therapy. Alternatively, β-blockade may diminish higher ACE activity associated with the ACE *D* allele through inhibition of norepinephrine-mediated renin release.

The β-blockers metoprolol, carvedilol, timolol, and propranolol are metabolized by the cytochrome P450 (CYP) 2D6 enzyme. This enzyme exhibits functional polymorphism resulting in the poor, extensive, and ultrarapid drug metabolizer phenotypes. The *CYP2D6*1/*1* genotype is considered the wild-type and is associated with the extensive metabolizer phenotype. A single copy of the variant *CYP2D6*2* allele does not appear to affect enzyme activity; however, two or more copies of the *CYP2D6*2* allele enhance enzyme activity and contribute to ultrarapid metabolism of CYP2D6 substrates. Theoretically, this could result in subtherapeutic plasma concentrations of drugs that are inactivated by the CYP2D6 enzyme. The *CYP2D6*3*, *CYP2D6*4*, and *CYP2D6*5* alleles are associated with absent enzyme activity and poor metabolism of CYP2D6 substrates. The *CYP2D6*10* allele occurs commonly in the Asian population and results in reduced enzyme activity. Studies have demonstrated significantly higher plasma concentrations of β-blockers that are CYP2D6 substrates in CYP2D6 poor metabolizers compared to extensive metabolizers. However, given that β-blockers have a wide therapeutic index, the presence of dysfunctional CYP2D6 alleles may or may not have significant clinical consequences. The initiation of β-blocker therapy in heart failure is the most likely scenario in which CYP2D6 genotype might influence drug response. The CYP2D6 genotype may contribute to β-blocker response in heart failure because in this setting, patient tolerability is significantly influenced by β-blocker plasma concentrations.

Digoxin

Digoxin reduces hospitalization rates for patients with heart failure and is recommended for those with symptomatic disease. Digoxin is a substrate for P-glycoprotein, the energy-dependent efflux pump expressed in many cell types, including intestinal enterocytes, hepatocytes, renal proximal tubule cells, and endothelial cells lining the blood-brain barrier. At these locations, P-glycoprotein may influence the amount of digoxin available for absorption and excretion, as shown in Figure 1, and limits access of the drug into the central nervous system. In addition, P-glycoprotein is believed to

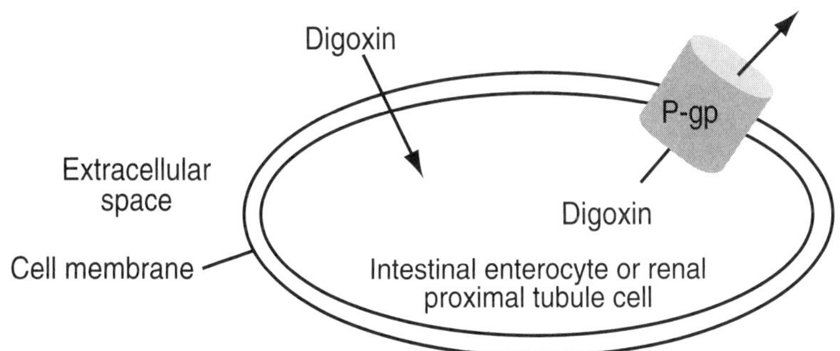

Figure 1. P-glycoprotein and its effects on digoxin concentrations.
P-gp = P-glycoprotein

mediate the drug interaction between digoxin and quinidine. Specifically, quinidine inhibits P-glycoprotein in the intestine and renal tubule, thus increasing digoxin absorption and reducing total body digoxin clearance.

P-glycoprotein is encoded by the multidrug resistance 1 (*MDR1*) gene, located on chromosome 7. Many polymorphisms have been identified in the promoter and coding regions of the *MDR1* gene, and their functional consequences has been explored by many investigators (Reference 16). The best characterized *MDR1* gene polymorphism is a synonymous SNP at nucleotide 3435 (*C* or T) in exon 26. The *3435T* allele has been associated with lower intestinal *MDR1* expression, reduced P-glycoprotein activity, and higher digoxin plasma concentrations in healthy volunteers. However, these findings have not been consistently replicated by other research groups. In fact, one group of investigators reported lower digoxin plasma concentrations with the *3435T* allele.

The *C3435T* polymorphism is in linkage disequilibrium with a nonsynonymous SNP in exon 21 (*G2677T*), resulting in either an alanine or serine at codon 893, and a synonymous SNP in exon 12 (*C1236T*). The *G2677T* polymorphism also has been associated with *MDR1* gene expression, although results to date are inconsistent. Evidence of linkage disequilibrium provides a possible explanation for the previously inconsistent data with *MDR1* gene polymorphisms. That is, the effects associated with the *C3435T* polymorphism may actually be a result of its linkage to one or more functionally significant variants in the *MDR1* gene. This hypothesis is supported by findings of higher serum drug concentrations after a single digoxin dose in healthy Japanese volunteers with the exon 21 *TT* genotype plus the exon 26 *TT* genotype (exon 21/26 *TT/TT* haplotype) compared to those with the exon 21/26 *GG/CC* haplotype (Reference 17). In this study, mean area under the curve (AUC) was 35.1 ng•h/ml with the *TT/TT* haplotype and 20.6 ng•h/ml with the *GG/CC* haplotype. Pharmacokinetic parameters for those with the heterozygous haplotype (*GT/CT*) were intermediate between the two homozygous haplotypes. With concomitant administration of clarithromycin, an inhibitor of P-glycoprotein, patients with *GG/CC*, but not patients with *TT/TT*, had a significant increase in digoxin bioavailability.

A European study also examined the influence of the exon 21/26 haplotype on digoxin pharmacokinetics (Reference 18). At a steady state, plasma digoxin AUC from 0 to 4 hours and the maximum plasma concentration (C_{max}) differed significantly among the *GG/CC* (n=6), *GT/CT* (n=7), and *GT/TT* (n=6) haplotypes, with the lowest values occurring in the *GG/CC* group. Too few patients with the exon 21/26 *TT/TT* haplotype were available for analysis.

Explanations for Inconsistent Data

There are several possible explanations for the discordant results from the RAS gene-RAS antagonist response studies, including differences in patient demographics and treatment durations. In addition, although not specifically discussed by the investigators, it is possible that drug adherence differed between genotype groups. A more likely explanation is that determinants of RAS antagonist responses are polygenic rather than monogenic; thus, a single polymorphism in one RAS gene contributes little to the overall response to an RAS antagonist. Indeed, the RAS has a complex signaling pathway, and numerous polymorphisms have been identified for various RAS proteins, as shown in Figure 2. Therefore, it is likely that genes for ACE, angiotensinogen, the AT_1 receptor, aldosterone synthase, and probably other RAS proteins interact to influence overall RAS antagonist response. Thus, future studies should examine combinations of RAS gene polymorphisms and the effects of these gene combinations on drug response.

The reasons for the inconsistencies between studies with the *MDR1* gene and digoxin pharmacokinetics are unclear. However, it is possible that the *MDR1* exon 12 polymorphism or a yet unrecognized polymorphism in

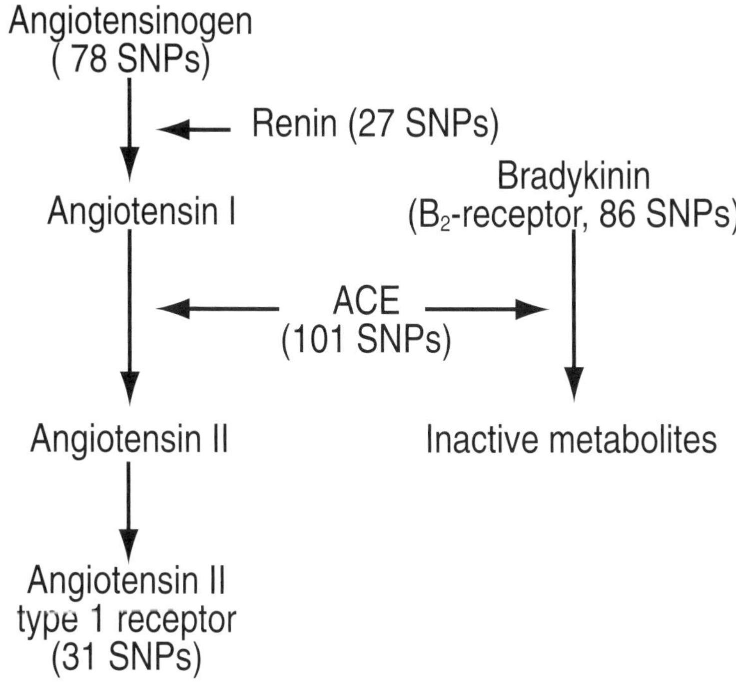

Figure 2. Single nucleotide polymorphisms for renin-angiotensin system genes that have been identified by The SNP Consortium Ltd as of March 3003. (*http://SNP.CSHL.ORG*). ACE = angiotensin-converting enzyme; SNP = single nucleotide polymorphism.

linkage disequilibrium with the exon 21 and 26 sites actually determines overall *MDR1* gene expression and functional consequences. Thus, studies analyzing the exon 12/21/26 haplotype and its effects on P-glycoprotein substrate pharmacokinetics may be necessary to more fully characterize *MDR1* gene-drug response associations. Further haplotype analyses may help to delineate whether the *MDR1* gene has clinically significant effects on digoxin pharmacokinetics in patients with cardiovascular diseases and may provide data to support or refute *MDR1* genotyping to manage diseases requiring digoxin treatment. In addition, results of future studies may enable us to predict the likelihood for significant drug interactions between digoxin and P-glycoprotein inhibitors or inducers based on *MDR1* genotype.

Application of these Data to Clinical Practice

The current pharmacological approach to treating hypertension involves one or more trials of various antihypertensive agents until a desired blood pressure response is achieved. Specifically, initial antihypertensive drug therapy is chosen for a patient. Then, the patient is monitored periodically for drug effectiveness and tolerance, while titrating the antihypertensive drug dose until blood pressure is reduced below a goal level. It is common for the initial therapy to either fail to lower blood pressure to goal or to produce intolerable adverse effects, as depicted in Figure 3. Thus, it may become necessary to institute additional or alternative agents until goal

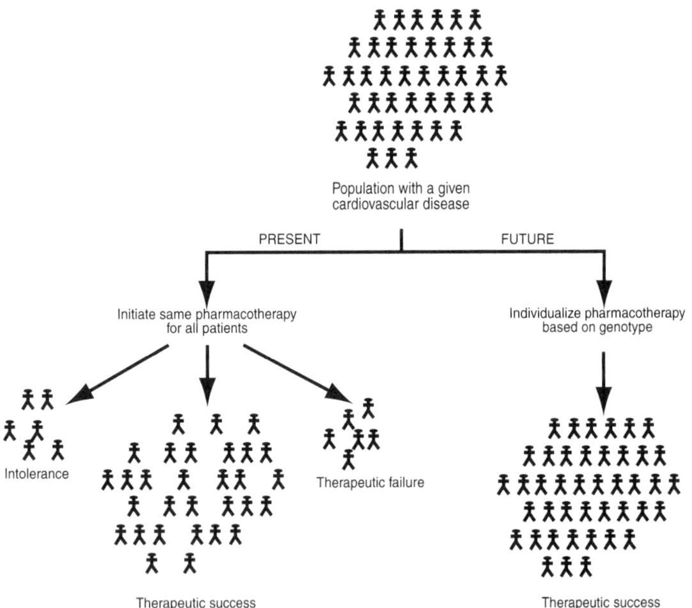

Figure 3. Current and potential future approach to cardiovascular disease management.

blood pressure is obtained with acceptable tolerability for the patient. While various agents are tried, the patient remains hypertensive and at risk for hypertension-related target organ damage. Pharmacogenomics has the potential to eliminate this trial-and-error approach to hypertension management. With pharmacogenomics, the drug expected to provide the greatest blood pressure response with the least toxicity may be chosen for a given patient based on his or her deoxyribonucleic acid (DNA). This approach could increase the likelihood of early therapeutic success.

As previously discussed, data to date with RAS antagonist responses are inconsistent. Before pharmacogenomics information can be incorporated into hypertension treatment decisions regarding ACE inhibitors and ARBs, the combination of genetic polymorphisms that best predict response to these agents must be elucidated. Data available to date on genetic influences on antihypertensive responses to β-blockers and diuretics are more promising and suggest that information about β-receptor and α-adducin genotypes may be helpful in deciding whether to institute β-blocker and diuretic therapy for hypertension management. For example, if an individual carries an α-adducin *460Trp* allele, the clinician may prefer therapy with a thiazide diuretic because evidence suggests that thiazide diuretics are effective antihypertensive agents and may improve clinical outcomes with this genotype. Conversely, if the individual has the α-adducin *460Gly/Gly* genotype, diuretic therapy may offer no advances over treatment with other agents. The presence of the β_1-receptor *389Arg/Arg* or *49Ser/Ser* genotype would support hypertension treatment with a β-blocker. Whether β_1-receptor genotype influences clinical outcomes during β-blocker treatment for hypertension remains to be examined.

For treating heart failure, pharmacogenomics may help to streamline drug therapy. Current guidelines advocate treating patients with heart failure with multiple agents, including ACE inhibitors, β-blockers, and spironolactone for morbidity- and mortality-reducing benefits; and diuretics and digoxin for symptom control. Thus, it is common for patients with heart failure to be taking four or more drugs for their heart failure alone, in addition to drugs they may be taking for concomitant diseases. Some patients may have difficulty managing such complicated regimens, and drug adherence may suffer as a result. In addition, complex multidrug regimens increase the risk for adverse drug effects and drug interactions. Some patients with heart failure may not have adequate blood pressure to safely take recommended doses of both ACE inhibitors and β-blockers. Thus, clinicians must decide which drug(s) to initiate and titrate upward and which drug(s) to withhold or continue albeit at lower doses than associated with beneficial outcomes in clinical trials. With pharmacogenomics, it may be possible to identify the combination of drugs that is expected to provide the greatest benefits for each heart failure patient based on genotype. This approach to pharmacotherapy would allow heart failure drug therapy to be tailored according to genotype, potentially simplifying drug regimens, improving drug adherence, and optimizing patient outcomes. For example, if associations between the ACE *I/D* genotype and β-blocker effects on transplant-free survival are confirmed in prospective studies, this association would support aggressive efforts to initiate and titrate β-blockers to target doses in patients with heart failure with the *D* allele of the ACE gene.

Prediction of Other Responses that Might Have a Genetic Basis

In the majority of the gene-drug response association studies previously discussed, the primary outcomes were related to drug efficacy. However, identifying genes associated with adverse effects is, in many instances, of even greater importance because serious adverse drug effects may result in substantial morbidity and even death. Angioedema is an example of a serious, potentially life-threatening effect from ACE inhibitor and ARB therapy that may have a genetic link. Given its infrequent occurrence, a large study population will be necessary to identify and validate genetic risk factors for angioedema. However, if a genetic link to this adverse effect can be identified, it may allow for the avoidance of ACE inhibitors and ARBs in patients genetically predisposed to developing angioedema.

Heart failure decompensation during β-blocker initiation is another serious adverse effect that may have a genetic link. Given its association with β_1-receptor down-regulation and adenylyl cyclase activity in vitro, it is possible that the β_1-receptor gene influences norepinephrine-mediated compensatory mechanisms in patients with heart failure. If this is the case, β_1-receptor genotype may consequently influence response to blockade of these compensatory mechanisms and the propensity for heart failure decompensation with β-blocker initiation. To date, no evidence of such an association has been reported. However, if a genetic risk factor for heart failure decompensation during β-blocker therapy were identified, it could have important clinical implications. Specifically, the ability to identify patients genetically predisposed to decompensation with β-blocker initiation could lead to improved monitoring during β-blocker initiation and dose titration. This ability could potentially decrease the incidence of emergency department visits and hospitalizations for worsening heart failure when β-blockers are started.

Pharmacogenomics of Anticoagulant and Antiplatelet Agents

Anticoagulant therapy with warfarin and heparin is widely prescribed to treat and prevent thromboembolic events. Antiplatelet agents, such as aspirin, ticlopidine, and clopidogrel, commonly are used to prevent and treat acute coronary syndromes and stroke. In addition, glycoprotein (GP) IIb/IIIa receptor antagonists reduce the risk of adverse clinical outcomes in the setting of unstable angina or non-ST-segment elevation myocardial infarction, particularly in adjunct with percutaneous coronary intervention. Examples of genetic polymorphisms that have been associated with effectiveness and risk for adverse effects with antithrombotic and antiplatelet agents are shown in Table 3 and discussed in detail in this section.

Warfarin

There is significant interpatient variability in warfarin dose requirements necessary to achieve optimal anticoagulation. Although factors, such as diet, concomitant drugs and diseases, body weight, and age, are known to influence the anticoagulant effects of warfarin, they do not account for all of the interpatient variability in warfarin dose requirements. The S-isomer of warfarin has 5 times the anticoagulant activity than the R-isomer and is metabolized by the polymorphic CYP2C9 enzyme. The variant *CYP2C9*2* (Cys144, Ile359) and *CYP2C9*3* (Arg144, Leu359) alleles result from single amino acid substitutions at CYP2C9 gene positions necessary for enzyme activity. The variant *CYP2C9*5* allele (Arg144, Ile359, Glu360), with reduced catalytic efficiency compared to the wild-type (*CYP2C9*1*), is expressed in about 3 percent of African Americans. Carriers of one or more variant CYP2C9 allele may have reduced clearance of S-warfarin and be at greater risk for overanticoagulation with usual warfarin doses compared to those with the wild-type *CYP2C9*1/*1* (Arg144, Ile359) genotype.

Many investigators have described increased bleeding risk and lower warfarin dose requirements with variant CYP2C9 alleles (References 17, 18). A retrospective analysis was conducted in 88 patients taking stable doses of warfarin for at least 3 months who were followed in a European anticoagulation clinic (References 19–21). The CYP2C9 genotypes were compared among patients requiring 1.5 mg/day or less of warfarin (low-dose group) and those requiring higher warfarin doses (standard-dose group) to maintain an international normalized ratio (INR) of

Table 3. Genes Linked to Effects of Anticoagulants and Antiplatelet Agents

Drug/Drug Class	Clinical Effect	Genes
Warfarin	Dose requirements	CYP2C9
	Bleeding risk	
	Difficulty with drug initiation	
Heparin	Thrombocytopenia	Platelet Fc gamma receptor
Aspirin + Ticlopidine	Subacute thrombosis	Glycoprotein IIIa

CYP = cytochrome P450.

2–3. Eighty-one percent of patients in the low-dose group versus 38 percent in the standard-dose group carried at least one variant *CYP2C9*2* or *CYP2C9*3* allele. Patients in the low-dose group had more difficulty with warfarin initiation, requiring longer hospitalizations and more frequent clinic visits for warfarin dose titration. In addition, patients in the low-dose group had a higher incidence of serious and life-threatening bleeding episodes than those in the standard-dose group (11 in 133 patient-years compared to seven in 311 patient-years), with a rate ratio of 3.68 (95% confidence interval = 1.43–9.50; p=0.007).

Similar findings were reported from a retrospective, cohort study that included 185 warfarin-treated Caucasian patients in two pharmacist-run anticoagulation clinics in the United States (Reference 20). Maintenance warfarin doses were recorded for those receiving consistent warfarin doses with an INR within therapeutic range for three consecutive clinic visits. Thirty-one percent of the study population carried at least one *CYP2C9*2* or *CYP2C9*3* allele, and 6 percent carried two variant alleles. There was a significant difference in mean maintenance doses of warfarin among the six CYP2C9 genotype groups (**1/*1, *1/*2, *1/*3, *2/*2, *3/*3, *2/*3*). The median daily warfarin doses were 5.27 mg with the wild-type genotype, 4.64 mg with one *CYP2C9*2* allele, and 2.92 mg with one *CYP2C9*3* allele. Carriers of a variant allele had a higher incidence of serious bleeding complications (10.92 vs. 4.89 per 100 patient-years), an increased risk of INR values higher than 4.0, and a slower rate of dose stabilization (median difference of 95 days) than those without a variant allele. In addition, the hazard ratio for bleeding within 90 days of warfarin initiation was 3.94 (95% confidence interval = 1.29–12.06) with the variant genotype.

A more recent study described the effects of the *CYP2C9* gene on warfarin dose requirements and metabolic clearance (Reference 21). In addition, investigators examined the effects of polymorphism in the CYP2C19 enzyme, which metabolizes the R-isomer of warfarin, on warfarin dose and pharmacokinetics. The study included 93 European Caucasians taking stable doses of warfarin with INR variations of 15 percent or less in the previous 3 months. Patients were divided into three groups based on their weekly warfarin requirements: low (less than 26.25 mg), medium (26.25–43.75 mg), and high (greater than 43.75 mg). Seventy percent of patients in the low-dose group, 37.5 percent in the medium-dose group, and only one of 24 patients in the high-dose group carried a variant CYP2C9 allele. Plasma S-to-R-warfarin ratio and S-warfarin clearance varied significantly by CYP2C9 genotype, with higher S-to-R-warfarin ratios and lower S-warfarin clearance with the variant genotypes. The CYP2C19 genotype was not associated with warfarin dose requirements or R-warfarin clearance. Of note, 30 percent of patients in the low-dose group had the *CYP2C9*1/*1* genotype, implying that nongenetic and/or other not yet identified genetic factors may be as important as CYP2C9 genotype in determining warfarin dose requirements for some patients.

Heparin

An immune-related thrombocytopenia is one of the most serious adverse reactions to heparin. Heparin-induced thrombocytopenia (HIT) can result in devastating thromboembolic complications, causing substantial morbidity and even death. The mechanism for type II HIT involves the recognition and binding of heparin-induced antibodies to platelet factor 4-heparin complexes with subsequent activation of platelets through the platelet Fc gamma receptor.

A nonsynonymous SNP (*Arg131His*) occurs commonly in the platelet Fc gamma receptor gene and appears to alter platelet aggregation. Several investigators have reported an association between the platelet Fc gamma receptor gene and the risk for HIT, whereas others have found no such association (Reference 22). In early positive studies, investigators reported an overrepresentation of the *131His* allele among patients with HIT. In contrast, a more recent study showed a higher frequency of the *Arg/Arg* genotype among patients with HIT (Reference 22). Specifically, in the largest study to date, *Arg131His* genotype was compared among 389 patients with a history of HIT type II, 351 patients with a history of thrombocytopenia from other causes or a thrombotic event unrelated to heparin, and 256 healthy blood donors. The frequency of the *Arg/Arg* genotype was significantly higher among those with HIT (27 percent) than in those without HIT (21 percent) and healthy blood donors (20 percent). Of 122 patients with HIT in whom data were collected prospectively, the *Arg/Arg* genotype was significantly overrepresented among 68 patients with thromboembolic complications compared to 54 individuals with isolated thrombocytopenia (37 percent vs. 17 percent). The reason for conflicting gene-HIT findings among studies is unclear. However, the discrepency may involve the differences among studies in the number of patients with thromboembolic complications versus isolated thrombocytopenia or the use of different assays to detect heparin-dependent antibodies.

Glycoprotein IIb/IIIa Inhibitors and Aspirin

The final common pathway of platelet aggregation involves the binding of fibrinogen to GP IIb/IIIa receptors expressed on the activated platelet surface and the cross-linking of adjacent platelets. The resultant thrombus may cause vessel occlusion at the site of plaque rupture and compromise blood flow to the myocardium often leading to an acute coronary event. A similar etiology underlies the pathophysiology of acute ischemic stroke. The ability of antiplatelet agents to inhibit platelet aggregation and prevent ischemic events varies considerably from patient to patient. Genetic polymorphisms for proteins involved in platelet activation and aggregation may influence response to antiplatelet therapy.

One such polymorphism is the $Pl^{A1/A2}$ variant of the platelet GP IIIa subunit gene, located on chromosome 17. This polymorphism results from a SNP at nucleotide 1565 (C or T) in exon 2 of the gene, causing a substitution of proline (Pl^{A2}) for leucine (Pl^{A1}) at amino acid position 33 and a change in the conformation of the receptor's extracellular domain. The Pl^{A2} allele occurs at a frequency of about 15 percent and is present in 20–30 percent of the population. Several in vitro studies demonstrated that platelets from Pl^{A2}-positive donors were more sensitive to inhibition by antiplatelet therapy compared to platelets from Pl^{A1} homozygotes. For example, in a study of platelets from 16 healthy donors, the concentration of aspirin required to reduce platelet aggregation by 50 percent (IC$_{50}$) was 2.7±0.6 µmol/L for Pl^{A2}-positive platelets and 23.4±3.3 µmol/L for Pl^{A2}-negative platelets (Reference 23).

The Pl$^{A1/A2}$ polymorphism has been associated with response to combination antiplatelet therapy after coronary artery stent implantation. However, findings to date are opposite of what might be expected based on the majority of in vitro data with antiplatelet response. For example, in a study that included 1150 patients who underwent coronary artery stent placement followed by treatment with aspirin plus ticlopidine, restenosis at 6 months was significantly higher in patients with the Pl^{A2} allele compared to homozygotes for the Pl^{A1} allele (47 percent vs. 38 percent) (Reference 24). Similarly, in a study of 318 patients with coronary stent implantation, the risk for subacute thrombosis was 5-fold greater in those with the Pl^{A2} polymorphism compared to homozygotes for the Pl^{A1} genotype, despite similar antiplatelet therapy (with aspirin plus ticlopidine) and clinical, angiographic, and procedural characteristics between genotype groups (Reference 25). The Pl^{A2} allele remained the only significant independent predictor of stent occlusion on multivariate analysis. These results suggest that Pl^{A2} carriers with ischemic disease may require more aggressive antiplatelet therapy for percutaneous coronary interventions to prevent subacute vessel closure or other vascular events after coronary artery stent implantation.

There are several possible explanations for the inconsistent findings with the in vitro and in vivo studies with the Pl$^{A1/A2}$ polymorphism. The most obvious is that the Pl$^{A1/A2}$ polymorphism interacts with other genetic and/or environmental factors to determine platelet aggregatibility and antiplatelet drug response. This interaction is supported by evidence that age, body weight, smoking status, lipoprotein concentrations, and the presence of diabetes mellitus influence platelet aggregation. Furthermore, a study from more than 2400 Framingham Heart Study participants revealed that although up to 30 percent of variability in platelet aggregation was attributed to genetic factors, the Pl$^{A1/A2}$ polymorphism contributed to less than 1 percent of the overall variation (Reference 26). Thus, future studies should attempt to identify the combination of genetic and environmental factors that best determines antiplatelet drug response.

Application of these Data to Clinical Practice

Data from these studies suggest that genotype may be useful in choosing oral anticoagulant doses, identifying patients at risk for serious complications with heparin therapy, and predicting response to oral and intravenous antiplatelet agents. Specifically, in the near future, it may be possible for clinicians to genotype individuals for CYP2C9 polymorphisms before warfarin initiation and start lower doses with more diligent follow-up in carriers of a variant CYP2C9 allele. Alternatively, clinicians may choose to withhold warfarin therapy for those whose anticipated benefit is low and risk for bleeding is high based on their DNA. These patients may be good candidates for therapy with oral direct thrombin inhibitors once they become available. However, before genotyping will be accepted as a guide to managing oral anticoagulant therapy, the clinical benefits and cost-effectiveness of warfarin dosing and monitoring based on *a priori* genotyping must first be evaluated.

If the association between the platelet Fc gamma receptor codon 131 polymorphism and thromboembolic complications from HIT is confirmed, information about the platelet Fc gamma receptor genotype could be an important consideration when initiating heparin therapy. In patients who carry the variant allele associated with increased risk of HIT, clinicians may choose to initiate alternative anticoagulant therapy with danaparoid or a direct thrombin inhibitor. Alternatively, the decision may be made to use heparin, but with close hematologic monitoring.

If the combination of genetic and environmental factors that best predicts response to antiplatelet therapy can be identified, it may have utility in predicting responses to antiplatelet drugs and tailoring therapy accordingly. For instance, in treating acute coronary syndromes, knowledge of genetic influences of antiplatelet drug response may be useful in identifying the best candidates for GP IIb/IIIa receptor antagonists. These agents are associated with considerable expense and bleeding risk and have questionable benefits for those not undergoing coronary interventions. In the future, these agents may be reserved for patients who are expected to derive their greatest benefits with the lowest risk of bleeding based on genotype.

Predicting Responses to Other Antiplatelet Agents and Newer Antithrombotic Agents that Might Have a Genetic Basis

Oral direct thrombin inhibitors currently are being investigated for treating and preventing venous thromboembolism. These drugs bind directly to thrombin and prevent activation of coagulation factors V and VIII and the conversion of fibrinogen to fibrin. Genetic polymorphisms commonly occur for proteins involved in the coagulation system that may influence risk for venous thromboembolism and response to anticoagulant treatment with warfarin or direct thrombin inhibitors. For example, genetic variability for the factor XIII and plasminogen activator inhibitor-1 proteins have been associated with risk for venous thrombosis. Whether these variants affect response to anticoagulant therapy remains to be determined, but could prove to be important markers for drug response. Direct thrombin inhibitors are associated with a high risk for bleeding. It is possible that genetic variations influence bleeding risk and that information about genotype could be useful in determining bleeding risks and drug doses of these agents in the future.

Pharmacogenomics of Lipid-lowering Drugs

In large clinical trials with lipid-modifying drugs for the primary or secondary prevention of coronary heart disease, a substantial number of participants experienced events despite drug therapy. The lack of a protective effect with statin therapy in some patients may be due, at least in part, to heritable factors. Substudies from several of these large trials, including the Regression Growth Evaluation Statin Study (REGRESS), Simvastatin Scandinavian Survival Trial (4S), Cholesterol and Recurrent Events (CARE) trial, and Veterans Affairs HDL Cholesterol Intervention Trial (VA-HIT), have demonstrated associations between genes for proteins involved in the progression of coronary heart disease and response to lipid-modifying drugs (Reference 27). The gene-drug response associations from these trials are summarized in Table 4.

Statins

The cholesteryl ester transfer protein (CETP) is involved in reverse cholesterol transport and the metabolism of high-density lipoprotein (HDL) cholesterol. A common polymorphism in intron 1 of the CETP gene is designated by the presence (*B1*) or absence (*B2*) of a restriction site for the *Taq*I restriction enzyme. The *B1B1* genotype has been associated with higher concentrations of CETP and lower concentrations of HDL cholesterol. The effect of the *Taq*IB genotype on coronary disease progression and statin response was examined in the REGRESS population. Participants in this trial were randomized to receive pravastatin or placebo for 2 years, at which point progression of atherosclerosis was determined by angiography. Overall, less progression of coronary atherosclerosis and fewer new cardiovascular events occurred in the pravastatin group. In the placebo group, the *Taq*IB genotype was associated with progression of coronary atherosclerosis, with the greatest progression observed in *B1B1* homozygotes. The decrease in mean luminal coronary artery diameter in the placebo group was 0.14 mm with the *B1B1* genotype, 0.10 mm with the *B1B2* genotype, and 0.01 mm with the *B2B2* genotype (p<0.03). Pravastatin therapy slowed the progression of coronary atherosclerosis in *B1B1* carriers but not in those with the *B2B2* genotype. In contrast to the placebo group, the decrease in mean luminal diameter in patients treated with pravastatin did not differ significantly among genotype groups

Table 4. Genetic Polymorphisms Linked to Drug Response in Coronary Heart Disease

Polymorphism	Drug	Follow-up	Outcome
CETP *B1/B2*	Pravastatin	2 years	Decreased progression of coronary atherosclerosis
	Gemfibrozil	7 months	Reduction of triglyceride levels
Stromelysin-1 *5A/6A*	Pravastatin	2 years	Decreased risk of clinical events and repeat angioplasty
β-Fibrinogen *G-455A*	Pravastatin	2 years	Decreased progression of atherosclerosis
Lipoprotein lipase *Asp9Asn*	Pravastatin	2 years	Decreased progression of atherosclerosis Decreased risk for clinical events
Apolipoprotein E ε4	Simvastatin	5.5 years	Decreased mortality
GP IIIa Pl[A1/A2], ACE *I/D*	Pravastatin	5 years	Decreased risk for coronary heart disease death or myocardial infarction

ACE = angiotensin-converting enzyme; CETP = cholesteryl ester transfer protein; GP = glycoprotein

(0.05 mm in *B1B1* carriers, 0.07 mm in *B1B2* carriers, and 0.09 mm in *B2B2* carriers). Thus, pravastatin therapy appeared to eliminate the adverse effect of the *B1B1* genotype on coronary atherosclerosis. Pravastatin produced similar changes in lipoprotein concentrations among genotype groups.

A second analysis of the REGRESS population focused on whether the stromelysin-1 genotype influenced coronary heart disease progression, clinical events, or response to pravastatin. Stromelysin-1 is a member of the matrix metalloproteinase family, which is involved in remodeling of the extracellular matrix of atherosclerotic plaques. There is a common polymorphism in the promoter region of the stromelysin-1 gene where 5 adenines (*5A*) are replaced by 6 adenines (*6A*). In in vitro studies, the *5A/6A* polymorphism was associated with stromelysin-1 activity, suggesting that it may influence degradation of the extracellular matrix in atherosclerotic lesions. Among 249 patients in REGRESS who were randomized to receive placebo, those with a *6A* allele experienced twice as many clinical events over 2 years of follow-up compared to *5A5A* homozygotes (26 percent vs. 12 percent). Treatment with pravastatin significantly reduced the risk of clinical events and the incidence of repeat angioplasty in patients with a *6A* allele, but not in those with the *5A5A* genotype. Again, these differential effects of pravastatin among genotype groups occurred despite similar changes in lipoprotein concentrations during therapy.

A third pharmacogenomic substudy of REGRESS examined the clinical consequences of the *G-455A* polymorphism of the β-fibrinogen gene. At baseline, the *-455AA* genotype was associated with higher plasma concentrations of fibrinogen, an independent risk factor for myocardial infarction and stroke. During the 2-year course of the study, patients in the placebo group with the *-455AA* genotype had significantly greater progression of their atherosclerotic disease as detected by angiography compared to those with other β-fibrinogen genotypes. In the pravastatin group, the differences between genotype groups were no longer evident, suggesting that pravastatin abolished the harmful effects associated with the *-455AA* genotype.

Participants in REGRESS also were genotyped for the *Asp9Asn* variation of the lipoprotein lipase enzyme, which is involved in triglyceride-rich lipoprotein breakdown. The *Asn9* allele was associated with lower HDL cholesterol concentrations. In the placebo group, carriers of the *Asn9* allele had greater progression of coronary atherosclerosis and a 2.16-fold greater risk for clinical events compared to noncarriers. These genetic differences in disease outcomes were no longer present after pravastatin therapy.

The influence of the apolipoprotein E gene on clinical outcomes with statin therapy was compared among 966 participants of the 4S trial, in which treatment with simvastatin for a median of 5.4 years reduced the risk for death and major coronary events in patients with coronary heart disease. In the placebo group of 4S, 16 percent of apolipoprotein E ε4 carriers died compared to 9 percent of non-ε4 carriers, corresponding to a risk ratio for all-cause mortality of 1.8 (95% confidence interval = 1.1–3.1) for the ε4 allele. Excess mortality risk with the ε4 allele was eliminated by simvastatin treatment. Specifically, among those with an ε4 allele, simvastatin treatment reduced the risk of dying to 0.33 (95% confidence interval = 0.16–0.69).

The contribution of the GP IIIa Pl[A1/A2] and the ACE *I/D* genotypes to clinical end points in secondary prevention of coronary heart disease was examined in 767 CARE participants (Reference 28). In the placebo group, neither genotype independently increased the risk for the primary end point after adjustment for differences in baseline characteristics. However, the combination of the Pl[A1/A2] genotype and ACE *D* allele (ACE *I/D* or ACE *D/D*) significantly increased the risk for coronary heart disease death or nonfatal myocardial infarction. The greatest effects with pravastatin occurred in those with the Pl[A1/A2] genotype and either the ACE *I/D* or ACE *D/D* genotype.

Fibrates

The association between the CETP *B1B2* genotype and response to gemfibrozil was examined in 852 participants of VA-HIT, in which treatment with gemfibrozil reduced the risk of major cardiovascular events in men with coronary heart disease and low HDL cholesterol concentrations as their primary lipoprotein abnormality (Reference 29). The CETP *B1B2* polymorphism previously had been linked to HDL cholesterol concentrations. *B1B1* carriers had greater increases in HDL cholesterol with gemfibrozil therapy compared to *B1B2* and *B2B2* carriers, although the differences between groups did not reach statistical significance. However, reductions in triglyceride concentrations with gemfibrozil differed significantly between genotype groups. Triglyceride concentrations decreased by 34 percent in *B1B1* carriers, 25 percent in *B1B2* carriers, and 23 percent in *B2B2* carriers.

Application of these Data to Clinical Practice

Overall, results from the statin studies suggest that genetic polymorphisms for proteins associated with coronary heart disease progression and risk for cardiovascular events are important determinants of statin response in individuals with coronary heart disease. In each study previously discussed, the greatest response to statin therapy was observed in the genotype group with the worst disease progression or clinical prognosis while receiving placebo. Although it currently is premature to withhold statin therapy from patients with certain genotypes, screening for polymorphisms associated with disease progression may have a future role in lipid management for patients with coronary heart disease.

Genetic associations with statin response in primary prevention of coronary heart disease have not yet been determined. However, if similar gene-statin response relationships are found to exist in primary prevention as in secondary prevention of coronary heart disease, they could have important implications because the number needed to prevent a single coronary event is much greater in primary compared to secondary prevention. Genotyping eventually may allow clinicians to identify individuals without established coronary heart disease who are at high risk for coronary events for whom a statin should be started. Individuals who would not be expected to derive significant clinical benefits from statin therapy based on genotype may be managed with alternative measures, such as aggressive dietary therapy. Because statins are expensive drugs and treatment is often continued indefinitely, statin use based on genotype may prove to be a cost-effective approach to dyslipidemia management.

The pharmacogenomic data regarding gemfibrozil that are available to date have little clinical utility. This is because changes in plasma cholesterol concentrations are surrogate end points and do not necessarily translate into improvements in clinical outcomes. As demonstrated in the pharmacogenomic studies with statins, genotype may be predictive of drug effects on disease progression and clinical outcomes without influencing drug effect on plasma lipoprotein concentrations. It is likely that the reverse also is true. That is, that genotype may be predictive of changes in plasma lipoprotein concentrations during drug therapy without influencing clinical outcomes. In the future, if genetic links to clinical outcomes during fibrate therapy are discovered, genotype may be a useful aid in choosing treatment strategies for meeting secondary goals in dyslipidemia management.

Prediction of Other Responses to Lipid-lowering Drugs that Might Have a Genetic Basis

Rhabdomyolysis is one of the most serious adverse reactions to lipid-modifying therapy with statin, niacin, and/or fibrates. In 2001, cerivastatin was removed from the market after several reports of severe rhabdomyolysis with its use. The risk of rhabdomyolysis increases when statins, niacin, and fibrates are used in combination. However, combination therapy is sometimes necessary to meet lipoprotein goals. Several genetic variants have been found in individuals with a history of exercise-induced myoglobinuria and rhabdomyolysis. It is possible that these polymorphisms also influence risk of myopathy and rhabdomyolysis with lipid-modifying agents. If so, they would be important screening tools to identify patients at risk for drug-induced rhabdomyolysis in whom combination therapies should be avoided or administered with careful monitoring.

Pharmacogenomics of Antiarrhythmic Agents

Proarrhythmia is the most serious adverse effect from antiarrhythmic therapy and significantly limits antiarrhythmic agent use. Factors such as structural heart disease, electrolyte abnormalities, and concomitant administration of interacting drugs increase the risk for proarrhythmic events. However, in many cases, drug-induced arrhythmias occur in the absence of such predisposing factors. Evidence suggests that genes for drug-metabolizing enzymes and cardiac ion channels may play a role in determining susceptibility for drug-induced proarrhythmia and other adverse effects with antiarrhythmic agents. These genes and their proarrhythmic effects are discussed in the specific antiarrhythmic agents sections.

Procainamide

Procainamide is an antiarrhythmic agent that exerts its effects through blockade of sodium channels in the cardiac cell membrane. The NAT-2 enzyme converts procainamide to the active metabolite,

N-acetylprocainamide (NAPA), which possesses potent potassium channel blocking activity. The NAT-2 enzyme exhibits genetic polymorphism, with at least 13 polymorphisms identified to date in the coding region of the NAT-2 gene. These polymorphisms contribute to at least 26 alleles and the rapid, intermediate, and slow acetylator phenotypes. The frequency of the slow acetylator phenotype differs among racial groups; about 50 percent of Caucasians, 40 percent of African Americans, and 10 percent of Asians are slow acetylators. Supratherapeutic plasma procainamide concentrations may occur with normal procainamide doses in slow acetylators, potentially increasing the risk for procainamide-induced systemic lupus erythematosus-like syndrome.

About 6 percent of Caucasians, 12 percent of African Americans, and up to 45 percent of Asians are homozygotes for the *NAT-2*4* allele and are considered rapid acetylators. Rapid acetylators may have increased conversion of procainamide to NAPA. This could potentially result in supratherapeutic NAPA concentrations with conventional procainamide doses, QT interval prolongation, and an increased risk for torsades de pointes, especially in patients with renal dysfunction. This is supported by evidence of a higher NAPA-procainamide ratio with the homozygous *NAT-2*4* genotype compared to other NAT-2 genotypes in a study of healthy volunteers (Reference 30). Given the relatively common occurrence of the rapid acetylator phenotype, particularly among the Asian population, these data suggest that screening for the homozygous *NAT-2*4* genotype may have a role in treating cardiac arrhythmias with procainamide. Specifically, presence of the homozygous *NAT-2*4* genotype could indicate a need for closer monitoring of serum drug concentrations and electrocardiographic changes or use of alternative agents for arrhythmia management.

Propafenone

The risk for proarrhythmia and many adverse effects with antiarrhythmic agents is dose-dependent. Thus, genetic polymorphisms resulting in reduced catalytic activity of metabolic pathways for antiarrhythmic drugs would be expected to increase the likelihood of proarrhythmia. The polymorphic CYP2D6 enzyme catalyzes the metabolism of the antiarrhythmic agent propafenone. At least 53 alleles have been identified in the CYP2D6 gene and contribute to the poor, extensive, and ultrarapid metabolizer phenotypes. Poor metabolizers may have higher plasma concentrations of propafenone compared to extensive metabolizers, potentially resulting in greater drug-related β blocking effects, including prolongation of the PR interval and bradycardia.

Drugs Causing QT Interval Prolongation

Long QT syndromes are characterized by abnormalities in ion flux across the cardiac cell membrane, resulting in an excess of intracellular positive ions and delayed ventricular repolarization. Congenital long QT syndromes are secondary to variations in genes for pore-forming channel proteins in the myocardial cell that affect potassium efflux (*KvLQT1*, *HERG*, *KCNE1*, and *KCNE2*) and sodium influx (*SCN5A*). Antiarrhythmic agents that block cardiac potassium channels (e.g., quinidine, procainamide, disopyramide, amiodarone, ibutilide, sotalol, and dofetilide) often are implicated as a cause of acquired long QT syndrome and increased the risk for torsades de pointes. In addition, there are noncardiovascular agents, such as macrolide antibiotics, trimethoprim-sulfamethoxazole, haloperidol, thioridazine, and many others, that may prolong the QT interval and provoke torsades de pointes. In recent years, several drugs have been withdrawn from the market because of their high propensity to induce torsades de pointes. These drugs include the antihistamines terfenadine and astemizole, the fluoroquinolone antibiotic grepafloxacin, and the antimotility agent cisapride.

There are several reports of the existence of otherwise clinically silent mutations in genes associated with congenital long-QT syndrome among individuals with a history of drug-induced torsades de pointes (Reference 31). Genetic associations with drug-induced proarrhythmia are listed in Table 5. In a recent study, investigators screened for variations in the cardiac potassium and sodium channel genes in a cohort of 92 individuals with a history of drug-associated torsades de pointes (Reference 32). Missense mutations in the *KvLQT1*, *HERG*, and *SCN5A* genes were found in five individuals who developed long-QT syndrome during treatment with class Ia or III antiarrhythmic agents.

Applying Data to Clinical Practice

Pharmacogenomics may have a role in identifying candidates for antiarrhythmic drugs who are at an increased risk for proarrhythmia based on their DNA. Clinicians may choose alternative therapeutic strategies in such patients. In addition, genetic information could prove to be of great

Table 5. Cardiac Channel Genes Associated with Drug-induced Long QT-syndrome

Gene	Drug
KVLQT111	Dofetilide
HERG	Amiodarone
	Clarithromycin
	Quinidine
	Procainamide
	Trimethoprim-sulfamethoxazole
SCN5A	Quinidine
	Sotalol
	Cisapride

importance in the prediction of proarrhythmic risk with noncardiovascular agents that have cardiac ion channel blocking activity. For example, in the future, before a patient is started on a macrolide antibiotic, the clinician may be able to first screen for cardiac ion channel gene variations associated with QT interval prolongation. For those found to carry gene variants linked to QT interval prolongation, an alternative antibiotic may be selected.

Prediction of Other Responses to Antiarrhythmic Drugs that Might Have a Genetic Basis

In addition to associations with proarrhythmia, there may be genetic links to other adverse effects with antiarrhythmic agents. Amiodarone is one of the most commonly used antiarrhythmic agents, but its use is limited by its propensity to cause serious organ toxicity, particularly to the lung and liver. Reasons that some patients develop these effects shortly after amiodarone initiation and others tolerate long-term amiodarone therapy are unclear but may be due in part to genetic factors. The ability to screen for genetic variations predisposing individuals to amiodarone-induced toxicity could have important implications. Specifically, those at a high risk for amiodarone-induced organ toxicity based on genotype may be treated with an alternative antiarrhythmic agent or treatment modality. To illustrate this point, suppose a patient presents with heart failure exacerbated by frequent recurrences of atrial fibrillation. This patient is a candidate for amiodarone therapy. If the patient has a genetic variant associated with a high risk for amiodarone-induced pulmonary fibrosis or hepatotoxicity, then dofetilide may be a safer alternative to amiodarone therapy for this patient.

Conclusion

Genetic polymorphisms influence the pharmacokinetic and pharmacodynamic properties of drugs used to treat a variety of cardiovascular diseases. Data with some polymorphisms, such as RAS polymorphisms, have been inconsistent and even conflicting. In other cases, several different polymorphisms have been positively correlated with drug response to a particular agent. For example, the stromelysin-1, β-fibrinogen, and apolipoprotein E genes have been independently associated with the effectiveness of statin therapy. These data suggest that for most cardiovascular agents, a combination of polymorphisms in multiple genes interact to influence overall drug response. However, to date, few studies have examined the influence of polymorphism combinations on drug response. Once the polymorphism combinations that best determine response to a cardiovascular agent are identified and rapid assays to identify these variations are available, clinicians may be able to screen patients before drug prescribing to identify the drug most likely to improve outcomes with the lowest risk of causing harm. Tests currently are commercially available for the detection of apolipoprotein E and CYP2D6 polymorphisms, but they have not yet been instituted to manage cardiovascular disease. Given the abundant research in the area of cardiovascular pharmacogenomics, it is likely that pharmacogenomics will become an important part of cardiovascular disease management within the next 10–20 years. Thus, a patient's genotype may be considered in addition to clinical trial data and consensus guidelines when making cardiovascular drug therapy decisions. As shown in Figure 3, this approach to cardiovascular disease management will likely improve pharmacotherapy by reducing the incidence of therapeutic failure and drug intolerance and improving the rate of therapeutic success.

References

1. Ferrari P, Bianchi G. Genetic mapping and tailored antihypertensive therapy. Cardiovasc Drugs Ther 2000;14:387–95.

2. Turner ST, Schwartz GL, Chapman AB, Boerwinkle E. *C825T* polymorphism of the G protein beta(3)-subunit and antihypertensive response to a thiazide diuretic. Hypertension 2001;37:739–43.

3. Baker EH, Duggal A, Dong Y, et al. Amiloride, a specific drug for hypertension in black people with *T594M* variant? Hypertension 2002;40:13–7.

4. Glorioso N, Manunta P, Filigheddu F, et al. The role of alpha-adducin polymorphism in blood pressure and sodium handling regulation may not be excluded by a negative association study. Hypertension 1999;34:649–54.

5. Psaty BM, Smith NL, Heckbert SR, et al. Diuretic therapy, the alpha-adducin gene variant, and the risk of myocardial infarction or stroke in people with treated hypertension. JAMA 2002;287:1680–9.

6. The ALLHAT Officers and Coordinators for the ALLHAT Collaborative Research Group. The Antihypertensive and Lipid-Lowering Treatment to Prevent Heart Attack Trial. Major outcomes in high-risk patients with hypertension randomized to angiotensin-converting enzyme inhibitor or calcium channel blocker vs diuretic: The Antihypertensive and Lipid-Lowering Treatment to Prevent Heart Attack Trial (ALLHAT-LLT). JAMA 2002;288:2981–97.

7. Sciarrone MT, Stella P, Barlassina C, et al. ACE and alpha-adducin polymorphism as markers of individual response to diuretic therapy. Hypertension 2003;41:398–403.

8. Turner ST, Schwartz GL, Chapman AB, Hall WD, Boerwinkle E. Antihypertensive pharmacogenetics: getting the right drug into the right patient. J Hypertens 2001;19:1–11.

9. Kurland L, Melhus H, Karlsson J, et al. Polymorphisms in the angiotensinogen and angiotensin II type 1 receptor gene are related to change in left ventricular mass during antihypertensive treatment: results from the Swedish Irbesartan Left Ventricular Hypertrophy Investigation versus Atenolol (SILVHIA) trial. J Hypertens 2002;20:657–63.

10. Tiago AD, Badenhorst D, Skudicky D, et al. An aldosterone synthase gene variant is associated with improvement in left ventricular ejection fraction in dilated cardiomyopathy. Cardiovasc Res 2002;54:584–9.

11. Johnson JA, Terra SG. Beta-adrenergic receptor polymorphisms: cardiovascular disease associations and pharmacogenetics. Pharm Res 2002;19:1779–87.

12. Sofowora GG, Dishy V, Muszkat M, et al. A common beta1-adrenergic receptor polymorphism (Arg389Gly) affects blood pressure response to beta-blockade. Clin Pharmacol Ther 2003;73:366–71.

13. Zineh I, Puckett BJ, McGorray SP, Pauly DF, Johnson JA. Beta 1-adrenergic receptor polymorphisms predict antihypertensive response to beta-blockers. Clin Pharmacol Ther 2003;74(1):44–52.

14. Jia H, Hingorani AD, Sharma P, et al. Association of the G(s)alpha gene with essential hypertension and response to beta-blockade. Hypertension 1999;34:8–14.

15. McNamara DM, Holubkov R, Janosko K, et al. Pharmacogenetic interactions between beta-blocker therapy and the angiotensin-converting enzyme deletion polymorphism in patients with congestive heart failure. Circulation 2001;103:1644–8.

16. Kim RB. *MDR1* single nucleotide polymorphisms: multiplicity of haplotypes and functional consequences. Pharmacogenetics 2002;12:425–7.

17. Kurata Y, Ieiri I, Kimura M, et al. Role of human *MDR1* gene polymorphism in bioavailability and interaction of digoxin, a substrate of P-glycoprotein. Clin Pharmacol Ther 2002;72:209–19.

18. Johne A, Kopke K, Gerloff T, et al. Modulation of steady-state kinetics of digoxin by haplotypes of the P-glycoprotein *MDR1* gene. Clin Pharmacol Ther 2002;72:584–94.

19. Aithal GP, Day CP, Kesteven PJ, Daly AK. Association of polymorphisms in the cytochrome P450 CYP2C9 with warfarin dose requirement and risk of bleeding complications. Lancet 1999;353:717–9.

20. Higashi MK, Veenstra DL, Kondo LM, et al. Association between CYP2C9 genetic variants and anticoagulation-related outcomes during warfarin therapy. JAMA 2002;287:1690–8.

21. Scordo MG, Pengo V, Spina E, Dahl ML, Gusella M, Padrini R. Influence of CYP2C9 and CYP2C19 genetic polymorphisms on warfarin maintenance dose and metabolic clearance. Clin Pharmacol Ther 2002;72:702–10.

22. Carlsson LE, Santoso S, Baurichter G, et al. Heparin-induced thrombocytopenia: new insights into the impact of the FcgammaRIIa-R-H131 polymorphism. Blood 1998;92.1526–31.

23. Andrioli G, Minuz P, Solero P, et al. Defective platelet response to arachidonic acid and thromboxane A(2) in patients with Pl(A2) polymorphism of beta(3) subunit (glycoprotein IIIa). Br J Haematol 2000;110:911–8.

24. Kastrati A, Koch W, Gawaz M, et al. PlA polymorphism of glycoprotein IIIa and risk of adverse events after coronary stent placement. J Am Coll Cardiol 2000;36:84–9.

25. Walter DH, Schachinger V, Elsner M, Dimmeler S, Zeiher AM. Platelet glycoprotein IIIa polymorphisms and risk of coronary stent thrombosis. Lancet 1997;350:1217–9.

26. O'Donnell CJ, Larson MG, Feng D, et al; Framingham Heart Study. Genetic and environmental contributions to platelet aggregation: the Framingham heart study. Circulation 2001;103:3051–6.

27. Maitland-van der Zee AH, Klungel OH, Stricker BH, et al. Genetic polymorphisms: importance for response to H MG-CoA reductase inhibitors. Atherosclerosis 2002;163:213–22.

28. Bray PF, Cannon CP, Goldschmidt-Clermont P, et al. The platelet Pl(A2) and angiotensin-converting enzyme (ACE) D allele polymorphisms and the risk of recurrent events after acute myocardial infarction. Am J Cardiol 2001;88:347–52.

29. Brousseau ME, O'Connor JJ Jr, Ordovas JM, et al. Cholesteryl ester transfer protein *Taq*I *B2B2* genotype is associated with higher HDL cholesterol levels and lower risk of coronary heart disease end points in men with HDL deficiency: Veterans Affairs HDL Cholesterol Intervention Trial. Arterioscler Thromb Vasc Biol 2002;22:1148–54.

30. Okumura K, Kita T, Chikazawa S, Komada F, Iwakawa S, Tanigawara Y. Genotyping of N-acetylation polymorphism and correlation with procainamide metabolism. Clin Pharmacol Ther 1997;61:509–17.

31. Abbott GW, Sesti F, Splawski I, et al. MiRP1 forms IKr potassium channels with HERG and is associated with cardiac arrhythmia. Cell 1999;97:175–87.

32. Yang P, Kanki H, Drolet B, et al. Allelic variants in long-QT disease genes in patients with drug-associated torsades de pointes. Circulation 2002;105:1943–8.

Self-Assessment Questions

1. A 64-year-old man with a history of hypertension, heart failure, and recurrent atrial fibrillation is started on warfarin 5 mg orally every day. A rapid single nucleotide polymorphism (SNP) test reveals the *CYP2C9*1/*3* genotype. Which one of the following can be predicted based on his genotype?

    A. Increased bleeding risk.
    B. Inadequate anticoagulant effects.
    C. Optimal anticoagulant effects.
    D. Low stroke risk.

2. A 58-year-old man arrives at the hospital with newly diagnosed heart failure and no other significant past medical history. The physician wishes to order a rapid SNP test to determine the patient's risk for developing a cough with angiotensin-converting enzyme (ACE) inhibitor therapy. He plans to use the genetic test results to choose initial vasodilator therapy. Which one of the following is the best response by the pharmacist?

    A. Recommend testing for the ACE *I/D* and bradykinin B_2-receptor *C-58T* genotypes and starting losartan if both the ACE *I* and bradykinin B_2-receptor *-58T* alleles are present.
    B. Recommend testing for the ACE *I/D* genotype only and starting enalapril if the patient has the *D/D* genotype.
    C. Recommend testing for the bradykinin B_2-receptor *C-58T* genotype only and starting losartan is the patient has the *-58C/C* genotype.
    D. Recommend against genetic testing as the results should not influence the choice of vasodilator therapy.

3. A 49-year-old woman with a history of chronic obstructive pulmonary disease and heart failure presents to your clinic. Her current drugs include lisinopril, furosemide, digoxin, and an albuterol/ipratropium inhaler. She has the ACE *DD* genotype. Based on current data regarding the ACE genotype, should treatment with a β-blocker be attempted and why or why not?

    A. No, her risk for bronchospasm is high.
    B. No, her expected benefit is low.
    C. Yes, her expected benefit is high.
    D. Yes, her risk for bronchospasm is low.

4. A 68-year-old man with coronary artery disease and a history of myocardial infarction currently is taking aspirin 325 mg every day, metoprolol XL 100 mg every day, and sublingual nitroglycerin as

needed. A fasting lipid profile shows a total cholesterol level of 207 mg/dl, low-density lipoprotein concentration of 135 mg/dl, high-density lipoprotein (HDL) concentration of 38 mg/dl, and a triglyceride concentration of 170 mg/dl. Genotyping reveals that the patient carries the apolipoprotein E ε4 allele and the cholesterol ester transfer protein *B1B1* genotype. Which one of the following responses to statin therapy can be predicted based on his genotype?

A. High risk for rhabdomyolysis.
B. Significant reduction in the risk of recurrent ischemic events.
C. Little effect on the progression of coronary atherosclerosis.
D. Large reductions in low-density lipoprotein cholesterol concentrations.

5. A 27-year-old woman is started on procainamide for Wolff-Parkinson-White syndrome. She has no other significant past medical history. She has the *N*-acetyltransferase-2 *4/*4 genotype and is heterozygous for the abnormal *HERG* gene allele. Which one of the following should be monitored particularly closely during procainamide therapy in this patient?

A. Antinuclear antibody titers.
B. QRS duration on the electrocardiogram.
C. Heart rate.
D. QT interval on the electrocardiogram.

6. The clinician wishes to initiate antihypertensive therapy in a 43-year-old patient with newly diagnosed hypertension and no other significant medical history. The patient carries duplicated copies of the *CYP2D6*2* allele and the G_S-protein α-subunit *FokI-/FokI-* and α-adducin *460Gly/Trp* genotypes. Which one of the following is the best initial antihypertensive therapy for this patient based on his genotype?

A. Atenolol.
B. Metoprolol.
C. Hydrochlorothiazide.
D. Lisinopril.

7. A 76-year-old woman is hospitalized for deep vein thrombosis. The decision is made to start warfarin and intravenous heparin therapy on hospital day 1 and continue heparin until a therapeutic international normalized ratio (INR) is reached. At that point, the patient will be discharged from the hospital and continued on warfarin at a target INR of 2–3 for at least 3 months. Basing antithrombotic therapy decisions on genotype may result in which one of the following?

A. Reduce the length of time to stable warfarin dosing.
B. Eliminate the need for INR monitoring during warfarin therapy.

C. Eliminate the need for activated partial thromboplastin time monitoring during heparin therapy.

D. Reduced the duration of anticoagulant therapy.

8. A 58-year-old postmenopausal woman is diagnosed with hypertension. She has no other significant past medical history. Genotyping reveals the angiotensinogen *235MM*, β_1-adrenergic receptor *Arg389Arg*, and the G protein β_3-subunit *825CC* genotypes. Which one of the following antihypertensives would be expected to provide the greatest blood pressure reduction based on her genotype?

A. Lisinopril.

B. Candesartan.

C. Atenolol.

D. Hydrochlorothiazide.

9. A 83-year-old man is admitted to the hospital for unstable angina. He is scheduled for coronary angioplasty the next morning. The interventional cardiologist is concerned about the increased bleeding risk in this elderly patient and asks your opinion about using abciximab at the time of catheterization. The presence of which one of the following alleles would favor abciximab use in this patient?

A. Platelet Fc gamma receptor *131Arg*.

B. Glycoprotein IIIa subunit Pl^{A2}.

C. Angiotensin-converting enzyme *I*.

D. Stromelysin-1 *5A*.

10. A 64-year-old man with a history of coronary artery disease presents to the clinic. A fasting lipid profile is done and reveals his total cholesterol is 180 mg/dl, low-density lipoprotein concentration is 115 mg/dl, HDL concentration is 36 mg/dl, and triglyceride concentration is 145 mg/dl. The physician in the clinic recently reviewed the Long-Term Intervention with Pravastatin in Ischemic Disease study, in which pravastatin reduced mortality and cardiovascular events in patients with coronary artery disease with a wide range of cholesterol concentrations. She asks whether this patient should be started on pravastatin. Which one of the following alleles would favor pravastatin use in this patient?

A. Cholesteryl ester transfer protein *B2*.

B. β-Fibrinogen *-455G*.

C. Apolipoprotein E ε1.

D. Stromelysin-1 *6A*.

Central Nervous System/ Psychiatry

Vicki L. Ellingrod, Pharm.D., BCPP
Jeff Bishop, Pharm.D.

Key Words

Serotonin receptors (5-HT1A, 5-HT1B, 5-HT1D, 5-HT1F, 5-HT2A, and 5-HT2C), serotonin transporter (5-HTT), P/Q-type calcium channel, apolipoprotein E (ApoE 1, 2, 3, and 4), *N*-acetyltransferase 2 (NAT2), cytochromes P450 (CYP), dopamine receptors (D1, D2, D3, and D4), histamine receptors (H1 and H2), β-3 receptors, α1A receptor, mu opioid receptor (OPRM1), P-glycoprotein (Pgp), multiple drug resistance gene (*MDR1*), microarray analysis, multiple sclerosis, Alzheimer's disease, Parkinson's disease, epilepsy, migraine headache, schizophrenia, pain, depression, polymorphisms, polymerase chain reaction (PCR), and microarray.

Abstract

The central nervous system is a vast frontier of synapses, signaling, and neurochemicals. Its complicated physical infrastructure intermingles to regulate body functions, sensory perceptions, emotions, and even influences an individual's personality. Knowledge of the genetic determinants of neurological and psychiatric disorders increases every year. Although the genetic factors influencing the responses of these disorders to drug therapy remain largely unknown, significant contributions to this area of research have been made throughout the past decade. Experimentation in this area continues to increase exponentially. This chapter reviews the pharmacogenetic research of drug response and side effects of neurological and psychiatric disorders. The overview of neurological pharmacogenetics focuses on multiple sclerosis, Alzheimer's disease, Parkinson's disease, migraine headache, epilepsy, and pain. The psychiatric conditions discussed include schizophrenia, major depression, and adverse effects of antipsychotic drugs (e.g., weight gain and tardive dyskinesia). The current and potential contributions of the technology for pharmacogenetic research (e.g., polymerase chain reaction [PCR], restriction fragment length polymorphism [RFLP], and microarray analysis) also are discussed to provide a comprehensive overview of the methods used to determine genetic predictors of drug response.

Outline

Learning Objectives

1. Discuss the role of pharmacogenetics in treating patients with central nervous system (CNS) disorders, including mental illness.
2. Describe how the use of deoxyribonucleic acid arrays can assist in the discovery and target selection of new drugs for treating CNS disorders.

Abbreviations in this Chapter

5-HT	Serotonin
5-HTT	Serotonin transporter
5-HTTLPR	Serotonin transporter gene promoter region
ApoE	Apolipoprotein E
CNS	Central nervous system
CYP	Cytochrome P450
DNA	Deoxyribonucleic acid
MDD	Major depressive disorder
MDR1	Multidrug resistance gene
NAT2	*N*-acetyltransferase 2
OPRM1	Mu opioid receptor gene
PCR	Polymerase chain reaction
Pgp	P-glycoprotein
RFLP	Restriction fragment length polymorphism
SNP	Single nucleotide polymorphism
SSRI	Selective serotonin reuptake inhibitor
VNTR	Variable nucleotide tandem repeat

Introduction

The human brain is one of the most complex organs known to man. Thus, it is not surprising that the knowledge of the genetic basis for central nervous system (CNS) diseases, and their treatment, is extremely small. The brain regulates a plethora of complex tasks, such as thought, affect, emotion, short- and long-term memory, coordination, and sensory functions (Reference 1). Of the more than 30,000 genes which have been discovered as part of the human genome project, the expression of several thousand of these have been found to occur in the brain or serve a role which enhances the brain's function (Reference 2).

Thus, with this in mind, this chapter is dedicated to the pharmacogenetics of CNS disorders. Despite all that is known about the pharmacotherapy of CNS disorders, little is still really known about why differences are seen in treatment response and the occurrence of side effects. Pharmacogenetics may be one of the parts of the puzzle needed to help explain these differences.

In addition to reviewing the literature on the pharmacogenetics of CNS disorders, this chapter strives to explain some of the newer techniques used in these investigations. Of the genetic techniques currently available for use, deoxyribonucleic acid (DNA) microarrays are some of the most powerful techniques available to simultaneously assess the expression of thousands of genes in a single sample. Thus, it is with this technology that scientists may be able to enhance the understanding of the genetics relating to CNS disorders, as well as the genetics principles underling response and treatment outcomes for the pharmacotherapy of CNS disorders. Despite all of the power associated with DNA microarrays, not every genetic investigation can use this technology. This chapter is dedicated to the pharmacogenetics of CNS disorders regardless of the technology used. Some of the techniques used are more traditional (i.e., polymerase chain reaction [PCR] and restriction fragment length polymorphism [RFLP]) and only allow for the determination of one or several genes at a time. More information of the use of microarrays and other genetics techniques used in the discovery and target selection of new drugs for treating CNS disorders is included in the microarray techniques and CNS section.

Central Nervous System Disorders

Multiple Sclerosis

Multiple sclerosis is a chronic disease involving demyelination of the white matter of the brain. In this illness, evidence points to the involvement of immune-mediated responses against components of the myelin sheath, which ultimately results in cell death and some of the clinical symptoms seen with this illness (i.e., unsteady gait and dementia). In a recent study (Reference 3), microarray analysis was used to examine genetic differences in patients with multiple sclerosis lesions compared to controls (patients without multiple sclerosis). In the patients with multiple sclerosis, there was an increased transcription of genes encoding inflammatory cytokines. Primarily, there was an increase in interleukin-6, interleukin-17, and interferon-γ and associated downstream pathways. In addition, differences in gene expression also were seen between patients with multiple sclerosis with acute lesions and inflammation versus those with "silent" lesions without inflammation. Thus, as researchers begin to understand the genetics behind multiple sclerosis and the immune effects of this illness on the brain, researchers can begin to target these gene products as well as search for effective ways to treat this illness.

Migraine

Migraine headache is a paroxysmal disorder of debilitating headache, afflicting more than 11 million Americans. Historically, numerous pharmaceutical agents have been used to treat acute migraine attacks (i.e., simple analgesics, caffeine, butalbital, and dihydroergotamine). However, since the 1990s, the class of drugs collectively known as the triptans has taken hold as the first-line treatment of acute migraine attacks. Pioneered by the drug sumatriptan, these drugs are thought to elicit their effects by vasoconstriction by serotonin (5-HT) 1B agonism; inhibition of neurogenic inflammation by 5-HT1D and/or 5-HT1F agonism; and/or central inhibition of pain transmission by agonizing 5-HT1B, 5-HT1D, or 5-HT1F receptors (Reference 4).

Up to 40 percent of patients responding to subcutaneous sumatriptan have headache recurrence within 48 hours, and 15 percent of patients never respond to the drug. It is thought that both genetic and environmental factors play roles in determining whether an individual will respond to sumatriptan. Polymorphisms have been identified in both the 5-HT1B and 5-HT1D receptors (References 6–10) and have been examined minimally for their relationship to drug response.

To date, only one study investigating whether gene polymorphisms correlate with clinical response to sumatriptan has been published (Reference 11). Specifically, two polymorphisms in the 5-HT1B receptor—G861C and T261G—were examined. Forty patients were classified as being responders, partial responders, or nonresponders to 6 mg subcutaneous sumatriptan. In addition, assessment of whether patients had chest symptoms as a result of sumatriptan therapy was analyzed and correlated with genotype.

The frequencies of the polymorphic and wild-type alleles did not differ in any of the patient groups. Furthermore, no difference in drug response or cardiovascular side effects was associated with genotype.

In addition to 5-HT receptor polymorphisms, P/Q-type calcium channel variants have received attention for their roles in familial migraine with aura. At least 13 missense mutations have been associated with inherited hemiplegic migraine. Fifty percent of the families with this inherited form of migraine headache have had mutations in this voltage-gated calcium channel α1A subunit on either chromosome 1 or 19 (Reference 5). Molecular analysis of these mutations has shown that these genetic variants likely alter calcium entry into cells (either decrease or increase) and may, therefore, play a role in drug response in these individuals. Studies examining drug response with calcium channel variants have not yet been conducted, and will likely differ with the functional alterations mediated by a specific mutation.

Alzheimer's Disease

Alzheimer's disease is a neurodegenerative disorder characterized by memory loss and dementia. The disease has a multifactorial etiology with numerous identified genetic components, including the β-amyloid precursor gene, presenilin 1, presenilin 2, and the E4 allele of apolipoprotein (ApoE) gene. Pharmacogenetic studies in Alzheimer's disease have primarily focused on the ApoE genotypes that correlate with drug response.

The ApoE4 allele is considered a risk factor for developing sporadic Alzheimer's disease (Reference 12). A study analyzing ApoE4 allele frequency in eight different Alzheimer's disease studies found that almost 57 percent of patients with available genotypes carried at least one E4 allele (Reference 13). Apolipoprotein E is a protein involved with cholesterol transport and is encoded by a gene on chromosome 19 (Reference 14). Three common alleles of ApoE exist; they are E2, E3, and E4 with respective frequencies being 8 percent, 77 percent, and 15 percent (Reference 14).

One study (Reference 15) was the first to associate a difference in clinical response to the cholinesterase inhibitor tacrine, in patients with different ApoE genotypes. Investigators studied patients with Alzheimer's disease who were involved in a 30-week clinical trial of tacrine that used the Alzheimer's Disease Assessment Scale Cognitive Component as the primary outcome variable. The 20 best and 20 worst responders of 202 participants were genotyped. Eighty-three percent of patients not carrying an E4 allele had a clinical response to tacrine therapy, whereas 60 percent of patients with at least one E4 allele were either unchanged or worse after completing the 30-week trial.

Other investigators (Reference 16) studied the effects of ApoE genotype and gender on clinical response in patients taking tacrine for mild to moderate Alzheimer's disease. This study analyzed 528 patients who completed a 30-week tacrine trial that also used the Alzheimer's Disease Assessment Scale Cognitive Component as the primary outcome measure. This study found that women who carried only E2 or E3 alleles were better responders than those who carried at least one E4 allele. This difference was not seen in men, as those with E4 alleles seemed to respond the same as those with only E2 or E3 alleles.

Researchers (Reference 17) studied 107 patients with probable Alzheimer's disease who were involved with a clinical trial for tacrine and a subsequent open-label trial with galantamine. Both of these trials used the Mini Mental Status Examination as the primary outcome measure. As a whole, more E4-negative patients responded to tacrine (79 percent vs. 59 percent) after 3 months of therapy. The presence of the E4 allele did not make a difference in response to galantamine (69 percent of E4-negative patients vs. 70 percent of E4-positive patients were responders after 3 months of therapy). When gender was analyzed for the 3-month treatment period, more E4-positive men responded than E4-negative men (81 percent vs. 71 percent) in the tacrine group, but an opposite trend was seen in the galantamine group with 63 percent of E4-negative men versus 100 percent of E4-positive men being classified as responders. More E4-negative women responded to both tacrine and galantamine (67 percent vs. 50 percent and 75 percent vs. 45 percent, respectively) after 3 months of therapy.

Selected patients underwent 3–9 additional months of therapy with tacrine (total of 6–9 months of tacrine therapy). Analysis of these patients showed that at 6 months, more E4-negative than E4-positive men responded to tacrine (70 percent vs. 50 percent) and at 12 months, 40 percent of E4-negative men were responders compared to 42 percent of E4-positive men. Fewer E4-negative than E4-positive women responded to tacrine at both the 6- and 12-month time points (67 percent vs. 80 percent and 33 percent vs. 71 percent, respectively). Small numbers could have potentially resulted in a type 2 error in both men and women after the 6- and 12-month time points (Reference 17).

Researchers (Reference 18) reported no effect of ApoE4 genotype on response to galantamine after a 6-month clinical trial using the Alzheimer's Disease Assessment Scale Cognitive Component as the primary outcome measure in 525 patients. Statistical details and gender breakdown were not provided.

Other researchers (Reference 19) describe a study of donepezil in which analyses of ApoE genotypes were conducted. This study evaluated 60 men and women (30 of each) using the Alzheimer's Disease Assessment Scale Cognitive Component as the primary outcome measure for this 6-week trial. There was no effect of ApoE genotype reported by investigators. Additional analysis of the data from this study suggests better improvements in Alzheimer's Disease Assessment Scale Cognitive Component scores were seen in E4-positive patients (Reference 20).

Other investigators (Reference 21) describe a study investigating whether ApoE genotype correlated with response to a new cholinesterase inhibitor, metrifonate. This study used the Alzheimer's Disease Assessment Scale Cognitive Component as the primary outcome variable in the 26-week study that procured genotypes from 585 of 959 participants. Although no significant difference was reported in this study, a trend toward a better response in E4-negative patients was seen.

A long-term study of metrifonate was analyzed for ApoE effects on response and found similar results to those presented previously (Reference 21) after 26 weeks, but observed a statistical separation (p<0.05) at 120 weeks between E4-positive carriers and E4-negative carriers. Patients with E4-negative were better responders, according to the Mini Mental Status Examination, which was the primary outcome measure for this study (Reference 20). These results were even more pronounced at 240 weeks with the non-E4 carriers responding the best (p<0.02) (Reference 20).

One analysis of a noncholinesterase inhibitor drug has been conducted (Reference 22). The study was of S12024, which facilitates brain noradrenergic and vasopressinergic activity. This dose-response trial involved 404 patients and used the Mini Mental Status Examination as the primary outcome measure. A higher frequency of responders was found in E4-positive patients.

From the studies conducted to date analyzing genotype correlations to drug response, it is evident that ApoE has an effect. The nature of this effect is well established for tacrine, with research showing that E4-negative patients with Alzheimer's disease respond better to this drug than those without an E4 allele. Subsequent studies investigating both cholinergic and noradrenergic drugs have mixed results, depending on the agent studied, treatment duration, and primary outcome measure used. Further long-term studies using the Alzheimer's Disease Assessment Scale Cognitive Component to assess patient response will determine which agents will be most beneficial to patients with or without an E4 allele.

Parkinson's Disease

The incidence of Parkinson's disease is about 1 percent in people older than 65 years of age. Clinically, it is characterized by tremor, rigidity, and bradykinesia. The cause of Parkinson's disease is unknown, although it is thought to result from an overall dopamine deregulation, which results in the loss of dopamine, its metabolites and precursor (tyrosine hydroxylase) as well as a loss of dopamine transporters (Reference 23). Recent discoveries about some of the mutations, which underlie the inheritability of this disorder, have shed light on aspects of its pathogenesis. α-Synuclein is a protein of unknown function that is located in the nerve terminals of the synaptic vesicles (Reference 24). Mutations within the gene for α-synuclein have been associated with the autosomal dominant form of Parkinson's disease. In addition to α-synuclein, homozygous mutations and point mutations in the parkin gene have been associated with an early-onset autosomal recessive Parkinson's disease occurring before 40 years of age, slow disease progression, and severe levodopa-induced dyskinesias in families of Japanese, European, and Middle Eastern origin (References 25, 26). Thus, there may be a link between these mutations and the polymorphisms, causing accumulations of α-synuclein. This link may be the first understanding into the true mechanism behind the occurrence of Parkinson's disease.

Despite the amount of evidence regarding the genetics of Parkinson's disease, the majority of studies conducted thus far have been in animals or have included a small number of humans. Recently, a meta-analysis (Reference 27) found that four polymorphisms are associated with Parkinson's disease. These include the slow acetylator genotypes for *N*-acetyltransferase 2 (NAT2) (odds ratio = 1.36), alleles more than 188 base pairs of the monoamine oxidase B, (GT)n polymorphism (odds ratio = 2.58); the deletion allele of glutathione transferase (odds ratio = 1.34); and A4336G of transfer ribonucleic acid glu (a mitochondrial gene) (odds ratio = 3.0). The authors concluded that although a causal relationship between these polymorphisms and the pathogenesis of Parkinson's disease cannot be implied, the polymorphisms' role and significance in treating Parkinson's disease needs to be further investigated. Despite the fact that three of these four polymorphisms have important roles in drug metabolism, little has been done to determine if they can functionally determine treatment outcome. Thus, the future for Parkinson's disease research needs to focus on these polymorphism as well as continue to develop new drugs to combat this illness. In addition, these polymorphisms can help researchers to better understand the pathogenesis of this illness and its current state of pharmacotherapy.

Epilepsy

Similar to many of the CNS disorders, epilepsy is a heterogeneous illness which also is reflected in the genetics of the disease. More than 33 chromosomes are related to epilepsy (Reference 28), which might indicate that this genetic variability also may have a relationship with treatment outcome for this disorder. Despite clear information that many of the cytochrome P450 (CYP) enzymes involved in the metabolism of the antiepileptic drugs are polymorphic, data only exist for phenytoin, which suggests a genetic-based response.

Phenytoin is primarily metabolized by the CYP isoenzymes CYP2C9 and CYP2C19 (References 29–32). Cytochrome P450 2C9 has two variant alleles (*2 and *3), which lead to amino acid substitutions, causing reduced enzyme activity (Reference 33). In patients with epilepsy, phenytoin's maximal elimination rate was significantly lower in those heterozygous for the *3 allele than in those homozygous for the *1 or normal allele. In addition, the average daily dose of phenytoin needed to obtain steady-state in the heterozygous subjects was lower, although this was not statistically significant (Reference 34). In a second study, similar results were found in that subjects with a *3 allele required lower daily doses of phenytoin compared to those with a *1/*1 genotype (Reference 35). Unfortunately, these studies were conducted with Japanese subjects who overall have a lower prevalence of the *2 and *3 alleles, resulting in studies that included small numbers of these genotypes. None of the subjects included in these studies was homozygous for the *2 or *3 allele and, as such, the full impact of these polymorphisms on phenytoin's metabolism and outcome from treatment may not be known. Thus, it is unknown if these results can be extrapolated to other ethnic groups. Cytochrome P450 2C19 also is involved in phenytoin's metabolism. This isoenzyme has two common polymorphisms (m1 and m2), both of which result in an inactive enzyme (Reference 36). In terms of phenytoin metabolism, subjects with a m^1/m^1 or m^2/m^2 genotype were found to eliminate phenytoin more slowly than those homozygous for the wild-type allele, although the differences were not statistically significant (References 34, 35). Thus, taken all together, these studies suggest that genotyping for the CYP2C9 and CYP2C19 polymorphisms in a Caucasian population, who have a higher expression of the variant alleles, could be a useful tool in predicting response to phenytoin.

Despite the number of drugs currently available to treat epilepsy-related disorders, about 10–20 percent of all patients are completely resistant to therapy (Reference 37). Of interest, the majority of these patients often have the ability to achieve therapeutic blood levels of the antiepileptic drug and, as such, the mechanism for this resistance has been speculated to be reduced CNS penetration, secondary to polymorphism related to the transporter proteins located on the blood-brain barrier. Recently, it was found that the expression of multidrug resistance gene (*MDR1*), cloned multidrug resistance-associated protein/MRP2, and MRP5 in the endothelial cells isolated from the temporal regions of the brain was much higher in subjects with refractory epilepsy, compared to controls (those without epliepsy) (Reference 38). Presence of these proteins suggests that subjects refractory to treatment for epilepsy may have a genetic disposition preventing the permeability of drug into the CNS.

Psychiatry

Depression

Major depressive disorder (MDD) has a lifetime prevalence of 10–25 percent for women and from 5–12 percent for men (Reference 39). Depression can be extremely debilitating and may involve changes in mood, sleep, weight, energy loss, decreased concentration, suicidal ideation, feelings of worthlessness, psychomotor agitation or depression, and/or an inability to experience pleasure.

The selective serotonin reuptake inhibitors (SSRIs; escitalopram, citalopram, fluoxetine, fluvoxamine, paroxetine, and sertraline) are important options available for treating depression and other psychiatric disorders. Although commonly prescribed for depressive disorders, 30–40 percent of users do not respond to SSRI therapy (Reference 40). Genetic determinants of SSRI response have been explored only recently and have focused primarily on polymorphisms in the serotonin transporter (5-HTT) gene SLC6A4 of patients with MDD. SLC6A4 is about 35 kilobases long and is located on chromosome 17 (Reference 41). Two polymorphisms have been described. The first is in the 5' promoter region (5-HTTLPR) of SLC6A4 and consists of the presence or absence of a 44 base pair repetitive sequence, resulting in either long (l) or short (s) 5-HTT transcripts. The "l" allele has higher levels of 5-HTT transcription than the "s" allele in in vitro studies, presumably resulting in reduced 5-HT uptake in s/s homozygotes (Reference 41). A second polymorphism involving a variable nucleotide tandem repeat (VNTR) in the second intron of SLC6A4 also has been described, but has been studied little for potential effects on SSRI response (Reference 42).

Human studies to date suggest that 5-HTTLPR variation likely influences response to SSRI therapy. Four studies have examined 5-HTT variation and SSRI response in patients with MDD, using the Hamilton Depression Rating Scale as the primary assessment of antidepressant response. Investigators (Reference 43) examined Italian patients presenting with MDD with psychotic features who were treated with fluvoxamine or fluvoxamine with pindolol augmentation to determine whether 5-HTT variability affected antidepressant response. Patients carrying at least one "l" allele had a more favorable response to fluvoxamine alone. Of interest, individuals who were augmented with pindolol (β-blocker with presynaptic somatodendritic

5-HT1A receptor inhibition) showed no variation in response to therapy correlating to genotype.

Responses to paroxetine or nortriptyline were examined in elderly patients (mean age = 72 years) with variations in the 5-HTTLPR (Reference 44). Patients with l/l genotypes responded faster (within 2 weeks) to paroxetine than l/s or s/s carriers (3–4 weeks). The number of responders after 12 weeks of treatment did not differ among genotypes. No variation in response to nortriptyline correlated with 5-HTTLPR genotype. Similarly, one study (Reference 45) showed that Italian patients with MDD who were treated with paroxetine responded more quickly if they were l/l homozygotes or l/s heterozygotes than if they were s/s homozygotes. However, in this study, carriers of at least one "l" allele had a larger reduction in Hamilton Depression Rating Scale scores at the end of the 4-week study.

Finally, a group of Korean patients with MDD who were treated with fluoxetine or paroxetine for 6 weeks were examined for genotypic variation in both the 5-HTTLPR and intron two loci for drug response correlations (Reference 46). Contrary to the previously discussed studies, there were more 5-HTTLPR s/s homozygotes in the SSRI responder group; furthermore, the l/l version of the VNTR produced a positive response correlation to SSRI treatment.

Most recently, a study (Reference 47) showed that a small number of healthy patients given a loading dose of citalopram exhibited a larger reduction in cortical inhibition as measured by paired pulse transcranial magnetic stimulation if they were l/l homozygotes than if they possessed l/s or s/s genotypes (Reference 47). This suggests that 5-HTT variability affects cortical responses to SSRI therapy even in the absence of disease.

Although 5-HTT polymorphisms have received the most attention in pharmacogenetic studies of SSRI response, clinicians should not forget the role of the CYP enzyme system in SSRI metabolism and the potential for genetic variability in these enzymes to affect drug response or drug-drug interactions. Briefly, fluoxetine has mild to moderate inhibitory effects on CYP2C9 and 2C19, and strong inhibition of 2D6; paroxetine also exhibits a strong inhibition of 2D6; sertraline has mild to moderate inhibitory effects on 2C19; finally, fluvoxamine has major inhibitory effects on 1A2 and 2C19, and moderate effects on both 2C9 and 3A (Reference 48). Because of the wide therapeutic range of the SSRIs, CYP variability alone is unlikely to affect drug response to these drugs, but may produce additive effects with other factors to determine response or potential interactions.

The etiology of MDD and consequently its response to therapy is likely multifactorial in nature. It is not known if the differences seen in the studies conducted to date are because of genotype alone or to other factors that may affect response in different patient populations. The previously discussed studies involved populations of European, and Korean descent and produced slightly different correlations of "l" allele effects of the

5-HTTLPR. More research involving patients of different ethnicities examining both the 5-HTTLPR and the VNTR of the second intron in SLC6A4 need to be conducted to further elucidate 5-HTT's role in SSRI response. Furthermore, it is not known if SSRI response in other disorders (i.e., obsessive-compulsive disorder, anxiety disorders, and eating disorders) is affected by 5-HTT polymorphisms. Similarly, side effects to SSRIs also may be influenced by 5-HTT variability, leaving many opportunities for further research in this area.

Schizophrenia

Schizophrenia often is a debilitating illness that affects about 1 percent of the population. The pharmacotherapy for schizophrenia primarily consists of antipsychotics. There is considerable variation in treatment response to these drugs. Pharmacologically, the typical antipsychotics exert their effect through the blockage of dopamine 2 receptors, whereas the atypical antipsychotics block additional dopamine receptors and also serve as antagonists at the 5-HT2A and 5-HT2C receptors. Clozapine was the first atypical antipsychotic available in the United States and is the antipsychotic on which most of the pharmacogenetic research has been conducted. Research suggests that response to the atypical antipsychotics, specifically clozapine and olanzapine, may be a function of polymorphisms, including the 5-HT2A and 5-HT2C receptors. In addition, research has suggested that two of the more common side effects seen with antipsychotic use (i.e., weight gain and tardive dyskinesia) have a genetic basis for their development.

Serotonin and Dopamine Receptors and Antipsychotic Response

The gene for the 5-HT2A receptor is located on chromosome 13 and a total of five polymorphisms have been identified (T102C, Thr25Asn, His452Tyr, T516C, and -G1438A) (Reference 49). Of these, there are two that result in protein alterations (i.e., His452Tyr and Thr25Asn). The T102C polymorphism has been the most widely studied and is associated with schizophrenia and antipsychotic response (References 49–52), although other researchers have been unable to verify this relationship (References 53–56). In 1995, one study (Reference 57) reported that homozygosity for the 102C allele was more frequent in nonresponders to clozapine (Reference 57) and in 1998, the same investigators (Reference 58) found that homozygosity for the -1438 G allele also was higher among nonresponders than responders (58 percent vs. 32 percent, p=0.001). The His452Tyr polymorphism also has been associated with clozapine response (References 59, 60) with the presence of the Tyr452 variant being tied to a poorer response (Reference 58). Although these results are interesting and point in the direction of a genetic basis for clozapine response, multiple researchers have been unable to replicate these findings (References 58, 61–63).

The gene for the 5-HT2C receptor is located on chromosome X, and a polymorphism resulting in a cysteine to serine substitution at codon 23 has been found (Reference 64). Similar to the 5-HT2A polymorphisms, previous reports are conflicting as to the role of this genotype in the clinical response to atypical antipsychotics for treating schizophrenia (Reference 64). One study (Reference 65) found a positive association between response to clozapine and 5-HT2C genotype, although other researchers were unable to confirm these results (References 62, 63, 66). In addition to the 5-HT2A and 5-HT2C receptors, various investigations into polymorphism of the 5-HT1A, 5-HT3, 5-HT5, 5-HT6, and 5-HT7 and response to clozapine have been conducted without finding any significant relationships (References 67–70).

Finally, for 5-HT transmission, polymorphisms of the 5-HTT also have been investigated in terms of antipsychotic response. The 5-HTT, 5-HTTLPR, has a polymorphic repetitive element upstream from the transcription start site, and a VNTR in intron two. No relationship between clozapine response and these polymorphisms have been found (Reference 71). Polymorphisms of the dopamine receptors also have been an area of pharmacogenetic study for antipsychotics and clozapine, given their ability to block dopamine receptors. Various authors have found no significant association between response and polymorphisms of the D2, D3, and D4 receptors (References 72–78).

More recently, olanzapine has become the focus of various pharmacogenetic investigations, given its similar structure to clozapine. One study (Reference 79) reported initial positive symptom response to olanzapine was dependent on the occurrence of therapeutic blood levels, whereas a statistical trend suggested a relationship between negative symptom response and a polymorphism of the 5-HT2A receptor, specifically the 102T/C allele. Subjects with the T/T genotype experienced a mean reduction of 46 percent ± 12 percent in Scale for the Assessment of Negative Symptoms of Schizophrenia score compared to those heterozygous or homozygous for the C allele who experienced only a mean reduction of 20 percent ± 6 percent (Reference 79). No other statistically significant relationships were found for these other polymorphism of the 5-HT2A and 5-HT2C receptors.

In addition to polymorphisms of 5-HT and dopamine receptors, the histamine receptors, cholinergic receptors, α-adrenergic receptors, and gamma aminobutyric acid receptors also contain polymorphisms. None of these polymorphisms has a significant relationship with response to clozapine in patients with schizophrenia (References 80, 81).

Cytochrome P450 Isoenzymes and Antipsychotic Pharmacokinetics

Polymorphisms also exist for the CYP isoenzymes, the primary isoenzymes which metabolize the antipsychotics. Large metabolic interindividual variability results in pronounced differences in steady-state plasma concentrations (Reference 82) for the antipsychotics. The CYP genes encode a multigene superfamily of mixed function monooxygenases responsible for Phase I metabolism of the antipsychotics and other drugs. This superfamily is divided into many subfamilies based on nucleotide sequence homology. The genes within a specific subfamily have a minimum of 40 percent sequence identity (Reference 83). The CYP proteins are found primarily in the liver, although specific isoenzymes also are expressed in many extrahepatic tissues, including the lung, kidneys, and gastrointestinal tract (Reference 84). Individual CYP isoenzymes have distinct substrate specificities, active site structures, and mechanisms of regulation (Reference 84). There is some degree of overlap in substrate specificity, particularly between members of the same family, as well as numerous examples of drugs that are substrates for more than one CYP isoenzyme. The best example of a polymorphic isoenzyme is CYP2D6 in which several mutations result in a poor metabolizer phenotype because of loss of functional protein production. Poor metabolizers constitute 5–10 percent of the population and are unable to metabolize compounds, which are CYP2D6 substrates (Reference 85). In terms of antipsychotic metabolism, there are six specific isoenzymes of interest (CYP1A2, CYP2D6, CYP3A4, CYP2E1, CYP2C9, and CYP2C19), all of which have specific genetic tests available to determine genetic polymorphisms. In looking at the antipsychotics individually, the exact CYP isoenzymes responsible for their metabolism often are not fully known, as the literature is conflicting. Table 1 lists atypical antipsychotics along with the specific isoenzymes hypothesized as being involved in their metabolism. Although studies are sometimes conflicting as to the degree of involvement for each isoenzyme, it is relatively clear that more than one isoenzyme is involved. Thus, individuals with allelic mutations in more than one CYP isoenzyme may have the highest risk for reduced antipsychotic metabolism.

Of these CYP enzymes, only polymorphisms of 1A2 have been linked to clinically relevant pharmacokinetic data with the antipsychotics. The CYP1A2 is highly involved in clozapine's metabolism. In a recent case report of clozapine nonresponders, who had higher levels of 1A2 after phenotyping with caffeine, the addition of fluvoxamine (a 1A2 inhibitor) to

Table 1. Cytochrome P450 Metabolism of Atypical Antipsychotics

Medication	CYP Isoenzymes	References
Clozapine	1A2, 3A4, 2D6, 2C19, 2C9, 2E1	86–94
Olanzapine	1A2, 2D6, 2C19, 3A4, 2C9	95, 96
Risperidone	2D6, 3A4	97, 98
Quetiapine	3A4, 2D6	99, 100
Ziprasidone	3A4	101, 102
Aripiprazole	3A4, 2D6	103

CYP = cytochrome P450.

their regimen resulted in higher clozapine serum concentrations and a reduction in psychiatric symptomatology (Reference 104). Recently, a C to A transversion in the first intron of CYP1A2 was found. This single nucleotide polymorphism (SNP) has been associated with variation in 1A2 induction in healthy volunteers who smoke. Investigators (Reference 105) found that the A/A genotype was more inducible than the C/A or C/C genotype. Thus, for patients with schizophrenia who smoke, it may be more difficult to reach acceptable clozapine serum concentrations if they have an A/A 1A2 genotype. In Japanese smokers, a G to A transversion in the 5' flanking region of 1A2 at position -2964 also has been associated with decreased 1A2 activity (Reference 106). Other authors have examined the role of these 1A2 polymorphisms on the pharmacokinetics of clozapine and were unable to find a relationship (Reference 107). In addition to 1A2, CYP2D6 has been implicated in the metabolism of clozapine, although it is thought to have a relatively minor role. In looking at the pharmacokinetics of clozapine in relation to polymorphisms of 2D6, no relationship has been found (Reference 57).

Finally, olanzapine also has been the focus of one pharmacokinetic study in which olanzapine pharmacokinetics was compared in individuals phenotyped for 1A2 and 2D6. Overall, no relationship was found between the phenotypes and olanzapine pharmacokinetics (Reference 108).

Pharmacogenetics and Weight Gain from Antipsychotics

The incidence and amount of weight gain from antipsychotics is highly variable. Retrospective chart reviews suggest that between 1 percent and 69 percent of patients receiving clozapine will experience significant weight gain (Reference 109), with most of the weight gain occurring within the first 6–12 months of treatment, although some patients continue to gain weight after 2–3years of treatment (References 110, 111). In one follow-up study (range = 3–90 months), the cumulative proportions of patients becoming 10, 20, 30, and 40 percent overweight were 86, 54, 23, and 13 percent, respectively (Reference 111). In 1999, a retrospective chart analysis was published (Reference 112) to compare the relative weight liabilities of clozapine, risperidone, olanzapine, sertindole, and haloperidol. Data on 92 men with schizophrenia were used to calculate measures of maximal weight gain, final weight, and duration to maximal weight. The mean duration of treatment was significantly longer for the olanzapine group compared to the others (73.1 ± 9.9 weeks vs. 24.7 ± 5.4–42.5 ± 12.6 weeks; p<0.01). Overall, clozapine and olanzapine had the highest maximal weight gains compared to the other groups (clozapine 6.9 ± 0.9 kg, olanzapine 6.8 ± 1 kg, risperidone 5 ± 0.6 kg, haloperidol 3.7 ± 0.6 kg, sertindole 3.1 ± 1.2 kg; p<0.05). This weight appeared to persist despite behavioral interventions, such as nutritional consultation and suggested exercise routine. In addition, a meta-analysis on weight gain from antipsychotics was published (Reference 113). Included in this article are 81 published reports.

Investigators found that after 10 weeks of treatment, the mean weight increases for patients taking antipsychotics were as follows: clozapine 4.45 kg, olanzapine 4.15 kg, sertindole 2.92 kg, risperidone 2.10 kg, and ziprasidone 0.04 kg, whereas both placebo and molindone showed weight decreases ranging from 0.39 kg to 0.74 kg. This translates into a weight gain of 0.5 kg/week, and based on previous data may translate into a total weight gain of up to 24 kg/year.

Antipsychotic-induced weight gain in this already stigmatized and undersocialized group is a common cause of drug noncompliance and discontinuation of treatment (References 114, 115). Recently, researchers (Reference 116), found that patients with a body mass index of more than 30 were 3 times as likely to miss their drugs (odds ratio = 2.9; 95 percent confidence interval = 1.1–7.3) than those with a body mass index of less than 30 and that this relationship was stronger in women (odds ratio = 13.8; 95 percent confidence interval = 2–95.4). Thus, the morbidities from the atypical antipsychotic are not just physical. Increased weight gain also can contribute significantly to drug noncompliance, which often is directly related to treatment discontinuation and ultimate failure.

There is a paucity of information available about the underlying mechanism and risk factors for antipsychotic morbidity. Recent pharmacogenetic investigations into antipsychotic-associated weight gain have shown that polymorphisms of the CYP isoenzymes, the 5-HT receptors, and other receptors may play a role. Given that clozapine has been associated with the largest amount of weight gain, it is only natural that this drug would be the center of these investigations. Results of a fairly comprehensive trial (Reference 117) investigating 10 polymorphisms for nine candidate genes for clozapine-induced weight gain were published recently. Investigators looked at SNPs of the 5-HT receptors (2A, 2C, and 1A), histamine receptors (H1 and H2), β-3 receptors, and the α1A receptor genes, as well as SNPs for CYP1A2 and tumor necrosis factor-α. Overall statistical trends were found between weight gain from clozapine and SNPs for the β receptors, α receptors, tumor necrosis factor-α, and 5-HT2C receptors. Recently, a polymorphism of the 5-HT2C receptor has been associated with the development of type 2 diabetes and obesity in a control population (patients without schizophrenia) (Reference 118). This polymorphism of the 5-HT2CR gene consists of a C to T substitution in the 5' flanking region, which contains regulatory and putative transcription factor-binding regions (Reference 119). As a result of this, polymorphisms in this region may result in alterations in the expression of the gene. Investigators (Reference 120) found the -759C/T polymorphism to be associated with the development of weight gain (more than 7 percent) over baseline in patients receiving primarily chlorpromazine and risperidone. Investigators estimated that both drugs were capable of inducing a weight gain of 2 kg over 10 weeks. Based on the subjects included in the study, a 10 percent increase in initial body weight translates into an 8 kg weight gain over 6 weeks (Reference 122).

In addition to clozapine, pharmacogenetic investigations involving olanzapine-induced weight gain also have been conducted. One of the CYP enzymes responsible for the metabolism of olanzapine is CYP2D6 (References 95, 96). Researchers (Reference 121) found that subjects with a heterozygous *1/*3, *4 genotype experienced a statistically significantly larger percentage change in body mass index than the homozygous *1/*1 group (28 percent vs. 12 percent). Thus, polymorphisms of CYP isoenzymes may be the trigger needed for excessive weight gain and other morbidity associated with olanzapine and other atypical antipsychotics. In addition, the same investigators (Reference 122) have found a relationship between the -759C/T polymorphism of the 5-HT2C receptor and significant weight gain (10 percent or more over baseline) during treatment for 6 weeks with olanzapine. The distribution of C alleles was higher in subjects gaining 10 percent or more of their body weight compared to those who did not gain significant weight (15/15 [100 percent] vs. 16/27 [59.3 percent]). All of the subjects, who gained more than 10 percent of their initial body weight over 6 weeks, had at least one C allele. Subjects with a C allele gained a mean of 12.2 percent ± 9.7 percent over their initial body weight compared to subjects with a T allele who gained a mean of 4.7 percent ± 4.2 percent. It has been hypothesized that this relationship may be because of higher transcription levels of this gene caused by the variant allele, which results in more resistance to obesity and diabetes.

Pharmacogenetics and Tardive Dyskinesia Development

The use of typical antipsychotics often is associated with the development of abnormal movements and tardive dyskinesia, which occurs in about 14 percent of patients receiving typical antipsychotics (Reference 123). Although the true mechanism behind tardive dyskinesia development is unknown, it has long been linked to a relative overactivity of the dopamine system (Reference 124). In addition to a genetic or familial predisposition associated with this condition (References 125, 126), antipsychotic exposure, cigarette smoking, and age also have been implicated in its development (References 127, 128).

Given dopamine's proposed role in tardive dyskinesia development, many of the polymorphisms associated with the dopamine receptors have been investigated as to their role. The human dopamine 3 receptor is located on chromosome 3q13.3 and contains a polymorphism in the first exon that gives rise to a serine (ser) to glycine (gly) substitution (Reference 129). In patients with schizophrenia, an excess of the gly/gly genotype has been found in patients with tardive dyskinesia (References 130–3), although this was not replicated in another study (Reference 134). In a more recent large multicenter study, this relationship between the Ser9Gly polymorphism of the dopamine 3 receptor and tardive dyskinesia development also was found

(Reference 135). In addition, a polymorphism of the dopamine 2 receptor also has been examined for its relationship to tardive dyskinesia. The dopamine 2 receptor is located on 11q23, and contains a *Taq-I* restriction polymorphism. One study (Reference 136) found an increased frequency of the A2 allele in patients with tardive dyskinesia. The results of this study have not yet been replicated.

Two studies have found a relationship between SNPs of the 5-HT2A receptor and tardive dyskinesia (References 137,138), although subsequent studies were unable to replicate these results (Reference 139). In one of the studies that found a relationship (Reference 137), there was a significant excess of the 102C and -1438G alleles in patients with tardive dyskinesia compared to patients without tardive dyskinesia and matched controls (patients without tardive dyskinesia) (62.7 percent vs. 41.1 percent and 45.9 percent, respectively). The 102C/C and -1438G/G genotypes also were significantly associated with higher Abnormal Involuntary Movement Scale trunk dyskinesia scores. None of the other 5-HT2A polymorphisms have shown a relationship with tardive dyskinesia. Similar to this, the relationship between the 5-HT2C receptor and tardive dyskinesia also has been investigated (Reference 140). One study (Reference 140) found the frequency of the 5-HT2C ser allele to be significantly higher in patients with tardive dyskinesia versus those without tardive dyskinesia and controls (patients without tardive dyskinesia) (27.2 percent vs. 14.6 percent and 14.2 percent, respectively). This was primarily because of the excess of Cyr/Ser and Ser/Ser genotypes in the women. In combining the analysis of the 5-HT2C and the dopamine 3 receptor polymorphisms, using a stepwise multiple regression, these authors then found that the 5-HT2C ser and dopamine 3 receptor gly alleles contributed to 4.2 percent and 4.7 percent of the variance seen in oralfacial dyskinesia scores. Thus, similar to other CNS disorders, tardive dyskinesia development is a multifactorial process of which polymorphisms of the 5-HT2C and dopamine 3 receptor may play a part.

Finally, the 5-HTTLPR also has been investigated in tardive dyskinesia development. An insertion/deletion polymorphism has been reported in the promoter region of this gene. The short variant of this gene has been associated with reduced 5-HTT expression, leading to reduced 5-HT uptake in lymphoblasts (Reference 41). No relationship has been found between this polymorphism of 5-HTTLPR, Abnormal Involuntary Movement Scale score, or the diagnosis of tardive dyskinesia (Reference 141).

Because the CYP isoenzymes are involved in the metabolism of antipsychotics, their role in tardive dyskinesia development also has been investigated. Both CYP1A2 and CYP2D6 have a relationship with tardive dyskinesia development (References 142, 143). For CYP2D6, several investigations were unable to find any significant association between poor metabolizer status for 2D6 and the occurrence of tardive dyskinesia (References 144–7), although there were some nonsignificant trends suggesting a relationship. Recently, it has been suggested that patients heterozygous for the CYP2D6 *3 or *4 alleles who smoke cigarettes may have the highest risk for developing abnormal movements and tardive dyskinesia compared to those homozygous for the *1 allele or nonsmokers (20 percent vs. 78 percent) (Reference 143). Thus, subjects with a CYP2D6 *3 or *4 allele may shunt antipsychotic metabolism through other pathways induced by cigarette smoke. This induction may result in formation of neurotoxic metabolites, leading to increased Abnormal Involuntary Movement Scale scores and a higher incidence of tardive dyskinesia, compared to subjects without these alleles.

In addition to CYP2D6, CYP1A2 also has been a focus of this research. One study (Reference 142) found that in patients with schizophrenia, the Abnormal Involuntary Movement Scale scores of subjects with a C/C genotype was 2.7–3.4-fold higher than those with a C/A or A/A genotype. When these subjects were examined based on their smoking status, this effect was even more pronounced with Abnormal Involuntary Movement Scale scores that were 5.4 –4.7-fold greater in smokers with a C/C genotype compared to the other groups. Thus, similar to the 2D6 data, it may be that patients with the correct combination of genetic and environmental factors may carry the largest risk for tardive dyskinesia.

Pain and Opioid Abuse

Opioid Receptors

Based primarily on clinical experience and case reports, it has been speculated that genetics play a role in an individual's pain relief response to opioids as well as their potential for the misuse and subsequent dependence on these agents. The majority of the information in the literature regarding opioid use has focused on dependence and addiction. Pharmacologically, the opioids exert their effects through the mu, delta, and kappa receptors. Of these three receptors, morphine preferentially acts through the mu opioid receptors. Currently, there have been more than 40 SNPs identified in the mu opioid receptor gene (OPRM1). The majority of these are in the 5' noncoding region of the receptor which indicates they might play a role in receptor regulation. Those found in the coding region might be associated with altered receptor binding, receptor function, or drug abuse (Reference 148). In looking at animal models, it can be shown that individual differences in opioid sensitivity exist (Reference 159).

One of the goals of pharmacogenomics as it relates to opiate use is to find relationships between various SNPs and an individual's risk of addition. In looking at the literature, two polymorphisms of the OPRM1 (17C/T and 118A/G) which result in amino acid changes have been associated with the occurrence of heroin abuse (References 150, 151), although subsequent replication studies did not find the same correlation (References 152, 153).

More recently, one study (Reference 154) found a significant characteristic pattern of sequence variants (-1793T/A, -1699Tins, -1320A/G, -111C/T, and 17C/T) for the OPRM1 and the existence of substance dependence. Among the SNPs included in these haplotypes, several are thought to affect gene regulation, although this has not yet been proven.

In looking at the pharmacology of the opioids, the mu receptor is the most logical candidate for pharmacogenetic study because it is believed to be the primary mediator of opioid analgesia. In reviewing the literature, little research on SNPs of the delta and kappa receptors has been conducted in humans. Previously, there were reports of a silent mutation in the delta receptor being associated with heroin abuse (Reference 155), but subsequent investigations were unable to find the same relationship (Reference 156).

Dopamine and Serotonin Receptors

In looking at other receptor polymorphisms, which may be associated with the occurrence of drug addiction, primarily the dopamine and 5-HT receptor and transporter have been investigated. Researchers (Reference 157) investigated a polymorphism of the dopamine 3 receptor, which leads to an amino acid substitution and opioid addiction. Overall, the investigators did not find a difference in the distribution of the SNP between case and control subjects but did find that homozygosity was more frequent in subjects who scored high on scales of sensation seeking. This personality trait has been linked to developing substance abuse. Unfortunately, two replication studies were able to confirm these results (References 157, 159). The same sort of association between personality traits and SNPs of the dopamine 4 receptor also has been suggested for opioid dependence. Individuals with longer alleles of several expressed repeat units in the third exon of dopamine 4 receptor are at higher risk for developing opioid dependence because of an increase in novelty seeking (References 158, 159). However, one study (Reference 160) examined this relationship as well as three other polymorphisms of dopamine 4 receptor and did not find this association. In addition, other investigators have been unable to find these associations (Reference 153).

In examining the 5-HT receptor and the 5-HTT, little association with opioid dependence has been found. Researchers (Reference 161) found an association between allele 10 of an intronic tandem repeat and the presence of opioid addiction in subjects of Chinese descent, but this could not be replicated (Reference 159). In addition, in the study that could not replicate results (Reference 159), no relationship between two of the 5-HT2A polymorphisms and opiate dependence was found.

Cytochrome P450

The primary isoenzyme responsible for the metabolism of the opioid is P2D6. Researchers (Reference 162) hypothesized that individuals homozygous for deletions of CYP2D6 would be at lower risk for developing opioid dependence. In comparing the distribution of CYP2D6 alleles, no homozygous deletions were found in the sample of opiate addicts, compared to 4 percent in the never dependent controls and 6.5 percent in the multidrug dependent group. Although these results were statistically significant and translated into an odds ratio of 7.2, the 95 percent confidence interval contained unity.

Drug Efflux from CNS and across the Blood-brain Barrier

P-glycoprotein

For many years, clinicians have known of the existence of a gene conferring drug resistance to multiple drugs. Recently, P-glycoprotein (Pgp) was found to be the product of the *MDR1* and, as such, polymorphisms of this gene have been associated with changes in drug absorption and elimination. P-glycoprotein is an adenosine triphosphate-dependent efflux transporter protein which translocates its substrates out of the cells. The *MDR1* gene is located on chromosome 7q21. P-glycoprotein is a 170-kilodalton phosphorylated and glycosylated protein that consists of 1280 amino acids. The distribution of Pgp within the body is fairly ubiquitous, with Pgp being present in the small intestine, kidney, pancreas, hepatocytes, and the blood-brain barrier. The location of Pgp in the body suggests an evolutionary role as a protective mechanism against naturally occurring toxins, which might be ingested.

Currently, 19 polymorphisms have been found for Pgp. Of these, only one in exon 26 at position 3435 is clinically relevant. Variations in the expression of this protein because of this polymorphism can potentially affect an individual's exposure to its substrates, including anticancer agents, human immunodeficiency virus protease inhibitors, immunosuppressants, cardiac drugs, β-adrenoceptor antagonists, loperamide, and cortisol (Reference 163). Currently, no relationship between the C3435T polymorphism of Pgp and CNS drugs have been found.

Microarray Techniques and CNS

Use of DNA arrays can assist in the discovery and target selection of new drugs for treating CNS disorders. Disturbances in the brain's functions underlie many of the CNS disorders. The ability of the brain to undertake complex tasks is mediated by multiple regions of the brain along wit complex biochemical systems (i.e., neurotransmitters). To understan alterations in these functions, which may result in altered gene expressic and protein production, it is necessary to have the capability simultaneously measure these changes in the brain. Deoxyribonucleic acid microarray technology is a tool currently available to investigate regional differences in gene expression for the brain (References 164, 165). Patterns of gene expression associated with specific illnesses (i.e., multiple sclerosis) may help identify specific diagnostic marks for these illnesses, as well as assist in the discovery and target selection of new drugs for treating CNS disorders.

Currently, there are two types of DNA microarrays. The first is an oligonucleotide array and the second is the cloned DNA-based array. The procedures for each of these assays is similar in that both operate using nucleic acid probes which are bound to a solid surface along with a hybridization of messenger ribonucleic acid, from the tissue or cell culture sample, to these probes. Once bound, the array can determine differences in messenger ribonucleic acid expression under different conditions. For the oligonucleotide array, this method involves the massive synthesis of oligonucleotides, which are placed on chips. These chips can then be used to investigate thousands of genes simultaneously (Reference 166). In contrast to this, the cloned DNA-based array couples DNA fragments to a glass surface (References 167, 168) which are then exposed to prepared messenger ribonucleic acid from two different tissue samples, which are labeled with two different fluorescent tags. Once hybridization of the messenger ribonucleic acid to the DNA fragments has taken place, the signal from each of the different probes is quantified and the ratio of the signal is used to determine differences in gene expression between the two samples.

In addition to microarray analysis, this technology also can be used to determine SNPs. This technology does not measure gene expression, rather it addresses the role of genomic variation in the function of genes and the treatment of disease. Use of SNP analysis may help to accelerate genetic association studies of diseases as well as pharmacogenetic studies of treatment. Millions of SNPs have been identified as a result of the recently completed human genome project (References 169, 170). The basis behind SNP analysis using microarray technology is amplification of the DNA sing PCR followed by fluorescent labeling of the variant base and then bridization of the SNP to a microarray chip for parallel detection. So, ilar to the previously discussed microarrays methods, this SNP analysis vs for detection of thousands of SNPs simultaneously.

us, DNA microarrays are some of the most powerful techniques ly available for pharmacogenetic investigations. These assays can global genetics functioning questions, allow for the expression of thousands of genes in a single experiment, and determine the role of genetic variants to human illness and ultimately treatment.

Conclusion

The area of CNS pharmacogenomics is rapidly changing. The majority of work conducted in this field has been accomplished within the past 10 years, and as such researchers are at the beginning in terms of knowing how genetic polymorphisms affect treatment response and the occurrence of side effects with CNS drugs. Currently, the majority of the work conducted in this area has been conducted in psychiatric illnesses, specifically schizophrenia and depression focusing on the dopamine and 5-HT receptors. Additional work in the CNS area includes the CYP system and more recently drug transporters. Regardless of the drug or disease state studied, the pharmacogenetic methods used often are similar and with recent advancements, such as microarrays, information regarding the pharmacogenetics of CNS disorders should be swiftly forthcoming.

References

1. Colantuoni C, Purcell AE, Bouton CM, Pevsner J. High throughput analysis of gene expression in the human brain. J Neurosci Res 2000;59:1–10.

2. Sutcliffe JG. mRNA in the mammalian central nervous system. Annu Rev Neurosci 1998;11:157–98.

3. Lock C, Hermans G, Bedotti R, et al. Gene-micro array analysis of multiple sclerosis lesions yields new targets validated in autoimmune encephalomyelitis. Nat Med 2002;8:500–8.

4. Ophoff RA, Van Den Maagdenberg AM, Roon KI, Ferrari MD, Frants RR. The impact of pharmacogenetics for migraine. Eur J Pharmacol 2001;413:1–10.

5. Ophoff RA, Terwindt GM, Vergouwe MN, et al. Familial hemiplegic migraine and episodic ataxia type-2 are caused by mutations in the Ca^{2+} channel gene CACNL1A4. Cell 1996;7:543–52.

6. Demchyshyn L, Sunahara RK, Miller K, et al. A human serotonin receptor variant (5-HT1B) encoded by an intronless gene on chromosome 6. Proc Natl Acad Sci U S A 1992;89:5522–6.

7. Lappalainen J, Dean M, Charbonneau L, Virkkunen M, Linnoila M, Goldman D. Mapping of the serotonin 5-HT1DB autoreceptor gene on chromosome 6 and direct analysis for sequence variants. Am J Med Genet 1995;60:157–61.

8. Nothen MM, Erdmann J, Shimrom-Abarbunell D, Propping P. Identification of genetic variation in the human serotonin 1DB receptor gene. Biochem Biophys Res Comm 1994;205:1194–200.

9. Ozaki N, Lappalainen J, Dean M, Virkkunen M, Linnoila M, Goldman D. Mapping of the serotonin 5-HT1D alpha autoreceptor gene (HTR1D) on chromosome 1 using a silent polymorphism in the coding region. Am J Med Genet 1995;60:162–4.

10. Sidenberg DG, Basett AS, Demchyshyn L, et al. New polymorphism for the human serotonin 1D receptor variant (5-HT1D) not linked to schizophrenia in five Canadian pedigrees. Hum Hered 1993;45:315–8.

11. Maassen VanDenBrink A, Vergouwe MN, Ophoff RA, Saxena PR, Ferrari MD, Frants RR. 5-HT1B receptor polymorphism and clinical response to sumatriptan. Headache 1998;38:288–91.

12. Lindsay J; the ApoE and Alzheimer's Disease Meta-Analysis Consortium. Effect of age, gender, and ethnicity on the association of apolipoprotein E genotype and Alzheimer's disease. JAMA 1997;278:1349–56.

13. Nalbantoglu J, Gilfix BM, Bertrand P, et al. Predictive value of apolipoprotein E genotyping in Alzheimer's disease. Ann Neurol 1994;36:889–95.

14. Zanis VI, Kardassis D, Zanis EE. Genetic mutations affecting human lipoproteins, their receptors, and their enzymes. Adv Hum Genet 1993;21:145–319.

15. Poirier J, Delisle ML, Quirion R, et al. Apolipoprotein E4 allele as a predictor of cholinergic deficits and treatment outcome in Alzheimer's disease. Proc Natl Acad Sci U S A 1995;92:12260–4.

16. Farlow MR, Lahiri DK, Poirier J, Davignon J, Schneider L, Hui SL. Treatment outcomes of tacrine therapy depends on apolipoprotein genotype and gender of subjects with Alzheimer's disease. Neurology 1998;50:669–77.

17. MacGowen SH, Wilcock GK, Scott M. Effects of gender and apolipoprotein E genotype on response to anticholinesterase activity in Alzheimer's disease. Int J Geriatr Psychiatry 1998;13:624–30.

18. Wilcock GK, Lilienfeld S, Gaens E. Efficacy and safety of galantamine in patients with mild to moderate Alzheimer's disease: a multicentre randomised controlled trial. BMJ 2000;321:1–7.

19. Greenberg SM, Tennis MK, Brown LB, et al. Donepezil in clinical practice: a randomized crossover study. Arch Neurol 2000;57:94–9.

20. Schappert K, Sevigny P, Poirier J. Apolipoprotein E in the treatment of Alzheimer's disease. In: Lerer B, ed. Pharmacogenetics of psychotropic drugs. Cambridge, UK: Cambridge University Press, 2002:360–71.

21. Farlow MR, Cyrus PA, Nadel A, Lahiri DK, Brashear A, Gulanski B. Metrifonate treatment of AD: influence of ApoE genotype. Neurology 1999;53:2010–6.

22. Richard F, Hetbecque N, Neuman E, Guez E, Levy R, Amouyel P. ApoE genotyping and response to drug treatment in Alzheimer's disease. Lancet 1997;349:539–40.

23. Price DL, Sisodia SS, Borchelt DR. Genetic neurodegenerative diseases: the human illness and transgenic models. Science 1998;282:1079–83.

24. Clayton DF, Georgy JM. Synucleins in synaptic plasticity and neurodegenerative disorders. J Neurosci Res 1999;58:120–9.

25. Kitada T, Asakawa S, Hattori N, et al. Mutations in the parkin gene cause autosomal recessive juvenile parkinsonism. Nature 1998;392:605–8.

26. Abbas N, Lucking CB, Ricard S, et al. A wide variety of mutations in the parkin gene are responsible for autosomal recessive parkinsonism in Europe. French

Parkinson's Disease Genetics Study Group and the European Consortium on Genetic Susceptibility in Parkinson's Disease. Hum Mol Genet 1999;8:567–74.

27. Tan EK, Khajavi M, Thornby JI, Nagamitsu S, Jankovic J, Ashizawa T. Variability and validity of polymorphism association studies in Parkinson's disease. Neurology 2000;55:533–8.

28. Prasad AN, Prasad C, Safstrom CE. Recent advances in the genetics of epilepsy: insights from human and animal studies. Epilepsia 1999;40:1329–52.

29. Veronese ME, Mackenzie PL, Doecke DJ, McManus ME, Miners JO, Birkett DJ. Tolbutamide and phenytoin hydroxylation by can-expressed human live cytochrome P4502C9. Biochem Biophys Res Comm 1991;172:1112–8.

30. Fritz S, Linder W, Roots I, Frey BM, Kupfer A. Stereochemistry of aromatic phenytoin hydroxylation in various drug hydroxylation phenotypes in humans. J Pharmacol Exp Ther 1987;241:615–22.

31. Bajpai B, Roskos LK, Shen DD, et al. Role of cytochrome P4502C9 and cytochrome P4502C19 in the stereoselective metabolism of phenytoin to its major metabolite. Drug Metab Dispos 1996;24:1401–3.

32. Hashimoto Y, Otsuki Y, Odani A, et al. Effect of CYP2C polymorphisms on the pharmacokinetics of phenytoin in Japanese patients with epilepsy. Biol Pharm Bull 1996;19(8):1103–5.

33. deMorias SMF, Wilkinson GR, Blaisdell J, et al. Identification of a new genetic defect for the polymorphism of (S)-mephenytoin metabolism in Japanese. Mol Pharmacol 1994;46:594–8.

34. Odani A, Hashimoto Y, Otsuki Y, et al. Genetic polymorphism of the CYP2C subfamily and its effects on the pharmacokinetics of phenytoin in Japanese patients with epilepsy. Clin Pharmacol Ther 1997;62:287–92.

35. Mamiya K, Ichiro I, Shimamoto J, et al. The effects of genetic polymorphism of CYP2C9 and CYP2C19 on phenytoin metabolism in Japanese adult patients with epilepsy: studies in stereoselective hydroxylation and population pharmacokinetics. Epilepsia 1998;12:1317–23.

36. Goldstein JA, de Morais SMF. Biochemistry and molecular biology of the human CYP2C subfamily. Pharmacogenetics 1994;4:285–99.

37. National Institutes of Health Consensus Conference. Surgery for epilepsy. JAMA 1990;264:729–33.

38. Dombrowski SM, Desai SY, Marroni M, et al. Overexpression of multiple drug resistance genes in endothelial cells from patients with refractory epilepsy. Epilepsia 2001;12:1501–6.

39. First MB. Diagnostic and Statistical Manual of Mental Disorders, 4th ed, Text Revision (DSM-IV-TR). Washington, D.C.: American Psychiatric Association; 2000.

40. United States Department of Health and Human Services. Mental Health: A Report of the Surgeon General—Executive Summary. Rockville, MD: United States Department of Health and Human Services, Substance Abuse and Mental Health Services Administration, Center for Mental Health Services, National Institutes of Health, National Institute of Mental Health; 1999.

41. Heils A, Teufel A, Petri S, et al. Allelic variation of human serotonin transporter gene expression. J Neurochem 1996;66:2621–4.

42. Ogilvie AD, Battersby S, Bubb VJ, et al. Polymorphism in serotonin transporter gene associated with susceptibility to major depression. Lancet 1996;347:731–3.

43. Smeraldi E, Zanardi E, Benedetti F, Di Bella D, Perez J, Catalano M. Polymorphism within the promoter of the serotonin transporter gene and antidepressant efficacy of fluvoxamine. Mol Psychiatry 2000;3:508–11.

44. Pollock BG, Ferrell RE, Mulsant BH, et al. Allelic variation in the serotonin transporter promoter affects onset of paroxetine treatment response in late-life depression. Neuropsychopharmacology 2000;23:587–90.

45. Zanardi R, Benedetti F, Di Bella D, Catalano M, Smeraldi E. Efficacy of paroxetine in depression is influenced by a functional polymorphism within the promoter of the serotonin transporter gene. J Clin Psychopharmacol 2000;20:105–6.

46. Kim DK, Lim SW, Lee S, et al. Serotonin transporter gene polymorphism and antidepressant response. Neuroreport 2000;11:215–9.

47. Eichhammer P, Langguth B, Wiegand R, Kharraz A, Frick U, Hajak G. Allelic variation in the serotonin transporter promoter affects neuromodulatory effects of a selective serotonin transporter reuptake inhibitor (SSRI). Psychopharmacology 2003;166:294–7.

48. Greenblatt DJ, von Moltke LL, Harmatz JS, Shader RI. Drug interactions with newer antidepressants: role of human cytochromes P450. J Clin Psychiatry 1998;59(suppl 15):19–27.

49. Erdmann J, Shimron-Abarbanell D, Reitschel M, et al. Systematic screening for mutations in the human serotonin-2A (5-HT2A) receptor gene: identification of two naturally occurring receptor variants and association analysis in schizophrenia. Hum Genet 1996;97:614–9.

50. Inayama Y, Yoneda H, Sakai T, et al. Positive association between a DNA sequence variant in the serotonin 2A receptor gene and schizophrenia. Am J Med Genet 1996;67:103–5.

51. Williams J, Spurlock G, McGuffin P, et al. Association between schizophrenia and T102C polymorphism of the 5-hydroxytryptamine type 2α-receptor gene. Lancet 1996;347:1294–6.

52. Williams J, McGuffin P, Nothen M, Owens MJ. Meta-analysis of association between the 5-HT$_{2a}$ receptor T102C polymorphism and schizophrenia. Lancet 1997;349:1221.

53. Ishigaki T, Xie DW, Liu JC, et al. Intact 5-HT2A receptor exons and the adjoining intron regions in schizophrenia. Neuropsychopharmacology 1996;14:339–47.

54. Jonsson E, Nothen MM, Bunzel R, Propping P, Sedvall G. 5-HT 2a receptor T102C polymorphism and schizophrenia. Lancet 1996;347(9018):1831.

55. Malhotra AK, Goldman D, Buchanan R, Breier A, Pickar D. 5-HT 2a receptor T102C polymorphism and schizophrenia. Lancet 1996;347(9018):1830–1.

56. Sasaki T, Hattori M, Fukuda R, Kunugi H, Nanko S. 5-HT 2a receptor T102C polymorphism and schizophrenia. Lancet 1996;347(9018):1832.

57. Arranz MJ, Dawnson E, Shaikh S, et al. Cytochrome P4502D6 genotype does not determine response to clozapine. Br J Clin Pharmacol 1995;39:417–20.

58. Arranz MJ, Munro J, Owen MJ, et al. Evidence for association between polymorphisms in the promoter and coding regions of the 5-HT2A receptor gene and response to clozapine. Mol Psychiatry 1998;3:61–6.

59. Arranz MJ, Collier DA, Munro J, et al. Analysis of the structural polymorphisms in the 5-HT2A receptor and clinical response to clozapine. Neurosci Lett 1996;217:177–8.

60. Badri F, Masellis M, Petronis A, et al. Dopamine and serotonin system genes may predict clinical response to clozapine. Am J Hum Genet 1996;59:A247.

61. Nothen MM, Rietschel M, Erdmann J, et al. Genetic variation of the 5-HT2A receptor and response to clozapine. Lancet 1995;346:908–9.

62. Malhotra AK, Goldman D, Ozaki N, et al. Clozapine response and the 5-HT2C Cys23Ser polymorphism. Neuroreport 1996;7:2100–2.

63. Masellis M, Basile VS, Meltzer HY, et al. Serotonin subtype 2 receptor genes and clinical response to clozapine in schizophrenia patients. Neuropsychopharmacology 1998;19:123–32.

64. Lappalainen J, Zhang L, Dean M, et al. Identification, expression, and pharmacology of Cys_{23}-Ser_{23} substitution in the human 5-HT_{2C} receptor gene (HTR2C). Genomics 1995;27:274–9.

65. Sodhi MS, Arranz MJ, Curtis D, et al. Association between clozapine response and allelic variation in the 5-HT2c receptor gene. Neuroreport 1995;7:169–72.

66. Rietschel M, Naber D, Fimmers R, Moller HR, Proppiing P, Nothen MM. Efficacy and side effects of clozapine not associated with variation in the 5-HT2c receptor. Neuroreport 1997;8:1999–2003.

67. Masellis M, Basile VS, Meltzer HY, et al. Lack of association between the T→C267 serotonin 5-HT6 receptor gene (HTR6) polymorphism and prediction of response to clozapine in schizophrenia. Schizopr Res 2001;47:49–58.

68. Arranz MJ, Munro J, Birkett J, et al. Pharmacogenetic prediction of clozapine response. Lancet 2000;355:1615–6.

69. Birkett JR, Arranz MH, Munro J, Osborne S, Kerwin RW, Collier DA. Association analysis of the 5-HT2A gene in depression, psychosis, and antipsychotic response. Neuroreport 2000;11:2017–20.

70. Yu YW, Tsai SJ, Lin CH, Hsu CP, Yang KH, Hong CJ. Serotonin-6 receptor variant (C267T) and clinical response to clozapine. Neuroreport 1999;10:1231–3.

71. Arranz MJ, Molonna AA, Munro J, Curtis CJ, Collier DA, Kerwin RW. The serotonin transporter and clozapine response. Mol Psychiatry 2000;5:124–5.

72. Arranz MJ, Li T, Munro J, et al. Lack of association between a polymorphism in the promoter region of the dopamine-2 receptor gene and clozapine response. Pharmacogenetics 1998;8:481–4.

73. Shaikh S, Collier DA, Sham P, et al. Analysis of clozapine response and polymorphisms of the dopamine D4 receptor gene (DRD4) in schizophrenic patients. Am J Med Genet 1995;60:541–5.

74. Shaikh S, Collier DA, Sham PC, et al. Allelic association between a Ser-9-Gly polymorphism in dopamine D3 receptor gene and schizophrenia. Hum Genet 1996;97:714–9.

75. Malhotra AK, Goldman D, Buchanan RW, et al. The dopamine D3 receptor (DRD3) Ser9Gly polymorphism and schizophrenia: a haplotypes relative risk study and association with clozapine response. Mol Psychiatry 1998;3:72–5.

76. Rao PA, Pickar D, Gejman PV, Ram A, Gershon ES, Gelernter J. Allelic variation in the D4 dopamine receptor (DRD4) gene does not predict response to clozapine. Arch Gen Psychiatry 1994;51:912–7.

77. Rietschel M, Naber D, Oberlander H, et al. Efficacy and side effects of clozapine: testing for association with allelic variation in the dopamine D4 receptor gene. Neuropsychopharmacology 1996;15:491–6.

78. Kohn Y, Ebstein RP, Heresco-Levy U, et al. Dopamine D4 receptor gene polymorphisms: relation to ethnicity, no association with schizophrenia and response to clozapine in Israeli subjects. Eur Neuropsychopharamcol 1997;7:39–43.

79. Ellingrod VL, Perry PJ, Lund BL, et al. 5-HT2A and 5-HT2C receptor polymorphism responsible for predicting clinical response to the antipsychotic agent olanzapine. J Clin Psychopharmacol 2002;22:554–60.

80. Mancama D, Arranz MJ, Munro J, Makoff A, Kerwin R. The histamine H1 and histamine H2 genes: candidates for schizophrenia and clozapine drug response. GeneScreen 2000;1:29–34.

81. Bolonna AA, Arranz MJ, Munro J, et al. No influence of adrenergic receptor polymorphism on schizophrenia and antipsychotic response. Neurosci Lett 2000;280:65–8.

82. Fang J, Gorrod JW. Metabolism, pharmacogenetics, and metabolic drug-drug interactions of antipsychotic drugs. Cell Mol Neurobiol 1999;19:419–510.

83. Nelson DR, Koymans L, Kamataki T, et al. P450 superfamily: update on new sequences, gene mapping, accession numbers and nomenclature. Pharmacogenetics 1996;6:1–42.

84. Raunio H, Pasanen M, Maenpaa J, Kakkola J, Peklonen O. Expression of extrahepatic cytochrome p450 in humans. In: Pacifici GM, Fracchia GN, eds. Advances in drug metabolism in man. Luxembourg: European Commission; 1995:233–88.

85. Gonzalez FJ. The molecular biology of cytochrome P450s. Pharmacol Rev 1990;40:243–88.

86. Fischer V, Vogel B, Maurer G, Tynes PE. The antipsychotic clozapine is metabolized by the polymorphic human microsomal and recombinant cytochrome P450 2D6. J Pharmacol Exp Ther 1992;260:1355–60.

87. Bertilsson L, Carrillo JA, Dahl ML, et al. Clozapine disposition covaries with CYP1A2 activity determined by a caffeine test. Br J Clin Pharmacol 1994;38:471–3.

88. Jerling M, Lindstrom L, Bondesson U, Bertilsson L. Fluvoxamine inhibition and carbamazepine induction of the metabolism of clozapine: evidence from a therapeutic drug monitoring service. Ther Drug Monit 1994;16:368–74.

89. Pirmohamed M, William D, Madden S, Templeton E, Park BK. Metabolism and bioactivation of clozapine by human liver in vitro. J Pharmacol Exp Ther 1995;272:984–90.

90. Fang J, Coutts RT, Mckenna KF, Baker GB. Elucidation of individual cytochrome P450 enzymes involved in the metabolism of clozapine. Naunyn Schmiedebergs Arch Pharmacol 1998;358:592–9.

91. Shader RI, Greenblatt DJ. Clozapine and fluvoxamine, a curious complexity. J Clin Psychopharmacol 1998;18:101–2.

92. Linnett K, Olesen OV. Metabolism of clozapine by cDNA-expressed human cytochrome P450 enzymes. Drug Metab Dispos 1997;25:1379–82.

93. Eiermann B, Engle G, Johnsson I, Zanger UM, Bertilsson L. The involvement of CYP1A2 and CYP2A4 in the metabolism of clozapine. Br J Clin Pharmacol 1997;44:439–46.

94. Raaska K, Neuvonen PJ. Serum concentrations of clozapine and N-desmethylclozapine are unaffected by the potent CYP3A4 inhibitor itraconazole. Eur J Clin Pharmacol 1998;54:167–70.

95. Ring BJ, Catlow J, Lindsay TJ, et al. Identification of human cytochrome P450 responsible for the in vitro formation of the major oxidative metabolite of the antipsychotic agent olanzapine in humans. J Pharmacol Exp Ther 1996;276:658–66.

96. Kassahun K, Mattiuz E, Nyhart E Jr, et al. Disposition and biotransformation of the antipsychotic agent olanzapine in humans. Drug Metab Dispos 1997;25:81–93.

97. Mannens G, Huang ML, Meuldermans W, Hendrickx J, Woestenborghs R, Heykants J. Absorption, metabolism, and excretion of risperidone in humans. Drug Metab Dispos 1993;21:1134–41.

98. Fang J, Bourin M, Baker GB. Metabolism of risperidone to 9-hydroxyrisperidone by human cytochromes P450 2D6 and 3A4. Naunyn Schmiedebergs Arch Pharmacol 1999;359:147–51.

99. Grimm SW, Stams KR, Bui K. In vitro prediction of potential metabolic drug interactions for seroquel. Schizophr Res 1997;24:198. Abstract.

100. Shen WW. The metabolism of atypical antipsychotic drugs: an update. Ann Clin Psychiatry 1999;11:145–58.

101. Prakash C, Kamel A, Cui D, Whalen RD, Miceli JJ, Tweedie D. Identification of the major liver cytochrome P450 isoform(s) responsible for the formation of the primary metabolites of ziprasidone and prediction of possible drug interaction. Br J Clin Pharmacol 2000;49(Suppl 1):35S–42S.

102. Prior TI, Baker GB. Interactions between the cytochrome P450 system and the second-generation antipsychotics. J Psychiatry Neurosci 2003;28:99–112.

103. Bowles TM, Levin GM. Aripiprazole: a new atypical antipsychotic drug. Ann Pharmacother 2003;37:687–94.

104. Bender S, Eap CB. Very high cytochrome P4501A2 activity and nonresponse to clozapine. Arch Gen Psychiatry 1998;55:1048–50.

105. Sachse C, Brockmoller J, Bauer S, Roots I. Functional significance of a C-->A polymorphism in intron 1 of the cytochrome P450 CYP1A2 gene tested with caffeine. Br J Clin Pharmacol 1999;47:445–9.

106. Nakajima M, Yokoi T, Mizutani M, Kinoshita M, Funayama M, Kamataki T. Genetic polymorphism of the 5'-flanking region of the human CYP1A2 gene: effect on the CYP1A2 inducibility in humans. J Biochem 1999;125:803–8.

107. Masellis M, Basile VS, Macciardi FM, et al. Genetic prediction of antipsychotic response following switch from typical antipsychotics to clozapine. In: XXIst Collegium Internationale Neuro Psychopharmacologicum (CINP) Congress. Glasgow, Scotland: 1998.

108. Hagg S, Spigest O, Lakso HA, Dahlqvist R. Olanzapine disposition in humans in unrelated to CYP1A2 and CYP2D6 phenotypes. Eur J Clin Pharmacol 2001;57:493–7.

109. Umbricht D, Kane JM. Medical complications of new antipsychotic drugs. Schizophr Bull 1996;22:475–83.

110. Lamberti JS, Bellnier T, Schwarzkopf SB. Weight gain among schizophrenic patients treated with clozapine. Am J Psychiatry 1992;149:689–90.

111. Umbricht DSG, Pollack S, Kane JM. Clozapine and weight gain. J Clin Psychiatry 1994;55(suppl B):157–60.

112. Wirshing DA, Wirshing WC, Kysar L, et al. Novel antipsychotics: comparison of weight gain liabilities. J Clin Psychiatry 1999;60:358–63.

113. Allison DB, Mentore JL, Moonseon H, et al. Antipsychotic-induced weight gain: a comprehensive research synthesis. Am J Psychiatry 1999;156:1686–96.

114. Berken GH, Weinstein Do, Stern WC. Weight gain: a side effect of tricyclic antidepressants. J Affect Disord 1984;7:133–8.

115. Bernstein JC. Psychotropic drug induced weight gain: mechanisms and management (review). Clin Neuropharmacol 1988;11(suppl 1):5194–206.

116 Weiden P, Mackel J, McDonnell DD. Obesity as a risk factor for antipsychotic noncompliance (abstract). Presented at the 40th New Clinical Drug Evaluation Unit Annual Meeting; May 30–June 2, 2000; Boca Raton, FL.

117. Basile VS, Masellis M, McIntrye RS, Meltzer HY, Lieberman JA, Kennedy JL. Genetic dissection of atypical antipsychotic-induced weight gain: novel preliminary data on the pharmacogenetic puzzle. J Clin Psychiatry 2001;62(suppl 23):45–66.

118. Yuan X, Yamada K, Ishiyama-Shigemoto S, Koyama W, Nonaka K. Identification of polymorphic loci in the promoter region of the serotonin 5-HT2C receptor gene and their association with obesity and type II diabetes. Diabetologia 2000;43:373–6.

119. Shih JC, Zhu Q, Chen K. Determination of transcription initiation sites and promoter activity of the human 5-HT2A receptor gene. Behav Brain Res 1996;73:59–62.

120. Reynolds GP, Zhang AJ, Zhang XB. Association of antipsychotic drug-induced weight gain with a 5-HT2C receptor gene polymorphism. Lancet 2002;359:2086–7.

121. Ellingrod VL, Miller DD, Schultz SK, Wehring H, Arndt S. CYP2D6 polymorphisms and atypical antipsychotic weight gain. Psychiatr Genet 2002;12:555–81.

122. Ellingrod VL, Perry PJ, Ringold JC, et al. Weight gain associated with the -759 C/T polymorphism of the 5-HT2C receptor and olanzapine. Am J Med Genet. In Press.

123. Casey DE, Hansen TE. Spontaneous dyskinesia. In: Jeste DV, Wyatt RJ, eds. Neuropsychiatric movement disorders. Washington, D.C.: American Psychiatric Press; 1984:68–95.

124. Tarsey D, Baldessarini RJ. The pathophysiologic basis of tardive dyskinesia. Biol Psychiatry 1977;12:431–50.

125. Mueller DJ, Ahle G, Alfter D, et al. Familiar occurrence of tardive dyskinesia. In: 6th World Congress on Psychiatric Genetics. Bonn, Germany; 1988.

126. O'Callaghan E, Larkin C, Kinsella A, Waddington JL. Obstetric complications, the putative familial-sporadic distinction and tardive dyskinesia in schizophrenia. Br J Psychiatry 1990;157:578–84.

127. Kirch DG, Alho AM, Wyatt RJ. Hypothesis: a nicotine-dopamine interaction linking smoking with Parkinson's disease and tardive dyskinesia. Cell Mol Neurobiol 1988;8:285–90.

128. Yassa R, Lal S, Korpassy A, Ally J. Nicotine exposure and tardive dyskinesia. Biol Psychiatry 1987;22:67–72.

129. Lannfelt L, Sokoloff P, Martres MP, et al. Amino acid substitution in the dopamine D3 receptor as a useful polymorphism for investigating psychiatric disorders. Psychiatr Genet 1993;2:249–56.

130. Steen VM, Lovelie R, MacEwan T, McCreadie RG. Dopamine D3 receptor gene variant and susceptibility to tardive dyskinesia in schizophrenic patients. Mol Psychiatry 1997;21:139–45.

131. Segman R, Neeman T, Heresco-Levy U, et al. Genotypic association between the dopamine D3 receptor gene and tardive dyskinesia in chronic schizophrenia. Mol Psychiatry 1999;4:247–53.

132. Basile VS, Masellis M, Badri F, et al. Association of the *MciI* polymorphism of the dopamine D3 receptor gene with tardive dyskinesia in schizophrenia. Neuropsychopharmacology 1999;21:17–27.

133. Lovlic R, Daly AK, Blennerhassett R, Ferrier N, Steen VM. Homozygosity for Gly-9 variant of the dopamine D3 receptor and risk for tardive dyskinesia in schizophrenia patients. Int J Neuropsychopharmacology 2000;3:61–6.

134. Rietschel M, Krauss H, Muller DJ, et al. Dopamine D3 receptor variant and tardive dyskinesia. Eur Arch Psychiatry Clin Neurosci 2000;250:31–5.

135. Lerer B, Segman RH, Fangerau H, et al. Pharmacogenetics of tardive dyskinesia: combined analysis of 780 patients supports association with dopamine D3 receptor gene Ser9Gly polymorphism. Neuropsychopharmacology 2002;27:105–19.

136. Chen CH, Wei FU, Koong FJ, Hsiao KJ. Association of the *Taq-I* A polymorphism of dopamine D2 receptor gene and tardive dyskinesia in schizophrenia. Biol Psychiatry 1997;41:827–9.

137. Segman RH, Heresco-Levy U, Finkel B, et al. Association between the serotonin 2A receptor gene and tardive dyskinesia in chronic schizophrenia. Mol Psychiatry 2001;6:225–9.

138. Tan EC, Chong SA, Mahendran R, Dong F, Tan CH. Susceptibility to neuroleptic-induced tardive dyskinesia and the T102C polymorphism in the serotonin type 2A receptor. Biol Psychiatry 2001;50:144–7.

139. Basile VS, Ozdemir V, Masellis M, et al. Lack of association between serotonin-2A receptor gene (5-HTR2A) polymorphisms and tardive dyskinesia in schizophrenia. Mol Psychiatry 2000;6:230–4.

140. Segman RH, Heresco-Levy U, Finkel B, et al. Association between the serotonin 2C receptor gene and tardive dyskinesia in chronic schizophrenia: additive contribution of the 5-HT2Cser and DRD3gly to susceptibility. Psychopharmacology (Berl) 2000;152:408–13.

141. Chong SA, Tan EC, Tan CH, Mahendren R, Tay AH, Chua HC. Tardive dyskinesia is not associated with the serotonin gene polymorphism (5-HTTLPR) in Chinese. Am J Med Genet 2000;96:712–5.

142. Basile VS, Ozdemir V, Masellis M, et al. A functional polymorphism of the cytochrome P450 1A2 (CYP1A2) gene: association with tardive dyskinesia in schizophrenia. Mol Psychiatry 2000;4:410–7.

143. Ellingrod VL, Schultz SK, Arndt SA. Cigarette smoking, CYP2D6, and abnormal movements. Pharmacotherapy 2002;22(11):1416–9.

144. Arthur H, Dahl ML, Siwers B, Sjoqvist F. Polymorphic drug metabolism in schizophrenic patients with tardive dyskinesia. J Clin Psychopharmacol 1995;15:211–6.

145. Armstrong M, Daly AK, Blennerhassett R, Ferrier N, Idle JR. Antipsychotic drug-induced movement disorders in schizophrenics in relation to CYP2D6 genotype. Br J Psychiatry 1997;170:23–6.

146. Andreasen OA, MacDwan T, Gulbandsen AK, McCreadie RG, Steen VM. Non-functional CYP2D6 alleles and risk for neuroleptic-induced movement disorders in schizophrenic patients. Psychopharmacology (Berl) 1997;131:174–9.

147. Ohmori O, Kojima H, Shinkai T, Terao T, Suzuki T, Abe K. Genetic association analysis between CYP2D6*2 allele and tardive dyskinesia in schizophrenic patients. Psychiatr Res 1999;87:239–44.

148. Lee NM, Smith AP. Opioid receptor polymorphisms and opioid abuse. Pharmacogenomics 2002;3:219–27.

149. Mogil JS. The genetic mediation of individual differences in sensitivity to pain and its inhibition. Proc Natl Acad Sci U S A 1999;6:7744–51.

150. Bond C, LaForge KS, Tian M, et al. Single nucleotide polymorphism in the human mu opioid receptor gene alters beta-endorphin binding and activity: possible implications for opiate addiction. Proc Natl Acad Sci U S A 1998;95:9608–13.

151. Szeto CY, Tang NL, Lee DT, et al. Association between mu opioid receptor gene polymorphism and Chinese heroin addicts. Neuroreport 2001;12:1103–6.

152. Gelernter J, Kranzler H, Cubells J. Genetics of two mu opioid receptor gene (OPRM1) exon 1 polymorphisms: population studies, and allele frequencies in alcohol- and drug-dependent subjects. Mol Psychiatry 1999;4:476–83.

153. Franke P, Nothen MM, Wang T, et al. DRD4 exon III VNTR polymorphism-susceptibility factor for heroin dependence? Results of a case-control and family based association approach. Mol Psychiatry 2000;5:101–4.

154. Hoehe M, Kopke K, Wendel B, et al. Sequence variability and candidate gene analysis in complex disease: association of the mu opioid gene variation with substance dependence. Hum Mol Genet 2000;9:2895–908.

155. Mayer P, Rochlitz H, Rauch E, et al. Association between a delta opioid receptor gene polymorphism and heroin dependence in man. Neuroreport 1997;8:2547–50.

156. Franke P, Nothen MM, Wang T, et al. Human delta-opioid receptor gene and susceptibility to heroin and alcohol dependence. Am J Med Genet 1999;88:462–4.

157. Duaux E, Gorwood P, Griffon N, et al. Homozygosity at the dopamine D3 receptor gene is associated with opiate dependence. Mol Psychiatry 1998;3:333–6.

158. Kotler M, Cohen H, Kremer L, et al. No association between the serotonin transporter promoter region (5-HTTLPR) and the dopamine D3 receptor (*BalI* D3DR) polymorphisms and heroin addiction. Mol Psychiatry 1999;4:313–4.

159. Li T, Liu X, Zhao J, Hu X, Sham PC, Collier DA. Allelic association analysis of dopamine D2, D3, 5-HT2A and GABA g2 receptors and the serotonin transporter genes with heroin abuse in Chinese subjects. Am J Med Genet 2000;96:520.

160. Gelernter J, Kranzler H, Coccaro E, Seiver L, New A, Mulgrew CL. D4 dopamine-receptor (DRD4) alleles and novelty seeking in substance-dependent, personality-disorder, and case control subjects. Am J Hum Genet 1997;61:1144–52.

161. Tan EC, Yeo BK, Ho BK, Tay AH, Tan CH. Evidence for an association between heroin dependence and a VNTR polymorphism at the serotonin transporter locus. Mol Psychiatry 1999;4:215–7.

162. Tyndale RF, Droll KP, Sellers EM. Genetically deficient CYP2D6 metabolism provides protection against oral opiate dependence. Pharmacogenetics 1997;7:375–9.

163. Fromm MF, Eichelabum M. The pharmacogenetics of human P-glycoprotein. In: Licinio J, Wong ML, eds. Pharmacogenomics. The search for individualized therapies. Germany: Wiley-VCH; 2002:159–78.

164. Lockhart DJ, S Barlow C. Expressing what's on your mind: DNA arrays and the brain. Nat Rev Neurosci 2001;2:63–8.

165. Sandberg R, Yasuda R, Pankratz DG, et al. Regional and strain-specific gene expression mapping in the adult mouse brain. Proc Natl Acad Sci U S A 2000;97:11038–43.

166. Shilling PD, Kelsoe JR. Functional genomics approaches to understanding brain disorders. Pharmacogenomics 2002;3:31–45.

167. Derisi JL, Iyer VR, Brown PO. Exploring the metabolic and genetic control of gene expression on genomic scale. Science 1997;278:680–6.

168. Marton MJ, Derisi JR, Bennett HA, et al. Drug target validation and identification of secondary drug target effects using DNA micro array. Nat Med 1998;4:1293–301.

169. Venter JC, Adams MD, Myers EW, et al. The sequence of the human genome. Science 2001;291:1304–51.

170. Sachidanandam R, Weissman D, Schmidt SC, et al. A map of human genomic sequence variation containing 1.42 million single nucleotide polymorphisms. Nature 2001;409:928–33.

Self-Assessment Questions

1. When looking at the pharmacogenetics of migraine headache, polymorphisms of which one of the following serotonin (5-HT) receptors have been investigated as to their relationship with sumatriptan response?

   A. 5-HT2A.
   B. 5-HT2C.
   C. 5-HT1B.
   D. 5-HT1D.

2. In looking at the effect of apolipoprotein E (ApoE) genotype on response to the acetylcholinesterase inhibitors, which one of the following has not been studied?

   A. Donepezil.
   B. Galantamine.
   C. Tacrine.
   D. Rivastigmine.

3. Which one of the following polymorphic cytochrome P450 (CYP) isoenzymes has a relationship with response to phenytoin?

   A. Cytochrome P450 2D6.
   B. Cytochrome P450 1A2.
   C. Cytochrome P450 2C9.
   D. Cytochrome P450 2E1.

4. Which one of the following best describes the relationship of serotonin transporter (5-HTT) variants to selective serotonin reuptake inhibitor (SSRI) response in major depressive disorders (MDDs)?

   A. The presence of an "s" allele of the serotonin transporter gene promoter region (5-HTTLPR) most consistently correlates with a positive response to SSRI therapy.
   B. The presence of an "l" allele of 5-HTTLPR most consistently correlates with a positive response to SSRI therapy.
   C. The variable nucleotide tandem repeat (VNTR) region of the 5-HTT promoter contains the polymorphisms most studied in SSRI response in patients with MDD.
   D. The 5-HTTLPR genotypes correspond more closely to SSRI adverse effects than they do to clinical response in patients with MDD.

5. Which one of the following best describes the relationship of SLC6A4
    gene variants to SSRI response?

    A. The correlation of polymorphisms of the SLC6A4 gene to SSRI
        response is similar in patients treated for MDD, anxiety disorders,
        obsessive-compulsive disorder, and eating disorders.
    B. The correlation of polymorphisms of the SLC6A4 gene to SSRI
        response is similar in patients of different ethnic backgrounds.
    C. Variations in the SLC6A4 gene are more useful in predicting drug
        interactions than they are for predicting response to SSRIs.
    D. There are studies showing that SLC6A4 genotype affects both
        magnitude of SSRI response and time to clinical response to SSRIs
        in patients with MDD.

6. Which one of the following pieces of information is most useful in
    assessing the potential for a drug-drug interaction in a patient taking
    fluoxetine for MDD?

    A. 5-HTTLPR genotype.
    B. Cytochrome P450 2D6 genotype.
    C. SLC6A4 VNTR genotype.
    D. Cytochrome P450 3A4 genotype.

7. Which one of the following alleles of the 5-HT2A receptor has been
    linked to clozapine response in schizophrenia?

    A. T102C.
    B. His452Tyr.
    C. Thr25Asn.
    D. T516C.

8. Which one of the following polymorphic CYP isoenzyme has a
    relationship with the induction of olanzapine's metabolism due to
    cigarette smoking?

    A. Cytochrome P450 2D6.
    B. Cytochrome P450 1A2.
    C. Cytochrome P450 2C9.
    D. Cytochrome P450 3A4.

9. For which one of the following polymorphisms does the strongest
    evidence regarding weight gain from atypical antipsychotics exist?

    A. Dopamine 3 receptor.
    B. Dopamine 4 receptor.
    C. 5-HTTLPR.
    D. 5-HT2C receptor.

10. The occurrence of tardive dyskinesia and abnormal movements because of antipsychotic drug use has been associated with which one of the following polymorphic receptors?

A. 5-HTC.
B. 5-HT2A.
C. Gamma aminobutyric acid.
D. Dopamine 4 receptor.

11. Polymorphisms of which one of the following opioid receptors have been associated with opioid dependence?

A. Mu.
B. Delta.
C. Kappa.
D. Sigma.

12. Which one of the following statements about P-glycoprotein (Pgp) is true?

A. High expression of Pgp in the central nervous system (CNS) results in high concentrations of Pgp substrates.
B. There are more than 19 clinically significant polymorphism of Pgp.
C. No relationship between polymorphism of the Pgp and CNS drugs has been found.
D. P-glycoprotein is only found in the blood-brain barrier.

13. Which one of the following explains why deoxyribonucleic acid (DNA) microarrays are a powerful technique for pharmacogenetic research?

A They are faster than other currently available genetic techniques.
B. They allow investigation of thousands of genes simultaneously.
C. They are easy to manipulate in the laboratory.
D. They do not require a lot of DNA and so these assays can be done on relatively small amounts of sample.

Respiratory Diseases

John J. Lima, Pharm.D.
Jianwei Wang, M.D.

Key Words

Asthma, chronic obstructive pulmonary disease (COPD), pharmacogenetics, polymorphisms, single nucleotide polymorphism (SNP), genotype, linkage disequilibrium, haplotype, and response variability.

Abstract

Asthma is a chronic, complex inflammatory disease that is associated with significant mortality and morbidity. Inhaled corticosteroids, leukotriene receptor antagonists (LTRAs) and long-acting β_2 adrenergic receptor (β_2 AR) agonists are used to control asthma symptoms. As many as 30–60 percent of patients with asthma fail to adequately respond to drug treatment, which is thought to be largely because of genetic variability. Numerous mutations in candidate genes encoding proteins that mediate response to inhaled corticosteroids and LTRAs have been identified but few have been associated with contributing to the interpatient variability in response to these drugs. Many studies have reported that several single nucleotide polymorphisms (SNPs) in the β_2 AR gene influence bronchodilator response to albuterol with conflicting results. Several β_2 AR polymorphisms are in tight linkage disequilibrium resulting in three or four common haplotypes, which associate better with bronchodilator response, compared to SNPs. The influence of β_2 AR haplotype on control of asthma symptoms evoked by long-acting beta agonists (LABAs) is less certain and requires more study. Several obstacles currently prevent the use of genetic information to individualize the drug treatment of asthma.

Chronic obstructive pulmonary disease (COPD) is a complex disease characterized by airflow obstruction because of chronic bronchitis or emphysema. Prevalence rates are increasing at an alarming rate worldwide partly because of increased rates of cigarette smoking. Cigarette smoking is the cause of COPD in 90 percent of patients with the disease. Yet only 15 percent of smokers get the disease, indicating a genetic component. Numerous candidate genes have been associated with COPD. Smoking cessation is the most effective way to reduce the progressive loss of lung function. Nicotine is the most addictive agent in cigarette smoking. Cytochrome P450 (CYP) 2A6 metabolizes 80 percent of nicotine to cotinine. Genetic variation in CYP2A6, CYP2D6, and dopaminergic pathways are thought to contribute to variability in cigarette consumption. Whether genetic variation contributes to variability in response to nicotine replacement requires study. Bronchodilators, including inhaled β_2 agonists, are central in the drug therapy of COPD. It is not clear if β_2 AR gene variants influence the bronchodilator response to short-acting beta agonists and LABAs. The contribution of genetic variants to interpatient variability in response requires extensive study.

Outline

Learning Objectives

1. Compare and contrast asthma and chronic obstructive pulmonary disease (COPD) symptoms and epidemiology.
2. List the drugs that are used to treat asthma and COPD symptoms and briefly describe mechanisms underlying the action of each drug class.
3. Briefly describe how the following polymorphisms influence response to montelukast or salmeterol: Sp-1 tandem repeats in 5-lipoxygenase (5-LO) gene; leukotriene C_4 synthase (LTC_4S) A-444→C single nucleotide polymorphism (SNP); the following β_2 receptor SNPs: cysteine (Cys)-19→arginine (Arg); glycine (Gly)16 Arg.
4. Explain the pharmacogenetic basis of the unimodal pattern of response to inhaled beclomethasone and montelukast.
5. List all possible haplotypes of β_2 receptor SNPs: Cys-19→Arg; Gly16→Arg; glutamine (Gln)27→glutamate (Glu)28, and briefly explain why only three haplotypes are common.
6. Assuming that the results of recombinant studies are correct, sketch the curves describing the relationship between response (percentage of change in forced expiratory volume in 1 second [FEV_1] over baseline) versus isoproterenol dose in individuals carrying the following genetic variants:
   - Gly16 homozygotes versus Arg16/Arg16 homozygotes;
   - Threonine (Thr)164 homozygotes versus Thr164/Iso164 heterozygotes.
7. Briefly describe a clinical trial that will advance β_2 receptor agonist pharmacogenetics to the clinic.
8. List and explain at least three pharmacogenetic interventions that would lead to alterations in cigarette smoking rates.

Abbreviations in this Chapter

β_2 AR	β_2 Adrenergic receptor
5-HPETE	5-hydroperoxyeicosatetraenoic
5-LO	5-Lipoxygenase
AAT	α-1-Antitrypsin
Ala	Alanine
Arg	Arginine
BHR	Bronchial hyperresponsiveness

cAMP	Cyclic adenosine monophosphate
CFTR	Cystic fibrosis transmembrane (conductance) regulator
COMT	Catecholamine-O-methyl transferase
COPD	Chronic obstructive pulmonary disease
CYP	Cytochrome P450
cysLT1R	Cysteinyl leukotriene 1 receptor
DA	Dopamine
DAT	Dopamine transporter
DR	Dopamine receptor
DZ	Dizygotic
FEV_1	Forced expiratory volume in one second
FVC	Forced vital capacity
GC	Glucocorticoid
Gln	Glutamine
Glu	Glutamate
Gly	Glycine
GM-CSF	Granulocyte-macrophage colony-stimulating factor)
GOLD	Global initiative for chronic obstructive lung disease
GRE	Glucocorticoid response element
GRK	G protein receptor kinase
G_S	Guanine stimulatory
ICS	Inhaled corticosteroid
IL	Interleukin
Ile	Isoleucine
LABA	Long-acting beta agonist
Leu	Leucine
LTA_4	Leukotriene A_4
LTA_4H	Leukotriene A_4 hydrolase
LTC_4S	Leukotriene C_4 synthase
LTRA	Leukotriene receptor antagonist
MAO	Monoamine oxidase
Met	Methionine
MMP	Matrix metalloproteinase
MRP	Multidrug resistance protein
MZ	Monozygotic
NOS	Nitric oxide synthase
PharmGKB	Pharmacogenetics knowledge base
PI	Protease inhibitor
PKA	Protein kinase A
SMART	Salmeterol Multicenter Asthma Research Trial
SNP	Single nucleotide polymorphism
TGF	Transforming growth factor
TH	Tyrosine hydroxylase
Thr	Threonine

TIMP   Tissue inhibitor of MMP
Val   Valine

Introduction

Asthma is a chronic inflammatory disease of the airways that is caused by a complex interaction between genetic and environmental factors. In the United States, more than 11 million individuals reported having at least one attack of asthma in 2002, and the number of people with asthma is expected rise to 29 million by 2020. The most common drugs used to control asthma symptoms fall into three pharmacological classes: inhaled corticosteroids (ICSs), leukotriene receptor antagonists (LTRAs) and long-acting β_2 adrenergic receptor (β_2 AR) agonists. Short-acting β_2 AR agonists are used as rescue drugs to provide rapid bronchodilation. Although effective, none of the drugs achieves a high degree of asthma control in all patients with asthma. Rather, response to drug therapy varies considerably. Genetic variability is thought to contribute to up to 80 percent of the interpatient variability in response. Knowledge of sequence variants that contribute to variability in response is important because it can lead to individualization of drug treatment according to genetic makeup and it can help enhance the understanding of drug targets, which can lead to the discovery of novel drugs.

In this chapter, the epidemiology and genetics of asthma and current treatment guidelines are reviewed. Next, the pharmacology of ICSs and LTRAs are reviewed, the interpatient variability in response to these drugs is discussed, and their pharmacogenetics is reviewed. The pharmacology and pharmacogenetics of short-acting β_2 agonists and long-acting beta agonist (LABAs) are summarized, and the obstacles that prevent the current use of genetic information in therapeutic decision-making are discussed.

A similar approach was adopted to chronic obstructive pulmonary disease (COPD), beginning with a review of epidemiology and genetics. Many of the drugs used in asthma are used to treat COPD. Yet, the degree of interpatient variability in response to drug treatment is not clear, and there are few, if any, pharmacogenetic studies performed in patients with COPD. Whether the available information from pharmacogenetic studies of asthma can be applied to COPD is not clear. Given the rising mortality and morbidity rates of COPD worldwide and the importance of drug therapy in improving the quality of life in afflicted patients, it is important in future studies to explore associations between genetic variation and drug-evoked outcomes in this patient population. Finally, the pharmacogenetics of nicotine is reviewed because of the role nicotine addiction plays in cigarette smoking.

It is important that the reader understand that the study of asthma (and possibly COPD) pharmacogenetics can be viewed a paradigm for the study of drug target pharmacogenetics. It appears that much of the interpatient variability in response to drugs currently used to treat asthma is because of sequence variants in drug targets and not drug metabolizing enzymes. (This does not rule out the possibility that existing or newly developed drugs for asthma may be substrates for one or more polymorphic drug metabolizing enzymes, which would contribute further to interpatient variability in response.) And unlike classical drug metabolism pharmacogenetics, polymorphisms in single drug target genes probably do not result in large differences in response. This may be related to the idea that one or more sequence variants in *multiple* genes encoding numerous proteins that mediate response to asthma drugs contributes to response variability.

Asthma

Epidemiology

Asthma is a chronic inflammatory disease characterized by airflow obstruction, recurrent bronchoconstriction of airways, and hyperresponsiveness to provocative stimuli (Reference 3). The pathophysiology of asthma has been reviewed elsewhere (References 4, 5) and is not covered herein. In the United States, more than 11 million individuals reported having at least one attack of asthma in 2002, and the number of people with asthma is expected rise to 29 million by 2020 (Reference 6). In 1999, asthma was responsible for 2 million emergency department visits, 478,000 hospitalizations, and 4426 deaths. The cost of asthma in 1998 was estimated to be $11.3 billion. Asthma mortality is almost 3 times higher in African Americans compared to Caucasians.

In preschool children, asthma prevalence increased 160 percent since 1980, resulting in more than 10 million missed school days per year. It is the No. 1 cause of hospitalizations and emergency department visits in children, and more than 5 percent of all children younger than 18 years of age reported having asthma (Reference 3). Although the specific etiology of asthma is not clear, the disease is thought to be multifactorial, involving complex interactions between environmental triggers and several genes (Reference 7).

Given the significant morbidity and mortality of asthma, and the fact that asthma occurrence is expected to increase worldwide (Reference 8), it is important to develop strategies that can safely and effectively control symptoms, minimize exacerbations, and improve the quality of life in patients with asthma. Currently, ICSs and LTRAs are used alone (monotherapy) or in combination with LABAs to manage asthma pharmacologically. The goals of therapy are to prevent and control asthma symptoms, reduce the frequency and severity of asthma exacerbations, reverse airflow obstruction, and prevent or reduce smooth cellular proliferation (Reference 3).

Asthma Genetics

Numerous candidate genes have been linked to asthma. The most investigated candidate location for asthma susceptibility has been the 5q31-5q33 region (Reference 9). Genes encoding interleukin (IL)-4, IL-5, IL-9, IL-13, and their receptors are located in this region (Reference 10). The granulocyte-macrophage colony-stimulating factor (GM-CSF) and the fibroblast growth factor acidic genes also are located in the region. In addition, the β_2 AR and the glucocorticoid receptor genes are located in 5q31-33 region, which has obvious pharmacogenetic implications. Other regions identified to influence asthma and atopy have been located in regions of chromosomes 4, 6, 11, 12, 13, and 16 (Reference 11).

Current Guidelines for Asthma Treatment

The stepwise pharmacological approach that is used to manage asthma in adults and children is based on asthma severity, daytime and nighttime symptoms, and the results of pulmonary function tests (Reference 3). High-dose ICS is the preferred treatment for mild persistent asthma with daytime symptoms less than once a day but more than twice a week, and with a forced expiratory volume in 1 second (FEV_1) of at least 80 percent. Though ICS monotherapy has been superior to LTRA monotherapy of asthma (References 12-15), LTRA monotherapy may be used in mild persistent asthma, thereby avoiding side effects of ICSs. For moderate and severe persistent asthma with more frequent symptoms and FEV_1 less than 80 percent, low- to high-dose ICSs and a LABA (salmeterol or formoterol) is the preferred treatment, with add-on LTRAs or higher doses of ICSs as alternatives. In general, ICSs combined with a LABA provides better control of asthma compared to ICSs combined with LTRAs (References 16, 17) or LTRA monotherapy (References 18, 19). Current guidelines do not recommend monotherapy with LABAs for any degree of asthma severity because of safety concerns (see the Long-acting Beta Agonist Use in Asthma section). In addition, short-acting inhaled β_2 agonists are used as bronchodilators in patients with acute asthma, but should not be used chronically to control asthma symptoms (see the β_2 Adrenergic Receptor Agonists section). Cromolyn sodium and nedocromil can be considered for treating persistent asthma, but they are not preferred therapies (Reference 3). Bronchodilator doses of theophylline are not used extensively for long-term control because of the risk of adverse events and the need for serum concentration monitoring. However, there is evidence to suggest that low-dose, sustained-release theophylline (300 mg/day) may have anti-inflammatory effects and may be beneficial as monotherapy in patients with mild persistent asthma or as add-on therapy in patients with moderate and severe persistent asthma (References 20, 21).

Zileuton, an inhibitor of 5-lipoxygenase (5-LO), is rarely used in this country because of the requirements for dosing 4 times/day and periodic monitoring of liver function test. Most pharmacogenetic studies in asthma have focused on the drugs commonly used in asthma as does this chapter.

Glucocorticoids

Glucocorticoids (GCs) are the most potent anti-inflammatory agents used to treat asthma, and ICSs are recognized as the most effective asthma controllers. Inhaled corticosteroids reduce airway inflammation and asthma symptoms; improve lung function; and reduce nocturnal symptoms, bronchial responsiveness, asthma exacerbations, and oral steroid dependence. They also improve quality of life and reduce hospital and emergency department admissions (References 3, 13, 22-23). Glucocorticoids exert their effects by binding to cytoplasmic GC receptors, which have three major domains: ligand, deoxyribonucleic acid and transcription factor regulatory domains (Figure 1) (Reference 24). The unbound, cytosolic GC receptor is thought to be a heterohexamer containing GC- and deoxyribonucleic acid-binding subunits and several heat shock proteins (Reference 25). There are numerous GC receptor isoforms, which are thought to be responsible for the diversity of GC-mediated responses (Reference 26). Activation results in GC receptor (α isoform) dephosphorylation, dissociation of heat shock proteins, dimerization with a second GC/receptor complex, and exposure of the deoxyribonucleic acid binding site. This is followed by translocation to the nucleus and binding of the GC receptor dimer to GC response elements (GREs) in the promoter region of the gene. This interaction leads to either induction or suppression of gene expression. Administration of GCs profoundly alters the expression of proinflammatory genes (References 1, 27). Proinflammatory genes trigger activation of transcription factors, including AP-1, NF-κB, NFAT, and STAT6, which induce chemoattractants, cytokines, cytokine receptor leukotrienes, and cell adhesion molecules that are involved in eosinophil and other leukocyte recruitment. Glucocorticoids evoke their anti-inflammatory effects directly and indirectly by altering gene transcription and post-transcriptional events. Given the number of proteins involved in signal activation of the GC receptor, signal transduction, and regulation of gene transcription, it is possible that genetic variation in one or several genes encoding these proteins could contribute to the interpatient variation in response to GCs.

Leukotriene Receptor Antagonists

Leukotriene receptor antagonists are thought to be the most innovative approach to asthma therapy in 20 years. They address one specific mechanism underlying inflammation that may not be affected by corticosteroids (Reference 28). Leukotriene receptor antagonists can improve lung function, significantly reduce β_2 agonist use, improve asthma

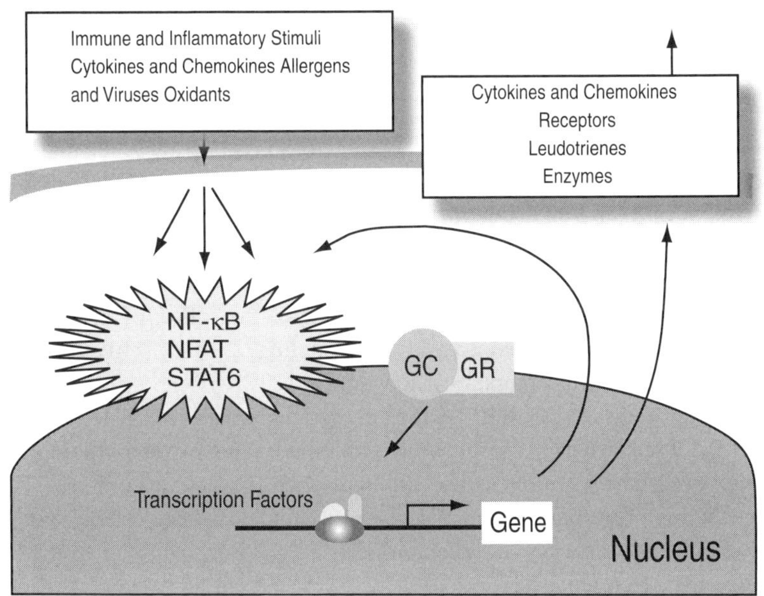

Figure 1. Glucocorticoid (GC) pathway. Glucocorticoids bind to the GC and other receptors where they directly and indirectly alter gene transcription. Polymorphisms in several candidate genes can influence response to GC. Reprinted with permission from Nature Publishing Group. Silverman ES, Liggett SB, Gelfand EW, et al. The pharmacogenetics of asthma: a candidate gene approach. Pharmacogenomics J 2001;1(1):27–37.
GR = glucocorticoid receptor.

symptoms, reduce the use of ICSs, improve quality of life, reduce circulating levels of blood eosinophils, reduce levels of exhaled nitric oxide, and evoke bronchoprotective effects (Reference 29-40). Leukotriene receptor agonists are indicated as an alternative to low-dose ICSs for patients with mild persistent asthma and are recommended as alternative add-on (to ICSs) treatment in patients with moderate persistent (step 3) and severe persistent (step 4) asthma (Reference 41).

Leukotriene receptor antagonists exert their beneficial effects in asthma by binding to the cysteinyl leukotriene receptor 1 (cysLT1R), thereby antagonising the detrimental effects of the cysteinyl leukotrienes in airways (Figure 2). Arachidonic acid is released from cell-membrane phospholipids by the action of phospholipase A_2. Arachidonic acid is converted to 5-hydroperoxyeicosatetraenoic (5-HPETE) and leukotriene A_4 (LTA$_4$) by membrane-bound 5-LO, which is activated by the action of 5-LO-activating protein (Reference 42). In human mast cells, basophils, eosinophils, and macrophages, LTA$_4$ is converted to LTB$_4$ by LTA$_4$ hydrolase (LTA$_4$H), and is conjugated with reduced glutathione by LTC_4 synthase (LTC_4S) to form LTC_4 (References 43, 44). Leukotriene C_4 is transported to the extracellular space by the ABC transport proteins, multidrug resistance protein 1 (MRP1) (Reference 45) and MRP2 (Reference 46).

The affinity of MRP1 for LTC_4 is 10-fold higher compared to MRP2 (Reference 47). In the extracellular space, LTC_4 is converted sequentially to the cysteinyl leukotrienes, LTD_4 and LTE_4 by γ-glutamyltransferase (Reference 48) and dipeptidase (Reference 49), respectively. The cysteinyl leukotrienes (LTC_4, LTD_4, and LTE_4) induce bronchoconstriction, enhance airway hyperresponsiveness and smooth muscle hypertrophy, cause mucus hypersecretion and mucosal edema, and induce the influx of eosinophils into airway tissue (Reference 41) by binding to and activating two G protein-coupled receptors, cysLT1R and cysLT2R (Reference 50). The relative affinities of the cysLT1R for the cys-leukotriene are $LTD_4 \gg LTC_4 > LTE_4$. Leukotriene 1 receptors are expressed in airway smooth muscle, tissue macrophages, monocytes, and eosinophils (Reference 51). The contribution of cys-leukotriene receptors to asthma has been established by the therapeutic efficacy of zileuton (5-LO inhibitor) and the cysLT1R antagonists (Reference 52).

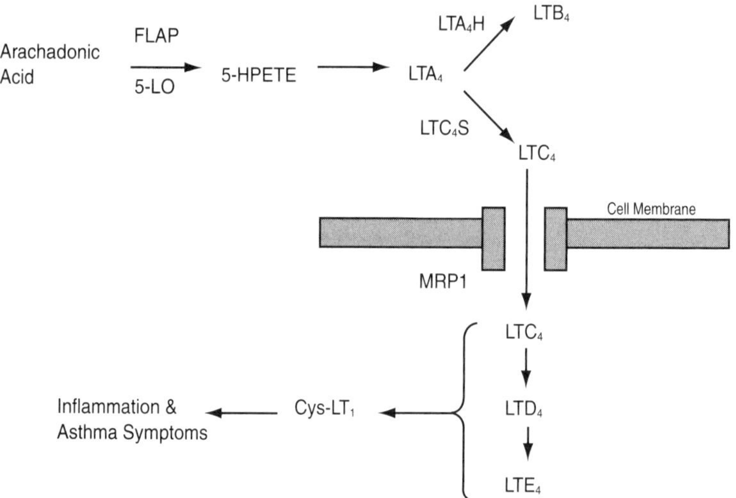

Figure 2. Simplified scheme of the leukotriene pathway, showing the formation and action of the cysteinyl leukotrienes (LTC_4, LTD_4, and LTE_4) and the proposed pharmacogenetic loci: 5-lipoxygenase (5-LO), leukotriene A_4 hydrolase (LTA_4H), LTC_4 synthase, multidrug resistance protein 1 (MRP1) and the cysteinyl leukotriene 1 receptor (Cys-LT_1). 5-HPETE = 5-hydroperoxyeicosatetraenoic.

Interpatient Variability in Response to ICSs and LTRAs

Despite their demonstrated efficacy and extensive use in treating asthma, both ICSs and LTRAs are associated with a significant degree of interpatient variability in response (Figure 3), which can limit their safety, efficacy, and cost-effectiveness (References 1, 12, 22, 53–55). In large clinical trials, 42–44 percent of patients receiving montelukast could be classified as good responders, whereas 34 percent could be classified as nonresponders (References 12, 55). Beclomethasone 200 µg 2 times/day improved FEV_1 by 11 percent or more in 50 percent of the patients, whereas 22 percent did not show improvement (References 12, 55). Thus, with respect to FEV_1 response to inhaled belcomethasone, 50 percent could be classified as good responders, 28 percent as marginal, and 22 percent as nonresponders.

The percentage of patients who were classifed as marginal or nonresponders to 200 µg 2 times/day inhaled beclomethasone (References 12, 55) and would have been classified as good responders had they received higher doses is unknown. From the results of a recent study (Reference 53), it can be inferred that dose rates of 400 µg/day beclomethasone used in other

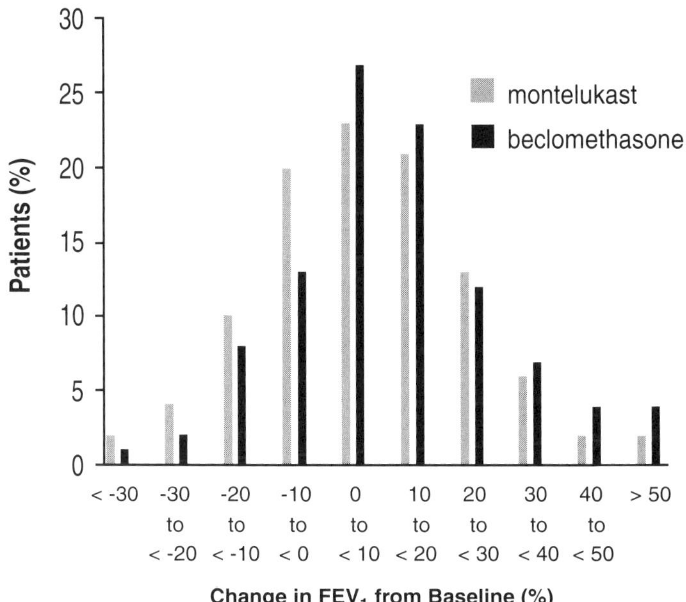

Figure 3. Distribution of treatment responses for FEV_1. Response distributions (% of patients) are shown as histograms for predefined intervals of % change in FEV_1. Shaded bars represent patients treated with montelukast and black bars represent patients treated with beclomethasone. Note wide variation in therapeutic response among patients. Reprinted with permission from Nature Publishing Group. Silverman ES, Liggett SB, Gelfand EW, et al. The pharmacogenetics of asthma: a candidate gene approach. Pharmacogenomics J 2001;1(1):27–37.

studies (References 12, 55) evoked a near maximal FEV_1 response, suggesting that dose rates of beclomethasone more than 400 µg/day would not have significantly changed the proprotion of patients classified as responders or nonresponders.

A small subset of patients with asthma appear to be steroid-resistant. Glucocorticoid-resistant asthma can be defined as the failure to improve baseline morning prebronchodilator FEV_1 more than15 percent following at least 7–14 days of 20 mg 2 times/day oral prednisolone or its equivalent (Reference 1). The mechanism of steroid resistance in asthma is not clear but may involve different expression of the β isoform of the GC receptor. Alternative splicing of the GC receptor pre-messenger ribonucleic acid results in the expression of α and β isoforms, which differ only at their carboxyl termini (Reference 56). In contrast to the α isoform, which functions as a ligand-dependent transcription factor, the β isoform does not bind the GC receptor and does not activate GC-responsive genes. Increased expression of the β isoform has been associated with GC-resistant asthma (References 57–59). Thus, it is possible that a fraction of marginal and nonresponders to beclamethasone (Figure 3) could be GC-resistant. However, because such a small fraction of patients is GC-resistant, this mechanism does not account for 50 percent of patients classified as marginal or nonresponders to beclomethasone (Reference 12).

Pharmacogenetics of ICSs

Given the number of proteins involved in signal activation of the GC receptor, signal transduction, and regulation of gene transcription (Figure 1), it is possible that genetic variation in one or several genes encoding these proteins could contribute to the interpatient variation in response to GCs. The gene encoding the GC receptor is located on chromosome 5q31, contains 10 exons and is 80 kilobases in size (Reference 60). A large number of varying mutations in the GC receptor gene have been identified including missense, nonsense, frameshift, and splice mutations (Reference 60). The pharmacogenetic significance of these mutations in asthma has not been investigated. The Pharmacogenetics of Asthma Treatment (PharmGKB) has genotyped candidate genes in the steroid pathway that might be influencing asthma treatment response to inhaled steroids and identified novel single nucleotide polymorphisms (SNPs), which strongly influenced response to ICSs (S. Weiss, personal communication, 2003). It is possible that these novel SNPs could lead to individualization of anti-inflammatory treatment in asthma according to genetic makeup.

Pharmacogenetics of Inhibitors and Antagonists of the Cys-Leukotriene Pathway

Several polymorphisms in genes that encode proteins in the leukotriene pathway have been identified (Figure 2). Polymorphisms in two genes are known or thought to influence response to leukotriene modifiers. A promoter polymorphism in 5-LO gene on chromosome 10q11.2, which contains 3-6 tandem repeats of the Sp1-binding motif GGGCGG has been linked to reduced response to ABT-761, a selective 5-LO inhibitor similar to zileuton (Reference 2). The average increase in FEV_1 in 64 wild-type (5 tandem Sp-1 repeats on both alleles) patients with asthma was 19 percent, whereas FEV_1 increased by 24 percent in 40 heterozygotes (five repeats on one allele, and 3, 4, or 6 tandem Sp-1 repeats on the other allele). In contrast, 10 patients with the mutant allele (no allele containing 5 tandem Sp-1 repeats) had no response (FEV_1 decreased by 1 percent) (Figure 4). These data established that 5-LO promoter genotype predicts response to ABT-761 and probably to LTRAs. However, the allele associated with diminished or no response to ABT-761 is found in only 6 percent of the population with asthma. Thus, only a small proportion of the interpatient variability to montelukast could be explained by the 5-LO promoter polymorphism.

The LTC_4S gene promoter (A-444C) polymorphism is thought to influence response to LTRAs. Several investigators have (References 61-63) found that response to LTRAs was greater in A/C heterozygotes compared to A/A homozygotes. These data are consistent with theoretical expectations (References 64–66). It is thought that the A-444C polymorphism creates an additional binding site for transcription factors, increasing transcription of LTC_4S, which results in higher

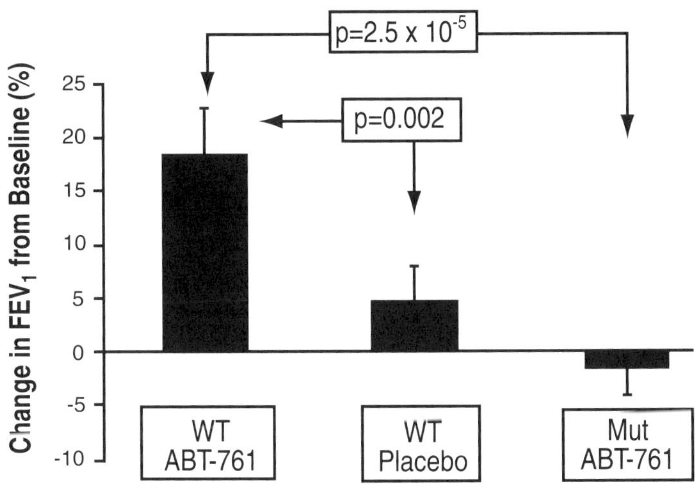

Figure 4. Polymorphism in the 5-LO gene predicts response to ABT-761. Reprinted with permission from Nature Publishing Group. Drazen JM, Yandava CN, Dube L, et al. Pharmacogenetic association between ALOX5 promoter genotype and the response to antiasthma treatment. Nat Genet 1999;22(2):168–70.
5-LO = 5-Lipoxygenase; WT = wild-type.

concentrations of leukotriene and increased inflammation (Reference 66). Therefore, LTRAs would evoke a greater anti-inflammatory effect in carriers of the C allele compared to A/A. To explore the association between response to LTRAs and the A-444C polymorphism, patients with moderate asthma (n=130) who had participated in previous studies were genotyped for the A-444C polymorphism (Reference 67). No associations between the A-444C polymorphism and the effect of montelukast on bronchial challenges by methacholine or adenosine monophosphate were found. However, for patients taking ICSs, carriers of the C allele had a higher FEV_1 response to LTRAs compared to A/A homozygotes (Reference 67). Taken together these data suggest that polymorphisms in the 5-LO and LTC_4S gene contribute to the observed interpatient variability in response to LTRAs. However, the contribution of these polymorphisms to the interpatient variability in response to LTRAs is modest. It is possible that polymorphisms in other leukotriene pathway genes also contribute to variability in response and a combination of polymorphisms in several genes, rather than a single gene, predicts response to LTRAs. Studies are under way to address this hypothesis.

Other Leukotriene Pathway Polymorphisms

Search of the National Center for Biotechnology Information Data Base SNP revealed that there are four polymorphisms in the LTA_4H gene at nucleic acid positions 99, 1377, 1552, and 1826. This gene encodes the enzyme that converts LTA_4 to LTB_4 (Figure 2). Leukotriene C_4 is transported to the extracellular space and converted to LTD_4 and LTE_4. The transport of LTC_4 is accomplished mainly by MRP1. Several polymorphisms in the MRP1 gene have been identified in a Japanese population, including 12 SNPs and four intron polymorphisms that could affect the transport of LTC_4 and, therefore, regulate the production of LTD_4 and LTE_4 and the response evoked by montelukast (Reference 68). The leukotriene 1 receptor is a G protein-coupled receptor that when activated stimulates phospholipase C, which enhances the formation of diacylglycerols and inositol1,4,5-triphophosphate, leading to increased cytosolic calcium (Reference 69). At least five polymorphisms in this gene have been identified. Whether these or other unidentified genetic variants have an important influence on response to LTRAs needs to be explored.

β_2 Adrenergic Receptor Agonists

β_2 Adrenergic receptor agonists exert their pharmacological effects by binding to and activating β_2 AR. β_2 Adrenergic receptors belong to the superfamily of G protein-coupled receptors, and are expressed on membranes in many different cells in the airways (Reference 70) (Figure 5). The β_2 AR spans the cell membrane 7 times; the N-terminus is extracellular, the C-terminus is intracellular (see Figure 6). Activation of β_2 AR initiates a cascade of events, which include dissociation of the α subunit from the guanine stimulatory (G_s)-binding protein and stimulation of adenlyly cyclase by $G_{s\alpha}$ to catalyze the conversion of adenosine triphosphate to cyclic adenosine monophosphate (cAMP). The second messenger, cAMP activates protein kinase A (PKA), which phophorylates several proteins, including myosin light chain kinase, sodium and potassium channels, phospholamban, and certain pumps that increase intracellular calcium uptake. Decreased intracellular calcium and protein phosphorylation of contractile proteins lead to smooth muscle relaxation and bronchodilation (Reference 71). Receptor-mediated function is rapidly desensitized by β_2 AR phosphorylation by PKA (heterologous desensitization) and G protein receptor kinases (GRKs) and arrestin (homologous desensitization), which leads to receptor uncoupling (References 70, 72, 73). Short- or long-term agonist exposure of β_2 AR results in a reduction of receptor density (down-regulation) and long-term desensitization β_2 AR-mediated function (References 72, 74).

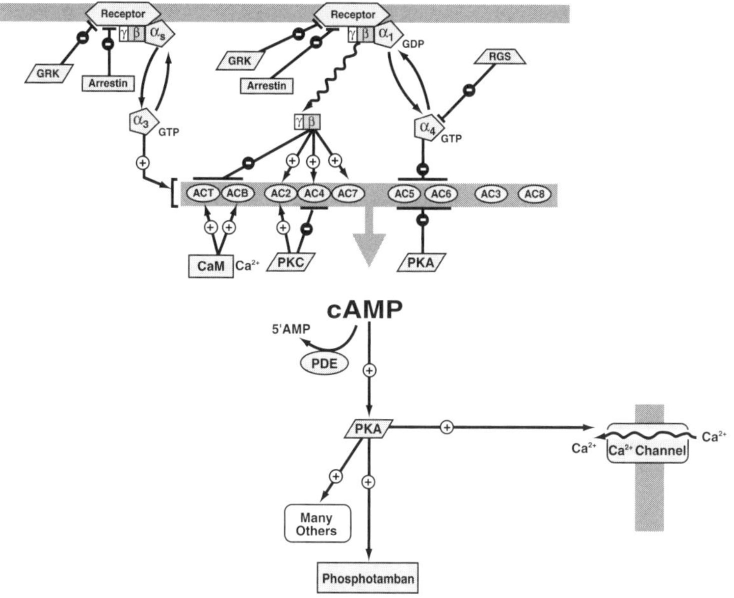

Figure 5. Simplified scheme of G-protein coupled receptors, showing stimulatory and inhibitory pathways. β_2 Agonists evoke their beneficial effects by coupling the β_2 AR and G$_{stimulatory}$ protein followed by dissociation of the α_s (stimulatory) subunit and stimulation of AC to stimulate cAMP. Shown are some proteins encoded by candidate genes that carry SNP, which can influence response to β_2 agonists.
AC = adenylyl cyclase; ACT = actinomycin; AR = agonist receptor; Ca²⁺ = calcium ions; CaM = calmodulin; cAMP = cyclic adenosine monophosphate; GRK = G-protein receptor kinase; PKA = protein kinase A; PKC = protein kinase C; PDE = phosphodiesterase; RGS = regulators of G protein signalling; SNP = single nucleotide polymorphism.

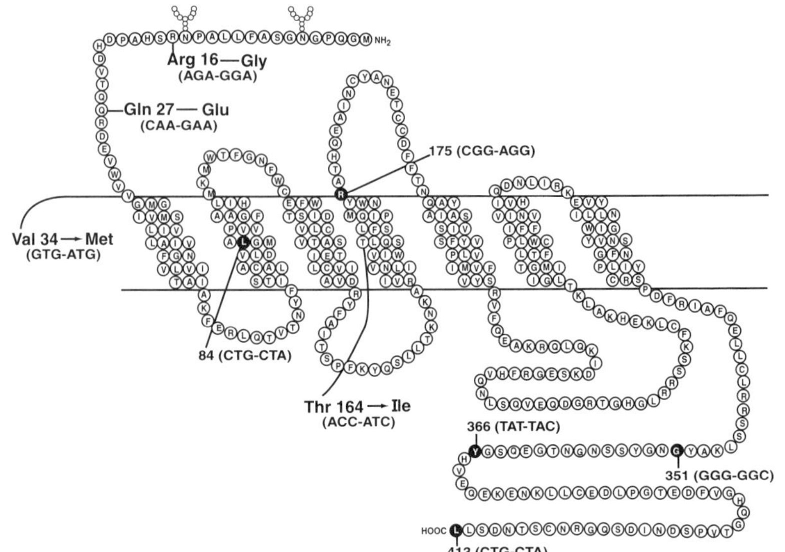

Figure 6. Polymorphisms of the human β₂ adrenergic receptor. Codons with nucleic acid changes are in parentheses; those that result in amino acid changes are indicated. Reprinted with permission from the American Lung Association. Liggett SB. Polymorphisms of the β₂ adrenergic receptor and asthma. Figure titled: Polymorphisms of the Human β₂ AR. In: Am J Respir Crit Care Med 1997;156:S156–62.
Arg = arginine; Gln = glutamine; Glu = glutanate; Gly = glycine; Ile = isoleucine; Met = methionine; Thr = threonine; Val = valine.

β₂ Adrenergic recpetor agonists include short-acting agents (e.g., albuterol and terbutaline), which are used as rescue drugs to treat acute symptoms in asthma, and LABAs (e.g., salmeterol and formoterol), which are used as add-on controllers. Short-acting agonists are not recommended as long-term monotherapy or as add-on controllers because chronic use can mask asthma deterioration.

Long-acting Beta Agonist Use in Asthma

Asthma treatment guidelines recommend that LABAs be added to drug regimens that include ICSs if ICS treatment alone fails to adequately control asthma symptoms (Reference 75). This is because addition of long-acting β₂ AR agonists was more effective in controlling asthma symptoms and improving lung function than doubling the dose of ICSs (References 76, 77). Continuous monotherapy with LABAs is not recommended because salmeterol monotherapy has been associated with higher rates of asthma exacerbations and treatment failures compared to ICSs (Reference 78), although this has not been a universal finding (Reference 79). Also, preliminary results of the Salmeterol Multicenter Asthma Research Trial

(SMART) showed in African Americans a statistically significant greater number of primary events and asthma-related events, including deaths in patients taking salmeterol compared to placebo. In addition, in the total population of patients not receiving ICSs, there was a statistically significant higher number of asthma-related deaths in patients taking salmeterol compared to placebo (Reference 80). Although not specifically studied, these outcomes are expected to apply to formoterol monotherapy.

Salmeterol is a partial agonist, which is thought to evoke its long-acting bronchodilating and bronchoprotective effects by binding to an exosite adjacent to the β_2 AR (Reference 81). Formoterol is a full agonist, which is thought to evoke its long-acting effects by forming stable complexes with the β_2 AR (Reference 82). As a partial agonist, salmeterol can antagonize the effects of other agonists at the β_2 AR, in contrast to the full agonist formoterol. On the other hand, as a full agonist, formoterol can promote agonist-induced tolerance or desensitization (receptor uncoupling and down-regulation) more rapidly and possibly to a greater extent than the partial agonist salmeterol. Theoretical differences between full and partial agonists notwithstanding, the results of head-to-head clinical studies revealed that the onset of action of formoterol is more rapid than salmeterol but that both drugs are comparable with respect to the control of asthma symptoms (References 83, 84–87).

Pharmacogenetics of β_2 Agonists in Asthma

The β_2 AR is probably the most extensively studied pharmacogenetic drug target. This is probably because the gene was one of the first drug targets to be cloned and sequenced (Reference 88), it is highly polymorphic, and several of the polymorphisms have functional significance that occur with common frequencies. The β_2 AR gene is intronless and is located on chromosome 5q31-33. It has 1239 nucleic acid bases, which encode a protein containing 413 amino acids. At least 13 SNPs in the β_2 AR gene have been identified (Reference 89). Four coding region mutations at nucleic acids 46, 79, 100, and 491 are nonsynonymous, resulting in the following amino acid changes: glycine (Gly)16→arginine (Arg), glutamine (Gln)27→glutamate (Glu), valine (Val) 34→methionine (Met) and threonine (Thr)164→isoleucine (Ile), respectively (Figure 6) (Reference 90). The allele frequencies of the Val34→Met and Thr164→Ile SNPs are low, whereas the Gly16→Arg and Gln27→Glu SNPs are common (Table 1). In addition, an open reading frame termed the 5' leader cistron located in the 5' region of receptor transcripts encode a 19-amino acid peptide (β_2 receptor upstream peptide) that reduces translation of messenger ribonucleic acid and regulates receptor expression (Reference 91). A Cys-19 Arg polymorphism has been identified and found to have a high allele frequency (Table 1) (Reference 92).

In addition, SNP at codons -19, 16, 27, and 164 are in tight linkage disequilibrium (References 92, 93) (Table 2). The Cys-19 allele is almost always coupled with Gln27 and the Arg-19 is almost always coupled with Gly16 and Glu27. In a recent study, the Ile164 allele was always coupled with the following SNPs: Cys-19, Gly16, and Gln27. Of the 16 possible haplotypes (combination of SNP), six have been identified and three are common: Cys-19 (C)/Arg16 (R)/Gln27 (Q)/Thr164 (T); Cys-19 (C)/Gly16 (G)/Gln27 (Q)/Thr164 (T); and Arg-19 (R)/Gly16 (G)/Glu27 (E)/Thr164 (T) (Table 2). Significant racial differences in allele frequencies of the common haplotypes have been found (Table 2).

Functional studies in recombinant cells have revealed that SNPs at loci -19, 16, and 27 influence receptor density in an agonist-dependent (References 94, 95) and agonist-independent manner (Reference 92). The -Cys19 allele is associated with a higher receptor density compared to the -Arg19 allele (Reference 92), the Arg16 allele is more resistant to agonist-promoted down-regulation compared to the Gly16 allele, and compared to the Gln27 allele, the Glu27 variant is not down-regulated at all (Reference 94). In contrast to the common SNPs that have functional significance, the Ile164 variant is uncommon (Table 1) and has a lower affinity for epinephrine compared to the wild-type (Reference 96).

Most pharmacogenetic studies of β_2 AR agonists have focused on short-acting agents. It is expected that the consequences of sequence variants on drug response apply equally to both short-acting agents and LABAs and a few studies have been reported (References 97–100). However, more pharmacogenetic studies of add-on LABAs using appropriate asthma-related outcomes are clearly needed (see the Moving Asthma Pharmacogenetics to the Clinic section). Early clinical studies were consistent with functional studies in that bronchodilator and bronchoprotective effects and resistance to desensitization evoked by albuterol were better associated with the Arg16 allele compared to Gly16 allele even if patients were taking ICSs (References 101-03). In contrast, more recent studies report that continuous use of inhaled albuterol is associated with deterioration in morning peak flow (Reference 104) and

Table 1. Distribution of Genotypes (%) at Amino Acid Positions -19, 16, 27, and 164 in 141 African Americans and 335 Caucasians with Physician-diagnosed Asthma

AMINO ACID LOCI											
-19			16			27			164		
Genotype	Race		Genotype	Race		Genotype	Race		Genotype	Race	
	AA	C		AA	C		AA	C		AA	C
Cys-Cys	68.8	36.1	Gly-Gly	28.4	37.9	Gln-Gln	68.8	36.1	Thr-Thr	99.3	97.3
Cys-Arg	28.4	45.7	Gly-Arg	48.2	45.1	Gln-Glu	28.4	45.7	Thr-Ile	0.7	2.67
Arg-Arg	2.8	18.2	Arg-Arg	23.4	17.0	Glu-Glu	2.8	18.2	Ile-Ile	0	0

AA = African Americas; Arg = ; C = Causasians; Cys = cysteine; Gln = glutamine; Glu = glutamate; Gly = glycine; Ile = isoleucine; Thr = threonine.

Table 2. Number and Allele Frequencies of β_2 AR Haplotypes in 143 African Americans and 336 Caucasians

HAPLOTYPE[a]	NUMBER, FREQUENCY (%) of ALLELES	
	AFRICAN AMERICAN	CAUCASIAN
CRQT	135 (47.2)	261 (38.8)
RGET	48 (16.8)	268 (39.9)[b]
CGQT	101 (35.3)	133 (19.8)[b]
CGQI	1 (0.35)	9 (1.34)
RGQT	1 (0.35)	0 (0)
RRQT	0 (0)	1 (0.15)

[a]Four letters refer to the amino acids at positions -19, 16, 27, and 164 of the β_2 AR.
[b]p<0.05, African American vs. Caucasian.
β_2 AR = β_2 adrenergic receptor; C = Cystine; E = Glutamate; G = Glycine; I = Isoleucine; Q = Glutamine; R = Arginine; T = Threonine

increased asthma exacerbations (Reference 98) in Arg16 homozygotes but not Gly16 homozygotes.

Conflicting data regarding the influence of β_2 AR genotype on 2 agonist-evoked response have led to the idea that haplotype (combination of SNPs on an allele) may be better associated with response than single-site SNPs or genotype. Recently, this hypothesis was tested (Reference 89), and it was reported that haplotype but not genotype predicted bronchodilator response to inhaled albuterol. Of interest, homozygous haplotypes carrying Arg and Gln at loci 16 and 27, respectively, had the poorest response to inhaled albuterol, whereas heterozygotes with Arg16/Gln27 and Gly16/Gln16 haplotypes responded the best. It was hypothesized that diplotypes carrying Gly16 and Gln27 would have the best response to inhaled albuterol. This study is important because it demonstrated that haplotype but not genotype predicted response to inhaled albuterol. The study also points to how pharmacogenetic information may be used in the clinic. Because individuals who carried the Arg16-Gln27 diplotype had the worst response to inhaled albuterol, patients with asthma carrying this diplotype may do better using ipratropium bromide (Atrovent) as rescue drugs compared to inhaled short-acting β_2 agonists, such as albuterol. This hypothesis needs to be tested.

It is probably more clinically relevant to explore phenotype/haplotype associations in studies of LABAs compared to short-acting β_2 agonists because LABAs are used as chronic add-on agents (to ICSs) to control asthma symptoms in moderate to severe persistent asthma. And the functional significance of β_2 AR SNPs lies in their sensitivity to agonist-promoted down-regulation, which is thought to require constant agonist occupation of the receptor (References 94, 95). Moreover, long-term treatment with inhaled LABAs may result in the development of tolerance (References 105, 106), which is consistent with agonist-promoted receptor down-regulation. The earliest pharmacogenetic data using LABAs have been reported (Reference 98). Of interest, although increased asthma exacerbations in Arg16 homozygotes were observed following continuous albuterol use, no differences in asthma exacerbations were observed between genotypes following continuous use of salmeterol (Reference 98). More recently, it has been reported that Arg 16 polymorphism predisposes patients with asthma to the bronchoprotective tolerance (Reference 100). Clearly, future pharmacogenetic studies of β_2 agonists must focus on LABAs.

Moving Asthma Pharmacogenetics to the Clinic

Notwithstanding the remarkable progress that has been made in exploring the functional and clinical significance of genetic variants on drug response, use of genetic information to individualize the drug treatment of asthma cannot be recommended. Currently, several obstacles prevent the use of genetic information (genotype/haplotype) to individualize drug treatment of asthma. First, though there is some progress (Reference 107), little has been published regarding the identity of sequence variants in candidate genes in the GC pathway, their frequencies, and racial and ethnic distributions. In addition, no studies have been published that explore associations between sequence variants and response to ICSs. More is known regarding sequence variants in the leukotriene pathway and their influence on response to LTRAs (see the Pharmacogenetics of Inhibitors and Antagonists of the Cys-Leukotriene Pathway section). However, all the important, functionally significant SNPs in the leukotriene pathway have not been identified, and it is still not clear if the substantial variation in response to LTRAs is because of genetic variants. Large clinical trials exploring associations between asthma-related outcomes and GC and leukotriene pathway sequence variants are needed before genetic information can be used to distinguish which patients should use ICSs or LTRAs to control asthma symptoms.

In contrast to ICSs and LTRAs, the identity, allele frequencies, and racial and ethnic distributions of most of the β_2 AR SNPs are known, and numerous pharmacogenetic studies have been published. Yet, several obstacles prevent the use of genetic information to individualize β_2 AR agonist treatment. First, most if not all pharmacogenetic studies of β_2 AR agonists in asthma have too few study participants and, therefore, lack statistical power to address the hypothesis that genetic variants are associated with a good or poor response. The β_2 AR gene is highly polymorphic with at least six common diplotypes, the frequencies of which differ by race. To test the hypothesis that a given diplotype associates with an asthma-related outcome, a well-controlled clinical trial would have to be designed with adequate numbers of participants in each of six groups corresponding to the common diplotypes.

Second, most pharmacogenetic studies have focused on albuterol or other short-acting β_2 agonists. There may even be a greater need to focus on LABAs as these drugs are used chronically as add-on therapy for moderate to severe persistent asthma. Does the knowledge gained from pharmacogenetic studies of albuterol apply to LABAs (e.g., salmeterol and formoterol)? Although pharmacogenetic studies of LABAs are now being pursued, so far only single-site SNPs have been studied. It is not clear if the influence of β_2 AR sequence variants on albuterol response is applicable to LABAs. Third, because LABAs should only be used as add-on therapy, do steroids alter the influence that genetic variants of the β_2 AR have on response to LABAs? Fourth, pulmonary function is the most common outcome in pharmacogenetic studies of β_2 agonists. Is this the appropriate outcome (phenotype) in pharmacogenetic studies of LABAs? Probably not, as asthma control is probably more clinically relevant.

Finally, for pharmacogenetic studies of β_2 agonists, it seemed reasonable to begin with the β_2 AR gene. However, there are dozens of genes that encode proteins (in addition to β_2 AR) that mediate response to β_2 agonists (Figure 5). These include G-binding proteins, adenylyl cyclase isoforms, phosphodiesterase isoforms, PKA, β arrestin, and GRKs, to name a few. Single nucleotide polymorphisms have already been identified for many of these, and it is possible that the interpatient variability in response to short-acting beta agonists and LABAs observed in the clinic is because of a combination of these SNPs.

Chronic Obstructive Pulmonary Disease

Epidemiology

Chronic obstructive pulmonary disease is characterized by expiratory airflow obstruction because of chronic bronchitis or emphysema and by inflammation of the airways. The worldwide prevalence of COPD in 1990 was estimated to be 9.34/1000 in men and 7.33/1,000 in women of all ages. About 24 million adults or 13.9 percent of the adult population in the United States were suffering from COPD during 2000 (Reference 108). Currently, COPD is a leading cause of hospitalization and the fourth leading cause of death. Among the top 10 killers of Americans, COPD is the only disease that continues to rise in prevalence, and is projected to be the third cause of death worldwide in 2020 (Reference 109).

The Global Initiative for Chronic Obstructive Lung Disease (GOLD) defines COPD as a disease state characterized by airflow limitation that is not fully reversible. The airflow limitation is usually both progressive and associated with an abnormal inflammatory response of the lungs to noxious particles or gases" (Reference 110). A diagnosis of COPD should be considered in any patient who has symptoms of cough, sputum production, or dyspnea, and/or a history of exposure to risk factors for the disease. The diagnosis can be confirmed by spirometry as a FEV_1-forced vital capacity (FVC) ratio less than 0.7 (70 percent) with FEV_1 80 percent of predicted or less, regardless of chronic symptoms. The severity of COPD is classified as in Table 3.

Asthma and COPD

About 90 percent of the COPD patients are current or former cigarette smokers (Reference 111). Smoking induces airway inflammation and destruction of the connective tissues of the lung, and inhibits bronchial epithelial cell repair processes (Reference 112). Many diseases, mostly emphysema, chronic bronchitis, and asthma, can lead to COPD, either independently or together (Reference 113). Asthma affects primarily the conducting airways, emphysema is a destructive process of the alveolar structures, and chronic bronchitis affects both the large and the small airways. The pathological processes differ with the disease that leads to COPD (Figure 7): smooth muscle contraction with narrowing of the airway lumen in asthma, destruction of alveolar walls associated with loss of lung elastic recoil in emphysema, mucus overproduction resulted from hypertrophy of glandular structures, and goblet cell metaplasia in chronic bronchitis.

Asthma and COPD coexist in a portion of patients, although asthma is usually not related to cigarette smoking, and is more common with bronchial hyperresponsiveness (BHR). However, some patients with asthma go on to develop irreversible airflow obstruction indistinguishable from COPD. Airway reactivity is associated with airway narrowing. Chronic airway narrowing over a long time period may cause fixed airflow limitation. Patients with asthma, smokers or not, had progressive loss of FEV_1 at a rate twice that of smokers without asthma (Reference 113). This observation indicates that BHR also plays a role in development of COPD.

Environmental Influence and Genetic Predisposition

Environmental, genetic, and socioeconomic factors contribute, independently or together, to the development of COPD. The prevalence of COPD is highest in countries where cigarette smoking has been common. Each puff of a cigarette contains 10^{17} free radicals, which cause lung

Table 3. Classification of Severity of COPD

Stage	FEV_1/FVC	FEV_1	Symptoms
0: At Risk	Normal	Normal	Chronic cough and sputum production
I: Mild	< 70%	> 80%	Usually with symptoms
II: Moderate	< 70%	50–79%	SOB
III: Severe	< 70%	30–49%	SOB with repeated exacerbation
IV: Very Severe	< 70%	< 30%	Chronic respiratory failure

COPD = chronic obstructive pulmonary disease; FEV_1 = forced expiratory volume in one second; FVC = forced vital capacity; SOB = shortness of breath.

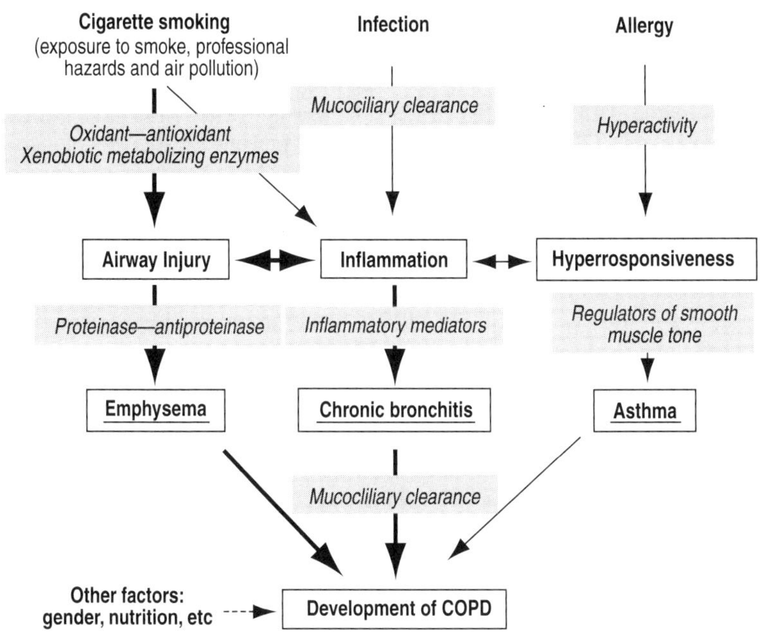

Figure 7. Pathology of asthma and COPD.
COPD = chronic obstructive pulmonary disease.

damage (Reference 114). The FEV_1 normally increases to a maximal value at young adulthood, remains stable for 10–15 years, and then decreases at a rate of 20 ml/year in healthy nonsmokers (Reference 113). Smokers have a more rapid decline, about twice that of normal nonsmokers (Reference 115). The decline is at an even more rapid pace in about 15 percent of smokers (Reference 113). This observation implies that genetic risk factors of COPD are likely present in these individuals. Familial aggregation studies indicated higher parent-children and sibling-sibling correlation in lung function, and a higher prevalence of COPD in relatives of cases than in relatives of controls (Reference 116). Familial resemblance studies revealed reduced FEV_1 and FEV_1-FVC values in the first-degree relatives of current or former cigarette smokers with severe early onset of COPD without α-1-antitrypsin (AAT) deficiency (Reference 117). The fact that no significant decrease in lung function was shown in the nonsmoking relatives of patients with early-onset COPD suggests that the genetic risk factors in these families only predispose to COPD in individual smokers. In another words, development of COPD is the combination of the interaction of genetic and environmental factors. Other risks include passive smoking, air pollution, occupational hazards, respiratory infection, allergy, nutrition, and alcohol ingestion.

Racial/Ethnic Differences in COPD Prevalence

Compared with African Americans, Caucasian Americans have a higher prevalence of COPD at similar age groups. In Hawaii, the prevalence of COPD in Japanese Americans smoking more than 20 cigarettes/day was 7.9 percent compared with 16.7 percent in a matched Caucasian-American group (Reference 111). The prevalence of COPD is low in China and this cannot be explained by lower tobacco consumption. The differences in the prevalence of COPD in different ethnic groups are difficult to separate from lifestyle factors. The fact that COPD is uncommon in Chinese Americans suggests that there are genetic differences. For example, the ZZ phenotype of AAT does not occur in African American patients and is rare in Asians, and abnormalities in cystic fibrosis transmembrane (conductance) regulator (CFTR) do not occur in the Japanese population. Because of the historically higher rates of cigarette smoking, men have higher prevalence of COPD than women do. However, women smokers may be more susceptible to severe, early-onset COPD (Reference 117). Thus, gender and ethnic differences also play roles in the development of COPD.

α-1-Antitrypsin Deficiency

Although the majority of COPD cases are attributed to cigarette smoking, a small number of cases of emphysema are caused by a genetic disorder, AAT deficiency. α-1-Antitrypsin is a serine protease inhibitor (PI) that primarily binds neutrophil elastase and, therefore, prevents the breakdown of elastic tissue, mainly in the lung. The wild-type allele of the AAT gene is designated the M allele. Alleles carrying polymorphisms in the coding region are designated S and Z. The S allele is a Glu264 Val polymorphism that accounts for intermediate AAT deficiency. The Z allele is mutation of Glu342 Lys, which resuls in severe AAT deficiency. The combination of these three alleles gives rise to several different genotypes: MM (Glu264Glu, Glu342Glu), MS (Glu264Val, Glu342Glu), MZ (Glu264Glu, Glu342Lys), SZ (Glu264Val, Glu342Lys), ZZ (Glu264Glu, Lys342Lys), and SS (Val264Val, Glu342Glu). α-1-Antitrypsin deficiency is associated with accelerated rate of development of emphysema in nonsmokers. The population prevalences for the MM, MS, and MZ genotypes of AAT among Caucasian are 86 percent, 9 percent, and 3 percent, respectively, the SZ, ZZ, and SS genotypes account for the remaining 2 percent. Protease inhibitor MM individuals have normal levels of AAT, whereas MS, MZ, SS, and ZZ individuals have mean levels of 75 percent, 57 percent, 52 percent, and 15 percent of normal, respectively. Protease inhibitor ZZ individuals have severe AAT deficiency and are at increased risk for COPD (Reference 118). Overall, AAT deficiency accounts for about 1–2 percent of all patients with COPD. Of importance, smoking is known to accelerate COPD in AAT deficiency (Reference 115). α-1-Antitrypsin binds to neutrophil elastase and inhibits the activity of neutrophil elastase. Met358 is located at the reactive center of AAT. Oxidation of Met358 and possibly other methionines in AAT by oxidants from cigarette smoke or other sources greatly decreases the elastase inhibitory activity of AAT. Replacing Met358 with leucine (Leu)358, Ile358, Val358, or alanine (Ala)358 by in vitro mutagenesis gives an effective neutrophil elastase inhibitor that is resistant to oxidants. Thus, the genetically engineered variants of AAT have therapeutic potential to treat destructive lung disorders. This indicates that gene-environment interaction may amplify the risk effects of each other.

α-1-Antitrypsin deficiency may become severe in individuals with moderate AAT deficiency when their production of matrix metalloproteinases (MMPs) is increased. Smokers with COPD exhibited greater activity of MMP-9 than healthy smokers and nonsmokers, whereas macrophages from the nonsmokers released more tissue inhibitor of MMP-1 (TIMP-1), an endogenous TIMP than that from smokers with or without COPD (Reference 119). Smokers with airway obstruction show increased MMP-1 (interstitial collagenase) and MMP-9 (gelatinase B) compared to smokers without COPD and nonsmokers. Transgenic mice overexpressing MMP-1 developed pulmonary emphysema. Compared to wild-type mice, MMP-12 (human macrophage elastase) null mice did not develop emphysema following exposure to cigarette smoke. A recent study of transforming growth factor (TGF)-beta in genetically engineered mice reveals a new molecular mechanism that leads to late-onset emphysema (Reference 120). Transforming growth factor-α strongly suppresses MMP-12 expression in macrophages and activates production of TIMP-1. Transforming growth factor-α also reduces the expression of nitric oxide synthases (NOS) that can amplify inflammation. These exciting results broaden the spectrum of factors involved in emphysema (a major component of COPD) to those that activate latent TGF-α in the lung. So, the actual contribution of AAT deficiency to the development of COPD may well exceed 1 percent. Clearly, measuring serum AAT level only is not enough to predict the severity of AAT deficiency. But it is unknown how to assert the protease-antiprotease balance among different individuals under different environments.

Cigarette smoking is a complex physiological addiction rather than a simple habit. Initiation of smoking is influenced both by social and environmental factors, such as advertising, peer influence, and family smoking, and by genetic factors. The latter may contribute more to persistence of smoking. A review of more than 17,500 monozygotic (MZ) and dizygotic (DZ) twins reared together from 14 studies revealed that genetic, familial-environmental, and individual-specific environmental factors accounted for 56 percent, 24 percent, and 20 percent of the variance in tobacco use, respectively (Reference 121). A higher concordance for smoking among the same sex MZ twins than in DZ twins suggests that smoking behavior is indeed genetically influenced (References 121, 122).

Other Genetic Factors in COPD

Linkage analysis and association studies have been widely used to identify genetic determinants of COPD and (reviewed in Reference 123). Chronic obstructive pulmonary disease, such as asthma, is a complex polygenic disorder. The candidate genes that influence the development of COPD are those involved in the pathogeneses of COPD (Table 4). The products of these genes are inflammatory mediators, xenobiotic enzymes, proteases, antiproteases, and other genetic markers, or those involved in BHR and nicotine metabolism (Figure 7). Segregation studies using MZ and DZ twins have indicated that the genetic risk is composed of several genes, each plays a small part rather than a major role in the development of COPD (Reference 116). It is quite possible that some genes lead to the development of airflow obstruction by loss of elastic recoil, resulting in emphysema, whereas others contribute to chronic airway inflammation, resulting in airway narrowing. Because of the extreme complexity and heterogeneity of COPD, there is a long list of candidate genes, which have been proposed to be involved in the development of COPD (Table 4). The presence of polymorphisms in a majority of the candidate genes has been reported and associations of COPD and many candidates have been established in recent years (References 111, 114–116, 124–127).

Guidelines for COPD Treatment

Because COPD, by definition, is not fully reversible with current therapy, management of COPD aims at preventing the progression of the disease and improving the quality of life. The current guidelines for therapy of all stages

Table 4. Candidate Genes of COPD

Candidate genes	COPD-related associations
Protease-antiprotease	
α-1-antitrypsin (AAT)	COPD (128), emphysema (129)
α-1-antichymotrypsin (AACT)	
α-2-macroglobulin (A2M)	
Matrix metalloproteinases (MMPs)	
Tissue inhibitor of metalloproteinase-1 (TIMP)	
Xenobiotic metabolism and oxidative stress	
Microsomal epoxide hydrolase-1 (EPHX1)	emphysema (130),
Glutathione S-transferases (GSTs)	COPD (131;132), asthma (132),
Heme oxygenase-1 (HMOX1)	rapid decline in lung
Cytochrome P450 (CYP) group enzymes	function (133), slower childhood lung function growth (134)

Table 4. Candidate Genes of COPD (continued)

Candidate genes	COPD-related associations
Inflammation mediators and chemoattractants	
Tumor necrosis factor (TNF)	bronchitis (135), asthma (135),
Interleukin-1 (IL-1) complex and	fibrosing alveolitis (136), rate of
other interleukines	decline in lung
Vitamin D-binding protein (VDBP)	function (137), COPD (138-141),
Leukotriene B4 (LTB$_4$)	BHR (142)
Interleukin-1 (IL-1) complex	
Vitamin D-binding protein (VDBP)	
Transforming growth factor-alpha (TGF-α)	
Airway smooth muscle and vasculature tone	
β-2-adrenergic receptor (B$_2$ AR)	BHR (143), reduced lung
Nitric oxide synthases (NOS)	function (144), emphysema
	(145), asthma (146;147)
Metabolism of nicotine and dopamine their signal pathway	
CYP group enzymes	Smoking habits (121;148),
(CYP2A6 and CYP2D6)	COPD (111)
Serotonin transporter (5-HTT)	
Dopamine receptors: DRD2, DRD4, and DRD1	
Dopamine transport gene: SLC6A3	
Monoamine oxidase: MAO-A and MAO-B	
Dopamine β-hydroxylase	
N-acetyltransferase 2 (NAT2)	
Mucociliary clearance.	
Cystic fibrosis transmembrane	COPD (149), asthma (149)
conductance regulator (CFTR)	
Other genetic markers	
Blood group antigen	COPD (150)
ABH secretor status	
immunoglobulin deficiency	
HLA	
Surfactant protein gene A, B, and D	

ABH = atypical bronchioloalveolar cellhyperplasia or blood group antigen H; BHR = bronchial hyperresponsiveness; COPD = chronic obstructive pulmonary disease; IILA = human leukocyte antigen.

of COPD are avoidance of risk factors and ensuring that patients receive vaccination against influenza and pneumococcus (*www.goldcopd.com*).

Smoking Cessation

Smoking cessation is the single most effective way to stop or at least slow the progressive loss of lung function (Reference 151). Unfortunately, only about 3 percent of the smokers will stop smoking simply on medical advice that smoking cessation is imperative. Smoking prevalence has remained essentially unchanged since 1990 after smoking prevalence rates in the United States declined to about 25 percent from almost 40 percent in 1965 (Reference 113).

Nicotine is the most active compound in cigarette smoke, contributing to addiction. Nicotine, acting on its receptors, increases the release of dopamine (DA) from presynaptic neurons (Figure 8). Dopamine is synthesized from L-tyrosine. Conversion of tyrosine to L-dopa by tyrosine hydroxylase (TH) is the rate-limiting step. Once released, DA can induce a euphoric sensation through dopaminergic receptors (DRs) located on postsynaptic neurons. Then, DA can be retaken back into presynaptic neurons by the dopamine transporter (DAT), or metabolized by catechol-O-methyl transferase (COMT) and monoamine oxidases (MAOs).

Nicotine is converted to the inactive metabolite cotinine by cytochrome P450 (CYP) enzymes, 80 percent by CYP2A6 (Reference 148). Dependent smokers adjust their smoking behavior to maintain their blood nicotine at a certain level. Nicotine-dependent individuals with defective CYP2A6 smoke fewer cigarettes than those with wild-type of CYP2A6. However, the

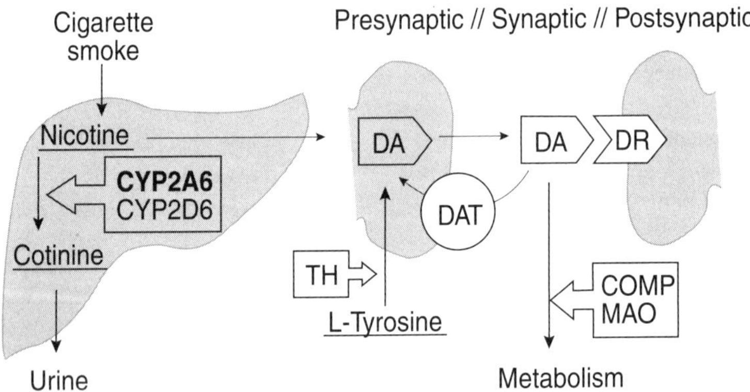

Figure 8. Disposition of nicotine and dopamine synthesis and disposition. Nicotine stimulates the release of dopamine (DA) from presynaptic nuerons where it synthesized for L-tyrosine by the action of tyrosine hydroxylase (TH). DA can bind to the dopamine receptor (DR) or be retaken up by the dopamine transporter (DAT) or metabolized.
COMT = catechol-O-methyl transferase; CYP = cytochrome P450; MAO = monoamine oxidase.

individuals with duplicated CYP2A6 smoked more, as evidenced by higher levels of breath carbon monoxide and blood cotinine (Reference 148). Methoxsalen, a CYP2A6 inhibitor, can reduce smoking by inhibiting nicotine first-pass metabolism. Cytochrome P450 2D6, another CYP member, also oxidizes nicotine to cotinine. Individuals can be grouped into poor, extensive, and ultrarapid metabolizers, respectively, according to their carrying of null alleles, one to two wild alleles, and more than two wild alleles of CYP2D6. There was a significant trend for the increased tobacco usage with increased metabolic capacity. Genetic differences in nicotinic receptors clearly play a role in smoking addiction (Reference 121). In addition, allelic variation in genes involved in dopaminergic pathway (the synthesis, release, retake, and metabolism of dopamine, and activation of its receptors) has implications for smoking cessation. Research in this area may lead to the identification of subgroups of individuals for whom pharmacological cessation aids may be most effective.

By providing a steady-state nicotine level, nicotine replacement can relieve some of the withdrawal symptoms. Any formulation of nicotine (e.g., gum, inhaler, nasal spray, and transdermal patch) reliably increases long-term smoking abstinence rates. However, whether there is a potential for addiction to nicotine in these formulations is not clear. The antidepressant bupropion also has increased long-term quit rates. The abstinence rates at 12 months were 16.4 percent, 30.3 percent, and 35.5 percent, respectively, after a 9-week treatment of nicotine-patch (21 mg/day), bupropion (150 mg 2 times/day), and the combination of both (Reference 152). There were observations that lower smoking rates were associated with better quitting rates and that women had more trouble quitting than men (Reference 121). The lack of genotype data from the clinical trials makes it impossible to explain the results pharmacogenetically.

Drug Treatment of COPD

Pharmacological treatment is used to prevent and control symptoms, reduce the frequency and severity of exacerbations, and improve health status and exercise tolerance. Pharmacological intervention does not modify long-term decline in lung function (*www.goldcopd.com*) (Reference 153). Bronchodilators are central in the drug therapy for COPD.

Rehabilitation and bronchodilators are administered for patients with stage II disease. Besides the treatments of stage II and for complications, inhaled GCs are recommended for stage III patients with repeated exacerbations. Long-term oxygen and surgical therapy should be considered for stage IV in the case of respiratory failure. The goals of COPD management are to prevent disease progression, relieve symptoms, improve exercise tolerance and health status, prevent and treat exacerbations and complications, reduce mortality, and minimize side effects from treatment.

Bronchodilators

Bronchodilator agents are central to symptom management in COPD. Inhaled therapy is preferred. All categories of bronchodilators, including β_2 AR agonists, anticholinergics, and theophylline, have increased exercise capacity in COPD. Short-acting bronchodilators are recommended, as needed for stage I COPD. For moderate to severe COPD, the GOLD update recommends the use of regular treatment with long-acting bronchodilators, including tiotropium rather than short-acting bronchodilators (Reference 153). Short-acting inhaled β_2 AR agonists, such as albuterol, fenoterol, and terbutaline, often are the preferred bronchodilators for treating acute exacerbation of COPD. The long-acting inhaled β_2 AR agonist, salmeterol, has improved health status significantly in doses of about 50 µg 2 times/day (Reference 154). Use of inhaled ipratropium 4 times/day also improves health status. Theophylline is less preferred because of its potential toxicity. Patients with COPD are frequently classified as "responders" or "nonresponders" to bronchodilators on the basis of lung function after acute challenge. This categorization is used to guide therapeutic intervention. However, the bronchodilator response of many individuals may vary day to day. In addition, the role genetic variation plays in classifying patients as responders or nonresponders to bronchodilator therapy is unknown and should be investigated.

Glucocorticoids

Systemic GCs are beneficial for managing acute exacerbation of COPD. They shorten recovery time and help to restore lung function more quickly (Reference 155). Long-term treatment with oral GCs is not recommended in COPD. Regular treatment with ICSs is only appropriate for severe COPD patients or with a documented spirometric response to ICSs.

Glucocorticoids have positive effects in asthma and a subpopulation of COPD patients (i.e., those with bronchial hyperresponsiveness and eosinophilia). Polymorphisms of the genes in the GC signal pathway probably do not explain the poor efficacy of GC therapy in COPD. The inflammatory process is different between COPD and asthma (Reference 156). In COPD, tobacco-induced airway inflammation is mediated by IL-8 and tumor necrosis factor-alpha from CD8+ lymphocytes, macrophages, and neutrophils. However, asthma involves IL-4, IL-5, and IL-13 from CD4+ lymphocytes, eosinophils, and mast cells. Glucocorticoids can reduce the eosinophilic inflammation in asthma, but they have little effect on inflammation of COPD. Genetic aberrations lead to abnormal production of many cytokines, chemokine, and proteases in COPD. Once the involvement of these factors in COPD inflammatory process and the genetic mechanism become clear, new therapies can be developed targeting at these factors and their receptors.

Chronic Obstructive Pulmonary Disease Pharmacogenetics

The role genetic variation plays in response to drug therapy in COPD has not been studied and is uncertain. Several facts support the idea to study the role genetic variation contributes to drug response variability. For example, bronchodilators (including short- and long-acting β_2 AR agonists) are used extensively in COPD. Polymorphisms in the β_2 AR have been associated with COPD (Reference 157), and asthma and cigarette smoking (Reference 93). Patients are classified as responders or nonresponders to bronchodilators (including albuterol) on the basis on pulmonary function after acute challenge (Reference 154). Taken together, along with a sizable asthma pharmacogenetic literature, it seems likely that genetic variation in the β_2 AR probably contributes to the variability in response to receptor-mediated bronchodilation in COPD. If a cohort of patients with COPD do not achieve the desired bronchodilator response using maximal doses of β_2 AR agonist because they carry a "nonresponsive" allele, then genotyping patients with COPD may beneficial. Based on the results of genetic tests, patients may be treated with β_2 AR agonists or anticholinergic agents. Future research in COPD should include studying the role genetic variation contributes to variability in response to bronchodilators and other therapeutic agents.

References

1. Silverman ES, Liggett SB, Gelfand EW, et al. The pharmacogenetics of asthma: a candidate gene approach. Pharmacogenetics J 2001;1(1):27–37.

2. Drazen JM, Yandava CN, Dube L, et al. Pharmacogenetic association between ALOX5 promoter genotype and the response to antiasthma treatment. Nat Genet 1999;22(2):168–70.

3. National Asthma Education and Prevention Program. Expert Panel Report: Guidelines for the Diagnosis and Management of Asthma Update on Selected Topics-2002.J Allergy Clin Immunol 2002;110(5):S141–S209.

4. Bousquet J, Jeffery PK, Busse WW, Johnson M, Vignola AM. Asthma. From bronchoconstriction to airways inflammation and remodeling. Am J Respir Crit Care Med 2000;161(5):1720–45.

5. Elias JA, Lee CG, Zheng T, Ma B, Homer RJ, Zhu Z. New insights into the pathogenesis of asthma. J Clin Invest 2003;111(3):291–7.

6. National Heart, Lung, and Blood Institute. Data Fact Sheet: Asthma Statistics. Washington, D.C.: United States Department of Health and Human Services, 1999.

7. Abramson MJ, Harrap SB. The new asthma genetics and its implications for public health. Public Health Rev 1998;26(2):127–44.

8. Beasley R, Crane J, Lai CK, Pearce N. Prevalence and etiology of asthma. J Allergy Clin Immunol 2000;105(2 Pt 2):S466–S72.

9. Palmer LJ, Cookson WO. Using single nucleotide polymorphisms as a means to understanding the pathophysiology of asthma. Respir Res 2001;2(2):102–12.

10. Meyers DA, Postma DS, Panhuysen CI, et al. Evidence for a locus regulating total serum IgE levels mapping to chromosome 5. Genomics 1994;23(2):464–70.

11. Cookson WO. Asthma genetics. Chest 2002;121(3 Suppl):7S–13S.

12. Malmstrom K, Rodriguez-Gomez G, Guerra J, et al. Oral montelukast, inhaled beclomethasone, and placebo for chronic asthma. A randomized, controlled trial. Montelukast/Beclomethasone Study Group. Ann Intern Med 1999;130(6):487–95.

13. Busse W, Raphael GD, Galant S, et al. Low-dose fluticasone propionate compared with montelukast for first-line treatment of persistent asthma: a randomized clinical trial. J Allergy Clin Immunol 2001;107(3):461–8.

14. Meltzer EO, Lockey RF, Friedman BF, et al. Efficacy and safety of low-dose fluticasone propionate compared with montelukast for maintenance treatment of persistent asthma. Mayo Clin Proc 2002;77(5):437–45.

15. Dempsey OJ, Kennedy G, Lipworth BJ. Comparative efficacy and anti-inflammatory profile of once-daily therapy with leukotriene antagonist or low-dose inhaled corticosteroid in patients with mild persistent asthma. J Allergy Clin Immunol 2002;109(1):68–74.

16. Nelson HS, Busse WW, Kerwin E, et al. Fluticasone propionate/salmeterol combination provides more effective asthma control than low-dose inhaled corticosteroid plus montelukast. J Allergy Clin Immunol 2000;106(6):1088–95.

17. Nelson HS, Nathan RA, Kalberg C, Yancey SW, Rickard KA. Comparison of inhaled salmeterol and oral zafirlukast in asthmatic patients using concomitant inhaled corticosteroids. MedGenMed 2001;3(4):3.

18. Calhoun WJ, Nelson HS, Nathan RA, et al. Comparison of fluticasone propionate-salmeterol combination therapy and montelukast in patients who are symptomatic on short-acting beta(2)-agonists alone. Am J Respir Crit Care Med 2001;164(5):759–63.

19. Fish JE, Israel E, Murray JJ, et al. Salmeterol powder provides significantly better benefit than montelukast in asthmatic patients receiving concomitant inhaled corticosteroid therapy. Chest 2001;120(2):423–30.

20. Sullivan P, Bekir S, Jaffar Z, Page C, Jeffery P, Costello J. Anti-inflammatory effects of low-dose oral theophylline in atopic asthma. Lancet 1994;343(8904):1006–8.

21. Evans DJ, Taylor DA, Zetterstrom O, Chung KF, O'Connor BJ, Barnes PJ. A comparison of low-dose inhaled budesonide plus theophylline and high-dose inhaled budesonide for moderate asthma. N Engl J Med 1997;337(20):1412–8.

22. Ind PW. Inhaled corticosteroids versus anti-leukotrienes: a literature review on the clinical effects. Allergy 1999;54 Suppl 50:43–6.

23. Stempel DA, Mauskopf J, McLaughlin T, Yazdani C, Stanford RH. Comparison of asthma costs in patients starting fluticasone propionate compared to patients starting montelukast. Respir Med 2001;95(3):227–34.

24. Bodwell JE, Hu JM, Hu LM, Munck A. Glucocorticoid receptors: ATP and cell cycle dependence, phosphorylation, and hormone resistance. Am J Respir Crit Care Med 1996;154(2 Pt 2):S2–S6.

25. Muller M, Renkawitz R. The glucocorticoid receptor. Biochim Biophys Acta 1991;1088(2):171–82.

26. Yudt MR, Cidlowski JA. The glucocorticoid receptor: coding a diversity of proteins and responses through a single gene. Mol Endocrinol 2002;16(8):1719–26.

27. Umland SP, Schleimer RP, Johnston SL. Review of the molecular and cellular mechanisms of action of glucocorticoids for use in asthma. Pulm Pharmacol Ther 2002;15(1):35–50.

28. Bisgaard H. Pathophysiology of the cysteinyl leukotrienes and effects of leukotriene receptor antagonists in asthma. Allergy 2001;56 Suppl 66:7–11.

29. Spector SL, Smith LJ, Glass M. Effects of 6 weeks of therapy with oral doses of ICI 204,219, a leukotriene D_4 receptor antagonist, in subjects with bronchial asthma. ACCOLATE Asthma Trialists Group. Am J Respir Crit Care Med 1994;150(3):618–23.

30. Fish JE, Kemp JP, Lockey RF, Glass M, Hanby LA, Bonuccelli CM. Zafirlukast for symptomatic mild-to-moderate asthma: a 13-week multicenter study. The Zafirlukast Trialists Group. Clin Ther 1997;19(4):675–90.

31. Noonan MJ, Chervinsky P, Brandon M, et al. Montelukast, a potent leukotriene receptor antagonist, causes dose-related improvements in chronic asthma. Montelukast Asthma Study Group. Eur Respir J 1998;11(6):1232–9.

32. Knorr B, Matz J, Bernstein JA, et al. Montelukast for chronic asthma in 6- to 14-year-old children: a randomized, double-blind trial. Pediatric Montelukast Study Group. JAMA 1998;279(15):1181–6.

33. Barnes PJ. Neural mechanisms in asthma: new developments. Pediatr Pulmonol Suppl 1997;16:82–3.

34. Tamaoki J, Kondo M, Sakai N, et al. Leukotriene antagonist prevents exacerbation of asthma during reduction of high-dose inhaled corticosteroid. The Tokyo Joshi-Idai Asthma Research Group. Am J Respir Crit Care Med 1997;155(4):1235–40.

35. Bratton DL, Lanz MJ, Miyazawa N, White CW, Silkoff PE. Exhaled nitric oxide before and after montelukast sodium therapy in school-age children with chronic asthma: a preliminary study. Pediatr Pulmonol 1999;28(6):402–7.

36. Christian VJ, Prasse A, Naya I, Summerton L, Harris A. Zafirlukast improves asthma control in patients receiving high-dose inhaled corticosteroids. Am J Respir Crit Care Med 2000;162(2 Pt 1):578–85.

37. Laviolette M, Malmstrom K, Lu S, et al. Montelukast added to inhaled beclomethasone in treatment of asthma. Montelukast/Beclomethasone Additivity Group. Am J Respir Crit Care Med 1999;160(6):1862–8.

38. Bisgaard H, Loland L, Oj JA. NO in exhaled air of asthmatic children is reduced by the leukotriene receptor antagonist montelukast. Am J Respir Crit Care Med 1999;160(4):1227–31.

39. Warner JO. The role of leukotriene receptor antagonists in the treatment of chronic asthma in childhood. Allergy 2001;56 Suppl 66:22–9.

40. Currie GP, Lipworth BJ. Bronchoprotective effects of leukotriene receptor antagonists in asthma: a meta-analysis. Chest 2002;122(1):146–50.

41. Salvi SS, Krishna MT, Sampson AP, Holgate ST. The anti-inflammatory effects of leukotriene-modifying drugs and their use in asthma. Chest 2001;119(5):1533–46.

42. Woods JW, Evans JF, Ethier D, et al. 5-lipoxygenase and 5-lipoxygenase-activating protein are localized in the nuclear envelope of activated human leukocytes. J Exp Med 1993;178(6):1935–46.

43. Dahlen SE, Hedqvist P, Hammarstrom S, Samuelsson B. Leukotrienes are potent constrictors of human bronchi. Nature 1980;288(5790):484–6.

44. Lewis RA, Austen KF, Soberman RJ. Leukotrienes and other products of the 5-lipoxygenase pathway. Biochemistry and relation to pathobiology in human diseases. N Engl J Med 1990;323(10):645–55.

45. Lam BK, Owen WF Jr, Austen KF, Soberman RJ. The identification of a distinct export step following the biosynthesis of leukotriene C_4 by human eosinophils. J Biol Chem 1989;264(22):12885–9.

46. Kawabe T, Chen ZS, Wada M, et al. Enhanced transport of anticancer agents and leukotriene C_4 by the human canalicular multispecific organic anion transporter (cMOAT/MRP2). FEBS Lett 1999;456(2):327–31.

47. Borst P, Kool M, Evers R. Do cMOAT (MRP2), other MRP homologues, and LRP play a role in MDR? Semin Cancer Biol 1997;8(3):205–13.

48. Anderson ME, Allison RD, Meister A. Interconversion of leukotrienes catalyzed by purified gamma-glutamyl transpeptidase: concomitant formation of leukotriene D_4 and gamma-glutamyl amino acids. Proc Natl Acad Sci U S A 1982;79(4):1088–91.

49. Lee CW, Lewis RA, Corey EJ, Austen KF. Conversion of leukotriene D_4 to leukotriene E_4 by a dipeptidase released from the specific granule of human polymorphonuclear leucocytes. Immunology 1983;48(1):27–35.

50. Drazen JM, Austen KF. Leukotrienes and airway responses. Am Rev Respir Dis 1987;136(4):985–98.

51. Lynch KR, O'Neill GP, Liu Q, et al. Characterization of the human cysteinyl leukotriene CysLT1 receptor. Nature 1999;399(6738):789–93.

52. Manning PJ, Watson RM, Margolskee DJ, Williams VC, Schwartz JI, O'Byrne PM. Inhibition of exercise-induced bronchoconstriction by MK-571, a potent leukotriene D_4-receptor antagonist. N Engl J Med 1990;323(25):1736–9.

53. Szefler SJ, Martin RJ, King TS, et al. Significant variability in response to inhaled corticosteroids for persistent asthma. J Allergy Clin Immunol 2002;109(3):410–8.

54. Drazen JM, Silverman EK, Lee TH. Heterogeneity of therapeutic responses in asthma. Br Med Bull 2000;56(4):1054–70.

55. Israel E, Chervinsky PS, Friedman B, et al. Effects of montelukast and beclomethasone on airway function and asthma control. J Allergy Clin Immunol 2002;110(6):847–54.

56. Encio IJ, Detera-Wadleigh SD. The genomic structure of the human glucocorticoid receptor. J Biol Chem 1991;266(11):7182–8.

57. Leung DY, Hamid Q, Vottero A, et al. Association of glucocorticoid insensitivity with increased expression of glucocorticoid receptor beta. J Exp Med 1997;186(9):1567–74.

58. Hamid QA, Wenzel SE, Hauk PJ, et al. Increased glucocorticoid receptor beta in airway cells of glucocorticoid-insensitive asthma. Am J Respir Crit Care Med 1999;159(5 Pt 1):1600–4.

59. Sousa AR, Lane SJ, Cidlowski JA, Staynov DZ, Lee TH. Glucocorticoid resistance in asthma is associated with elevated in vivo expression of the glucocorticoid receptor beta-isoform. J Allergy Clin Immunol 2000;105(5):943–50.

60. Bray PJ, Cotton RG. Variations of the human glucocorticoid receptor gene (NR3C1): pathological and in vitro mutations and polymorphisms. Hum Mutat 2003;21(6):557–68.

61. Whelan GJ, Blake K, Kissoon N, et al. Effect of montelukast on time-course of exhaled nitric oxide in asthma: influence of LTC_4 synthase A(-444)C polymorphism. Pediatr Pulmonol 2003;36(5):413–20.

62. Sampson AP, Siddiqui S, Buchanan D, et al. Variant LTC(4) synthase allele modifies cysteinyl leukotriene synthesis in eosinophils and predicts clinical response to zafirlukast. Thorax 2000;55 Suppl 2:S28–S31.

63. Asano K, Shiomi T, Hasegawa N, et al. Leukotriene C_4 synthase gene A(-444)C polymorphism and clinical response to a CYS-LT(1) antagonist, pranlukast, in Japanese patients with moderate asthma. Pharmacogenetics 2002;12(7):565–70.

64. Sanak M, Simon HU, Szczeklik A. Leukotriene C_4 synthase promoter polymorphism and risk of aspirin-induced asthma. Lancet 1997;350(9091):1599–600.

65. Sanak M, Sampson AP. Biosynthesis of cysteinyl-leukotrienes in aspirin-intolerant asthma. Clin Exp Allergy 1999;29(3):306–13.

66. Sanak M, Pierzchalska M, Bazan-Socha S, Szczeklik A. Enhanced expression of the leukotriene C(4) synthase due to overactive transcription of an allelic variant associated with aspirin-intolerant asthma. Am J Respir Cell Mol Biol 2000;23(3):290–6.

67. Currie GP, Lima JJ, Sylvester JE, Lee DK, Cockburn WJ, Lipworth BJ. Leukotriene C_4 synthase polymorphisms and responsiveness to leukotriene antagonists in asthma. Br J Clin Pharmacol 2003;56(4):422–6.

68. Ito S, Ieiri I, Tanabe M, Suzuki A, Higuchi S, Otsubo K. Polymorphism of the ABC transporter genes, MDR1, MRP1 and MRP2/cMOAT, in healthy Japanese subjects. Pharmacogenetics 2001;11(2):175–84.

69. Halushka PV, Mais DE, Mayeux PR, Morinelli TA. Thromboxane, prostaglandin and leukotriene receptors. Annu Rev Pharmacol Toxicol 1989;29:213–39.

70. Barnes PJ. Beta-adrenergic receptors and their regulation. Am J Respir Crit Care Med 1995;152(3):838–60.

71. Hakonarson H, Grunstein MM. Regulation of second messengers associated with airway smooth muscle contraction and relaxation. Am J Respir Crit Care Med 1998;158(5 Pt 3):S115–S22.

72. Lohse MJ. Molecular mechanisms of membrane receptor desensitization. Biochim Biophys Acta 1993;1179(2):171–88.

73. Billington CK, Penn RB. Signaling and regulation of G protein-coupled receptors in airway smooth muscle. Respir Res 2003;4(1):2.

74. Hardin A, Lima JJ. Beta 2-adrenoceptor agonist-induced down-regulation after short-term exposure. J Recept Signal Transduct Res 1999;19:835–52.

75. National Asthma Education and Prevention Program. Expert panel report: guidelines for the diagnosis and management of asthma-updated on selected topics 2002. Bethesda, MD: United States Department of Health and Human Services, Public Health Service, National Institutes of Health, National Heart, Lung, and Blood Institute, 2002. Publication No. 02-5075.

76. Woolcock A, Lundback B, Ringdal N, Jacques LA. Comparison of addition of salmeterol to inhaled steroids with doubling of the dose of inhaled steroids. Am J Respir Crit Care Med 1996;153(5):1481–8.

77. Pauwels RA, Lofdahl CG, Postma DS, et al. Effect of inhaled formoterol and budesonide on exacerbations of asthma. Formoterol and Corticosteroids Establishing Therapy (FACET) International Study Group. N Engl J Med 1997;337(20):1405–11.

78. Lazarus SC, Boushey HA, Fahy JV, et al. Long-acting beta2-agonist monotherapy vs continued therapy with inhaled corticosteroids in patients with persistent asthma: a randomized controlled trial. JAMA 2001;285(20):2583–93.

79. Nathan RA, Pinnas JL, Schwartz HJ, et al. A six-month, placebo-controlled comparison of the safety and efficacy of salmeterol or beclomethasone for persistent asthma. Ann Allergy Asthma Immunol 1999;82(6):521–9.

80. GlaxoSmithKline. Serevent Safety Alert. Research Triangle Park, NC: GlaxoSmithKline; 2003.

81. Johnson JA. Racial differences in lymphocyte beta-receptor sensitivity to propranolol. Life Sci 1993;53(4):297–304.

82. Lemoine H, Overlack C, Kohl A, Worth H, Reinhardt D. Formoterol, fenoterol, and salbutamol as partial agonists for relaxation of maximally contracted guinea pig tracheae: comparison of relaxation with receptor binding. Lung 1992;170(3):163–80.

83. Rabe KF, Jorres R, Nowak D, Behr N, Magnussen H. Comparison of the effects of salmeterol and formoterol on airway tone and responsiveness over 24 hours in bronchial asthma. Am Rev Respir Dis 1993;147(6 Pt 1):1436–41.

84. Campbell LM, Anderson TJ, Parashchak MR, Burke CM, Watson SA, Turbitt ML. A comparison of the efficacy of long-acting beta 2-agonists: eformoterol via Turbohaler and salmeterol via pressurized metered dose inhaler or Accuhaler, in mild to moderate asthmatics. Force Research Group. Respir Med 1999;93(4):236–44.

85. van Noord JA, Smeets JJ, Raaijmakers JA, Bommer AM, Maesen FP. Salmeterol versus formoterol in patients with moderately severe asthma: onset and duration of action. Eur Respir J 1996;9(8):1684–8.

86. Vervloet D, Ekstrom T, Pela R, et al. A 6-month comparison between formoterol and salmeterol in patients with reversible obstructive airways disease. Respir Med 1998;92(6):836–42.

87. Condemi JJ. Comparison of the efficacy of formoterol and salmeterol in patients with reversible obstructive airway disease: a multicenter, randomized, open-label trial. Clin Ther 2001;23(9):1529–41.

88. Kobilka BK, Dixon RA, Frielle T, et al. cDNA for the human beta 2-adrenergic receptor: a protein with multiple membrane-spanning domains and encoded by a gene whose chromosomal location is shared with that of the receptor for platelet-derived growth factor. Proc Natl Acad Sci U S A 1987;84(1):46–50.

89. Drysdale CM, McGraw DW, Stack CB, et al. Complex promoter and coding region beta 2-adrenergic receptor haplotypes alter receptor expression and predict in vivo responsiveness. Proc Natl Acad Sci U S A 2000;97(19):10483–8.

90. Reihsaus E, Innis M, MacIntyre N, Liggett SB. Mutations in the gene encoding for the beta 2-adrenergic receptor in normal and asthmatic subjects. Am J Respir Cell Mol Biol 1993;8(3):334–9.

91. Parola AL, Kobilka BK. The peptide product of a 5' leader cistron in the beta 2 adrenergic receptor mRNA inhibits receptor synthesis. J Biol Chem 1994;269(6):4497–505.

92. McGraw DW, Forbes SL, Kramer LA, Liggett SB. Polymorphisms of the 5' leader cistron of the human beta2-adrenergic receptor regulate receptor expression. J Clin Invest 1998;102(11):1927–32.

93. Wang J, Mougey EB, David CJ, et al. Determination of human β_2-adrenoceptor haplotypes by denaturation selective amplification and subtractive genotyping. Am J Pharmacogenomics 2001;1(4):1175–2203.

94. Green SA, Turki J, Innis M, Liggett SB. Amino-terminal polymorphisms of the human beta 2-adrenergic receptor impart distinct agonist-promoted regulatory properties [published erratum appears in Biochemistry 1994 Nov 29;33(47):14368]. Biochemistry 1994;33(32):9414–9.

95. Green SA, Turki J, Bejarano P, Hall IP, Liggett SB. Influence of beta 2-adrenergic receptor genotypes on signal transduction in human airway smooth muscle cells. Am J Respir Cell Mol Biol 1995;13(1):25–33.

96. Green SA, Cole G, Jacinto M, Innis M, Liggett SB. A polymorphism of the human beta 2-adrenergic receptor within the fourth transmembrane domain alters ligand binding and functional properties of the receptor. J Biol Chem 1993;268(31):23116–21.

97. Lipworth BJ, Hall IP, Aziz I, Tan KS, Wheatley A. Beta2-adrenoceptor polymorphism and bronchoprotective sensitivity with regular short- and long-acting beta2-agonist therapy [see comments]. Clin Sci (Lond)1999;96(3):253–9.

98. Taylor DR, Drazen JM, Herbison GP, Yandava CN, Hancox RJ, Town GI. Asthma exacerbations during long term beta agonist use: influence of beta(2) adrenoceptor polymorphism. Thorax 2000;55(9):762–7.

99. Lipworth BJ, Dempsey OJ, Aziz I, Wilson AM. Effects of adding a leukotriene antagonist or a long-acting beta(2)-agonist in asthmatic patients with the glycine-16 beta(2)-adrenoceptor genotype. Am J Med 2000;109(2):114–21.

100. Lee DKC, Currie GP, Hall IP, Lima JJ, Lipworth BJ. Differences in bronchoprotective subsensitivity between formoterol (FM) and salmeterol (SM) are associated with β_2-adrenoceptor polymorphism. Eur Respir J 2002;20:38.

101. Martinez FD, Graves PE, Baldini M, Solomon S, Erickson R. Association between genetic polymorphisms of the beta2-adrenoceptor and response to albuterol in children with and without a history of wheezing. J Clin Invest 1997;100(12):3184–8.

102. Lima JJ, Mohamed M, Eberle LV, Self TH, Johnson JA. Impact of genetic polymorphisms of the β_2-adrenergic receptor on albuterol bronchodilator pharmacodynamics. Clin Pharmacol Ther 1999;65:519–25.

103. Tan S, Hall IP, Dewar J, Dow E, Lipworth B. Association between beta 2-adrenoceptor polymorphism and susceptibility to bronchodilator desensitisation in moderately severe stable asthmatics [see comments]. Lancet 1997;350(9083):995–9.

104. Israel E, Drazen JM, Liggett SB, et al. The effect of polymorphisms of the beta(2)-adrenergic receptor on the response to regular use of albuterol in asthma. Am J Respir Crit Care Med 2000;162(1):75–80.

105. Newnham DM, McDevitt DG, Lipworth BJ. Bronchodilator subsensitivity after chronic dosing with eformoterol in patients with asthma [see comments]. Am J Med 1994;97(1):29–37.

106. Ramage L, Lipworth BJ, Ingram CG, Cree IA, Dhillon DP. Reduced protection against exercise induced bronchoconstriction after chronic dosing with salmeterol. Respir Med 1994;88(5):363–8.

107. Davis AF, Long RM. Pharmacogenetics Research Network and Knowledge Base third scientific meeting. Pharmacogenetics 2003;13(7):437–40.

108. Mannino DM. Chronic obstructive pulmonary disease: definition and epidemiology. Respir Care 2003 Dec;48(12):1185–91.

109. Rennard SI, Farmer SG. COPD in 2001: a major challenge for medicine, the pharmaceutical industry, and society. Chest 2002;121(90050):113S.

110. Pauwels RA, Buist A, Calverley P, Jenkins C, Hurd SS; GOLD Scientific Committee. Global strategy for the diagnosis, management, and prevention of chronic obstructive pulmonary disease. NHLBI/WHO Global Initiative for Chronic Obstructive Lung Disease (GOLD) Workshop Summary. Am J Respir Crit Care Med 2001;163(5):1256–76.

111. Barnes PJ. Genetics and pulmonary medicine. 9. Molecular genetics of chronic obstructive pulmonary disease. Thorax 1999;54(3):245–52.

112. Wang H, Liu X, Umino T, et al. Cigarette smoke inhibits human bronchial epithelial cell repair processes. Am J Respir Cell Mol Biol 2001;25(6):772–9.

113. Rennard SI. COPD: overview of definitions, epidemiology, and factors influencing its development. Chest 1998;113(4):235S–41S.

114. Lomas D, Silverman E. The genetics of chronic obstructive pulmonary disease. Respir Res 2001;2(1):20–6.

115. Senior R, Anthonisen N. Chronic obstructive pulmonary disease (COPD). Am J Respir Crit Care Med 1998;157(4):139S–47S.

116. Chen Y. Genetics and pulmonary medicine. 10: Genetic epidemiology of pulmonary function. Thorax 1999;54(9):818–24.

117. Silverman EK, Chapman HA, Drazen JM, et al. Genetic epidemiology of severe, early-onset chronic obstructive pulmonary disease. Risk to relatives for airflow obstruction and chronic bronchitis. Am J Respir Crit Care Med 1998;157(6 Pt 1):1770–8.

118. Sandford AJ, Weir TD, Spinelli JJ, Pare PD. Z and S mutations of the alpha1-antitrypsin gene and the risk of chronic obstructive pulmonary disease. Am J Respir Cell Mol Biol 1999;20(2):287–91.

119. Russell RE, Culpitt SV, DeMatos C, et al. Release and activity of matrix metalloproteinase-9 and tissue inhibitor of metalloproteinase-1 by alveolar macrophages from patients with chronic obstructive pulmonary disease. Am J Respir Cell Mol Biol 2002;26(5):602–9.

120. Roberts AB. Medicine: smoke signals for lung disease. Nature 2003;422(6928):130–1.

121. Batra V, Patkar AA, Berrettini WH, Weinstein SP, Leone FT. The genetic determinants of smoking. Chest 2003;123(5):1730–9.

122. Rennard SI, Daughton DM. Smoking cessation. Chest 2000;117(90052):360S–4S.

123. Sandford AJ, Silverman EK. Chronic obstructive pulmonary disease. 1: Susceptibility factors for COPD the genotype-environment interaction. Thorax 2002;57(8):736–41.

124. Hill A, Gompertz S, Stockley R. Factors influencing airway inflammation in chronic obstructive pulmonary disease. Thorax 2000;55(11):970–7.

125. Sandford AJ, Silverman EK. Chronic obstructive pulmonary disease. 1: susceptibility factors for COPD the genotype-environment interaction. Thorax 2002;57(8):736–41.

126. Silverman EK, Mosley JD, Barth M, et al. Genomewide linkage analysis of quantitative spirometric phenotypes in severe early-onset chronic obstructive pulmonary disease.Genomewide linkage analysis of quantitative spirometric phenotypes in severe early-onset chronic obstructive pulmonary disease. Am J Hum Genet 2002;70(5):1229–39.

127. Joos L, Pare PD, Sanford AJ. Genetic risk factors for chronic obstructive pulmonary disease. Swiss Med Wkly 2002;132:27–37.

128. Asthma mortality and hospitalization among children and young adults-United States, 1980-1993. MMWR Morb Mortal Wkly Rep 1996 May 3;45(17):350–3.

129. Eriksson S. A 30-year perspective on alpha 1-antitrypsin deficiency. Chest 1996;110(6):237S–42S.

130. Smith CA, Harrison DJ. Association between polymorphism in gene for microsomal epoxide hydrolase and susceptibility to emphysema. Lancet 1997;350:630–3.

131. Koyama H, Geddes DM. Genes, oxidative stress, and the risk of chronic obstructive pulmonary disease. Thorax 1998;53(90002):10S–14S.

132. Ishii T, Matsuse T, Teramoto S, et al. Glutathione S-transferase P1 (GSTP1) polymorphism in patients with chronic obstructive pulmonary disease. Thorax 1999;54(8):693–6.

133. He JQ, Ruan J, Connette JE, Anthonisen NR, Pare PD, Sandford AJ. Antioxidant gene polymorphisms and susceptibility to a rapid decline in lung function in smokers. Am J Respir Crit Care Med 2002;166(3):323–8.

134. Gilliland FD, Gauderman WJ, Vora H, Rappaport E, Dubeau L. Effects of glutathione-S-transferase M1, T1, and P1 on childhood lung function growth. Am J Respir Crit Care Med 2002;166(5):710–16.

135. Huang S, Su C, Chang S. Tumor necrosis factor-alpha gene polymorphism in chronic bronchitis. Am J Respir Crit Care Med 1997;156(5):1436–9.

136. Whyte M, Hubbard R, Meliconi R, et al. Increased risk of fibrosing alveolitis associated with interleukin-1 receptor antagonist and tumor necrosis factor-alpha gene polymorphisms. Am J Respir Crit Care Med 2000;162(2):755–8.

137. Joos L, McIntyre L, Ruan J, et al. Association of IL-1beta and IL-1 receptor antagonist haplotypes with rate of decline in lung function in smokers. Thorax 2001;56(11):863–6.

138. Schellenberg D, Pare PD, Weir TD, Spinelli JJ, Walker BA, Sandford AJ. Vitamin D binding protein variants and the risk of COPD. Am J Respir Crit Care Med 1998;157(3 Pt 1):957–61.

139. Ishii T, Keicho N, Teramoto S, et al. Association of Gc-globulin variation with susceptibility to COPD and diffuse panbronchiolitis. Eur Respir J 2001;18:753–7.

140. Keatings VM, Cave SJ, Henry MJ, et al. A polymorphism in the tumor necrosis factor-alpha gene promoter region may predispose to a poor prognosis in COPD. Chest 2000;118(4):971–5.

141. Takizawa H, Tanaka M, Takami K, et al. Increased expression of transforming growth factor-beta1 in small airway epithelium from tobacco smokers and patients with chronic obstructive pulmonary disease (COPD). Am J Respir Crit Care Med 2001;163(6):1476–83.

142. Kuhn C 3rd, Homer RJ, Zhu Z, et al. Airway hyperresponsiveness and airway obstruction in transgenic mice. Morphologic correlates in mice overexpressing interleukin (IL)-11 and IL-6 in the lung. Am J Respir Cell Mol Biol 2000;22(3):289–95.

143. D'amato M, Vitiani LR, Petrelli G, et al. Association of persistent bronchial hyperresponsiveness with beta 2-adrenoceptor (ADRB2) haplotypes. A population study. Am J Respir Crit Care Med 1998;158(6):1968–73.

144. Summerhill E, Leavitt SA, Gidley H, Parry R, Solway J, Ober C. beta 2-adrenergic receptor Arg16/Arg16 genotype is associated with reduced lung function, but not with asthma, in the Hutterites. Am J Respir Crit Care Med 2000;162(2):599–602.

145. Novoradovsky A, Brantly ML, Waclawiw MA, et al. Endothelial nitric oxide synthase as a potential susceptibility gene in the pathogenesis of emphysema in alpha 1-antitrypsin deficiency. Am J Respir Cell Mol Biol 1999;20(3):441–7.

146. Wang Z, Chen C, Niu T, et al. Association of asthma with beta(2)-adrenergic receptor gene polymorphism and cigarette smoking. Am J Respir Crit Care Med 2001;163(6):1404–9.

147. Wechsler ME, Grasemann H, Deykin A, et al. Exhaled nitric oxide in patients with asthma. Association with NOS1 genotype. Am J Respir Crit Care Med 2000;162(6):2043–7.

148. Rao Y, Hoffmann E, Zia M, et al. Duplications and defects in the CYP2A6 gene: identification, genotyping, and in vivo effects on smoking. Mol Pharmacol 2000;58(4):747.

149. Tzetis M, Efthymiadou A, Strofalis S, et al. CFTR gene mutations-including three novel nucleotide substitutions-and haplotype background in patients with asthma, disseminated bronchiectasis and chronic obstructive pulmonary disease. Hum Genet 2001;108(3):216–21.

150. Guo X, Lin HM, Lin Z, et al. Surfactant protein gene A, B, and D marker alleles in chronic obstructive pulmonary disease of a Mexican population. Eur Respir J 2001;18(3):482–90.

151. Pride NB. Smoking cessation: effects on symptoms, spirometry and future trends in COPD. Thorax 2001;56(90002):ii7–10.

152. Jorenby DE, Leischow SJ, Nides MA, et al. A controlled trial of sustained-release bupropion, a nicotine patch, or both for smoking cessation. N Engl J Med 1999;340(9):685–91.

153. Fabbri LM, Hurd SS; GOLD Scientific Committee. Global Strategy for the Diagnosis, Management and Prevention of COPD: 2003 update. Eur Respir J 2003;22:1–2.

154. Rennard SI, Anderson W, ZuWallack R, et al. Use of a long-acting inhaled beta2-adrenergic agonist, salmeterol xinafoate, in patients with chronic obstructive pulmonary disease. Am J Respir Crit Care Med 2001;163(5):1087–92.

155. Burge PS, Calverley PM, Jones PW, Spencer S, Anderson JA, Maslen TK. Randomised, double blind, placebo controlled study of fluticasone propionate in patients with moderate to severe chronic obstructive pulmonary disease: the ISOLDE trial. BMJ 2000;320(7245):1297.

156. Barnes P, Pedesen S, Busse WW. Efficacy and safety of inhaled corticosteroids. New developments. Am J Respir Crit Care Med 1998;157(3):1S–53S.

157. Ho LI, Harn HJ, Chen CJ, Tsai NM. Polymorphism of the beta(2)-adrenoceptor in COPD in Chinese subjects. Chest 2001;120(5):1493–9.

Self-Assessment Questions

Questions 1 and 2 pertain to the following case.

R.J. is a 22-year-old African American with a 5-pack-year history of smoking presenting with cough, chest tightening, wheezing, and difficulty in breathing. His forced expiratory volume in one second-forced vital capacity (FEV_1-FVC) = 0.7, FEV_1 is 60 percent of predicted, and two puffs of albuterol increases FEV_1 to 80 percent predicted.

1. R.J. probably has which one of the following?

    A. Asthma.
    B. Bronchitis.
    C. Emphysema.
    D. Asthma, bronchitis, and emphysema.

2. The best therapy for R.J. is which one of the following?

    A. Daily salmeterol and inhaled albuterol as needed.
    B. Daily low-dose inhaled corticosteroid (ICS) and inhaled albuterol as needed.
    C. Daily low-dose ICS and salmeterol and inhaled albuterol as needed.
    D. Inhaled albuterol as needed.

3. Which one of the following is the most likely pharmacogenetic explanation for the unimodal distribution of FEV_1 associated with montelukast treatment (see Figure 3 of this chapter)?

    A. Genetic variation in drug metabolizing enzymes.
    B. The tandem repeat polymorphism in the 5-lipoxygenase (5-LO) gene.
    C. The leukotriene C_4 synthase (LTC_4S) A-444C polymorphism.
    D. Multiple polymorphisms in one or more genes encoding leukotriene pathway proteins.

4. The wild-type β_2 adrenergic receptor (β_2 AR) haplotype in African Americans is which one of the following?

    A. Cysteine (Cys)-19/arginine (Arg)16/glutamine (Gln)27/threonine (Thr)164 (CRQT).
    B. Cys-19/glycine (Gly)16/Gln27/Thr164 (CGQT).
    C. Arg-19/Gly16/glutamate (Glu)27/Thr164 (RGET).
    D. Arg-19/Gly16/Gln27/Thr164 (RGGT).

5. According to Table 2 of this chapter, the allele frequency of the β_2 AR Gly16 genotype in Caucasians is which one of the following?

    A. 38.8 percent.

B. 39.9 percent.
C. 61.0 percent.
D. 19.8 percent.

6. The better response versus dose curve in the figure below is best exemplified by patients with asthma carrying which one of the following β_2 AR diplotypes?

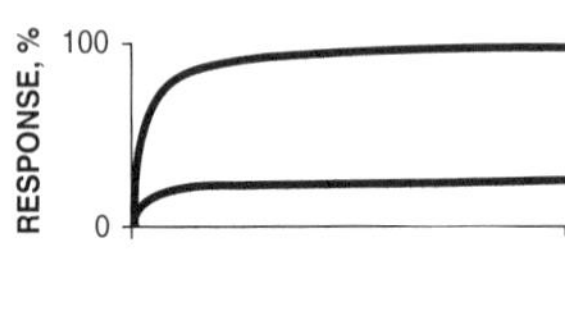

Bronchodilator response (percent above baseline) following inhalation of increasing doses of albuterol

A. Arg16/Gln27/Thr164.
B. Gly16/Gln27/Thr164.
C. Gly16/Glu27/Thr164.
D. Gly16/Gln27/Ile164.

7. The emboldened response versus dose curve in the figure is best exemplified by patients with asthma carrying which one of the following β_2 AR haplotypes?

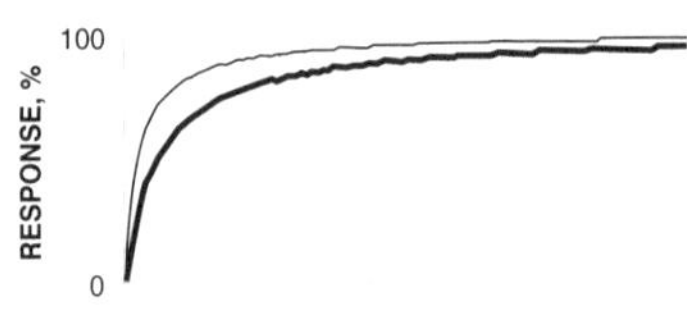

Bronchodilator response (percent above baseline) following inhalation of increasing doses of albuterol

A. Arg16/Gln27/Thr164.
B. Gly16/Gln27/Thr164.
C. Gly16/Glu27/Thr164.
D. Gly16/Gln27/Ile164.

8. In a clinical trial comparing montelukast versus low-dose ICS as asthma controllers, which of the following is the least important outcome?

A. Asthma exacerbation rate.
B. Inhaled albuterol use.

C. Forced expiratory volume in 1 second.
D. Emergency department visit.

9. The mechanism underlying agonist-induced, long-term desensitization of β_2 AR-mediated function is which one of the following?

    A. Homologous receptor phosphorylation.
    B. Receptor uncoupling.
    C. Receptor sequestration.
    D. Receptor down-regulation.

10. Genetic variation in drug targets can influence the pharmacodynamics of drugs. Three classes of drug targets are receptors, enzymes, and transporters. An example of a polymorphism in a drug transporter is which one of the following?

    A. Number of Sp-1 tandem repeats in 5-LO gene.
    B. A-444→C polymorphism in the LTC$_4$S gene.
    C. C924→T single nucleotide polymorphism in cysteinyl leukotriene 1 receptor gene.
    D. Arg723→Gln single nucleotide polymorphism in multidrug resistance protein 1.

Transplantation

HongXia Zheng, M.D., Ph.D.,
Gilbert J. Burckart, Pharm.D., FCCP

Keywords

Transplant, P-glycoprotein (Pgp), multidrug resistance gene (*MDR1*), cytochrome P450 (CYP) 3A5, thiopurine methyltransferase (TPMT), cytokines, chemokines, adhesion molecules, corticosteroids, tacrolimus, cyclosporine (CsA), ethnicity, rejection.

Abstract

Organ transplantation is a complex clinical science combining the technical skills of the surgeon with the most advanced knowledge of immunology and pharmacology. Although organ transplantation has made tremendous advances throughout the past 20 years, improving the patient's outcome through drug therapy remains more of an art than it does a science. Two major advances will soon change the effect of immunosuppression in organ transplantation: clinical pharmacogenomics and the availability of a whole new set of biotechnology-derived immunosuppressive agents. Clinical pharmacogenomics will allow the selection of the pharmacological regimen, which can be individualized based on a wide range of available agents with diverse actions and adverse effects. This individualization of therapy may be the next significant advance in treating organ transplant patients.

The current understanding of genetic variation in relation to response in organ transplant patients can be divided into drug disposition markers and drug targets. The membrane pump P-glycoprotein (Pgp) may have the largest impact of any of the factors studied to date. The genetic polymorphism of the gene that encodes for Pgp, multidrug resistance gene (*MDR1*), has been associated with improved steroid weaning, tacrolimus dosage requirement, renal function after organ transplantation, and patient survival after transplantation. The drug metabolizing enzymes, such as cytochrome P450 (CYP) 3A5 and thiopurine methyltransferase (TPMT) for the calcineurin antagonists and azathioprine, respectively, have an impact on drug dosage requirement and adverse effects for organ transplant patients.

The polymorphic drug targets for the immunosuppressant agents include cytokines, such as tumor necrosis factor (TNF) and interleukin-10 (IL-10); chemokines; adhesion molecules; and growth factors, such as vascular endothelial growth factor (VEGF). Although none of these factors has the direct impact of *MDR1* polymorphisms, each has demonstrated an association with transplantation outcome in a specific patient population. The impact of this group of genetic variants will most certainly be in their cumulative effect on the immune and inflammatory process, and they must be designed into any risk calculation that is to be calculated for an individual patient.

Treatment algorithms dependent upon pharmacogenomic variables will be designed in the near future for transplant patients. A simplified example is provided related to *MDR1*. The process of testing these algorithms for safety and efficacy may be an extended process, but the end result will be the improvement of transplant patient outcomes based on better prospective choices regarding drug therapy regimens.

Outline

Learning Objectives

1. Describe the current understanding of clinical pharmacogenomics in the pharmacotherapy of transplant patients in relation to drug disposition markers and drug targets.
2. Describe the candidate genes, outcome markers, and analysis of this information in transplant patients.
3. Discuss the future use of clinical pharmacogenomic data in individualizing immunosuppressive therapy for transplant patients.

Abbreviations in this Chapter

6-MP	6-Mercaptopurine
CAD	Coronary artery disease
CD31	Platelet-endothelial-cell adhesion molecule
CsA	Cyclosporine
CYP	Cytochrome P450
GVHD	Graft-versus-host disease
ICAM-1	Intercellular adhesion molecule-1
IL	Interleukin
LFA-1	Lymphocyte function-associated antigen-1
MDR1	Multidrug resistance gene
PECAM	Platelet-endothelial-cell adhesion molecule
Pgp	P-glycoprotein
SNP	Single nucleotide polymorphism
TGF-β	Transforming growth factor-beta
TNF-α	Tumor necrosis factor-alpha
TPMT	Thiopurine methyltransferase
VEGF	Vascular endothelial growth factor

Pharmacogenomics in Transplantation

Introduction

Organ transplant patients are among the most complex patient populations, which require intense immunosuppressive therapy The complexity of these patients is secondary to many complicating factors, such as long-standing organ failure preoperatively, the surgical intervention that is necessary and its technical complications, the donor-recipient considerations that not only include tissue antigenicity but also extend to infectious disease susceptibility, and the large number of adverse effects of the transplant and drug therapy on organ systems peripheral to the transplant. Consequently, health care professionals' ability to optimize the drug therapy in an organ transplant patient has a major impact on the survival of the transplant and of the patient.

Adverse Effects are a Problem in Transplantation

If preemptive monitoring of a patient's genotype is to be attempted, the objective should not only be improved graft function but also avoidance of adverse drug effects. Adverse drug effects presently represent a substantial portion of the morbidity encountered by an organ transplant patient. These adverse effects include nephrotoxicity, occasionally to the extent of renal failure requiring dialysis and/or kidney transplantation, hypertension, diabetes mellitus, hepatotoxicity, and neurotoxicity. Because these adverse effects are not directly related to drug concentrations of the immunosuppressive agents, then an inherent sensitivity to the production of the adverse effect based on pharmacogenomic differences among patients is most likely part of this process.

Drug and Dose Individualization is Needed in Organ Transplantation

The tools available to the pharmacotherapist to manage the organ transplant patient are still quite crude. One of the reasons for this is the nature of the primary immunosuppressive agents (presently the calcineurin antagonists cyclosporine and tacrolimus) used in transplantation. Both of these agents have very unique biopharmaceutic profiles; they require monitoring blood concentrations and multiple changes to the assay techniques for these agents have taken place throughout the past 20 years. Despite thousands of publications on monitoring these agents, every clinician knows that the results of the blood assays provide only a general guide to dosing and avoidance of adverse effects. From an immunologic viewpoint, the blood concentrations of cyclosporine and tacrolimus only provide useful information at the extremes of the observed values (very low or very high values). In general, both acute and chronic rejection routinely occur in the face of "therapeutic" blood concentrations of cyclosporine and tacrolimus.

Immunologic monitoring in organ transplant patients currently is an art that has been advanced only modestly throughout the past 20 years. Many immunologic tests have taken their turns at being touted as the answer to immunologic monitoring, and have included blood concentrations of cytokines, cytokine receptors, or changes in cell markers monitored by flow cytometry. The failure of routine immunologic monitoring is not surprising in view of the complexity and redundancy of the immune system. Effective immunologic monitoring requires the measurement of a large number of interacting substances and monitoring within the milieu of the transplanted organ. Given these restrictions on effective monitoring post-transplantation, a preemptive program of assigning patients to a drug regimen based on pharmacogenomic principles in combination with postoperative monitoring appears to hold the most promise for improving graft and patient survival.

Multiple Types of Drugs are used in Organ Transplant Patients

The use of pharmacogenomic information prospectively for transplant patient management will require a substantial amount of research to become a reality. Working against this concept are the number of genes involved because drug effects are most commonly polygenic in nature, and the number of different drugs that transplant patients receive. Although the initial impression is that the complexity of these drug effects may be impossible to elucidate and predict prospectively, the initial research in the area of clinical pharmacogenomics and organ transplantation has been exceptionally fruitful. As discussed in the Drug Disposition Markers section, the major candidate drug disposition marker genes have proven to have definite associations with drug use and dosing, adverse drug effects, and patient outcomes in many small series of transplantation. Therefore, if a few major candidate genes can explain a significant amount of the variability observed clinically in a transplant patient response to therapy and adverse effects, then trials of prospective randomization of transplant patients are a realistic possibility.

The next section addresses the current experience with the drug disposition markers and drug targets in organ transplantation, and then discusses the use of this information in treating patients now and in the future.

Drug Disposition Markers

P-glycoprotein

The human multidrug resistance gene (*MDR1*) encodes for P-glycoprotein (Pgp), a 170-kDa transport membrane glycoprotein consisting of more than 1200 amino acids, which is responsible for resistance to many structurally and functionally unrelated types of clinically used drugs. P-glycoprotein acts as an adenosine 5'-triphosphate-dependent pump expelling the drug to the outside, thereby reducing drug accumulation within the cell.

P-glycoprotein and Drug Absorption

P-glycoprotein plays an important role in the absorption, distribution, and elimination of drugs that are substrates for the pump. The primary immunosuppressive agents used in organ transplantation are substrates for Pgp and include cyclosporine (CsA), tacrolimus, sirolimus, and corticosteroids. In living-donor liver transplantation, intestinal *MDR1* expression was found to predict both tacrolimus pharmacokinetics and patient survival (Reference 16). Therefore, Pgp may play a major role in the effectiveness and toxicity of drug therapy in transplant patients. Recent studies have demonstrated that genetic polymorphisms lead to functional alterations and phenotypic variation in Pgp expression, and at least 16 polymorphisms of the *MDR1* gene have been characterized (References 8, 18, 19, 54, 56). These previous studies have focused on the functional outcomes of the single nucleotide polymorphisms (SNPs) C3435T and G2677T. The C3435T SNP is a silent mutation at a wobble position in exon 26. The *MDR1* G2677T mutation is in tight linkage disequilibrium with the C3435T mutation (Reference 54), and some investigators have suggested the C3435T mutation might be related to Pgp function through its linkage to the amino acid-encoding G2677T mutation (Reference 27). The *MDR1* C3435T has been associated with changes in the function of Pgp both in vitro (Reference 18), as demonstrated by higher Pgp function in CD56+ natural killer cells from 3435 CC patients (the wild-type), and in vivo (References 19, 26), where the 3435 CC genotype was associated with lower plasma levels of phenytoin or digoxin in healthy volunteers. The relationship between the *MDR1* C3435T polymorphisms at exon 26 and Pgp effect on drug absorption is illustrated in Figure 1. The figure shows a cartoon of how *MDR1* polymorphisms at C3435T (exon 26) can affect Pgp function in the process of drug absorption. The *MDR1* 3435 CC wild-type genotype on the left is associated with greater Pgp function and less drug absorption into the blood compared to the *MDR1* 3435 TT

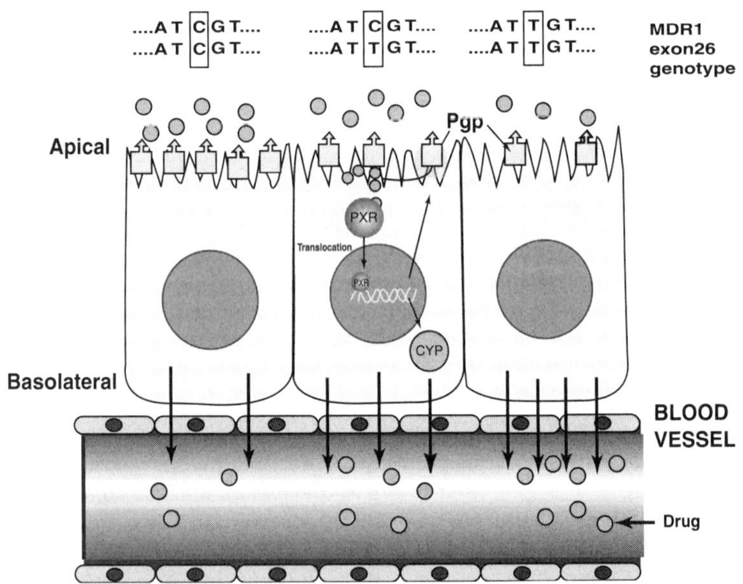

Figure 1. Illustration of *MDR1* polymorphisms at C3435T (exon 26).
The *MDR1* 3435 CC wild-type genotype on the left is associated with greater P-glycoprotein function and less drug absorption into the blood in comparison to the *MDR1* 3435 TT genotype on the right, which allows more drug to be absorbed.
CYP = cytochrome P450; *MDR1* = multidrug resistance; PXR = pregnane x receptor.
Reprinted with permission from Stan Louie, Pharm.D., University of Southern California.

genotype on the right, which allows more drug to be absorbed. The exact relationships between *MDR1* polymorphisms and Pgp function are controversial, and further prospective studies on the role that *MDR1* polymorphisms play in drug absorption are warranted.

Cyclosporine/Tacrolimus Absorption and MDR1 *Genotype*

The calcineurin antagonists have enabled solid organ transplantation to obtain its current place as a therapeutic option for end-stage renal, liver, heart, and lung disease. Both tacrolimus and its predecessor CsA have contributed to the understanding of T-cell activation and immunosuppression in solid organ transplant patients. These immunosuppressive agents have a narrow therapeutic index and poor bioavailability when given by the oral route. Although some manipulation of the dosage forms may influence the pattern and extent of drug absorption, absorption of CsA and tacrolimus is highly variable and unpredictable. The relationship between *MDR1* genotypic markers and the clinical response to a drug may vary considerably, depending on the disease state. In a study in renal transplant patients, CsA trough blood concentrations did not differ between *MDR1* 3435 genotypes in renal transplant patients, even though CsA is a substrate for and potent inhibitor of Pgp (Reference 56). A study of 14 healthy patients reported that there were no statistical differences in CsA pharmacokinetics among different *MDR1* 3435 genotypes, although the maximum concentration of drug and the area under the curve in the CT and TT group were larger than those in CC group (Reference 40). Previous observations have associated tacrolimus absorption in small bowel transplant patients with *MDR1* expression (References 25, 36). A recent study reported that the polymorphisms of *MDR1* are weakly associated with dose-adjusted blood concentrations of tacrolimus 3 months after renal transplantation (Reference 35), whereas another study (Reference 66) found a significant association between tacrolimus blood levels per dose/kg/day and the *MDR1* 2677 and 3435 genotypes in pediatric heart transplant patients. At 3, 6, and 12 months post-transplantation, patients with 2677 GG genotype required a higher dosage of tacrolimus to achieve similar blood levels compared with the GT/TT patients (see Figure 2). The figure shows the tacrolimus level in blood (ng/ml) per dose (mg/kg/day) at 3, 6, and 12 months post-transplantation in the pediatric heart transplant patients separated into their *MDR1* G2677T GG and GT/TT genotypes. Although the difference was not significant at 3 months (p=0.26), the GG patients have a significantly lower tacrolimus level/dose than the GT/TT patients at 6 months (p=0.017) and 12 months (p=0.014). The same observation is true for the *MDR1* 3435 CC wild-type patients compared to the CT/TT patients. In contrast to the findings in pediatric heart transplant patients, one study (Reference 70) did not find a relationship between tacrolimus dosing and *MDR1* genotypes in adult lung transplant patients. In summary, Pgp and *MDR1* genotypes probably play a role in the absorption of tacrolimus, but

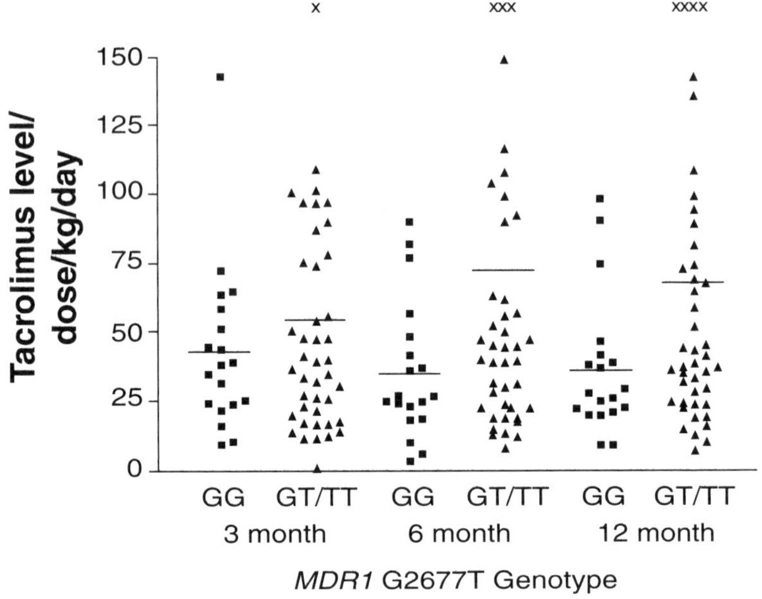

Figure 2. The tacrolimus level in blood (ng/ml) per dose (mg/kg/day) at 3, 6, and 12 months post-transplantation in the pediatric heart transplant patients separated into their *MDR1* G2677T GG and GT/TT genotypes.
Although the difference was not significant at 3 months (p=0.26), the GG patients have a significantly lower tacrolimus level/dose than the GT/TT patients at 6 months (p=0.017) and 12 months (p=0.014).

this relationship in adult organ transplant patients is clouded by other factors and by the overriding importance of CYP3A5 polymorphisms to the absorption of these agents (see Cytochrome P450 3A 4/5). Cyclosporine absorption does not appear to share this relationship, but external factors such as the solubilizers used in the oral preparations of CsA may directly influence Pgp function (Reference 57).

P-glycoprotein and Renal Function

Various normal epithelial and endothelial tissues exhibit Pgp function. Renal tubular cells express Pgp on their apical membranes and its drug transport function is unidirectional and acts to extrude drug out into urine. Other tissues which express the protein include cerebral vascular endothelium as a component of the blood-brain barrier, intestinal epithelium, and biliary tubular epithelial cells. The renal elimination of digoxin has been used as a marker of renal Pgp function in previous publications, although there is no consensus on the role of Pgp in the renal elimination of drugs (Reference 57).

Two studies have now linked renal dysfunction after organ transplantation with the *MDR1* genotype. One study (Reference 67) found that nephrotoxicity, one of the adverse effects of tacrolimus, and tacrolimus dosing in organ transplant patients was related to *MDR1* genotype in lung transplant patients. Seventy of 79 patients continued taking tacrolimus for the entire year, and their highest serum creatinine was significantly different between the *MDR1* 2677 GG and the GT/TT patients. Study investigators concluded that tacrolimus nephrotoxicity is partially mediated through Pgp-related renal processes (see Figure 3). The figure shows the highest serum creatinine measured during the first postoperative year in adult lung transplant patients separated by *MDR1* exon26, 21 and CYP3A5 genotypes.

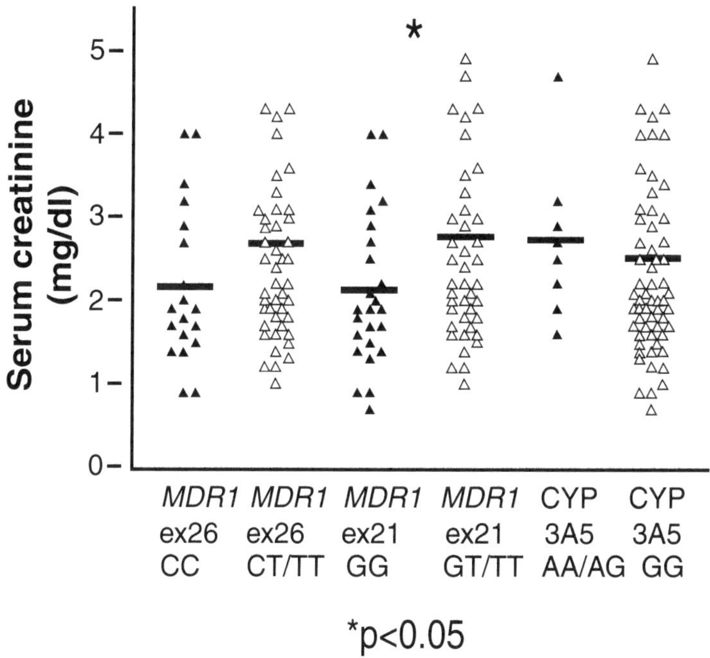

*p<0.05

Figure 3. The highest serum creatinine measured during the first postoperative year in adult lung transplantation patients separated by *MDR1* exon26, 21 and CYP3A5 genotypes.
For clarification, *MDR1* ex26 = *MDR1* 3435, *MDR1* ex21 = *MDR1* 2677, and CYP3A5 A = *1 and G = *3. The only significant difference was between the *MDR1* 2677 GG and the GT/TT patients.
CYP = cytochrome P450; *MDR1* = multidrug resistance gene.

The only significant difference was between the *MDR1* 2677 GG and the GT/TT patients.

Another observation of *MDR1* genotype and renal dysfunction was published based on a study at the University of Washington in liver transplant patients (Reference 17). Investigators found that patients followed for 3 years post-transplant who were genotyped as *MDR1* 2677 TT had less renal dysfunction, as defined by a serum creatinine of 1.6 mg/dl or lower. The mechanism by which *MDR1* genotypes result in long-term differences in serum creatinine remains to be determined.

P-glycoprotein and Blood-brain Barrier

Neurotoxicity is one of the adverse effects associated with CsA and tacrolimus therapy. Several studies reported that a high blood concentration of tacrolimus is not correlated with neurotoxicity because these events happen even if the blood concentration of tacrolimus is within the therapeutic range (Reference 4). Despite the high lipophilic properties of tacrolimus, the transport of the drug through the blood-brain barrier into the brain is restricted by Pgp. The concentration of tacrolimus in the brain was dramatically increased by depleting the *MDR1* gene in mice (Reference 29), which supports Pgp involvement in tacrolimus distribution to the brain. Tacrolimus is a substrate for Pgp and is pumped out from the brain to prevent accumulation, a process which should reduce the neurotoxicity. Recently, a study of 17 patients who received living-donor liver transplants reported that blood concentrations, liver function, graft weight, and polymorphism in the *MDR1* gene are important predictors of tacrolimus-induced neurotoxicity (Reference 64). However, the small patient population and conflicting results between *MDR1* G2677T and C3435T make the study conclusions questionable. The importance of *MDR1* polymorphisms in other central nervous system diseases, such as in drug-resistant epilepsy (Reference 52) suggest that Pgp should have an effect on central nervous system adverse drug effects, but additional studies in organ transplant patients are needed to clearly make this association.

P-glycoprotein and Steroid Effect

Although most of these immunosuppressive agents are administered for the life of the transplant patient, corticosteroids frequently are weaned from the drug regimen in patient populations at high risk for steroid adverse effects. A recent study (Reference 65) demonstrated that a significantly larger number of the *MDR1* 3435 CC genotype pediatric heart transplant patients remain on steroids at 1 year after transplantation compared to CT/TT patients (Figure 4), and linkage occurs between the *MDR1* 3435 genotype and the 2677 genotype in these patients. The figure shows pediatric heart transplant patients who had to remain on corticosteroids after 1 year post-transplantation (first block) and patients who did not require corticosteroids after 1 year (second block). The patients are divided into the

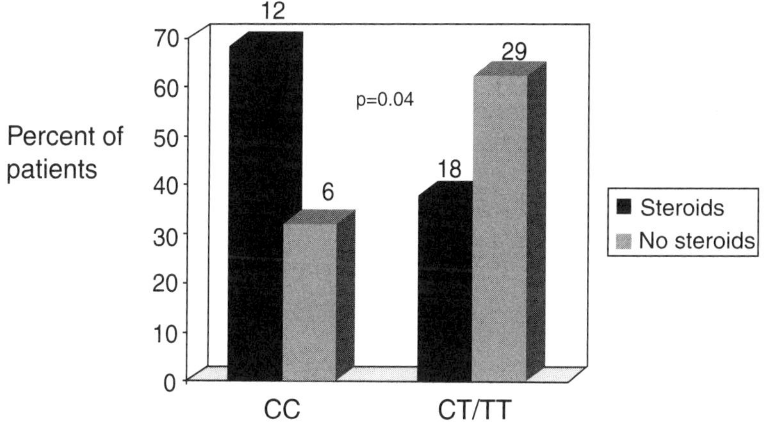

Figure 4. Pediatric heart transplantation patients who had to remain on/off corticosteroids after 1 year post-transplantation separated by the *MDR1* 3435 CC and CT/TT genotypes.

MDR1 3435 CC patients and the CT/TT patients. A significant difference was observed between the two groups (p=0.04, Chi-square). These observations are timely in that transplant centers are now actively attempting to minimize and quickly wean corticosteroid agents because of their long-term detrimental effects in organ transplant patients. This report suggests that patients with the *MDR1* 3435 CC genotype and the 2677 GG genotype may require more aggressive alternative therapy if corticosteroids are going to be weaned from the immunosuppressive regimen.

P-glycoprotein and Ethnic Differences in Acute Rejection/Graft Survival

The frequency of polymorphisms of *MDR1* has shown that there is a significant variability among various ethnic groups. The African-American group has a 68–83 percent frequency of the *MDR1* 3435 CC genotype, compared to 21–25 percent in Caucasian patients (References 2, 8, 48). The racial disparity in renal transplant outcomes between Caucasian and African-American patients has been recognized throughout the past 20 years. A recent review (Reference 23) of data from the United Network for Organ Sharing Renal Transplant Registry for patients undergoing living-related renal allografting shows that African-American patients are 1.8 times as likely as Caucasians to suffer graft failure during the 9-year study period. This report discounted the poor human leukocyte antigens matching for African-American patients suggested in earlier reports (References 31, 47), and concluded that nonhuman leukocycle antigen mechanisms must contribute to the poor renal transplant outcomes in African-American patients. The higher rates of acute rejection and graft failure in African-American patients results in a poorer quality of life for

African-American transplant patients (Reference 24). These observations about African-American patients and poor renal transplant outcomes have now been extended to pediatric (Reference 15) and adult liver transplantation (Reference 43) and to pediatric heart transplantation. In summary, the differences observed in acute rejection and graft survival in African-American renal transplant patients could possibly be attributed to genetic polymorphisms, including the high frequency of the *MDR1* 3435 CC genotype associated with poor drug absorption and steroid resistance.

P-glycoprotein and Rejection/Graft Survival

As previously discussed, Pgp is involved in many different physiological processes. The exact mechanism by which these processes impact graft survival is not clear, but increasing evidence suggests that Pgp and the *MDR1* genotype may have an impact on overall graft survival. One of the first indicators for this was a study (Reference 16) in living-donor liver transplantation. During the operative procedure, mucosal cells of the upper jejunum were obtained to assess messenger ribonucleic acid for *MDR1* and cytochrome P450 (CYP) 3A4. High levels of expression of *MDR1*, but not CYP3A4, were strongly associated with a reduction in the survival rate of patients after liver transplantation. Although the intestinal *MDR1* was inversely related to the tacrolimus concentration-dose ratio, the results suggest that additional factors may link *MDR1* and Pgp to patient survival.

More recently, one study (Reference 68) genotyped lung transplant patients for *MDR1* 2677 and 3435 variants. In a study of 132 adult lung transplant patients, only *MDR1* C3435T was independently associated with acute persistent rejection. Sixty-seven percent of patients in the CC wild-type group had acute persistent rejection, compared to 42 percent in the TT homozygous mutant group (p=0.03). Study investigators also found that in the 52 patients who had died at the time of the assessment, the long-term survivors were the patients who expressed the mutant allele for each of the genes assessed. Because the calcineurin antagonists (tacrolimus and CsA) blood concentrations are routinely monitored and adjusted, the overall effect on patient survival of Pgp may be because of some overriding influence (e.g., Pgp in T cells) or some combinations of factors yet to be determined.

Cytochrome P450 3A4/5

The CYP3A enzymes represent one of the most important families of the CYP superfamily. The CYP3A family comprises the most abundantly expressed CYP enzymes in human liver. In humans, four isoforms of the CYP3A superfamily, CYP3A4, CYP3A5, CYP3A7 (Reference 44), and CYP3A43 (Reference 61), have been identified and known to account for as much as 30 percent of total CYP content in the liver (Reference 51). These enzymes are responsible for the metabolism of more than 50 percent of all currently prescribed drugs, including agents as diverse as steroids, antidepressants, immunosuppressive agents, and macrolide antibiotics

(Reference 9). The four CYP3A genes are localized in a cluster on chromosome 7q21-q22.1 (Reference 53) and are characterized by a high structural similarity and protein sequence identity. Cytochrome P450 3A4 has been considered to be the dominant CYP3A in the intestine followed by CYP3A5. Cytochrome P450 3A5 and CYP3A7, but not CYP3A4, also are expressed in the adrenal gland and in the prostate, whereas only CYP3A5 is detected in the kidney (Reference 30). The third CYP3A, CYP3A7, was originally described in the human fetal liver where it accounts for at least 50 percent of the total CYP protein, but its expression is usually silenced after birth (Reference 63). Similarly, protein expression is very low in adult livers for the recently identified fourth member of the family, CYP3A43 (Reference 61).

Interindividual variation in the activity and levels of expression of CYP3A is considerable. This variation is manifested by differences greater than 10-fold in the in vivo metabolism of drugs that are substrates for the CYP3As (Reference 28) and a 31-fold variation in CYP3A4 activity in vitro (Reference 50). Furthermore, such differences can be increased significantly by induction and inhibition of CYP3A4. A 400-fold variation of the area under the curve has been observed between patients receiving rifampicin as an inducer and itraconazole as an inhibitor of CYP3A4 (Reference 5). Such variation can cause clinically important differences in drug toxicity and response. Aside from the effects of drugs as inducers and inhibitors, genetic, pathological, hormonal, and dietary factors also may contribute to variability in CYP3A4 activity. Of these, it appears that genetic factors are of great importance for the interindividual variability in constitutive expression and activity of the CYP3A subfamily, accounting for 70–90 percent of the variation, although the underlying genetic factors are essentially unknown (Reference 45). In the search for such factors, the functional polymorphism of the CYP3A4 gene has been investigated, and 19 different polymorphic CYP3A4 alleles carrying missense mutations have been found. In general, variants in the coding regions of CYP3A4 occur at allele frequencies less than 5 percent and appear as heterozygous with the wild-type allele. These coding variants may contribute to but are not likely to be the major cause of interindividual differences in CYP3A-dependent clearance, because of the low allele frequencies and limited alterations in enzyme expression or catalytic function. Thus, additional factors that control the genetically determined differences in CYP3A4 expression remain to be identified. The variable expression of other CYP3A enzymes most likely contributes to the overall differences in CYP3A enzyme activity. The CYP3A5 protein has been expressed in 10–97 percent of human livers at levels varying by up to an order of magnitude. A recent study (Reference 32) challenged the prevailing view that CYP3A4 forms the bulk of the hepatic CYP3A protein and activity, suggesting that CYP3A5 contributes substantially to the CYP3A-dependent drug metabolism because of very high hepatic expression in about 30 percent of Caucasian livers.

Study investigators described two functional SNPs in CYP3A5 and provided a molecular explanation for the absence of the CYP3A5 protein from some people. The CYP3A5*3 (22893A→G) allele in intron 3 resulted in a truncated protein with loss of CYP3A5 expression, whereas the CYP3A5*6 (30597G→A) allele in exon 7 causes deletion of exon 7 from the splice variant and was associated with lower CYP3A5 catalytic activity. Patients with the polymorphic *3 allele have lower hepatic expression and decreased hepatic CYP3A5 activity than patients with at least one *1 allele. An illustration of how the CYP3A5 *1 and *3 polymorphisms could affect the bioavailability of an immunosuppressant is shown in Figure 5. The figure shows a cartoon of how the polymorphisms of CYP3A5 can affect the bioavailability of a drug that is a substrate for the enzyme. The *1/*1 and the *1/*3 patients are the enzyme expressors, and the *3/*3 patients are the nonexpressors of the enzyme. Furthermore, although no inter- or intraethnic group differences in CYP3A4 content were detected in the samples of 47 livers from Caucasians and African Americans, the amount of total CYP3A content in these ethnic groups was found to be 3-fold higher in patients with the *1 allele. The CYP3A5 protein was found to account for more than 50 percent of total hepatic CYP3A protein in about 30 percent of

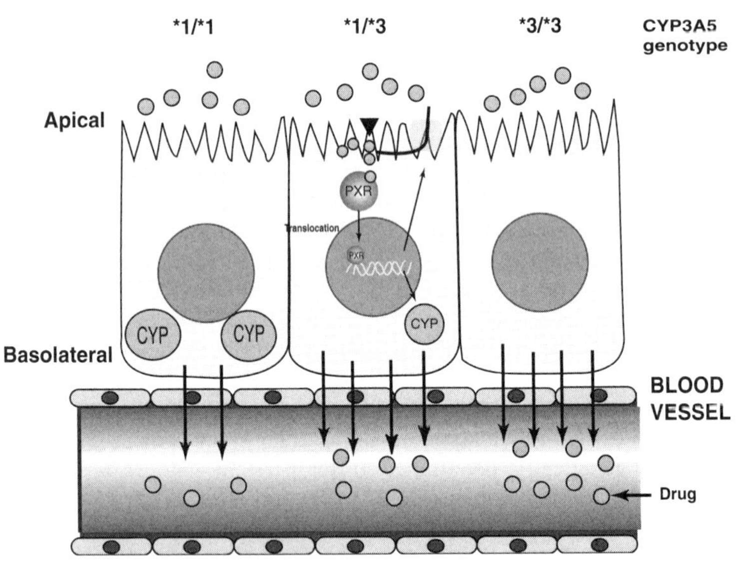

Figure 5. Illustration of how the polymorphisms of CYP3A5 can affect the bioavailability of a drug that is a substrate for the enzyme.
The *1/*1 and the *1/*3 patients are the enzyme expressors, and the *3/*3 patients are the nonexpressors of the enzyme.
CYP = cytochrome P450; PXR = pregnane X receptor.
Reprinted with permission from Stan Louie, Pharm.D., University of Southern California.

Caucasian livers and in more than 50 percent of African-American livers. One study (Reference 62) compared the in vitro relative metabolic capabilities of three different CYP3A isoforms (CYP3A4, CYP3A5, and CYP3A7) on the clearance of a wide range of CYP3A substrates. Investigators found that CYP3A5 metabolic activity was equal to or reduced compared with CYP3A4, and also found a significantly lower activity for CYP3A7. These findings as well as those of a previously cited study (Reference 32) suggest that CYP3A5 may be the most important genetic contributor to interindividual as well as interethnic differences in clearance of CYP3A substrates. This position also was strongly supported in a recent review of these systems (Reference 12).

One study (Reference 66) has established that the tacrolimus blood concentration per dose of drug is clearly associated with the CYP3A5 genotype. Cytochrome P450 3A5 expressors (*1/*1 and *1/*3) require more tacrolimus to achieve the same blood concentrations than do the enzyme nonexpressors (*3/*3) at all points in the first year after transplantation (see Figure 6). The figure shows the tacrolimus level in blood (ng/ml) per dose (mg/kg/day) at 3, 6, and 12 months post-transplantation in the pediatric heart transplant patients separated into their *1/*3 and *3/*3 genotypes of

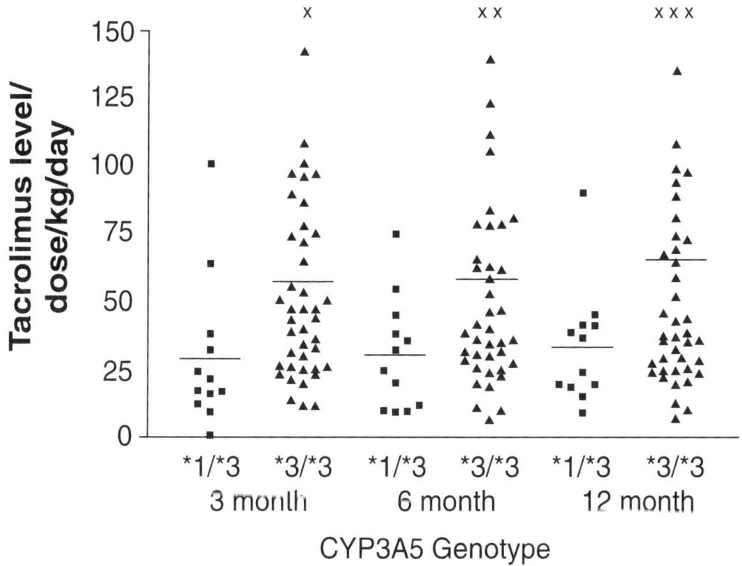

Figure 6. The tacrolimus level in blood (ng/ml) per dose (mg/kg/day) at 3, 6, and 12 months post-transplantation in the pediatric heart transplant patients separated into their *1/*3 and *3/*3 genotypes of CYP3A5.
The *1/*3 patients have a significantly lower tacrolimus level/dose than the *3/*3 patients at 3 months (p=0.014), 6 months (p=0.017), and 12 months (p=0.015).
CYP = cytochrome P450.

CYP3A5. The *1/*3 patients have a significantly lower tacrolimus level/dose than the *3/*3 patients at 3 months (p=0.014), 6 months (p=0.017), and 12 months (p=0.015). Another study (Reference 70) has confirmed this observation in adult lung transplant patients. Yet another study (Reference 35) also reported recently that the CYP3A P1 pseudogene in CYP3A5, which is strongly correlated with CYP3A5 activity, is associated with the tacrolimus dosage requirement at 3 months after renal transplantation. Investigators found that this SNP of CYP3A5 is a more important factor than ethnicity in determining tacrolimus pharmacokinetics. As CYP3A5 is the primary extrahepatic CYP3A isoform, its polymorphic expression may be implicated in disease risk and in the metabolism of endogenous steroids or xenobiotics.

In summary, CYP3A5 polymorphism has been demonstrated to have a significant effect on tacrolimus dosing in organ transplant patients. Patients with the CYP3A5 *1/*1 and *1/*3 genotype express more metabolic activity than those with the *3/*3 nonexpressor genotype and, therefore, would require larger dosages of CYP3A5 drug substrates. The higher frequency of expression of CYP3A5 activity in African-American patients (Reference 32) also may contribute to the poorer renal transplant outcomes previously discussed.

Thiopurine Methyltransferase

The genetic polymorphism displayed by thiopurine methyltransferase (TPMT) has a major effect on the metabolism of purines, such as 6-mercaptopurine (6-MP) and azathioprine. A more detailed discussion of this polymorphism is found in the Oncology and Hematology chapter, where 6-MP has primarily found its usage. Even though mycophenolate has taken over as the antiproliferative agent of choice in the United States, TPMT polymorphism is still critically important in the large number of transplant patients throughout the world who receive azathioprine.

Azathioprine has been used in organ transplantation for 25 years. The low incidence (about 0.3 percent) of the homozygous mutant for TPMT has probably not allowed the detection of transplant patients who were prone to develop severe leukopenia secondary to absent TPMT activity. This is particularly true in the transplant patient population where multiple causes of leukopenia are possible. Nevertheless, as testing for pharmacogenetic alterations becomes more frequent, the screening for TPMT genotypes in transplant patients should be considered critical information in individualizing therapy.

The TPMT genotypes in 30 heart transplant patients were studied (Reference 49) and four patients were found to have mutation of the TPMT gene. Neutrophils were significantly lower in the four heart transplant patients with the mutant TPMT gene, and two of those patients developed severe neutropenia. Severe neutropenia did not occur in any of the 26 patients with the reference TPMT genotype. Discontinuation of azathioprine in the four patients resulted in an increase in the neutrophil count. However, azathioprine therapy also was discontinued in nine of the 26 wild-type patients for reasons varying from a low leukocyte or platelet count after antithymocyte globulin administration to hepatitis B or C.

Alternative means of monitoring azathioprine therapy has been attempted with blood concentration monitoring of 6-thioguanine nucleotides or by measuring TPMT activity in red blood cells. Erythrocyte TPMT activity was measured in 82 renal transplant patients at 0, 7, and 30 days post-transplantation (Reference 55). Investigators found that patients who had increased TPMT activity during this time period also were the patients who had less delayed graft function and a significantly improved graft survival. The patients who did not have an induction of TPMT activity also had a somewhat lower white blood cell count. If a homozygous mutant for the TPMT gene was given full doses of azathioprine, the potential to produce severe neutropenia exists. Therefore, prospective genotyping remains one way to identify transplant patients who may be at risk for severe neutropenia and infection after the administration of full doses of azathioprine. Because TPMT genotyping is now commercially available, this approach should be considered in transplantation centers using azathioprine as part of the immunosuppressive protocol.

Drug Targets

Cytokines

Cytokines play a key role in mediating the immune response and acute rejection, and regulating cytokine production is a therapeutic strategy that can minimize rejection. Cytokine production has a genetic predisposition, which may contribute to the substantial interindividual differences in immune response (Reference 3). Promoter region polymorphism may influence the binding of transcription factors, consequently increasing or decreasing the production of messenger ribonucleic acid, thus regulating cytokine production. Several polymorphisms in the regulatory regions of cytokine genes have been identified and correlated with the production of those cytokines (see Table 1). Some cytokine genes have multiple polymorphisms, although not all have been associated with actual changes in the production of the cytokine (References 20–22). Many previous investigations have demonstrated the association between cytokine gene polymorphisms and disease pathogenesis, including infection (Reference 42), allergies (Reference 41), and autoimmune diseases (Reference 46). These studies support the potential relationship between cytokine gene polymorphisms and either the frequency and severity of allograft rejection or the ability to induce tolerance.

One investigation found that a (tumor necrosis factor-alpha (TNF-α) low phenotype combined with an interleukin-10 (IL-10) high/intermediate phenotype was associated with the lowest incidence of rejection after pediatric heart transplantation (Reference 3). Similarly, children

Table 1. Cytokine Genotypes and their Associated Phenotypes

Cytokine Polymorphism	Genotype	Phenotype Producer
TNF-α (-308)	G/G	Low
	G/A, A/A	High
TGF-β1 (codons 10-25)	T/T-G/G, T/C-G/G	High
	T/C-G/C, C/C-G/G, T/T-G/C	Intermediate
	C/C-G/C, C/C-C/C, T/T-C/C,	
	T/T-C/C, T/C-C/C	Low
IL-10 (-1082, -819, -592)	GCC/GCC	High
	GCC/ACC	Intermediate
	GCC/ATT	
	ACC/ACC	Low
	ACC/ATA	
	ATA/ATA	
IL-6 (-174)	G/G, G/C	High
	C/C	Low
INF-γ (+874)	T/T, T/A	High
	A/A	Low

IL = interleukin; INF-γ = interferon-gamma; TGF-ß1 = transforming growth factor-beta-1; TNF-α = tumor necrosis factor-alpha.

successfully maintained off immunosuppression were more likely to have a combination of a TNF-α low, IL-10 high/intermediate cytokine phenotype (Reference 37). Previous studies of transforming growth factor-beta (TGF-β) have demonstrated a correlation between the development of lung fibrosis and death in lung transplant recipients (References 10,11). One study (Reference 69) found that the IL-10 genotype for high cytokine production provides protection from acute persistent rejection compared to the intermediate/low phenotypes in lung transplant patients. The lung transplant patients with the IL-10 intermediate phenotype vary in haplotype response with the patients with GCC/ACC having more acute persistent rejection compared to patients with GCC/ATA genotype.

The immunomodulatory effects of IL-6 are differentiated in the G/C and G/G alleles, both of which are correlated with high producers of IL-6. Interleukin-6 is produced by monocytes and T cells and promotes the differentiation of B cells similar to IL-10. The increased production of IL-6 depends on the G allele, and in 102 healthy patients the C allele was associated with significant lower levels of plasma levels of IL-6 (Reference 14). Diseases that are characterized by hyperactivation of B cells, such as systemic lupus erythematosus and rheumatoid arthritis, are associated with IL-10 high and IL-6 high phenotypes. In lung transplant patients, the IL-6 G/C genotype had more acute persistent rejection in conjunction with the IL-10 GCC/ACC haplotype than did the G/G genotype (Reference 69). Interleukin-10 polymorphism effects may be differential, depending on the transplanted organ. High levels of both IL-10 and IL-6 are associated with renal transplant rejection, whereas in lung allografts, the presence of high phenotypes of IL-10 and IL-6 seems to confer a protective effect. A study of 93 lung transplant patients (Reference 34) found that the presence of high expression polymorphisms of the IL-6 gene and of the interferon-gamma gene significantly increases the risk for developing bronchiolitis obliterans syndrome after lung transplantation.

Chemokines

Chemokines are the chemoattractants that draw leukocytes to a sight of action. Several types of chemokines exist, and their complex interaction determines the leukocyte population that is attracted into a site of inflammation. Chemokine receptors also can be used by viruses as an entry site into the cell. Clearly chemokines can be targeted for immunosuppressive therapy as evidenced by the development of FTY-720. Although a full discussion of chemokines and chemokine receptors is beyond the scope of this chapter, the importance of chemokines with regard to transplant rejection and infection cannot be minimized.

Presently, two studies have examined the human chemokine receptor polymorphic variants and outcome in renal transplant patients. One of those studies (Reference 13) examined the CCR5 chemokine receptor where 1 percent of the Caucasian population is homozygous carriers of a deletion which leads to an inactive chemokine receptor. Out of 576 renal transplant recipients, 21 patients who were homozygous for CCR5Δ32 were identified. Only one of these patients lost his graft, whereas 78 of the remaining 555 patients lost their renal graft. Therefore, graft survival was significantly longer in the homozygous CCR5Δ32 group than it was in the other genotypes. Although this genotype is uncommon, it does demonstrate the potential for targeting this chemokine receptor in organ transplantation.

The other study (Reference 1) examined 163 renal transplant patients for variants of chemokine receptors. Unfortunately, these investigators did not identify any homozygous CCR5Δ32 patients, so they could not confirm the previous study's result. However, they did identify two additional alleles that were associated with a reduction in the risk of acute renal transplant rejection. Recipients who possessed the CCR2-64I allele or the CCR5-59029-A allele had a lower risk of acute transplant rejection. These relationships were supported by animal studies in knockout mice. Therefore, many subtle effects from variations in chemokine receptors may play a role as a risk factor for transplant rejection, and may eventually be factored into a complex equation that directs drug therapy.

Chemokines also may play a role in many auxiliary processes that are important for transplant patients. These processes would include infection, recurrence of autoimmune disease, or development of chronic rejection. For example, one study (Reference 38) recently identified a CX3CR1 chemokine receptor which is protective against coronary artery disease

(CAD). Although it is unknown whether this genotype also might be protective against the accelerated CAD associated with chronic rejection in heart transplant patients, these relationships remain to be established.

Adhesion Molecules

The adhesion molecules are involved in the movement of leukocytes from blood into tissue. Several types of adhesion molecules are involved in this process, including the integrins on T cells, such as leukocyte function-associated antigen-1 (LFA-1); the immunoglobulin supergene family, including intercellular adhesion molecule-1 (ICAM-1); and the selectins. These molecules already have been proven to be very effective targets for immunosuppressive drug therapy, so it is no surprise that gene polymorphisms that change the effectiveness of these molecules also will have an immunomodulatory effect. In transplantation, this effect has been demonstrated in renal transplant patients, in the chronic vasculopathy associated with heart transplantation and with graft-versus-host disease (GVHD) after bone marrow transplantation.

One study (Reference 39) genotyped renal allograft recipients for five polymorphisms in ICAM-1, E-selectin, and L-selectin. Study investigators compared the results of 62 patients who experienced chronic allograft failure with 110 patients who experienced long-term graft survival, and found that the ICAM R241 variant allele was more common in the chronic allograft failure patients. The time to allograft failure also was associated with the ICAM E469 variant, where patients experienced more rapid graft failure. No associations with the polymorphisms of the selectins were found.

Another study (Reference 7) examined heart transplant patients and their donors for the development of CAD in the post-transplant period. The donors whose recipients did not develop CAD for the first 2 years after transplant had the ICAM E469 allele more frequently compared with donors whose recipients did develop CAD or with controls. The ICAM E469 allele also was associated with a decreased frequency of acute rejection episodes. This information appears to be in contrast to a previously cited study of renal transplant patients (Reference 39), but the exact involvement of ICAM-1 in the varying pathophysiological processes of heart transplant CAD and renal chronic allograft failure is unknown. No association with the other polymorphisms of the adhesion molecules E-selectin, L-selectin and platelet-endothelial-cell adhesion molecule (PECAM) were found with post-transplant CAD.

The involvement of the PECAM-1 (also called CD31) polymorphism in GVHD after bone marrow transplantation was studied (Reference 6). In the 46 bone marrow transplant patients with CD31 genotyping, they found that a donor-recipient CD31 mismatch was associated with 71 percent of patients developing GVHD, whereas only 22 percent of recipients developed GVHD when CD31 was matched for donor and recipient. This report points out the importance of considering both donor and recipient genetic polymorphisms in fully understanding the complex interactions between recipient and donor tissue.

Growth Factors

Macrophages and lymphocytes produce the growth factor vascular endothelial growth factor (VEGF), which is a potent stimulator of angiogenesis. Vascular endothelial growth factor also can activate the transcription factor nuclear factor-kB, which turns on the production of inflammatory cytokines and chemokines. The promotor region contains five polymorphisms, and a recent study examined VEGF polymorphisms in 173 renal transplant patients (Reference 50). They found that the VEGF -1154*G and -2578*C genotypes encode for a higher VEGF production and are strongly associated with an increased risk of acute rejection, as defined by either the clinical response to corticosteroids or by biopsy. Although these results should be extended to larger patient groups and other types of transplants, VEGF and the other growth factor polymorphisms may play a role in graft rejection and response to therapy.

Applications to Transplant Patients in the Future

Figure 7 shows a future picture of applying the pharmacogenomic information in clinical therapeutic regimens. Genetic polymorphisms have a profound effect on the response of a patient to drug therapy, and the importance of this field of genetic study is just beginning to be appreciated. The most significant effects currently are believed to be on drug metabolizing enzymes or on the targets of drugs. The models for the future use of this information in developing treatment algorithms may be quite complex. If a human leukocyte antigen mismatch on a molecular typing level is considered in addition to drug disposition markers and drug targets, then a statistical model could be developed which assesses risk of post-transplant adverse events. The relationship of this assessment to drug therapy will then depend on the drugs that are available and the testing of the safety or efficacy of a combined regimen in a patient population.

Although acknowledging the complexity of future situations, how the current information could be used can still be assessed. For example, *MDR1* genotyping will soon be readily available and could be used in a treatment algorithm for organ transplant patients. The selection of steroid weaning regimens could then be chosen based on *MDR1* genotype. Also, the initial dosage of tacrolimus may be predicted based on the *MDR1* genotype. Figure 7 gives the example of using this type of information in a treatment algorithm.

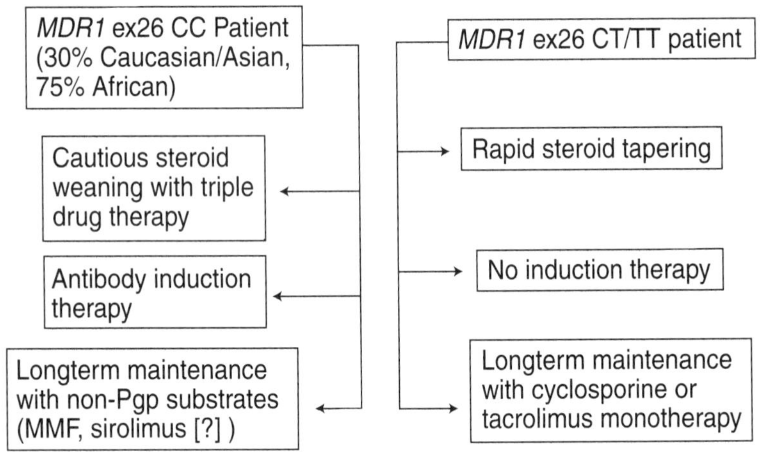

Figure 7. An example of how patient genotyping for *MDR1* exon26 could be used in a prospective transplant patient treatment algorithm.
MMF = mycophenolate mofetil; Pgp = P-gyucoprotein; [?] = sirolimus if questionable as a traditional substrate for Pgp.

The addition of each drug disposition or drug target polymorphism to this algorithm substantially increases its complexity. If all of the above polymorphisms were to be factored into a drug regimen that either initiates or continues long-term graft survival, then a computer model would be necessary to guide the clinician in making decisions based on the odds ratios for the observation of a therapeutic or adverse effect. The development of this model requires both a large database of patient observations, and large controlled trials that could confirm the validity of the proposed treatment algorithm.

Many factors that are presently unknown must be eventually factored into these processes. The critical pathophysiological process that is yet to be understood in extending graft and patient survival is that of chronic rejection of the transplanted organ. Additional genes and their associated polymorphisms related to this process will be identified and then maybe integrated into this model to improve patient outcome.

References

1. Abdi R, Tran TB, Sahagun-Ruiz A, et al. Chemokine receptor polymorphism and risk of acute rejection in human renal transplantation. J Am Soc Nephrol 2002;13(3):754–8.

2. Ameyaw MM, Regateiro F, Li T, et al. *MDR1* pharmacogenetics: frequency of the C3435T mutation in exon 26 is significantly influenced by ethnicity. Pharmacogenetics 2001;11(3):217–21.

3. Awad MR, Webber S, Boyle G, et al. The effect of cytokine gene polymorphisms on pediatric heart allograft outcome. J Heart Lung Transplant 2001;20(6):625–30.

4. Backman L, Nicar M, Levy M, et al. FK506 trough levels in whole blood and plasma in liver transplant recipients. Correlation with clinical events and side effects. Transplantation 1994;57(4):519–25.

5. Backman JT, Kivisto KT, Olkkola KT, Neuvonen PJ. The area under the plasma concentration-time curve for oral midazolam is 400-fold larger during treatment with itraconazole than with rifampicin. Eur J Clin Pharmacol 1998;54(1):53–8.

6. Behar E, Chao NJ, Hiraki DD, et al. Polymorphism of adhesion molecule CD31 and its role in acute graft-versus-host disease. N Engl J Med 1996;334(5):286–91.

7. Borozdenkova S, Smith J, Marshall S, Yacoub M, Rose M. Identification of ICAM-1 polymorphism that is associated with protection from transplant associated vasculopathy after cardiac transplantation. Hum Immunol 2001;62(3):247–55.

8. Cascorbi I, Gerloff T, Johne A, et al. Frequency of single nucleotide polymorphisms in the P-glycoprotein drug transporter *MDR1* gene in white subjects. Clin Pharmacol Ther 2001;69(3):169.

9. Cholerton S, Daly AK, Idle JR. The role of individual human cytochromes P450 in drug metabolism and clinical response. Trends Pharmacol Sci 1992;13(12):434–9.

10. El-Gamel A, Sim E, Hasleton P, et al. Transforming growth factor beta (TGF-beta) and obliterative bronchiolitis following pulmonary transplantation. J Heart Lung Transplant 1999;18(9):828–37.

11. El-Gamel A, Awad MR, Hasleton PS, et al. Transforming growth factor-beta (TGF-beta1) genotype and lung allograft fibrosis. J Heart Lung Transplant 1999;18(6):517–23.

12. Evans WE, McLeod HL. Pharmacogenomics-drug disposition, drug targets, and side effects.[comment]. N Engl J Med 2003;348(6):538–49.

13. Fischereder M, Luckow B, Hocher B, et al. CC chemokine receptor 5 and renal-transplant survival. Lancet 2001;357(9270):1758–61.

14. Fishman D, Faulds G, Jeffery R, et al. The effect of novel polymorphisms in the interleukin-6 (IL-6) gene on IL-6 transcription and plasma IL-6 levels, and an association with systemic-onset juvenile chronic arthritis. J Clin Invest 1998;102(7):1369–76.

15. Gupta P, Hart J, Cronin D, Kelly S, Millis JM, Brady L. Risk factors for chronic rejection after pediatric liver transplantation. Transplantation 2001;72(6):1098–102.

16. Hashida T, Masuda S, Uemoto S, Saito H, Tanaka K, Inui K. Pharmacokinetic and prognostic significance of intestinal *MDR1* expression in recipients of living-donor liver transplantation. Clin Pharmacol Ther 2001;69(5):308–16.

17. Hebert MF, Dowling AL, Gierwatowski C, et al. Association between *MDR1* (multiple resistance transporter) genotype and after liver transplantation renal dysfunction in patients receiving calcineurin inhibitors. Pharmacogenetics 2003;13:1–14.

18. Hitzl M, Drescher S, van der Kuip H, et al. The C3435T mutation in the human *MDR1* gene is associated with altered efflux of the P-glycoprotein substrate rhodamine 123 from CD56+ natural killer cells. Pharmacogenetics 2001;11(4):293.

19. Hoffmeyer S, Burk O, von Richter O, et al. Functional polymorphisms of the human multidrug-resistance gene: multiple sequence variations and correlation of one allele with P-glycoprotein expression and activity in vivo. Proc Natl Acad Sci U S A 2000;97(7):3473.

20. Hutchinson IV, Turner DM, Sankaran D, Awad MR, Sinnott PJ. Influence of cytokine genotypes on allograft rejection. Transplant Proc 1998;30(3):862–3.

21. Hutchinson IV, Turner D, Sankaran D, Awad M, Pravica V, Sinnott P. Cytokine genotypes in allograft rejection: guidelines for immunosuppression. Transplant Proc 1998;30(8):3991–2.

22. Hutchinson IV, Pravica V, Perrey C, Sinnott P. Cytokine gene polymorphisms and relevance to forms of rejection. Transplant Proc 1999;31(1-2):734–6.

23. Isaacs RB, Lobo PI, Nock SL, Hanson JA, Ojo AO, Pruett TL. Racial disparities in access to simultaneous pancreas-kidney transplantation in the United States. Am J Kidney Dis 2000;36(3):526–33.

24. Johnson CD, Wicks MN, Milstead J, Hartwig M, Hathaway DK. Racial and gender differences in quality of life following kidney transplantation. Image J Nurs Sch 1998;30(2):125–30.

25. Kaplan B, Lown K, Craig R, et al. Low bioavailability of cyclosporine microemulsion and tacrolimus in a small bowel transplant recipient: possible relationship to intestinal P-glycoprotein activity. Transplantation 1999;67(2):333–5.

26. Kerb R, Aynacioglu AS, Brockmoller J, et al. The predictive value of *MDR1*, CYP2C9, and CYP2C19 polymorphisms for phenytoin plasma levels. Pharmacogenomics J 2001;1(3):204–10.

27. Kim RB, Leake BF, Choo EF, et al. Identification of functionally variant *MDR1* alleles among European Americans and African Americans. Clin Pharmacol Ther 2001;70(2):189.

28. Kleinbloesem CH, van Brummelen P, Faber H, Danhof M, Vermeulen NP, Breimer DD. Variability in nifedipine pharmacokinetics and dynamics: a new oxidation polymorphism in man. Biochem Pharmacol 1984;33(22):3721–4.

29. Kochi S, Takanaga H, Matsuo H, Naito M, Tsuruo T, Sawada Y. Effect of cyclosporin A or tacrolimus on the function of blood-brain barrier cells. Eur J Pharmacol 1999;372(3):287–95.

30. Koch I, Weil R, Wolbold R, et al. Interindividual variability and tissue-specificity in the expression of cytochrome P450 3A mRNA. Drug Metab Dispos 2002;30(10):1108–14.

31. Koyama H, Cecka JM, Terasaki PI. Kidney transplants in black recipients. HLA matching and other factors affecting long-term graft survival. Transplantation 1994;57(7):1064–8.

32. Kuehl P, Zhang J, Lin Y, et al. Sequence diversity in CYP3A promoters and characterization of the genetic basis of polymorphic CYP3A5 expression. Nat Genet 2001;27(4):383–91.

33. Liu Z, Colpaert S, D'Haens GR, et al. Hyperexpression of CD40 ligand (CD154) in inflammatory bowel disease and its contribution to pathogenic cytokine production. J Immunol 1997;163(7):4049–57.

34. Lu KC, Jaramillo A, Lecha RL, et al. Interleukin-6 and interferon-gamma gene polymorphisms in the development of bronchiolitis obliterans syndrome after lung transplantation. Transplantation 2002;74(9):1297–302.

35. Macphee IA, Fredericks S, Tai T, et al. Tacrolimus pharmacogenetics: polymorphisms associated with expression of cytochrome p4503A5 and P-glycoprotein correlate with dose requirement. Transplantation 2002;74(11):1486–9.

36. Masuda S, Uemoto S, Hashida T, Inomata Y, Tanaka K, Inui K. Effect of intestinal P-glycoprotein on daily tacrolimus trough level in a living-donor small bowel recipient. Clin Pharmacol Ther 2000;68(1):98–103.

37. Mazariegos GV, Reyes J, Webber SA, et al. Cytokine gene polymorphisms in children successfully withdrawn from immunosuppression after liver transplantation. Transplantation 2002;73(8):1342–5.

38. McDermott DH, Halcox JP, Schenke WH, et al. Association between polymorphism in the chemokine receptor CX3CR1 and coronary vascular endothelial dysfunction and atherosclerosis. Circ Res 2001;89(5):401–7.

39. McLaren AJ, Marshall SE, Haldar NA, et al. Adhesion molecule polymorphisms in chronic renal allograft failure. Kidney Int 1999;55(5):1977–82.

40. Min D, Ellingrod VL. C3435T mutation in exon26 of the human *MDR1* gene and cyclosporine pharmacokinetics in healthy subjects. Ther Drug Monit 2002;24:400–4.

41. Moffatt MF, Cookson WO. Tumour necrosis factor haplotypes and asthma. Hum Mol Genet 1997;6(4):551–4.

42. Nadel S, Newport MJ, Booy R, Levin M. Variation in the tumor necrosis factor-alpha gene promoter region may be associated with death from meningococcal disease. J Infect Dis 1996;174(4):878–80.

43. Nair S, Eustace J, Thuluvath PJ. Effect of race on outcome of orthotopic liver transplantation: a cohort study. Lancet 2002;359:287–93.

44. Nelson DR, Koymans L, Kamataki T, et al. P450 superfamily: update on new sequences, gene mapping, accession numbers and nomenclature. Pharmacogenetics 1996;6(1):1–42.

45. Ozdemir V, Kalowa W, Tang BK, et al. Evaluation of the genetic component of variability in CYP3A4 activity: a repeated drug administration method. Pharmacogenetics 2000;10(5):373–88.

46. Rood MJ, van Krugten MV, Zanelli E, et al. TNF-308A and HLA-DR3 alleles contribute independently to susceptibility to systemic lupus erythematosus. Arthritis Rheum 2000;43(1):129–34.

47. Ross W, Solomon H, Reese J, Fairchild R, Garvin P, Kurtz M. Beneficial effects of HLA-DR3 gene expression on renal allograft survival in black recipients. Transplant Proc 1993;25(4):2408–10.

48. Schaeffeler E, Eichelbaum M, Brinkmann U, et al. Frequency of C3435T polymorphism of *MDR1* gene in African people. Lancet 2001;358(9279):383–4.

49. Sebbag L, Boucher P, Davelu P, et al. Thiopurine S-methyltransferase gene polymorphism is predictive of azathioprine-induced myelosuppression in heart transplant recipients. Transplantation 2000;69(7):1524–7.

50. Shahbazi M, Fryer AA, Pravica V, et al. Vascular endothelial growth factor gene polymorphisms are associated with acute renal allograft rejection. J Am Soc Nephrol 2002;13(1):260–4.

51. Shimada T, Yamazaki H, Mimura M, Inui Y, Guengerich FP. Interindividual variations in human liver cytochrome P-450 enzymes involved in the oxidation of drugs, carcinogens and toxic chemicals: studies with liver microsomes of 30 Japanese and 30 Caucasians. J Pharmacol Exp Ther 1994;270(1):414–23.

52. Siddiqui A, Kerb R, Weale ME, et al. Association of multidrug resistance in epilepsy with a polymorphism in the drug-transporter gene ABCB1. N Engl J Med 2003;348(15):1442–8.

53. Spurr NK, Gough AC, Stevenson K, Wolf CR. The human cytochrome P450 CYP3 locus assignment to chromosome 7q22-qter. Hum Genet 1989;81(2):171–4.

54. Tanabe M, Ieiri I, Nagata N, et al. Expression of P-glycoprotein in human placenta: relation to genetic polymorphism of the multidrug resistance (MDR)-1 gene. J Pharmacol Exp Ther 2001;297(3):1137.

55. Thervet E, Anglicheau D, Toledano N, et al. Long-term results of TMPT activity monitoring in azathioprine-treated renal allograft recipients. J Am Soc Nephrol 2001;12(1):170–6.

56. von Ahsen N, Richter M, Grupp C, Ringe B, Oellerich M, Armstrong VW. No influence of the MDR-1 C3435T polymorphism or a CYP3A4 promoter polymorphism (CYP3A4-V allele) on dose-adjusted cyclosporin A trough concentrations or rejection incidence in stable renal transplant recipients. Clin Chem 2001;47(6):1048.

57. Wandel C, Kim RB, Stein CM. "Inactive" excipients such as Cremophor can affect in vivo drug disposition. Clin Pharmacol Ther 2003;73(5):394–6.

58. Wakasugi H, Yano I, Ito T, et al. Effect of clarithromycin on renal excretion of digoxin: interaction with P-glycoprotein. Clin Pharmacol Ther 1998;64(1):123–8.

59. Webber SA, Naftel DC, Parker J, et al. Late rejection episodes greater than 1 year after pediatric heart transplantation: risk factors and outcomes. J Heart Lung Transplant 2003;22(8):869–75.

60. Westlind A, Lofberg L, Tindberg N, Andersson TB, Ingelman-Sundberg M. Interindividual differences in hepatic expression of CYP3A4: relationship to

genetic polymorphism in the 5'-upstream regulatory region. Biochem Biophys Res Commun 1999;259(1):201–5.

61. Westlind A, Malmebo S, Johansson I, et al. Cloning and tissue distribution of a novel human cytochrome p450 of the CYP3A subfamily, CYP3A43. Biochem Biophys Res Commun 2001;281(5):1349–55.

62. Williams JA, Ring BJ, Cantrell VE, et al. Comparative metabolic capabilities of CYP3A4, CYP3A5, and CYP3A7. Drug Metab Dispos 2002;30(8):883–91.

63. Wrighton SA, Molowa DT, Guzelian PS. Identification of a cytochrome P-450 in human fetal liver related to glucocorticoid-inducible cytochrome P-450HLp in the adult. Biochem Pharmacol 1988;37(15):3053–5.

64. Yamauchi A, Ieiri I, Kataoka Y, et al. Neurotoxicity induced by tacrolimus after liver transplantation: relation to genetic polymorphisms of the ABCB1 (*MDR1*) gene. Transplantation 2002;74(4):571–2.

65. Zheng H, Webber S, Zeevi A, et al. The *MDR1* polymorphisms at exons 21 and 26 predict steroid weaning in pediatric heart transplant patients. Hum Immunol 2002;63:765–70.

66. Zheng HX, Webber S, Zeevi A, et al. Tacrolimus dosing in pediatric heart transplant patients is related to CYP3A5 and *MDR1* gene polymorphisms. Am J Transplant 2003;3:1–7.

67. Zheng HX, Zeevi A, Lamba J, et al Tacrolimus nephrotoxicity is predicted by *MDR1* Exon21 gene polymorphism whereas dosing is predicted by cytochrome P4503A5 polymorphism in adult lung transplant patients. American Transplant Congress, Washington, D.C. Transplantation 2003;3:S(5):426.

68. Zheng HX, Zeevi A, McCurry K, et al *MDR1* exon26 genotype predicts treatment-resistant rejection in lung transplant patients as assessed by logistic regression analysis. American Society of Histocompatibility and Immunogenetics 29th Annual Meeting, Miami Beach, FL. Hum Immunol 2003;64:S42.

69. Zheng HX, Burckart GJ, McCurry K, et al. IL-10 gene polymorphisms are associated with acute rejection after lung transplantation. J Heart Lung Transplant [In Press].

70. Zheng HX, Zeevi A, Lamba J, et al. Tacrolimus nephrotoxicity is predicted by *MDR1* exon21 gene polymorphism whereas dosing is predicted by cytochrome P4503A5 polymorphism in adult lung transplant patients. J Clin Pharmacol [In Press].

Self-Assessment Questions

1. Which one of the following is true regarding current drug therapy monitoring for transplant patients and future monitoring with pharmacogenomic considerations?

    A. The current monitoring scheme can minimize or avoid calcineurin antagonist-induced renal dysfunction.
    B. Precise measurement of immune function will be possible in the future with better pharmacogenomic information.
    C. Drug level monitoring will still have an important place in monitoring even after there is good pharmacogenomic information on transplant patients.
    D. Drug levels of steroids and steroid receptor function will be predictable based on pharmacogenomic information.

2. Which one of the following is a correct definition for clinical pharmacogenomics?

    A. The study of drug metabolism.
    B. The exploration of how drugs work.
    C. The study of how the human genomic profile can influence the full spectrum of drug disposition and drug effect in producing a clinical outcome.
    D. The correlation between drug formulation and drug absorption.

3. A postoperative heart transplant patient is on prednisone after transplantation. Which one of the following will the pharmacotherapist have to consider when weaning the patient from steroids using current pharmacogenomic published information?

    A. Currently, there have not been any correlations between multidrug resistance gene (*MDR1*) genotyping and P-glycoprotein (Pgp) protein expression. Pharmacotherapists do not have to consider any influence of *MDR1* genotyping.
    B. The pharmacotherapist should test the *MDR1* C3435T genotype as previous work has demonstrated that it determines Pgp expression.
    C. The pharmacotherapist should stop steroids as they have many adverse effects and should prescribe tacrolimus to prevent rejection.
    D. The pharmacotherapist should test the *MDR1* C3435T genotype as it has been associated with ability to discontinue steroids.

4. Based on previous studies, which one of the following statements is true related to the role of cytokine polymorphisms in transplant patients?

A. In pediatric heart transplantation, patients with high tumor necrosis factor-alpha (TNF-α) production will do better than those with lower production.

B. In lung transplantation, TNF-α is the most important cytokine in post-transplant rejection.

C. In lung transplantation, transforming growth factor-beta (TGF-β) has been more likely correlated with the development of pulmonary fibrosis.

D. Patients with high interleukin-10 (IL-10) production always have longer survival than those with low IL-10 production.

5. Which one of the following is true regarding the effect of ethnic variations in the frequency of *MDR1* polymorphisms?

A. Asian patients have a different profile than Caucasian patients and require higher dosages of tacrolimus.

B. African-American transplant patients will have a higher percentage of the population having the wild-type of *MDR1* 3435CC.

C. African-American patients have less steroid resistance than Caucasian transplant patients, which could be related to their distribution of *MDR1* genotypes.

D. Even though African Americans differ in their frequency of the *MDR1* genotype, their overall outcome after organ transplantation is the same because of drug level monitoring.

6. As a pharmacotherapist, which one of the following pharmacogenomic pieces of information should you consider in drug dosing for a post-transplant patient taking tacrolimus?

A. Previous studies have found that *MDR1* and cytochrome P450 (CYP) 3A5 genotypes are correlated with tacrolimus dose requirement. The patient should be tested for both *MDR1* and CYP3A5 genotypes.

B. *MDR1* 3435 CC patients and 2677 GG patients require a lower tacrolimus dose to achieve the same level as other patients.

C. Cytochrome P450 3A5 *1/*1 genotype is a rare mutation and patients with *1/*1 genotype are nonexpressors.

D. Tacrolimus is an immunosuppressant with a wide therapeutic index and so the pharmacotherapist does not have to consider patient's genomic profile.

7. Which one of the following is incorrect for adhesion molecules?

A. The adhesion molecules are involved in the movement of leukocytes from blood into tissue. Several types of adhesion molecules are involved in this process, including the integrins on T cells, such as leukocyte function-associated antigen-1 (LFA-1); the immunoglobulin supergene family, including intracellular adhesion molecule-1 (ICAM-1); and the selectins.

B. These molecules have been proven to be very effective targets for immunosuppressive drug therapy, but there have not been any single nucleotide polymorphisms (SNPs) identified that correlate with transplant outcomes.

C. The involvement of the platelet-endothelial-cell adhesion molecule (PECAM-1; also called CD31) polymorphism in graft-versus-host disease (GVHD) after bone marrow transplantation points out the importance of considering both donor and recipient genetic polymorphisms in fully understanding the complex interactions between recipient and donor tissue.

D. The goal of exploring the SNPs of adhesion molecules is to develop drugs that either reduce their production or modify their function.

8. A post-transplant patient with *MDR1* exon26 C3435C genotype is on an immunosuppressive regimen, including tacrolimus. Which one of the following would you recommend the physician do based on your knowledge of pharmacogenomics?

A. Because *MDR1* 3435 CC patients may have a higher Pgp activity, then a higher dosage of tacrolimus should be recommended.

B. Nothing should be done except following the standard therapeutic protocol.

C. An alternative drug should be recommended.

D. Although *MDR1* 3435 CC patients are high Pgp expressors, the relative importance that the *MDR1* and CYP3A5 genotypes contribute to tacrolimus dosing is unclear. The patient's tacrolimus blood concentrations and clinical outcome should guide the immunosuppressive dosage.

9. The thiopurine methyltransferase (TPMT) genetic polymorphism has been critically important in cancer patients being treated with 6-mercaptopurine (6-MP) related to adverse effects. Which one of the following explains why this is not true in transplant patients being treated with azathioprine?

A. 6-MP is much more dependent on TPMT for metabolism than is azathioprine.

B. No one uses azathioprine any more.

C. Transplant patients always have leukopenia so the effect is not evident.

D. The frequency of the genetic variant and the number of other effects on blood leukocyte count in a transplant patient limits identification of the transplant patients affected.

10. Although *MDR1* polymorphisms clearly have been associated with differences in drug absorption, which one of the following other body processes may NOT be affected by alterations in Pgp function?

    A. Neurotoxicity or response to anticonvulsant agents.
    B. Renal elimination of Pgp substrates or renal toxicity.
    C. Pulmonary secretion of Pgp substrates.
    D. T-cell resistance to immunosuppressive agents.